AUTOIMMUNITY
Physiology and Disease

EDITORS

ANTONIO COUTINHO

Unité d'Immunobiologie
Institut Pasteur
Paris, France

MICHEL D. KAZATCHKINE

Unité d'Immunopathologie
Hôpital Broussais
Paris, France

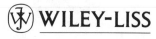

A JOHN WILEY & SONS, INC., PUBLICATION
NEW YORK • CHICHESTER • BRISBANE • TORONTO • SINGAPORE

Address All Inquiries to the Publisher
Wiley-Liss, Inc., 605 Third Avenue, New York, NY 10158-0012

Copyright © 1994 Wiley-Liss, Inc.

Printed in the United States of America

While the authors, editor, and publisher believe that drug selection and dosage and the specification and usage of equipment and devices, as set forth in this book, are in accord with current recommendations and practice at the time of publication, they accept no legal responsibility for any errors or omissions, and make no warranty, express or implied, with respect to material contained herein. In view of ongoing research, equipment modifications, changes in governmental regulations and the constant flow of information relating to drug therapy, drug reactions, and the use of equipment and devices, the reader is urged to review and evaluate the information provided in the package insert or instructions for each drug, piece of equipment, or device for, among other things, any changes in the instructions or indication of dosage or usage and for added warnings and precautions.

Library of Congress Cataloging-in-Publication Data

Autoimmunity : physiology and disease / editors, Antonio Coutinho,
 Michel D. Kazatchkine.
     p.   cm.
   Includes index.
   ISBN 0-471-59227-7
   1. Autoimmune diseases.   2. Autoimmunity.   I. Coutinho, Antonio,
 II. Kazatchkine, M. (Michel)
   [DNLM: 1. Autoimmunity—physiology.   2. Autoimmune Diseases-
 -immunology.   3. T-Lymphocytes—immunology.   WD 305 A9397 1993]
 RC600.A854 1993 1994
 616.97´8—dc20
 DNLM/DLC
 for Library of Congress   93-12816

The text of this book is printed on acid-free paper.

CONTENTS

Contributors   ix

Preface   xiii
Antonio Coutinho and Michel D. Kazatchkine

SECTION I: PHYSIOLOGICAL AUTOREACTIVITY

1   Autoimmunity Today   3
    Antonio Coutinho and Michel D. Kazatchkine

2   Kadishman's Tree, Escher's Angels, and the
    Immunological Homunculus   7
    Irun R. Cohen

3   Light Chain Variable Region Gene Repertoire in
    Human Autoantibodies   19
    Kimberly D. Victor and J. Donald Capra

4   Role of the Major Histocompatibility Complex in
    T-Cell Receptor Repertoire Selection   35
    Charles A. Janeway, Jr.

5   Stimulation of T and B Cells   45
    Jan Andersson, Yves Modigliani, and Alf Grandien

6   B-1 (CD5 B) Cells   57
    Paolo Casali, Marion T. Kasaian, and Geoffrey Haughton

7 Selection of the B-Cell Repertoire and
  Natural Autoantibodies   89
  Dan Holmberg and John Kearney

8 Human Natural Self-Reactive Antibodies   107
  Gilles Dietrich and Michel D. Kazatchkine

9 Autoantibodies and Autoimmune Network: The
  Evolving Paradigm   129
  Maurizio Zanetti

10 Lymphocyte Population Kinetics: A Cellular
   Competition Model   143
   António A. Freitas and Benedita B. Rocha

11 Postthymic T-Lymphocyte Population Dynamics in
   Mouse and Man   161
   Lisa J. Glickstein and Osias Stutman

12 Quantification of Autoreactive Lymphocytes in
   Health and Disease   173
   *Rudolf H. Zubler, Alessandra Tucci, Robert Rieben, Thomas
   Matthes, and Urs E. Nydegger*

13 Tolerance and Autoimmunity in the Peripheral
   T-Cell Repertoire   191
   J.F.A.P. Miller

14 Thymus, T Cells, and Autoimmunity: Various Causes
   But a Common Mechanism of Autoimmune Disease   203
   Shimon Sakaguchi and Noriko Sakaguchi

15 Autoimmunity and Idiotypic Networks   229
   John Stewart

SECTION II: AUTOIMMUNE DISEASE

16 Boundaries Between Physiological Autoreactivity and
   Pathological Autoimmunity   243
   Michel D. Kazatchkine and Antonio Coutinho

17 New Insights on the Physiological and Pathological
    Rheumatoid Factors in Humans   247
    Pojen P. Chen and Dennis A. Carson

18 Human and Experimental Myasthenia Gravis   267
    Ann Kari Lefvert

19 Immunoregulation of Autoimmune Responses in
    Systemic Vasculitis   307
    C.M. Lockwood

20 Immunological Disturbances Responsible for
    Graves' Disease   315
    John M. Dwyer

21 Specific Regulation of Experimental Autoimmune
    Thyroiditis: Toward a New Conception of
    Autoimmune Reactivity   339
    *Karine Mignon-Godefroy, Marie-Pierre Brazillet, and
    Jeannine Charreire*

22 Is Experimental Allergic Encephalomyelitis
    a Model of Multiple Sclerosis?   353
    Ellen Heber-Katz

23 Autoimmunity and Autoimmune Diabetes Mellitus   365
    Alan G. Baxter and Anne Cooke

24 Natural and Therapeutic Control of Ocular
    Autoimmunity: Rodent and Man   377
    Rachel R. Caspi and Robert B. Nussenblatt

25 Cellular and Molecular Aspects of
    Systemic Autoimmunity   407
    Michel Goldman and Paul-Henri Lambert

26 Immunodeficiency and Autoimmunity   423
    Fred S. Rosen

27 Autoimmunity Tomorrow   433
   Antonio Coutinho and Michel D. Kazatchkine

Index   439

CONTRIBUTORS

Jan Andersson, Department of Immunology, University of Uppsala Biomedical Center, S-751 23 Uppsala, Sweden

Alan G. Baxter, Department of Pathology, Division of Immunology, Cambridge University, Cambridge CB2 1QP, United Kingdom

Marie-Pierre Brazillet, INSERM U.283, Hôpital Cochin, 27 rue du Faubourg St. Jacques, 75674 Paris Cedex 14, France

J. Donald Capra, Department of Microbiology, University of Texas Southwestern Medical Center, Dallas, TX 75235-9048

Dennis A. Carson, Department of Medicine, University of California, San Diego, La Jolla, CA 92093-0663

Paolo Casali, Department of Pathology and Kaplan Comprehensive Cancer Center, New York University School of Medicine, New York, NY 10016

Rachel R. Caspi, Laboratory of Immunology, National Eye Institute, NIH, Bethesda, MD 20892

Jeannine Charreire, INSERM U.283, Hôpital Cochin, 27 rue du Faubourg St. Jacques, 75674 Paris Cedex 14, France

Pojen P. Chen, Department of Medicine, University of California, San Diego, La Jolla, CA 92093-0663

Irun R. Cohen, Department of Cell Biology, Weizmann Institute of Science, Rehovot 76100, Israel

Anne Cooke, Department of Pathology, Division of Immunology, Cambridge University, Cambridge CB2 1QP, United Kingdom

Antonio Coutinho, Unité d'Immunobiologie, CNRS URA 359, Institut Pasteur, 25 rue du Docteur Roux, 75724 Paris Cedex 15, France

Gilles Dietrich, Service d'Immunologie and INSERM U.28, Hôpital Broussais, 75674 Paris Cedex 14, France

John M. Dwyer, Division of Medicine, Prince of Wales Hospital, High Street, Randwick, NSW 2031, Australia

António A. Freitas, Unité d'Immunobiologie, CNRS URA 359, Institut Pasteur, 25 rue du Docteur Roux, 75724 Paris Cedex 15, France

Lisa J. Glickstein, Immunology Program, Memorial Sloan-Kettering Cancer Center, New York, NY 10021

Michel Goldman, Service d'Immunologie, Hôpital Erasme, 808 route de Lennik, B-1070 Brussels, Belgium

Alf Grandien, Department of Immunology, University of Uppsala Biomedical Center, S-751 23 Uppsala, Sweden

Geoffrey Haughton, Department of Microbiology and Immunology, University of North Carolina, Chapel Hill, NC 27599

Ellen Heber-Katz, The Wistar Institute, 3601 Spruce Street, Philadelphia, PA 19104

Dan Holmberg, Institute for Cell and Molecular Biology, University of Umeå, S-901 85 Umeå, Sweden

Charles A. Janeway, Jr., Section of Immunobiology, Howard Hughes Medical Institute, Yale University School of Medicine, New Haven, CT 06511

Marion T. Kasaian, Department of Pathology and Kaplan Comprehensive Cancer Center, New York University School of Medicine, New York, NY 10016

Michel D. Kazatchkine, Unité d'Immunopathologie, Hôpital Broussais, 96 rue Didot, 75674 Paris Cedex 14, France

John Kearney, Division of Developmental and Clinical Immunology, Department of Microbiology, University of Alabama at Birmingham, Birmingham, AL 35294

Paul-Henri Lambert, WHO Immunology Research and Training Center, Geneva/Lausanne, Switzerland

Ann Kari Lefvert, Department of Medicine and Immunological Research Laboratory, Karolinska Hospital, S-104 01 Stockholm, Sweden

C.M. Lockwood, Department of Medicine, Addenbrooke's Hospital, Cambridge CB2 1QP, United Kingdom

Thomas Matthes, Division of Hematology, Department of Medicine, Hôpital Cantonal Universitaire, 1205 Genève, Switzerland

Karine Mignon-Godefroy, INSERM U.283, Hôpital Cochin, 27 rue du Faubourg St. Jacques, 75674 Paris Cedex 14, France

J.F.A.P. Miller, The Walter and Eliza Hall Institute of Medical Research, Post Office Royal Melbourne Hospital, Victoria 3050, Australia

Yves Modigliani, Unité d'Immunobiologie, CNRS URA 359, Institut Pasteur, 25 rue du Docteur Roux, 75724 Paris Cedex 15, France

Robert B. Nussenblatt, Laboratory of Immunology, National Eye Institute, NIH, Bethesda, MD 20892

Urs E. Nydegger, Central Laboratory of Hematology, University of Bern, 3010 Bern, Switzerland

Robert Rieben, Central Laboratory of Hematology, University of Bern, 3010 Bern, Switzerland

Benedita B. Rocha, INSERM U.345, CHU Necker, Paris, France

Fred S. Rosen, Department of Pediatrics, Harvard Medical School, The Center for Blood Research and Children's Hospital, Boston, MA 02115

Noriko Sakaguchi, Institute of Physical and Chemical Research, Tsukuba Life Science Center, 3-1-1 Koyadai, Tsukuba, Ibaraki 305, Japan

Shimon Sakaguchi, Institute of Physical and Chemical Research, Tsukuba Life Science Center, 3-1-1 Koyadai, Tsukuba, Ibaraki 305, Japan

John Stewart, Unité d'Immunobiologie, Institut Pasteur, 28 rue du Docteur Roux, 75724 Paris Cedex 15, France

Osias Stutman, Cellular Immunology Section, Memorial Sloan-Kettering Cancer Center, New York, NY 10021

Alessandra Tucci, Division of Hematology, Department of Medicine, Hôpital Cantonal Universitaire, 1205 Genève, Switzerland

Kimberly D. Victor, Department of Microbiology, University of Texas Southwestern Medical Center, Dallas, TX 75235-9048

Maurizio Zanetti, Department of Medicine and Cancer Center, University of California, San Diego, La Jolla, CA 92103-0612

Rudolf H. Zubler, Division of Hematology, Department of Medicine, Hôpital Cantonal Universitaire, 1205 Genève, Switzerland

PREFACE

Concepts of autoimmunity have changed drastically over the last few years. Thus, it is now recognized that autoreactive antibodies and T cells exist in healthy individuals; that autoreactive repertoires are selected predominantly early in ontogeny; and that the autoreactive repertoire embodies V region-dependent interactions which, under normal conditions, determine expression and dynamics characteristic of natural tolerance. It has therefore become common to speak of the physiology of autoreactivity, although the boundaries between autoreactivity in healthy individuals and pathological autoimmunity (i.e., autoimmune disease) remain elusive. Novel views go as far as suggesting that autoreactivity is not only necessary for the establishment and maintenance of self-tolerance but actually underlies molecular homeostasis in the whole organism. We are thus experiencing major shifts in paradigms that should have consequences for most of our views on the function and evolutionary significance of the immune system. This progress is already having a significant impact at very pragmatic levels on the nature of therapeutic strategies in autoimmune disease.

Thus far, the molecular and cellular bases of autoimmune diseases usually have been approached independently of progress in the analysis of autoreactive repertoire selection under physiological conditions. Work in this area often has been split between experimentalists analyzing normal mice and clinicians attempting to correlate autoimmune manifestations with structural and genetic markers. Both basic and clinical investigators have invested primarily in analyzing isolated components, rather than in evaluating the entire immune system, be it normal or diseased. This probably reflects the predominance of the "clonal" view over the "network" perspective of tolerance, and usually corresponds to the split between those favoring inactivation or deletion of autoreactive clones and those concerned with regulatory and suppressive mechanisms. This dichotomy is also reflected in therapeutic approaches to autoimmune diseases, namely, conventional immunosuppressive strategies becoming increasingly more targeted to specific autoreactive pathogenic clones and novel approaches, including idiotypic vaccination and infusion of normal immunoglobulins, that aim to stimulate physiological mechanisms of natural tolerance.

For these reasons, we have been enthusiastic about the prospect of putting together in a single volume the views of some investigators who have contributed critically to progress in these areas. The principal purpose of this endeavor has been to blend the experience and ideas of experts in aspects of physiological autoreactivity and autoimmune disease in mouse and in man; to derive basic unifying concepts in physi-

2

KADISHMAN'S TREE, ESCHER'S ANGELS, AND THE IMMUNOLOGICAL HOMUNCULUS

Irun R. Cohen

Department of Cell Biology, The Weizmann Institute of Science,
Rehovot, Israel

KADISHMAN'S TREE

On the grounds of the Weizmann Institute, near the Graduate School building, stands a statue of a tree done by the Israeli sculptor Menashe Kadishman (Fig. 1). It is a statue of a tree despite the fact that there is no material image of a tree. The tree is virtual; it is made of air. The virtual image of the tree was created when Kadishman cut out the silhouette of a tree from five plates of steel. Some of the steel plates intersect at right angles, giving the virtual tree a virtual three-dimensional shape. The plates are so artfully joined that the tree silhouette changes as it is viewed from different angles; so a moving observer sees a changing, vegetating image of a tree. In essence Kadishman has presented us with a picture of a tree formed by materializing its background: the plates of steel exist on the grounds of the Institute; the tree exists only in the mind of the beholder. The sculpture is named "Continuum"; but it might be called "Boundary."

Autoimmunity: Physiology and Disease, Pages 7–18
© *1994 Wiley-Liss, Inc.*

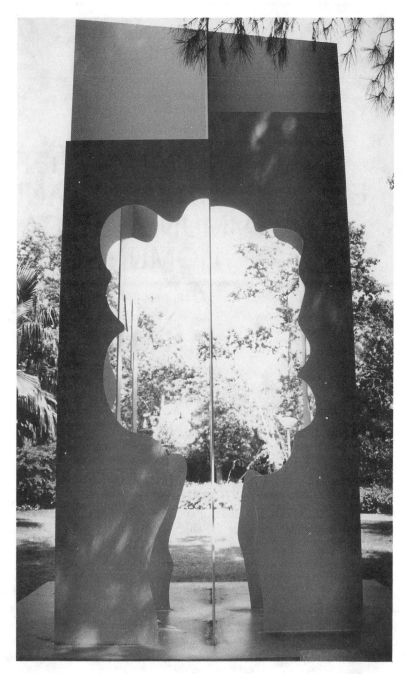

FIGURE 1. ''Continuum'' by Menashe Kadishman. A sculpture of a virtual tree; the background of the tree is made of steel, but the tree itself has no material existence. Real trees can be seen through Kadishman's virtual tree.

ESCHER'S ANGELS

The idea of creating a virtual object by portraying its ground is an old device that did not originate with Kadishman. Escher has put the subject–ground distinction to work by making the ground a subject too. A telling example is the print entitled "Circle Limit IV" (Fig. 2). In this picture, dark devils alternate with light angels, each serving as a ground for the other subject. Escher's image pulsates as the angels and the devils compete for our attention. We cannot have both angels and devils at the same instant; one form must recede into ground for its opposite to become subject. Kadishman's tree becomes animated by the orbiting movement of its observer; but Escher's image comes alive through the observer's oscillation of mind between angels and devils.

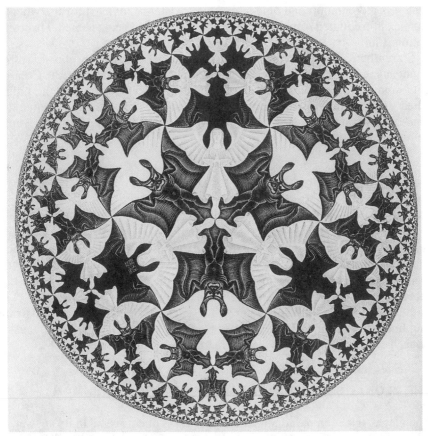

FIGURE 2. "Circle Limit IV" by M.C. Escher. A print done in 1960 in which angels and devils wage a subject–ground war for our attention. (Reproduced with permission of M. C. Escher Foundation, Baarn, Holland.)

CREATION BY DISTINCTION

Along with its lessons for the psychophysiology of human perception, Escher's picture of the cosmic conflict between subject and ground calls attention to a principle of existence: the angels emerge from the continuum of the picture and exist only when separated from the devils (and vice versa). To recognize an object in essence is to separate it from its surround, to establish its boundaries and thus define it. In fact, the word *define* derives from the Latin *definire,* to set a boundary.

Definition as establishment of boundaries is even older than is Latin. Religious literature states that the Creator spent the first six days separating one thing from another: earth from heaven, light from darkness, dry land from water, and so forth (Gen. 1:1–19). To crown the act of separation it was only necessary to give names, to conceptualize in mind the distinctions in matter: the darkness was named *night* and the light was named *day.* Since reality is a continuum, an object achieves existence, at least for us, when it can be differentiated from its neighbors to the point of being named. Discrimination is all.

(Parenthetically, note that Adam is charged with the responsibility of giving names to the animals [Gen. 2:19–20]; his first job is to help the Creator with some of the residual details of creation. It would seem that the unfinished, perhaps unfinishable, business of creation is to continue to refine the nameable distinctions among the creatures. Scientists, among others, would so have it.)

THE IMMUNOLOGICAL DISTINCTION

Now we are taught that immunology is the science of self–nonself discrimination [Klein, 1982]. This implies that the immune system exists to establish the boundary between the self and all the rest; this distinction defines the self and thus establishes the self. We could equally well put it the other way: the self–nonself distinction defines and creates the foreign. Either way, self-integrity requires discrimination between self and other.

But let us return to Kadishman and Escher. Granted that there exists an immunological boundary between self and nonself, which of them, self or nonself, is the subject and which of them is the ground?

THE CLONAL SELECTION PARADIGM FAVORS KADISHMAN

The clonal selection paradigm [Burnet, 1959] is unequivocal in its answer to the question: The foreign is the subject, and the self is the ground. The job of the immune system is to attack; and the subject of attack is the foreign. In other words, if there exists in the mind of the immune system a picture of the

PREFACE

Concepts of autoimmunity have changed drastically over the last few years. Thus, it is now recognized that autoreactive antibodies and T cells exist in healthy individuals; that autoreactive repertoires are selected predominantly early in ontogeny; and that the autoreactive repertoire embodies V region-dependent interactions which, under normal conditions, determine expression and dynamics characteristic of natural tolerance. It has therefore become common to speak of the physiology of autoreactivity, although the boundaries between autoreactivity in healthy individuals and pathological autoimmunity (i.e., autoimmune disease) remain elusive. Novel views go as far as suggesting that autoreactivity is not only necessary for the establishment and maintenance of self-tolerance but actually underlies molecular homeostasis in the whole organism. We are thus experiencing major shifts in paradigms that should have consequences for most of our views on the function and evolutionary significance of the immune system. This progress is already having a significant impact at very pragmatic levels on the nature of therapeutic strategies in autoimmune disease.

Thus far, the molecular and cellular bases of autoimmune diseases usually have been approached independently of progress in the analysis of autoreactive repertoire selection under physiological conditions. Work in this area often has been split between experimentalists analyzing normal mice and clinicians attempting to correlate autoimmune manifestations with structural and genetic markers. Both basic and clinical investigators have invested primarily in analyzing isolated components, rather than in evaluating the entire immune system, be it normal or diseased. This probably reflects the predominance of the "clonal" view over the "network" perspective of tolerance, and usually corresponds to the split between those favoring inactivation or deletion of autoreactive clones and those concerned with regulatory and suppressive mechanisms. This dichotomy is also reflected in therapeutic approaches to autoimmune diseases, namely, conventional immunosuppressive strategies becoming increasingly more targeted to specific autoreactive pathogenic clones and novel approaches, including idiotypic vaccination and infusion of normal immunoglobulins, that aim to stimulate physiological mechanisms of natural tolerance.

For these reasons, we have been enthusiastic about the prospect of putting together in a single volume the views of some investigators who have contributed critically to progress in these areas. The principal purpose of this endeavor has been to blend the experience and ideas of experts in aspects of physiological autoreactivity and autoimmune disease in mouse and in man; to derive basic unifying concepts in physiology and disease; and to open prospects for new therapeutic approaches to autoimmunity. Our hope is that this volume will help mark this period of transition in concepts and will reflect the shifts in paradigms related to understanding autoimmune disease and deriving relevant therapeutic approaches. We are particularly grateful to our colleagues who generously invested their time in sharing their ideas with the readers of this book.

We thank Peter Brown, Senior European Editor for Wiley-Liss, for having encouraged us to undertake this effort.

ANTONIO COUTINHO
MICHEL D. KAZATCHKINE

I

PHYSIOLOGICAL AUTOREACTIVITY

1

AUTOIMMUNITY TODAY

Antonio Coutinho and Michel D. Kazatchkine

Unité d'Immunobiologie, Institut Pasteur (A.C.); Unité d'Immunopathologie,
Hôpital Broussais (M.D.K.), Paris, France

During this century, the evolution of concepts on autoimmunity could be summarized by "never, sometimes, always." Thus from the early "horror autotoxicus" to the 1960s, immune autoreactivity was simply not considered. As Silverstein points out, this was the result of Ehrlich's consideration that autoantibodies are "dysteleological," and of the dominance of that school of thought over the next 50 years. This is surprising because the "side chain theory," by assuming that antibodies are the secretory form of cellular receptors, implies that they must have complementarities inside the body and thus that all antibodies are necessarily autoreactive.

With the first identification of autoreactive antibodies in patients and the subsequent conceptual association with autoaggressive immune behaviors, the "sometimes" phase was entered, necessarily equated with disease. By this time, immunology had laid its foundation on the clonal selection theory, which forbids autoreactive clones in normal individuals. Immunologists thereafter devoted 30 years discovering ways by which autoreactive lymphocyte clones can be deleted and why they fail to be deleted in autoimmune patients. On the clinical side, the logical consequence of this framework was that autoimmune disease had to be treated by suppression or elimination of the abnormally expressed clones. Lacking specific tools, the therapy of autoimmune disease employed aggressive cytostatic regimens, and only more recently has it become possible to suppress lymphocytes with some degree of cell type selectivity. As lymphocyte physiology has become better

Autoimmunity: Physiology and Disease, Pages 3–5
© *1994 Wiley-Liss, Inc.*

understood, much effort has been invested in a variety of novel strategies to suppress specific clonal activities. Most of the recent experimental therapeutic approaches therefore are new only in the methods used to suppress single clones and persist in considering that autoreactivity necessarily is associated with disease, driven by abnormal recognition of autoantigens.

In the 1970s at least three sets of observations and ideas began to alter this course of events and to herald the "always" period. First, multiple indications of the existence of autoreactive lymphocytes in normal individuals were obtained: for example, it was possible to induce autoimmune disease readily by immunization with cross-reactive antigens by injecting allogeneic T cells or a polyclonal mitogen. Second, T-cell-dependent specific and nonspecific suppression was demonstrated and seemed directly relevant to autoimmune disease mechanisms. Third, Jerne proposed the idiotypic network theory, which implied that immune repertoires and all lymphocyte activities are essentially autoreactive. Although originally it did not address the question directly, the network theory seemed particularly relevant to autoimmunity. Thus it is based on the notions that the immune system contains and recognizes all possible antigens, ignoring the dichotomy between self- and nonself-antigens (at least structurally), and therefore the need to ensure natural tolerance by repertoire purging. Furthermore, the theory explicitly stated that the immune system regulates itself into a "suppressed state" that is compatible, therefore, with physiological autoreactivity. These concepts rapidly gained attention, and for some time autoimmune disease was considered the consequence of the failure of "suppressor" cells or of the "lack of anti-idiotypes". With time, however, these expectations have faded, largely confounded by the degree of complication that such models reached, possibly related to incompatibility between the desire for linear causality by immunologists and the conceptual and empirical difficulties imposed by complex systems with nonlinear dynamics.

It is only over the last 10 years that the concept of physiological autoreactivities has become established, and such a short time actually may justify current controversies. Thus there is today much evidence for the existence of autoreactive antibodies, B cells and T cells at quite high frequencies in healthy individuals. Furthermore, it is accepted widely that autoreactivities are positively selected in early ontogeny and activated in the adult. The concepts of "control" and "anergy" have retaken some ground from clonal deletion in the current explanations for tolerance. Finally, novel nonsuppressive therapeutic measures for autoimmune disease have been introduced, after some striking and unexpected successes. While today many immunologists are still not in agreement with the general idea that autoimmune reactivity is normal, others have even postulated that autoreactivity is actually necessary for natural self-tolerance. We believe therefore that we are experiencing a major shift in the central paradigm of immunology, namely, that the immune system is selected somatically to fail to recognize self. This shift should have consequences for most of our views on the function and evolutionary significance of the immune system as well as for our approaches to autoimmune disease, with respect both to hypotheses on the mechanisms of their emergence and to very pragmatic attitudes of treatment strategies.

The new paradigm faces great difficulties in several aspects. First, there is a difference in interests and approaches between basic immunologists experimenting with animals and clinicians treating autoimmune patients. Second, the new paradigm requires a conceptual approach that is incompatible with the dominant views in modern biology, for it disposes of simple, lineal causality. Also related to approach, this framework requires more than genetic, biochemical, or cellular analyses of components and demands the development of systemic strategies. Finally, even for some adherents to the new paradigm the weight of history and the importance (fear) of infection continue to impose the view that all immune activities are necessarily aggressive and destructive of their targets. According to this view, the evolution of the immune system is related to adaptation to selective pressures of pathogens rather than to building a molecular identity of self.

We often forget that, to be infected, vertebrates must first exist. For this, they must ensure an homeostasis of their internal molecular environment, a coherence of all organ systems. Vertebrate evolution is characterized by the development of centralized and/or centralizing control systems (brain, heart and circulation, neuroendocrine systems); similarly, the immune system ensures the homeostasis of all molecular shapes (configurations) in the organism. Its ability to protect vertebrates from microbial invasion is only another expression of this primary function to maintain the molecular composition of self, most obviously manifested by natural tolerance in the physiology of normal individuals. Immune disorders represent failures of homeostasis, whether they are manifested as microbial invasion, as tissue destruction by immune-mediated inflammation, or as organ dysfunction, by altered ratios of receptor/antireceptor antibody, for example. In our view, immunodeficiencies and autoimmune diseases are two faces of the same coin, involving essentially the same fundamental mechanisms, namely, impairment of the immune potential to maintain homeostasis.

self, then that picture, like Kadishman's tree, is virtual and without substance. (My application of the term *mind* to the immune system is obviously a metaphor for the mind of the immunologist; by immune *substance,* I here refer to the functional repertoires of the antigen receptors, T and B, and the antibodies.)

According to the clonal selection paradigm, the immune system is born with a clean slate; the primal immune system consists of an astronomical number of potential receptors and a set of rules that oversees the realization of the receptor potential by the process of antigen selection. The antigens write on the slate and so organize the system: Receptors that see self-antigens are cut out (deleted or anergized), while receptors that see foreign antigens germinate and flourish. Like Kadishman, the immune system erases from the slate of its repertoire the silhouette of the self while realizing that part of the repertoire that constitutes its image of all the rest, the foreign [Burnet, 1969]. According to clonal selection, only the picture of nonself has substance; the picture of the self must be virtual. The immunological self can exist legitimately only as that which bounds the foreign; in health, the self-antigens are an empty class. Autoimmune disease must result when for any reason or accident there appear elements of the repertoire that can recognize self [Burnet, 1969]. In other words, autoimmune disease must result whenever a virtual self-antigen becomes an actual self-antigen, that is, when a self-antigen becomes an antigen recognized by clones of lymphocytes.

However, in contradiction of the paradigm, healthy immune systems are replete with T and B cells that recognize self-antigens [Avrameas, 1991; Cohen and Young, 1991]. In other words, the immune picture of the healthy self is substantial, not virtual. Finding itself obliged to climb out on a limb of Kadishman's tree, the clonal selection paradigm falls short.

THE IMMUNOLOGICAL HOMUNCULUS FAVORS ESCHER

Elsewhere I have developed the concept of the immunological homunculus to face up to the truth of natural autoimmunity and to describe how the immune system really views the self [Cohen, 1989, 1991a; Cohen and Young, 1991]. The term *immunological homunculus* was borrowed from the neurological homunculus; both homunculi constitute physiological images of the self encoded by specific networks of cells, neurons if neurological and lymphocytes if immunological. Happily, many of the ideas implicit in the immunological homunculus metaphor can be exposed to view by Escher's "Circle Limit IV" (Fig. 2).

Let us suppose for the sake of self-respect that the angels represent the self and that the devils represent the foreign. Which features of Escher's picture express the immune system's view of self and nonself? What is common to both angels and devils, and what is unique to each class? Let us consider four attributes of the Escher forms: substance, essence, origin, and harmony.

Substance

Escher forms the angels and the devils out of identical substances, which are merely the paper and ink he uses to draw them. Both images, angel and devil, have the same material reality and are equally recognizable. Where they may differ, in fact where ideally they *must* differ, is in the type of response they arouse. We can recognize them both, but for our own good we respond to each differently.

Likewise does the immune system construct the images of the self and the foreign. Both the self and the foreign antigens are recognized by the same classes of elements: antibodies and T- and B-cell receptors. These elements inscribe images of the antigens within the immune system [Jerne, 1974]. The internal images of self-antigens are as substantial as are the internal images of the foreign antigens. Fortunately, however, like Escher's images of angels and devils, we usually respond differently to self and foreign antigens; we cherish and protect the former, and we attack and reject the latter.

Self-antigens and foreign antigens are made of similar chemicals and are apprehended by the same receptor machinery [Cohen, 1988]. The immunological difference between self and foeign antigens, like the psychological difference between angels and devils, is a matter of interpretation. The observer of Escher's picture will appreciate its meaning only if he can recognize and interpret its forms as those of angels and devils before he actually views the picture. In fact, I imagine that an observer from another culture knowing nothing of angels and devils would not even see the oscillation between subject and ground which is the heart and soul of the work; apprehending the print as a single comprehensive subject, he might imagine it to be one of those exercises in tiling devised by topologists. Likewise, the selfness or foreignness of an antigen depends on the interpretation given it by the immune system. Interpretation requires you to know the essence of what you see; otherwise you will not see it at all, or seeing it, you will not know how to respond. Just as Escher's viewer has to know the essence of angel (or of devil), the immune system has to know the essence of self (or of foreign) to interpret what it sees and then respond in an appropriate manner.

Essence

The quiddity or "whatness" of an entity is its unique attribute or set of attributes that allows us to identify the entity and define it apart from its surroundings. Kadishman's tree, made of air, can be discriminated physically from its surround, made of steel; but it cannot be identified as a tree unless the observer has had previous experience with trees and knows what the form of a tree is. Escher's angels and devils are made physically of the same material and so the difference between them is absolutely dependent on the set of preformed ideas of the observer.

The immunological homunculus is the preformed set of autoimmune B and

T cells that the immune system has formed about the dominant self-antigens: basic protein (BP), insulin, heat shock proteins, nucleic acids, various critical enzymes, and so forth [Cohen, 1989, 1991a; Cohen and Young, 1991]. These particular self-antigens are immunologically dominant because of the natural autoimmunity that anticipates them. The autoimmunity to these antigens is benign because the system knows that they are self and has prepared regulatory machinery ahead of time to handle them.

Other elements, in addition to the observer's foreknowledge, are of the essence in both the immunological homunculus and Escher's picture. The images of angel and devil are minimalistic; only a few features suffice to signify them. The signature of an angel is a winged humanoid with an angelically serene expression. A devil is a horned humanoid expressing devilish malice and the power to harm: teeth, claws, muscles. Wings are optional for devils. Any more detail is superfluous.

The images of angels and devils are universal in our culture: anyone will recognize the forms with fidelity. The images are public conventions that supersede most individual differences between observers.

Similarity, the immunological homunculus is a minimalisitic, conventional picture of the self. A relatively few antigens, the same limited set of dominant antigens mentioned above, comprise the system's image of the self. Moreover, different individuals, even different species, recognize similar sets of self-antigens: Humans and mice have natural autoimmunity to BP, to the antigens associated with lupus, to thyroglobulin, and so on. The homunculus image is a shared, public convention.

Note that the immune system image of foreign invaders also may be quite minimalistic and stereotypic. A bacterium with 10^4 genes and consequently with at least 10^4 potential antigens may be recognized and repulsed by antibodies to one or two of them: enteric bacteria by O antigens, group A streptococci by M protein, and so on. Also note that different individuals (and different species too) may focus their responses on the same limited set of foreign antigens. This is despite an astronomical repertoire potentially able to recognize any organic structure. Escher can depict the essence of an angel without drawing in all the feathers, a devil without copying the hooves or scales. The immune system can interpret and dispose of a microbe with no greater detail in memory than a few epitopes.

Origins

What is the origin of the uniformity of conventions defining trees, angels, devils, and antigens? Why does the immunological homunculus consist of just that particular set of self antigens? How are the standard forms revealed to the systems that have to recognize and interpret them? How does a system know which entities to see as its subjects and which entities are merely background? One thing is sure, experience is critical.

Would Kadishman's tree be recognized by an Eskimo who never saw a tree? Would Escher's angels be recognized by one who never saw an angel? Except for uncommon revelation, few have ever seen real angels. (Devils would seem to be more abundant.) Nevertheless, all have seen representations of angels and devils, and the idea alone is enough for one to experience the subject–ground conflict and to interpret "Circle Limit IV."

What experience endows the immune system with the capacity to interpret whether an antigen is self or foreign? Obviously this question applies to the antigens for which the repertoire has receptors, antigens to which the system is not blind. Mammalian immune systems are outfitted with T cells that can recognize self-BP [Schluesener and Wekerle, 1985], but each system tends to behave in a benign way to the BP it sees. The immune system does not attack BP unless the BP comes with adjuvants (signals of infection), and even then the autoimmune encephalomyelitis (EAE) attack is usually self-limited and usually cannot be induced a second time, at least in rats in which the experiment can be done [Ben-Nun and Cohen, 1982]. The immune system knows that BP is self; it knows how to behave differently to foreign antigens.

There are two sources of experience that help an individual immune system distinguish between self and foreign antigens: the evolutionary experience encoded in the germline of the species and the somatic experience of the individual.

The germline has been selected to survive infection by parasites of all kinds, and thus it has evolved elaborate sets of cells and molecules that enable it to identify and respond to infection and inflammation without recourse to recognition of specific antigens. Bacterial products (lipopolysaccharide, cell walls, muramyldipeptide) and viral products (nucleic acids) are recognized by germline-encoded elements expressed in cells (e.g., macrophages, polymorphonuclear leukocytes, natural killer cells) or in molecules (complement components, acute phase proteins). The presence of these signals of infection triggers cell migrations, the expression of adhesion molecules, the secretion of various cytokines, and so forth. Antigens seen in this complicated context are rejected; they are interpreted functionally as foreign. Antigens seen without all of these adjuvant signals are left alone; they are interpreted functionally as self, even if they have a foreign origin. Foreign antigens encoded by the major histocompatibility complex (MHC) elicit powerful immune responses; but it is not clear why allogeneic MHC signals are so compelling.

Note that there are various functional options for carrying out rejection of the foreign; the effector repertoire includes all kinds of T cells (CD8, CD4–TH1, CD4–TH2, double negatives, double positives, $\alpha\beta$, $\gamma\delta$, and so forth) and their cytokines and all kinds of B cells and their antibody isotypes. Also note that there are various options for tolerating self: nonreactivity (anergy) of different types, active suppression (antigen specific, nonspecific, CD8 mediated, CD4 mediated, anti-idiotypic, antiergotypic), blocking antigen, and blocking antibody. Some of these elements overlap and some compete; indeed, some are thought actually not to exist in vivo. What matters here is that the particular mix of regulatory elements is surely the product of somatic experience with self-antigens and with foreign antigens. Somatic experience, guided by germline experience, organizes the internal structure of the immune system so that the arrival of a particular antigen can be properly interpreted and an appropriate response can be carried out. Among the outcomes of this internal organization is the formulation of the immunological homunculus; the focus of special networks on a particular set of self-antigens.

Each self-antigen represented in the homunculus must have a good reason for being there; otherwise we (including mice) would not tend to form similar homunculus sets. The reasons are yet unknown, but are probably different for each antigen. Self-heat shock proteins (hsp) are likely to be important for resisting infection [Cohen, 1991b]. Buy why is BP in the homunculus? I would guess that the germline, physiological functions of antigens are likely to influence the way the immune system organizes the homunculus.

To complete this brief discussion of origins, we must ask whether human evolution has helped the nervous system formulate its somatic images of trees, angels, and devils. At the level of sensory input, evolution certainly has programmed the brain to apprehend boundaries; the retina is hard-wired to see lines [Young, 1988] and the brain will even invent lines to complete pictures [Ramachandran, 1992]. More than that, the brain may be programmed at the cognitive level to recognize certain entities.

Jung and his followers claim that particular primal images are shared by humankind, as a whole and irrespective of a particular culture [Jung, 1968]. I do not know of a definitive cross-cultural study of the images of trees, angels, and devils, but it is clear that humans are very receptive to such images. I doubt if the forms are encoded in human DNA; the receptivity might be. Note that trees are no less mythic symbols than are angels and devils; there are trees of life, of knowledge, of creation. Even the logo of the Weizmann Institute is a tree. Perhaps the Eskimo we supposed never to have seen a tree would still recognize Kadishman's tree; the human germline, we are told, did originate in Africa [Cavalli-Sforza, 1991]. To use an outmoded term, humans, like other primates, may have an *instinctive* affinity for trees.

In any case, all systems, including those neurological and those immunological, can recognize and interpret actual somatic experience only if they have a built-in image, however primitive, of what they are looking for. The immune system, not only the brain, needs paradigms.

Harmony

Escher's "Circle Limit IV" comprises an orb (the world) paved in angels (the good) and in devils (the bad). The observer's retina transmits all the forms simultaneously to the brain for processing. The brain interprets the input in the light of its past experience (germline and somatic) and grasps the picture either as light angels on a dark ground or as dark devils on a light ground. Unless experience dictates a pervasive preference, the brain will alternate between the two possible subjects to the delight of the little man (consciousness) who watches the brain processing Escher's picture.

Behind the picture we may infer a lesson in deportment: To experience the orb fully, there is a time to see the angels and a time to see the devils. Total preoccupation with one or the other produces an incomplete, unbalanced picture. The price for such neglect is esthetic in "Circle Limit IV" and may be disastrous beyond. The devils, like the angels, demand due attention. Harmony in and beyond the picture is proper attention to the right subject at the right time, combined with a suitable response.

Harmony is the concern of the immune system: recognition of the right self-antigens and the right foreign antigens, interpretation of the context of recognition and a suitable response. Immunological disease results more often from a defect in interpretation than from a defect in recognition. Everyone has T cells that recognize BP naturally; rats develop EAE (and people may develop multiple sclerosis) when BP is interpreted as deserving of an aggressive response [Cohen and Young, 1991]. Likewise, lepromatous leprosy develops, not when *Mycobacterium leprae* is ignored, but when it is interpreted to be deserving of a copious antibody response on the interleukin (IL)-4 pathway [Bloom et al., 1992]. The picture loses harmony when an angel is painted darkly (an aggressive response to self) or when a devil is painted lightly (a tolerant response to foreign). If the angels represent the dominant self-antigens encoded in the homunculus, then an inappropriate response (a dark angel) may culminate in an autoimmune disease targeted precisely to the same self-antigen characteristic of benign natural autoimmunity [Cohen and Young, 1991].

Immunologically dominant, but regulated responses to homunculus self-antigens may produce tolerance to the other self-antigens not represented in the homunculus, the nondominant self-antigens. Tissue inflammation caused by infection or infarction can expose self-antigens in a context demanding an immune response; however, the one or two dominant homunculus self-antigens preempt the response to themselves and automatically protect the many nondominant self-antigens [Gammon et al., 1991] from being attacked. We find that strongly activated T cells have the capacity to inhibit the activation of adjacent T cells (Cohen, in preparation). Thus the first clones to be activated can dominate the entire response and determine its specificity. As the first autoimmune clones are likely to be members of the homunculus set, the response is regulated and the autoimmunity remains benign. "Circle Limit IV" illustrates this principle well: A dominant subject makes other potential subjects disappear into the background. In this way, the immunological homunculus can function as a guardian angel against the dangers of random, unregulated autoimmunity.

CONCLUSION

Now that immunology has deciphered the molecular biology of how the immune system gathers antigenic data, it can free itself of the clonal selection paradigm, a fallen angel [Coutinho et al., 1984; Cohen, 1992a–c], and begin the task of learning how the system inteprets its data.

ACKNOWLEDGMENTS

I thank Mrs. Anna Mecheh of the Photographic Department for photographing Kadishman's tree for Figure 1 and Mrs. Doris Ohayon for helping prepare the manuscript. I am the incumbent of the Mauerberger Chair of Immunology and the director of the Robert Koch-Minerva Center for Research in Autoimmune Diseases.

REFERENCES

Avrameas, S (1991): Natural autoantibodies: From "honor autotexicus" to "gnothi seaton." Immunol Today 12:154–159.

Ben-Nun A, Cohen IR (1982): Spontaneous remission and acquired resistance to autoimmune encephalomyelitis (EAE) are associated with suppression of T cell reactivity: Suppressed EAE effector T cells recovered as T cell lines. J Immunol 128:1450–1457.

Bloom BR, Modlin RL, Salgame P (1992): Stigma variations: Observations on suppressor T cells and leprosy. Annu Rev Immunol 10:453–488.

Burnet FM (1959): "The Clonal Selection Theory of Acquired Immunity." Cambridge: Cambridge University Press.

Burnet FM (1969): "Self and Non-Self." Cambridge: Cambridge University Press.

Cavalli-Sforza LL (1991): Genes, peoples and languages. Sci Am 265:72–78.

Cohen IR (1988): The self, the world and autoimmunity. Sci Am 258:52–60.

Cohen IR (1989): Natural id–anti-id networks and the immunological homunculus. In Atlan H, Cohen IR (eds): "Theories of Immune Networks." Berlin: Springer-Verlag, pp 6–12.

Cohen IR (1991a): The immunological homunculus and autoimmune disease. In Talal N (ed): "Molecular Autoimmunity." San Diego: Academic Press, pp 438–453.

Cohen IR (1991b): Autoimmunity to chaperonins in the pathogenesis of arthritis and diabetes. Annu Rev Immunol 9:567–589.

Cohen IR (1992a): Autoimmunity to hsp65 and the immunologic paradigm. Adv Intern Med 37:295–311.

Cohen IR (1992b): The cognitive principle challenges clonal selection. Immunol Today 13:441–444.

Cohen IR (1992c): The cognitive paradigm and the immunological homunculus. Immunol Today 13:490–494.

Cohen IR, Young DB (1991): Autoimmunity, microbial immunity and the immunological homunculus. Immunol Today 12:105–110.

Coutinho A, Forni L, Holmberg D, Ivars F, Vaz N (1984): From an antigen-centered, clonal perspective of immune responses to an organism-centered, network perspective of autonomous activity in a self-referential immune system. Immunol Rev 79:151–168.

Gammon G, Sercarz EE, Benichou G (1991): The dominant self and the cryptic self: shaping the autoreactive T-cell repertoire. Immunol Today 12:193–195.

Jerne NK (1974): Towards a network theory of the immune system. Ann Immunol (Inst Pasteur) 125c:373–389.

Jung CG (1968): "The Archetypes and the Collective Unconscious." Bollingen Series XX. Princeton, NJ: Princeton University Press.

Klein J (1982): "Immunology: The Science of Self-Nonself Discrimination." New York: John Wiley.

Ramachandran VS (1992): Blind spots. Sci Am 266:44–49.

Schluesener HJ, Wekerle H (1985): Autoaggressive T lymphocyte lines recognizing the encephalitogenic region of myelin basic protein: In vitro selection from unprimed rat T lymphocyte populations. J Immunol 135:3128–3133.

Young JZ (1988): "Philosophy and the Brain." Oxford: Oxford University Press.

3

LIGHT CHAIN VARIABLE REGION GENE REPERTOIRE IN HUMAN AUTOANTIBODIES

Kimberly D. Victor and J. Donald Capra

Department of Microbiology, University of Texas Southwestern Medical Center, Dallas, Texas

INTRODUCTION

The ability to generate an infinite array of antigenic specificities is directly related to the structure of the immunoglobulin gene complex and the mechanisms of recombination that are unique to the immune system. Utilization of germline-encoded information, combined with somatic processes, generates the diversity in the immunoglobulin or antibody molecule. Inherent in this process is the capacity to generate specificities that are capable of recognizing self-determinants [Koopman and Schrohenloher, 1980; Prabhakar et al., 1984]. The main task of immune regulation is to endow the immune system with the ability to distinguish between foreign components and self-components. The ability to modulate an immune response directed against a self-antigen, or immunological tolerance, is believed to be induced during fetal development as immature lymphocytes are exposed to self-antigens during differentiation.

Autoimmunity: Physiology and Disease, Pages 19–34
© *1994 Wiley-Liss, Inc.*

Unlike T cells, the generation of the B-cell repertoire occurs in two stages. Immunoglobulin variable region rearrangement in the bone marrow produces a preimmune repertoire consisting of relatively low affinity B-cell receptors. As mature peripheral B cells are exposed to antigen, clonal expansion and somatic mutation lead to the development of a repertoire of B cells bearing receptors with increased affinity for antigen [Tonegawa, 1983; Alt et al., 1988; French et al., 1989]. As self-reactive B cells may be produced during each phase of development, tolerance must be induced not only during B-cell differentiation in the bone marrow but also as an ongoing process in mature B cells within peripheral lymphoid organs [Goodnow et al., 1990].

There are at least three mechanisms involved in regulating self-recognition. Immature lymphocytes expressing receptors for self antigens are deleted during differentiation and maturation (in the thymus for T cells or in the bone marrow for B cells), providing that the self-antigen is present in that environment [Marrack et al., 1988; Nemazee and Buerki, 1989; Hartley et al., 1991]. Autoreactive lymphocytes that escape deletion during development are controlled in the periphery by clonal inactivation or anergy, which does not necessarily involve receptor modulation or cell death but is thought to take place if exposure to antigen occurs in the absence of appropriate co-stimulatory signals [Goodnow et al., 1988; Nossal, 1989]. Finally, self-reactive lymphocytes can be functionally inactivated by either suppressor T cells or anti-idiotypic antibodies.

Autoantibody production is a characteristic of many autoimmune diseases, but the role of these antibodies in the pathogenesis of disease is unclear. Such antibodies may contribute to the induction or maintenance of disease and may influence the severity. To delineate the genetic basis for autoantibody synthesis, the variable regions of approximately 40 human antibodies with defined specificities have been studied. The molecular analysis of a diverse group of human autoantibodies was designed to examine variable gene expression in human antibodies and to assess the contribution of somatic mutation and antigenic selection in the generation of autoreactivity. An understanding of the genetic origin of autoantibodies may provide insight into the development or regulation of autoimmunity.

HUMAN LIGHT CHAIN ORGANIZATION

The structural organization of the human κ locus has been well characterized. The major gene complex has been localized to the short arm of chromosome 2 and is composed of approximately 85 V_κ gene segments, 5 J_κ gene segments, and a single constant region gene [Hieter et al., 1982; Zachau, 1990]. This locus accounts for nearly 90% of the germline V_κ gene segments, as to date 25 additional V_κ gene segments or "orphons" have been mapped to other chromosomes. The contribution of these orphon gene segments to the repertoire is limited, as the majority of these gene segments (20 of 25) are pseudogenes.

Based on sequence homology, the V_κ gene segments have been classified into six families that are separated into clusters of 1 to 15 kb [Straubinger et al., 1988; Pargent et al., 1991; Marks et al., 1991]. Analogous to the heavy chain locus, the V_κ gene families are interdigitated [Pech and Zachau, 1984; Lotscher et al., 1986], and approximately 50% are pseudogenes [Zachau, 1990]. The actual number of V_κ gene segments in each family is not precisely known, but the $V_\kappa I$ and $V_\kappa II$ families are the largest, with approximately 20–30 members. The $V_\kappa III$ family is slightly smaller, with approximately 15 members [Pech et al., 1984; Klobeck et al., 1985a; Pohlenz et al., 1987]. The $V_\kappa IV$ family consists of a single member, which is the most J_κ proximal gene segment [Klobeck et al., 1985b, 1987]. The size of the $V_\kappa V$ and $V_\kappa VI$ families has not been determined, but they are probably small.

The configuration of the human κ locus resulted from a gene duplication event as genes that are highly homologous are present in different regions of the complex, with the transcriptional polarities within the duplications being largely identical but opposite between the copies [Pech et al., 1985]. There are seven main V_κ gene groups located on the short arm of chromosome 2, termed B, L_p, A_p, O_p, O_d, A_d, and L_d (where p stands for J_κ proximal and d indicates gene segments that are more J_κ distal). Additionally, a second group of V_κ gene segments have been localized to the long arm of chromosome 2, referred to as W_a, W_b, and W_c, but many of these gene segments are pseudogenes. Recent studies have shown that some of the V_κ gene segments are polymorphic while others are relatively nonpolymorphic. Even more striking is the observation that the majority of the population (70%) does not possess the duplicated region of this locus (O_d, A_d, and L_d) and do not contain the entire locus within the germline [Zachau, 1990]. Thus, the κ locus is highly polymorphic in both the V_κ gene segments and the single C_κ gene, which has been shown to consist of three polymorphic alleles.

The human λ light chain locus, whose structure is more complicated than that of the κ locus, has been studied relatively little, even though λ light chains constitute 40% of all human immunoglobulins. The major gene complex is on chromosome 22 and is composed of approximately the same number of V_λ gene segments as the κ locus. It can be divided into six families. There are seven constant region gene segments, three of which are pseudogenes ($C_\lambda 4$, $C_\lambda 5$, and $C_\lambda 6$), each associated with a single J_λ gene segment [Hieter et al., 1981; Udey and Blomberg, 1987; Vasicek and Leder, 1990; Combriato and Klobeck, 1991].

Four λ isotypes, termed Mcg^+, Ke^-Oz^-, Ke^-Oz^+, and Ke^+Oz^-, have been described on the basis of reactivity with the Oz, Kern, and Mcg antisera [Hess et al., 1971]. Isolation and nucleotide sequence analysis of the C_λ gene segments has shown that $C_\lambda 1$ encodes the Mcg specificity, $C_\lambda 2$ is responsible for the Ke^-Oz^- phenotype, $C_\lambda 3$ generates the Ke^-Oz^+ reactivity pattern, and $C_\lambda 7$ represents the Ke^+Oz^- specificity [Hieter et al., 1981; Vasicek and Leder, 1990]. Amino acid analysis of λ proteins has revealed 10 additional, unique C_λ sequences [Frangoine et al., 1985]. It is not known whether these proteins represent the products of distinct C_λ genes or whether these differences represent polymorphisms within the C_λ complex. Limited analysis of V_λ gene segments suggests that the λ locus also contains a significant number of pseudogenes [Combriato and Klobeck, 1991] and is polymorphic [Paul et al., 1991]. The organization of the C_λ gene segments provides further evidence for the processes of gene conversion and gene duplication in the evolution of the immunoglobulin loci.

LIGHT CHAIN REPERTOIRE IN HUMAN AUTOANTIBODIES

Table I describes the human autoantibodies that have been sequenced in our laboratory. This study summarizes the molecular characterization of the light chain variable regions of autoantibodies isolated from patients with various autoimmune diseases including monoclonal rheumatoid factors (RF), polyreactive antibodies (PR), cold agglutinins (CA), striational antibodies (SA), antiacetylcholine receptor (AChR) antibodies, antithyroglobulin (Tg) antibodies, and C3 nephritic factors (C3NeF). This analysis is unlike most previous studies with monoclonal paraproteins resulting from a transformation event or naturally occurring autoreactive antibodies, as these autoantibodies are more representative of pathogenic antibodies.

The majority of the cell lines were produced by Epstein-Barr virus (EBV) transformation of B cells isolated from the synovium (RF and PR) that were stabilized by back fusion to a murine myeloma or by EBV transformation of B cells isolated from thymic tissue (SA) that were fused to a human myeloma. The remaining antibodies were isolated by EBV transformation of peripheral blood lymphocytes (CA, AChR, Tg, and C3NeF) or by direct fusion with a human myeloma. The specificities for each of the antibodies was determined by our collaborators [Randen et al., 1989; Victor et al., 1991; Stevenson et al., 1989; Spitzer et al., 1991; McLachlan et al., 1987; Lefvert and Holm, 1987; Williams and Lennon, 1986].

V_L Gene Segment Utilization in Autoantibodies Is Diverse

The opportunity to analyze over 40 distinct human autoantibodies at the molecular level has provided important insights into the structures of these antibodies. As the only selection bias was antigenic specificity, we believe the utilization of the various V_H, D, J_H, V_L, and J_L gene segments in these antibodies reflects the genetic origin of autoantibodies. The most striking observation among this group of antibodies is that V_L gene usage is very diverse (Table II). There appears to be no preferential utilization of specific V_L gene families or overrepresentation of certain V_L gene segments in autoantibodies. Although it appears that the $V_\kappa I$ and $V_\kappa III$ gene families are overrepresented in our samples, the observed frequencies of these families within autoantibodies parallels the observed frequency of expression of these particular V_L families in peripheral blood [Guigou et al., 1990] and does not

TABLE I. Human autoantibodies characterized

Clone	Source	Specificity	Isotype	$V_H{}^a$	V_L	J_L
RF–KES1	SLE	RF	IgM_κ	III	I	5
RF–KL1	RA	RF	IgM_κ	III	I	5
RF–KL2	RA	RF	IgM_κ	III	I	5
RF–KL3	RA	RF	IgM_κ	III	I	5
RF–TS5	RA	RF	IgM_κ	III	I	4
RF–SJ5	RA	RF	IgG_κ	III	I	4
RF–SJ6	RA	RF	IgG_κ	III	I	4
RF–SJ7	RA	RF	IgG_κ	III	I	4
RF–TS3	RA	RF	IgM_κ	I	II	5
RF–TS1	RA	RF	IgM_κ	I	IIIb	1
RF–TS2	RA	RF	IgM_κ	III	IIIa	5
RF–TMC1	N	RF	IgM_κ	IV	III	4
RF–SJ3	RA	RF	IgM_κ	III	IIIb	2
RF–SJ4	RA	RF	IgM_κ	IV	IIIb	5
RF–KL5	RA	RF	IgG_κ	III	VI	2
RF–SJ1	RA	RF	IgM_λ	III	λI	λ2
RF–SJ2	RA	RF	IgM_λ	III	λI	λ2
PR–TS1	RA	PR–RF	IgM_λ	III	λI	λ2
PR–SJ2	RA	PR–RF	IgM_λ	III	λII	λ2
PR–TS2	RA	PR–RF	IgM_λ	IV	λIV	λ2
PR–SJ1	RA	PR–RF	IgM_λ	IV	λV	λ2
PR–SJ3	RA	PR–RF	IgM_λ	IV	λV	λ2
FS–5	CA	i	IgM_κ	IV	I	1
FS–7	CA	I	IgM_κ	IV	I	1
FS–1	CA	I	IgM_κ	IV	II	2
FS–2	CA	I	IgM_κ	IV	IIIb	5
FS–4	CA	I	IgM_κ	IV	IIIa	2
FS–6	CA	I	IgM_κ	IV	IIIb	1
FS–3	CA	i	IgM_λ	IV	λI	λ1
SA–1A	MG	SM	IgM_κ	V	I	4
SA–1D	MG	SM	IgM_κ	V	I	4
SA–4B	MG	SM	IgG_κ	III	I	1
SA–4A	MG	SM	IgG_κ	IV	IIIb	3
AChR–19	MG	AChR	IgG_κ	II	I	1
AChR–37	MG	AChR	IgM_κ	V	IIIb	2
AChR–29	MG	AChR	IgM_κ	V	IIIb	2
$V\beta5$	GD	Tg	IgG_λ	IV	λI	λ1
ID3	GD	Tg	IgG_λ	IV	λI	λ2
CK	SLE	C3NeF	IgG_κ	IV	I	2

[a] V. Pascual, personal communication.

TABLE II. V$_L$ utilization in human autoantibodies

Specificity	V$_\kappa$I	V$_\kappa$II	V$_\kappa$III	V$_\kappa$IV	V$_\kappa$V	V$_\kappa$VI	V$_\lambda$I	V$_\lambda$II	V$_\lambda$III	V$_\lambda$IV	V$_\lambda$V	V$_\lambda$VI	Total
RF	8	1	5	—	—	1	3	1	—	1	2	—	22
CA	2	1	3	—	—	—	1	—	—	—	—	—	7
SA	3	—	1	—	—	—	—	—	—	—	—	—	4
α-AChR	1	—	2	—	—	—	—	—	—	—	—	—	3
α-Tg	—	—	—	—	—	—	2	—	—	—	—	—	2
C3NeF	1	—	—	—	—	—	—	—	—	—	—	—	1
Total	15	2	11	0	0	1	6	1	0	1	2	0	39

differ significantly from the predicted frequency based on the number of gene segments within each family in the genome. The $V_\kappa II$ family is under-represented in comparison with the size of the family, but does not differ significantly from the frequency seen in the peripheral blood. None of the antibodies studied expressed a $V_\kappa IV$ gene segment that was unexpected based on the frequency observed in peripheral blood. The $V_\kappa V$ and $V_\kappa VI$ families and the λ locus in general have not been fully defined; therefore it is difficult to address the issue of restriction in terms of these particular families in autoantibodies, although it appears to be random.

V_H and V_L Association Is Unrestricted

The utilization of the various variable gene families in autoantibodies is random and demonstrates a lack of restriction of V_H and V_L association (Table III). Although the $V_H III$ gene family is used in over one-third of these antibodies, based on the size of this family, which contains some 30 members, the large proportion of antibodies using a member of the $V_H III$ gene family is expected. It is obvious that certain V_H gene families such as $V_H IV$ and $V_H V$ are overrepresented in autoreactive antibodies. As the $V_H IV$ family contains approximately 15 members and the $V_H V$ gene family consists of only two functional gene segments, the $V_H IV$ and $V_H V$ gene families are used at a frequency greater than expected based on the small portion of the genome these families represent. As CA activity is restricted to the expression of the $V_H 4–21$ gene segment, this may introduce a slight bias into the data. The $V_H I$ and $V_H II$ families appear to be underutilized in this group of antibodies based on the size of these families.

J_L Usage Is Random

The J_L gene segments used by this group of antibodies is heterogeneous (Table IV). Each of the germline J_κ gene segments are represented at expected frequencies with the exception of the $J_\kappa 3$ gene segment. The question

TABLE III. V_H and V_L utilization in human autoantibodies

	$V_H I$	$V_H II$	$V_H III$	$V_H IV$	$V_H V$	$V_H VI$	Total
$V_\kappa I$	0	1	9	3	2	0	15
$V_\kappa II$	1	0	0	1	0	0	2
$V_\kappa III$	1	0	2	6	2	0	11
$V_\kappa VI$	0	0	1	0	0	0	1
$V_\lambda I$	0	0	3	3	0	0	6
$V_\lambda II$	0	1	0	0	0	0	1
$V_\lambda IV$	0	0	0	1	0	0	1
$V_\lambda V$	0	0	0	2	0	0	2
Total	2	2	15	16	4	0	39

TABLE IV. V_L and J_L utilization in human autoantibodies

V_κ Family	$J_\kappa 1$	$J_\kappa 2$	$J_\kappa 3$	$J_\kappa 4$	$J_\kappa 5$	Total	V_λ Family	$J_\lambda I$	$J_\lambda 2/3$	$J_\lambda 7$	Total
$V_\kappa 1$	4	1	0	6	4	15	$V_\lambda I$	2	4	0	6
$V_\kappa II$	0	1	0	0	1	2	$V_\lambda II$	0	1	0	1
$V_\kappa III$	2	4	1	1	3	11	$V_\lambda IV$	0	1	0	1
$V_\kappa VI$	0	1	0	0	0	1	$V_\lambda V$	0	2	0	2
Total	6	7	1	7	8	29	Total	2	8	0	10

of restriction among the J_λ gene segments is complicated by the fact that several of the J_λ gene segments are identical at the nucleotide level and cannot be distinguished from one another. Overall, it appears that J_λ gene usage is also random.

SOME AUTOANTIBODIES ARE DIRECT COPIES OF GERMLINE GENES

In every group of autoantibodies studied, there is at least one example of an antibody that expresses a germline V_H or V_L gene segment, illustrating that at some autoantibodies are direct copies of germline genes. Upon comparison of the expressed variable gene segments with the most homologous germline gene (Table V), there is good correlation between the structures of the heavy and light chains. For example, if one chain expresses a direct copy of a germline gene, such as in RF–TS3, the second chain is also in germline configuration. As both heavy and light chain genes generally mutate at approximately the same rate, in those instances in which there appears to be a discrepancy (RF–TS5, RF–TS1, RF–TMC1, RF–SJ4, RF–SJ2, RF–SJ1, PR–SJ1, and FS–7) it is likely that the appropriate germline counterpart of the expressed V_H or V_L gene segment has not been identified. Most of these antibodies use a direct copy of a germline V_H or V_L gene segment or differ at most by two nucleotides from a known germline gene. These nucleotide substitutions may reflect either genetic polymorphism or somatic mutation. This suggests that the majority of autoantibodies derived from patients with autoimmune diseases are in nearly germline configuration.

THE VARIABLE REGIONS OF SOME AUTOANTIBODIES ARE CLEARLY MUTATED, SUGGESTIVE OF AN ANTIGEN-DRIVEN RESPONSE

While the majority of the autoantibodies appear to be germline or nearly germline in configuration, there are clear examples of somatic mutation and antigenic selection among them (Table V). This conclusion is supported by

TABLE V. Comparison of the V_H and V_L gene segments to germline genes

Clone	V_H Family	GL Donor (% NT homology)		V_L Family	GL Donor (% NT homology)	
RF–KES1	III	ND		I	V52	(96.1)
RF–KL1/2/3	III	VH26	(96.0)	I	Vd	(97.5)
RF–TS5	III	222B	(99.2)	I	HK102	(97.9)
RF–SJ5/6/7	III	ND		I	IGK14	(94.4)
RF–TS3	I	4.16	(100.0)	II	A23	(100.0)
RF–TS1	I	51P1	(95.0)	IIIb	325	(99.3)
RF–TS2	III	1.9III	(97.8)	IIIa	328	(97.2)
RF–TMC1	IV	4–21	(99.6)	III	38K	(94.0)
RF–SJ3	III	1.9III	(99.4)	IIIb	325	(98.6)
RF–SJ4	IV	71.2	(95.4)	IIIb	305	(100.0)
RF–KL5	III	ND		VI	A10	(73.0)
RF–SJ1	III	56P1	(95.3)	λI	FOG-B	(92.9)
RF–SJ2	III	56P1	(99.4)	λI	FOG-B	(96.3)
PR–TS1	III	3005	(99.6)	λI	FOG-B	(98.3)
PR–SJ2	III	1.9III	(94.7)	λII	Vλ21	(90.8)
PR–TS2	IV	4–21	(100.0)	λIV	V3S1	(100.0)
PR–SJ1/3	IV	71-4	(99.6)	λV	PAG-1	(82.7)
FS–5	IV	4–21	(100.0)	I	16K	(100.0)
FS–7	IV	4–21	(100.0)	I	HK102	(97.9)
FS–1	IV	4–21	(94.4)	II	GM607	(96.0)
FS–2	IV	4–21	(94.8)	IIIb	305	(97.5)
FS–4	IV	4–21	(95.0)	IIIa	KAP	(96.5)
FS–6	IV	4–21	(96.0)	IIIb	305	(97.9)
FS–3	IV	4–21	(99.6)	λI	VIS2	(100.0)
SA–1A/1D	V	VH251	(100.0)	I	16K	(100.0)
SA–4B	III	VH152	(84.0)	I	HK102	(93.0)
SA–4A	IV	4–21	(97.0)	IIIb	305	(97.2)
AChR–19	II	L1-1	(94.3)	I	Vd	(94.7)
AChR–37/29	V	VH32	(100.0)	IIIb	325	(100.0)
Vβ5	IV	71-2	(86.0)	λI	FOG-B	(92.2)
ID3	IV	4–21	(87.0)	λI	FOG-B	(87.8)
CK	IV	12G-1	(90.0)	I	HK102	(92.6)

GL, germline; ND, not determined; NT, nucleotide.

the analysis of replacement (R) and substitution (S) mutations in the light chains. Table VI presents the combined R/S ratios for the FW1–4 regions and CDR1–3. A V_L region that has a high replacement to silent mutation ratio (R/S) and a nonrandom distribution of mutations in the V_L region argues that antigenic selection has occurred. Random mutations in regions of the immunoglobulin molecule that are not essential to maintain structure, such as in a CDR, should yield an R/S ratio of 2.9. In regions such as FW, which need to be conserved in order to maintain proper structure, the ratio is expected to be

TABLE VI. Comparison of the V_L gene segment to closest germline gene

Clone	V_L Family	GL Donor	% Homology (nucleotide)	R/S Mutations FW	R/S Mutations CDR	J_L
RF–KES1	I	V52	96.1	0.5	1.5	5
RF–KL1/2/3	I	Vd	97.5	1.0	2.0	5
RF–TS5	I	HK102	97.9	0.0	1.5	4
RF–SJ5/6/7	I	IGK14	94.4	2.0	3.5	4
RF–TS3	II	A23	100.0	—	—	5
RF–TS1	IIIb	325	99.3	0.0	0.0	1
RF–TS2	IIIa	328	97.2	2.0	0.5	5
RF–TMC1	III	38K	94.0	1.0	3.0	4
RF–SJ3	IIIb	325	98.6	>1.0	0.5	2
RF–SJ4	IIIb	305	100.0	—	—	5
RF–KL5	VI	A10	73.0	ND	ND	2
RF–SJ1	λI	FOG-B	92.9	4.0	1.7	λ2
RF–SJ2	λI	FOG-B	96.3	2.3	1.2	λ2
PR–TS1	λI	FOG-B	98.3	1.0	2.0	λ2
PR–SJ2	λII	Vλ21	90.8	0.67	2.0	λ2
PR–TS2	λIV	V3S1	100.0	—	—	λ2
PR–SJ1/3	λV	PAG-1	82.7	1.2	2.4	λ2
FS–5	I	16K	100.0	—	—	1
FS–7	I	HK102	97.9	>1.0	1.0	1
FS–1	II	GM607	96.0	1.0	1.0	2
FS–2	IIIb	305	97.5	>4.0	1.4	5
FS–4	IIIa	KAP	96.5	1.0	1.5	2
FS–6	IIIb	305	97.9	0.0	5.0	1
FS–3	λI	VIS2	100.0	—	—	λ1
SA–1A/1D	I	16K	100.0	—	—	4
SA–4B	I	HK102	93.0	1.0	1.6	1
SA–4A	IIIb	305	97.2	2.0	2.3	3
AChR–19	I	Vd	94.7	1.0	4.5	1
AChR–37/29	IIIb	325	100.0	—	—	2
Vβ5	λI	FOG-B	92.2	0.86	1.0	λ1
ID3	λI	FOG-B	87.8	1.4	1.7	λ2
CK	I	HK102	92.6	0.57	2.0	2

GL, germline; ND, not determined.

lower and is about 1.5 for the light chain [Shlomchik et al., 1987a,b]. As most of the antigen contact residues occur within the CDRs, antigenic selection should exert a greater influence on the R/S ratio within the CDRs and select against R mutations in FW.

The data presented in Table VI illustrate that the variable regions of the IgG autoantibodies are extensively mutated, with the pattern of mutations distributed within the V_L region being consistent with a model of antigenic selection (RF–SJ5/6/7, RF–KL5, AChR–19). The structures of several IgM autoantibodies are also mutated (RF–TMC1, FS–6), with R/S ratios within the CDRs compatible with an antigen-driven response. Interestingly, the R/S ratios within the FW regions of several autoantibodies (RF–SJ5/6/7, RF–TS2, RF–SJ3, RF–SJ1, RF–SJ2, FS–7, FS–2, SA–4A) are greater than 1.5, providing evidence that the FW regions may be actively involved in antigen binding and subject to antigenic selection.

The process of antigenic selection can be best illustrated in the analysis of the clonally related rheumatoid factors RF–SJ1 and RF–SJ2. The structure of RF–SJ2 is in germline configuration, while the structure of RF–SJ1 is mutated. Measurements of the affinity for human IgG of these two rheumatoid factors illustrate that RF–SJ1 ($K_d = 2.4 \times 10^{-8}$ M) has a hundredfold higher affinity for IgG than RF–SJ2 ($K_d = 2.7 \times 10^{-6}$ M) [Randen et al., 1992]. These findings indicate that IgM rheumatoid factors in rheumatoid arthritis can undergo affinity maturation and that certain rheumatoid factors may be the product of an antigen-driven immune response.

ADDITIONAL MECHANISM OF ANTIBODY DIVERSITY IS CENTERED AT THE V_L–J_L JOINT

The joining of various V (D) and J gene segments during DNA rearrangement of the antigen receptor genes is one of the principle mechanisms responsible for the generation of antibody diversity. In the absence of N-segment variation, the structures of the coding joints formed during light chain rearrangement are less complex than their heavy chain counterparts. Consequently, the V_L–J_L joint formed during recombination is thought to account for all of the junctional diversity seen within the third CDR. The CDR3 of the light chain is typically nine amino acid residues in length, the first seven amino acids contributed by a particular V_L gene segment and the last two amino acid residues encoded by the J_L gene segment.

This study identified a number of autoantibodies that contained additional amino acids within CDR3. In the analysis of variable gene usage of rheumatoid factors isolated from the synovial fluid of patients with rheumatoid arthritis, four rheumatoid factors were characterized that contained one or two additional amino acid residues within CDR3 (RF–TS5, RF–TS2, RF–TMC1, and RF–SJ3). Similarly, two other autoantibodies, a striational antibody (SA-4B) and an anti-acetylcholine receptor antibody (AChR-37) isolated from patients with myasthenia gravis expressed a variation in the length of CDR3. This variation in the length of CDR3 has been seen in 35% of the autoantibodies presented in this study.

There are very few examples in the literature of either murine or human antibody systems in which variations in the length of CDR3 have been described. In the human system, many examples can be found in lymphomas involving translocations within either the κ or λ light chain loci [Roth et al., 1989]. To date, there are only a few human antibodies characterized that contain additional residues at the V_L–J_L joint [Ledford et al., 1983; Heller et al., 1987; Scott et al., 1989; Marks et al., 1991].

Randomly generated κ light chain transcripts from human fetal liver and peripheral blood lymphocytes demonstrated that approximately one-third contain additional nucleotides at the V_κ–J_κ joint independent of the J_κ gene segment utilized. While it appears that variation in the length of CDR3 occurs more frequently with V_κIII gene segments, the process occurs in all V_κ gene families. Analysis of the structures of the V_κ–J_κ joints suggests that both germline derived and nongermline encoded nucleotides (N segments) contribute to the junctional diversity of the immunoglobulin light chain variable region. Nearly 20% of the transcripts contain N-segment additions, consistent with Tdt-like activity. These observations suggest that Tdt or an analogous enzyme must be active in a significant percentage of human B cells during light chain rearrangement. Length variation in light chain CDR3 expands the potential repertoire and thus contributes an additional means of generating diversity in the antibody molecule.

CONCLUSION

The initial step toward defining the mechanisms involved in the development of human autoimmune disease began with the molecular characterization of variable gene repertoires encoding autoantibodies. There is an overwhelming amount of evidence in the literature that supports a model of oligoclonality or restriction of variable gene utilization in the B-cell repertoire of autoreactive antibodies such as mixed cryoglobulin rheumatoid factors, anti-DNA antibodies, and cold agglutinins based on serological and molecular analysis [Mageed and Jefferies, 1988; Chen et al., 1986; Spatz et al., 1990; Pascual et al., 1991]. These data clearly demonstrate that autoreactive antibodies are derived from a diverse repertoire of V_L gene segments. In addition, many autoantibodies are directly encoded by variable genes with little evidence of somatic mutation. However, the structures of some autoreactive antibodies are the product of somatic mutation and antigenic selection.

This analysis has documented that variation in the length of CDR3 of the light chain is a common element of human antibodies. Many of the additional residues are encoded by the germline V_κ and J_κ gene segments involved in recombination. In addition, there is evidence for N-segment addition at the V_κ–J_κ joint. Based on the composition of the N segments, in addition to the activity of Tdt, a second enzyme with a similar function may be implicated. Such length variations in CDR3 of the light chain add yet another dimension to the generation of antibody diversity.

REFERENCES

Alt F, Blackwell T, Yancopoulos G (1988): Development of the primary antibody repertoire. Science 238:1079–1087.

Chen PP, Albrandt K, Orida NK, Radoux V, Chen EY, Schrantz R, Liu F, Carson DA (1986): Genetic basis for the cross-reactive idiotypes of the light chains of human IgM anti-IgG autoantibodies. Proc Natl Acad Sci USA 83:8318–8322.

Combriato G, Klobeck H (1991): V_λ and J_λ–C_λ gene segments of the human immunoglobulin λ light chain locus are separated by 14 kb and rearrange by a deletion mechanism. Eur J Immunol 21:1513–1522.

Frangoine B, Moloshok T, Prelli F, Solomon A (1985): Human λ light chain constant region gene $C\lambda^{Mor}$: The primary structure of lambda VI Bence-Jones protein Mor. Proc Natl Acad Sci USA 82:3415–3419.

French DL, Laskov R, Scharff MD (1989): The role of somatic hypermutation in the generation of antibody diversity. Science 244:1152–1157.

Goodnow CC, Crosbie J, Adelstein S, Lavoie TB, Smith-Gill SJ, Brink RA, Pritchard-Briscoe H, Wotherspoon JS, Loblay RH, Raphael K, Trent RJ, Basten A (1988): Altered immunoglobulin expression and functional silencing of self-reactive B lymphocytes in transgenic mice. Nature 334:676–682.

Goodnow CC, Adelstein S, Basten A (1990): The need for central and peripheral tolerance in the B-cell repertoire. Science 248:1373–1379.

Guigou V, Cruisinier AM, Tonnelle C, Moinier D, Fougereau M, Fumoux F (1990): Human immunoglobulin V_H and V_κ repertoire revealed by in situ hybridization. Mol Immunol 27:935–940.

Hartley SB, Crosbie J, Brink R, Kantor AB, Basten A, Goodnow CC (1991): Elimination from peripheral lymphoid tissues of self-reactive B lymphocytes recognizing membrane-bound antigens. Nature 353:765–769.

Heller M, Owens JD, Mushinski JF, Rudikoff S (1987): Amino acids at the site of V_κ–J_κ recombination not encoded by germline sequences. J Exp Med 166:637–646.

Hess M, Hilschmann N, Rivat L, Rivat C, Ropartz C (1971): Isotypes in human immunoglobulin λ chains. Nature 234:58–61.

Hieter P, Hollis G, Korsmeyer S, Waldmann T, Leder P (1981): Clustered arrangement of immunoglobulin λ constant region genes in man. Nature 294:536–540.

Hieter PA, Maizel J, Leder P (1982): Evolution of human immunoglobulin light chain kappa J region genes. J Biol Chem 257:1516–1522.

Klobeck H, Meindl A, Combriato G, Solomon A, Zachau HG (1985a): Human immunoglobulin kappa light chain genes of the subgroups II and III. Nucleic Acids Res 13:6499–6513.

Klobeck H, Bornkamm GW, Combriato G, Mocikat R, Pohlenz H, Zachau HG (1985b): Subgroup IV of human immunoglobulin kappa light chain is encoded by a single germline gene. Nucleic Acids Res 13:6515–6529.

Klobeck HG, Zimmer FJ, Combriato G, Zachau HG (1987): Linkage of human V_κ and J_κ/C_κ regions by chromosomal walking. Nucleic Acids Res 15:9655–9665.

Koopman J, Schrohenloher RA (1980): In vitro synthesis of IgM rheumatoid factor lymphocytes from healthy donors. J Immunol 2:934–938.

Ledford DK, Goni F, Pizzolato M, Franklin EC, Solomon A, Frangoine B (1983): Preferential association of V$_\kappa$IIIb light chains with monoclonal IgM$_\kappa$ autoantibodies. J Immunol 131:1322–1325.

Lefvert AK, Holm G (1987): Idiotypic network in myasthenia gravis demonstrated by human monoclonal B-cell lines. Scand J Immunol 26:573–579.

Lotscher E, Grzeschik K, Bauer HG, Pohlenz H, Straubinger B, Zachau HG (1986): Dispersed human immunoglobulin kappa light-chain genes. Nature 320:456–458.

Mageed RA, Jefferies R (1988): Analysis of rheumatoid factor autoantibodies in patients with essential mixed cryoglobulinemia and rheumatoid arthritis. Scand J Rheumatol Suppl 75:172–178.

Marks JD, Tristem M, Karpas A, Winter G (1991): Oligonucleotide primers for polymerase chain reaction amplification of human immunoglobulin variable genes and design of family specific oligonucleotide probes. Eur J Immunol 21:985–991.

Marrack P, Lo D, Brinster R, Palmiter R, Burkly L, Flavell RH, Kappler J (1988): The effect of the thymus environment on T-cell development and tolerance. Cell 54:627–634.

McLachlan SM, Feldt-Rasmussen U, Young ET, Middleton SL, Blichert-Taft M, Siersboek-Nielson K, Date J, Carr D, Clark F, Smith BR (1987): IgG subclass distribution of thyroid autoantibodies: A fingerprint of an individual's response to thyroglobulin and thyroid microsomal antigen. Clin Endocrinol 26: 335–346.

Nemazee DA, Buerki K (1989): Clonal deletion of B-lymphocytes in a transgenic mouse bearing anti-MHC class I antibody genes. Nature 337:562–566.

Nossal GJV (1989): Immunologic tolerance: Collaboration between antigen and lymphokines. Science 245:147–153.

Pargent W, Schable KF, Zachau HG (1991): Polymorphisms and haplotypes in the human immunoglobulin κ locus. Eur J Immunol 21:1829–1835.

Pascual V, Victor KD, Lelsz D, Spellerberg MB, Hamblin TJ, Thompson KM, Randen I, Natvig J, Capra JD, Stevenson FK (1991): Nucleotide analysis of the variable regions of two cold agglutinins: Evidence that the VH4-21 gene segment is responsible for the major cross-reactive idiotype. J Immunol 146:4385–4391.

Paul E, Livneh A, Manheimer-Lory A, Diamond B (1991): Characterization of the human immunoglobulin VλII gene family and analysis of VλII and Cλ polymorphism in systemic lupus erythematosus. J Immunol 147:2771–2776.

Pech M, Zachau HG (1984): Immunoglobulin genes of different subgroups are interdigitated within the Vκ locus. Nucleic Acids Res 12:9229–9236.

Pech M, Jaenichen H, Pohlenz H, Neumaier P, Klobeck H, Zachau HG (1984): Organization and evolution of a gene cluster for human immunoglobulin V regions of the kappa type. J Mol Biol 176:189–204.

Pech M, Smola H, Pohlenz H, Straubinger B, Gerl R, Zachau HG (1985): A large section of the gene locus encoding the human immunoglobulin variable regions of the kappa type is duplicated. J Mol Biol 183:291–299.

Pohlenz H, Straubinger B, Thiebe R, Pech M, Zimmer F, Zachau HG (1987): The human Vκ locus: Characterization of extended immunoglobulin gene regions by cosmid cloning. J Mol Biol 193:241–253.

Prabhakar BG, Segusa J, Onodera T, Notkins AL (1984): Lymphocytes capable of making monoclonal autoantibodies that react with multiple organs are a common feature of the normal B-cell repertoire. J Immunol 133:2815–2817.

Randen I, Thompson KM, Natvig JB, Forre O, Waalen K (1989): Human monoclonal rheumatoid factors from the polyclonal repertoire of rheumatoid synovial tissue: Production and characterization. Clin Exp Immunol 78:13–18.

Randen I, Brown D, Thompson KM, Hughes-Jones N, Pascual V, Victor K, Capra JD, Forre O, Natvig JB (1992): Clonally related IgM rheumatoid factors undergo affinity maturation in rheumatoid synovial inflammation. J Immunol 148:3296–3301.

Roth DB, Chang X, Wilson JH (1989): Comparison of filler DNA at immune, nonimmune, and oncogenic rearrangements suggests multiple mechanisms of formation. Mol Cell Biol 9:3049–3057.

Scott MG, Crimmins DL, McCourt DW, Zoucher I, Thiebe R, Zachau HG, Nahm MH (1989): Clonal characterization of the human IgG antibody repertoire to *H. influenzae* type b polysaccharide. III. A single V$_\kappa$II gene and one of several J$_\kappa$ genes are joined by an invariant arginine to form the most common light chain variable region. J Immunol 143:4110–4116.

Shlomchik MJ, Marshak-Rothstein A, Wolfowicz CB, Rothstein TL, Weigert MG (1987a): The role of clonal selection and somatic mutation in autoimmunity. Nature 328:805–811.

Shlomchik MJ, Aucoin AH, Pisetsky DS, Weigert MG (1987b): Structure and function of anti-DNA autoantibodies derived from a single autoimmune mouse. Proc Natl Acad Sci USA 84:9150–9154.

Spatz LA, Wong KK, Williams M, Desai R, Golier J, Berman JE, Alt FW, Latov N (1990): Cloning and sequence analysis of the V$_H$ and V$_L$ regions of an anti-myelin/DNA antibody from a patient with peripheral neuropathy and chronic lymphocytic leukemia. J Immunol 144:2821–2828.

Spitzer RE, Stitzel AE, Tsokos GC, Pascual V, Victor K, Capra JD (1991): DNA sequence of C3NeF from a patient with membrane-proliferative glomerulonephritis (MPGN): Evidence for antigen driven affinity maturation. Am Soc Neurol (in press).

Stevenson FK, Smith GJ, North J, Hamblin TJ, Glennie MJ (1989): Identification of normal B-cell counterparts which secrete cold agglutinins of anti-I and anti-i specificity. Br J Haematol 72:9–15.

Straubinger B, Thiebe R, Huber C, Osterholzer E, Zachau HG (1988): Two unusual human immunoglobulin V-kappa genes. Hoppe-Seyler 369:601–608.

Tonegawa S (1983): Somatic generation of antibody diversity. Nature 302:575–581.

Udey J, Blomberg B (1987): Human λ light chain locus: Organization and DNA sequences of three genomic J regions. Immunogenetics 25:63–70.

Vasicek T, Leder P (1990): Structure and expression of the human immunoglobulin λ genes. J Exp Med 172:609–620.

Victor KD, Randen I, Thompson K, Forre O, Natvig JB, Fu SM, Capra JD (1991): Rheumatoid factors isolated from patients with autoimmune disorders are derived from germline genes distinct from those encoding the Wa, Po and Bla cross-reactive idiotypes. J Clin Invest 87:1603–1613.

Williams CL, Lennon VA (1986): Thymic B-lymphocyte clones from patients with myasthenia gravis secrete monoclonal striational antibodies reacting with myosin, α-actinin or actin. J Exp Med 164:1043–1059.

Zachau HG (1990): The human immunoglobulin kappa locus and some of its acrobatics. Hoppe-Seyler 371:1–6.

4

ROLE OF THE MAJOR HISTOCOMPATIBILITY COMPLEX IN T-CELL RECEPTOR REPERTOIRE SELECTION

Charles A. Janeway, Jr.

Section of Immunobiology, Howard Hughes Medical Institute, Yale University School of Medicine, New Haven, Connecticut

INTRODUCTION

Autoimmune diseases require that an immune response persist over long periods of time. All persistent immune responses require a specific T cell, and there is evidence from many different systems documenting the central role of T cells in autoimmunity. Therefore the development of the T-cell receptor repertoire, and the subsequent activation of T cells by antigens in the periphery, are among the central concerns in studying autoimmunity. Central to the process of T-cell activation is the presentation of peptide fragments of protein by major histocompatibility complex (MHC) molecules at the cell surface. Likewise, MHC molecules are central in repertoire selection of T cells. The role of the MHC in these two processes is analyzed in this chapter.

Autoimmunity: Physiology and Disease, Pages 35–43
© *1994 Wiley-Liss, Inc.*

MHC MOLECULES ARE THREE-CHAIN STRUCTURES THAT DISPLAY BOTH POLYMORPHISM AND HYPERVARIABILITY

T cells always recognize MHC molecules. The MHC molecule has two very interesting characteristics. First, MHC molecules are the most polymorphic structures known, there being as many as 100 alleles at loci encoding them. Second, the mature MHC molecule at the cell surface that is recognized by the T-cell receptor is always a three-chain structure, with the third chain being an extremely variable peptide. MHC molecules are designed to fold around their associated peptide, whose nature is determined by the polymorphic residues on the MHC molecule, which control binding, and the availability of the peptide in the compartment where folding is accomplished; for MHC class I molecules, this is the endoplasmic reticulum, and for MHC class II molecules it is an acidified post-Golgi vesicle whose precise nature is still being defined. The two MHC molecules present peptides from two distinct cellular domains separated by a lipid bilayer membrane, the MHC class I molecules from the cytosol and MHC class II molecules from cellular vesicles.

In a healthy individual, the peptides presented by MHC molecules at the cell surface are all derived from self-proteins [Jardetzky et al., 1991; Rudensky et al., 1991b]. During infection, peptides derived from the pathogen's protein are added to the set of self-peptides presented and ideally elicit a protective immune response. However, self-peptides are presented by MHC molecules at all times. It is likely that these MHC molecules containing self peptides are the targets of T cell recognition in autoimmunity.

An interesting feature of most autoimmune diseases is how specific and reproducible they are, so that they can be named and their character anticipated: insulin-dependent diabetes mellitus, Grave's disease, ankylosing spondylitis, and so forth. This strongly suggests that very specific responses directed at a particular self-peptide are involved. This impression is reinforced by the finding that individual diseases are associated with MHC genotype. As MHC polymorphism focuses on the peptide binding cleft, different allelic variants of MHC molecules bind and present very different self-peptides. Thus MHC control of susceptibility to particular autoimmune diseases implies that only rare and very specific combinations of MHC and self-peptide can trigger disease.

Peptide binding to MHC molecules involves a few specific amino acid side chains spaced at intervals along the peptide [Jardetzky et al., 1991; Falk et al., 1991; Madden et al., 1991; Rudensky et al., 1992]. These amino acid side chains enter deep pockets in the MHC structure, allowing tight binding of the peptide [Madden et al., 1991]. The MHC molecule actually folds around the peptide, so that binding is nearly irreversible. The amino acid side chains that bind in the pockets and anchor the peptide to the MHC molecule have been called *anchor residues*. The pattern of anchor residues that allows binding to a given MHC molecule is called a *peptide motif*. Each MHC molecule defines a distinct peptide motif, implying that each MHC molecule will present a unique set of self-peptides. Thus one would expect each autoimmune syndrome to be associated with one or a few MHC alleles that can bind the relevant autoantigenic peptide.

A second factor that controls the peptides presented by MHC molecules is the abundance of the peptide in the compartment where the MHC proteins fold [Jardetzky et al., 1991; Rudensky et al., 1991b]. Thus highly abundant peptides will be presented at higher levels than rare peptides that bind an MHC molecule with equivalent affinity. Three factors control abundance of peptides: the amount of precursor protein, its rate of breakdown into peptide, and the ability of a peptide to be generated by processing. Some peptides within a protein, while able to bind MHC and elicit a response, cannot be generated by the processing machinery [Mamula, 1992; Lehmann et al., 1992]. These have been termed *cryptic epitopes*. They elicit neither tolerance nor immunity to the whole protein. Thus self will be defined by the peptides presented by an individual's MHC molecules, and these in turn are influenced by MHC polymorphism and by peptide abundance.

HOW COMPLEX IS SELF?

The ability of T cells to respond to self-peptides presented by self-MHC molecules, leading to autoimmunity requires that the self-peptide be presented. However, T cells specific for abundant self-peptides are eliminated during T-cell development, rendering the host self-tolerant. How many different self-peptides play a role in this latter process?

It is estimated that humans have about 10^5 genes encoding proteins of an average of 300 amino acids, capable of generating $\sim 3 \times 10^7$ peptides of 10 amino acids, the minimum length required for MHC binding. As there are roughly 10^{13} peptides of 10 amino acids possible, self defines a minute subset of the total available. Thus there is about one chance in a million that one could be tolerant to a selected non-self peptide. This means that recognition of peptides from pathogens is unlikely to be significantly impeded by self-tolerance.

The complexity of self in terms of T-cell responsiveness, however, is actually far less than the theoretical number of 3×10^7. First, only a small fraction of these peptides will contain suitable sequences for MHC binding— roughly 1% based on specifying two anchor positions, each of which can be fulfilled by two amino acids. Second, most genes are either not expressed or are expressed at a very low level, yielding too little peptide to bind MHC molecules. Third, and probably most important, it requires about 100 MHC molecules on a single cell, all binding the same peptide, to signal a T cell [Demotz et al., 1990; Harding and Unanue, 1990]. As there are $\sim 10^5$ MHC molecules of a given type on a cell, not more than 10^3 different peptides can be presented by one cell at levels detectable by a T-cell, assuming all are present in equal abundance. However, some peptides are very abundantly bound in cells; in one case, one MHC class II molecule in eight was binding the same self-peptide [Rudensky et al., 1991a]. Moreover, this peptide was presented at this level by all cells examined. Thus self is likely represented by a few hundred peptides to which T cells must be tolerant.

One mechanism for increasing the complexity of self-peptides presented for tolerance induction may be the resting B cell. Peptides presented by resting B cells lead to tolerance of specific T cells [Eynon and Parker, 1992]. B cells can bind and internalize protein with their specific Ig receptor [Lanzavecchia, 1985; Rock et al., 1984; Davidson and Watts, 1989]. This leads to high levels of peptide presentation by MHC class II molecules on the B cell. As each B cell will internalize different proteins, individual B cells may present different self-peptides, leading to a broader range of self-tolerance. However, the importance of this is unclear as B-cell-deficient animals and people have not been reported to have an elevated rate of autoimmunity. Finally, the tissue cells that are the target of autoimmune diseases express lower levels of MHC molecules than lymphoid cells, so one would expect only rare cases in which specific peptide–MHC complexes on tissue cells would achieve levels of expression worthy of a T cell's attention. These facts may explain the rarity of autoimmune disease, its specificity, and its relationship to MHC genotype.

MHC AND T-CELL RECEPTOR REPERTOIRES

The MHC not only presents antigens in the periphery, but also plays a key role in selecting the repertoire of T-cell receptors. The MHC plays a role in two different selective processes in the thymus, called *positive* and *negative selection*. Positive selection is the selection for further maturation of immature T cells whose receptor is specific for foreign peptides bound to self-MHC molecules. This is required because, of 100 possible MHC molecules at a given locus, an individual will express only one or two, and T cells that can recognize foreign peptides presented only by non-self MHC molecules will be useless. Negative selection is the removal of T cells whose receptor can be bound by self-peptide–self-MHC complexes.

There is a paradox here; all MHC molecules in the thymus are believed to bind self-peptides. Would not the same self-peptide–self-MHC complexes inform cells to mature and then delete them? Obviously not, as a repertoire of T cells is generated that is both self-MHC restricted and self-tolerant [von Boehmer et al., 1989]. What distinguishes these two processes and allows T-cell maturation?

Two main hypotheses have been proposed to explain how positive and negative selection differ [Janeway et al., 1992]. One states that the affinity threshold for positive selection is lower than that for deletion, so that cells with an affinity for self-MHC too low for activation will be selected for further maturation but not deleted [Janeway et al., 1976]. The other states that the peptides presented by the thymic cortical epithelium, the cells involved in positive selection, differ from those on antigen-presenting cells that control deletion [Marrack and Kappler, 1988]. Evidence for either hypothesis is weak. Thymic cortical epithelial cells may have unique features that allow positive selection that cannot be mimicked by other cell types [Cosgrove et al., 1992]; the nature of these features is unclear.

Some years ago, Janeway et al. [1989] presented data suggesting that T-cell receptors require both aggregation and conformational change for optimal signalling. Recent data showing that analogue peptides can specifically inhibit T-cell activation may be interpreted the same way (De Magistris et al., 1992]. Thus it is possible that positive selection involves T-cell receptor aggregation with peptides that do not alter T-cell receptor conformation and thus only partially signal. This could account for the distinction in the two types of selection. A requirement for conformational change in signalling for activation or deletion might also account for the low affinity of T-cell receptors for their activating ligands [Matsui et al., 1991; Weber et al., 1992], as induced changes in conformation are usually energetically unfavorable. It is possible that the inhibitory analogue peptide binds far better than the stimulatory native peptide, but does not activate as no conformational change is induced. The aggregation signal, presented on cortical epithelial cells, may be sufficient for maturation but not for eliciting signals that lead to activation and hence to deletion.

EXPRESSION OF AUTOANTIGENS IS NECESSARY BUT NOT SUFFICIENT FOR AUTOIMMUNE DISEASE

It is clear that autoantigens, in the form of self-peptide–self-MHC complexes, must be expressed on the target tissue or on antigen-presenting cells at levels sufficient to signal a T cell in order for autoimmune disease to ensue. However, there is strong evidence that mere presence of an autoantigen is not sufficient to elicit autoimmunity (see Chapter 13). Rather, it is clear that the activation of autoreactive T cells is the conditional feature required for autoimmune disease. For instance, cloned, autoreactive T cells can readily induce a wide range of autoimmune diseases upon adoptive transfer to perfectly normal recipients, provided the recipients express the correct peptide–MHC ligand [Zamvil et al., 1985; Reich et al., 1989]. Thus autoantigen expression, while necessary for disease induction, is not sufficient to explain the occurrence of autoimmune disease.

Why, then, do autoimmune diseases occur? Although a complete answer is obviously not available (otherwise this book would be much shorter and less speculative), the likely answer comes from an analysis of the requirements for T-cell activation. T cells must receive a signal from their receptor, which requires binding to a specific peptide–MHC complex. This gives the response its specificity. They must also receive an additional signal from the same cell presenting the specific ligand [Jenkins et al., 1987; Liu and Janeway, 1992]. This signal, known as the *costimulatory* signal, does two things to the T cell that may simply be different faces of the same coin. First, the costimulatory signal allows the T cell to undergo clonal expansion. This is usually driven by autocrine stimulation by interleukin (IL)-2. Second, this signal permits the T cell to remain responsive to antigen; in its absence, the T cell becomes nonresponsive or anergic. This strongly suggests that the regulation of the costimulatory signal in an individual whose MHC genotype allows presentation of autoantigen is the key factor determining whether autoimmune disease occurs. Therefore, in addition to the analysis of MHC binding of autoantigen peptides, an understanding of the regulation of costimulation is crucial to understanding autoimmunity.

Many different molecules on T cells have been shown to have a role in T-cell activation, and some have been said to deliver costimulatory signals [van Seventer et al., 1991; Damle et al., 1992]. These, however, fall into two sets. Some aid the T-cell receptor in recognizing antigens; others actually provide not only signals that lead to clonal expansion of the specific T cells but also block the induction of anergy [Liu et al., 1992; Harding et al., 1992]. Among the latter, CD28 has received the most attention. CD28 binds B7, a molecule found on potent antigen-presenting cells but not elsewhere in the body [Linsley et al., 1991]. B7 expression is induced by a variety of infectious agents and their purified products [Liu and Janeway, 1991; Liu et al., 1993]. Blocking B7 inhibits T-cell activation and leads to anergy [Linsley et al., 1991; Liu et al., 1993], while stimulating CD28 prevents anergy induction [Liu and Janeway, 1991; Harding et al., 1992]. Thus the regulation of B7 expression may play a key role in initiating autoimmune T-cell responses. Once initiated, it is possible that cytokines produced by the responding cells maintain B7 expression and thus sustain the response. This may explain the association of recent infection with autoimmune disease and the requirement for bacterial adjuvants in experimental autoimmune disease induction.

CONCLUSION

T cells recognize the hypervariable peptides that make up the central part of the outer end of an MHC molecule. Apparently, only rare combinations of self-peptides with self-MHC molecules can lead to autoimmune disease. However, expression of autoantigens is not the only requirement for autoimmunity to occur. Responsive T cells must be present in an activatable state, requiring positive but not negative selection during development in the thymus. The nature of these two processes, and their necessary distinction, is unclear at present. However, different mechanisms of signalling via the T-cell receptor may lead to the distinctive outcome of these two processes. Finally, T cells specific for expressed autoantigens must be induced into a sustained immune response. This last step is crucial, and it may be triggered by infection, which activates expression of costimulatory signals on antigen-presenting cells.

ACKNOWLEDGMENTS

This work was supported by grants NIH Al-14579, Al-26810, and the Howard Hughes Medical Institute.

REFERENCES

Cosgrove D, Chan SH, Waltzinger C, Benoist C, Mathis D (1992): The thymic compartment responsible for positive selection of CD4$^+$ T cells. Int Immunol 4:707–710.

Damle NK, Klussman K, Linsley PS, Aruffo A (1992): Differential costimulatory effects of adhesion molecules B7, ICAM-1, LFA-3, and VCAM-1 on resting and antigen-primed CD4$^+$ T lymphocytes. J Immunol 148:1985–1992.

Davidson HW, Watts C (1989): Epitope-directed processing of specific antigen by lymphocytes. J Cell Biol 109:85–92.

De Magistris MT, Alexander J, Coggeshall M, Altman A, Gaeta FCA, Grey HM, Sette A (1992): Antigen analog–major histocompatibility complexes act as antagonists of the T cell receptor. Cell 68:625–634.

Demotz S, Grey HM, Sette A (1990): The minimal number of class II MHC–antigen complexes needed for T cell activation. Science 249:1028–1030.

Eynon EE, Parker DC (1992): Small B cells as antigen-presenting cells in the induction of tolerance to soluble protein antigens. J Exp Med 175:131–138.

Falk K, Rotzschke O, Stevanovic S, Jung G, Rammensee H-G (1991): Allele-specific motifs revealed by sequencing of self-peptides eluted from MHC molecules. Nature 351:290–296.

Harding FA, McArthur JG, Gross JA, Raulet DH, Allison JP (1992): CD28-mediated signalling co-stimulates murine T cells and prevents induction of anergy in T-cell clones. Nature 356:507–609.

Harding CV, Unanue ER (1990): Quantitation of antigen-presenting cell MHC class II/peptide complexes necessary for T-cell stimulation. Nature 346:574–576.

Janeway CA Jr, Rudensky A, Rath S, Murphy D (1992): It is easier for a camel to pass the needle's eye. Curr Biol 2:26–28.

Janeway CA Jr, Dianzani U, Portoles P, Rath S, Reich E-P, Rojo J, Yagi J, Murphy DB (1989): Cross-linking and conformational change in T-cell receptors: Role in activation and in repertoire selection. Cold Spring Harbor Symp Quant Biol LIV:657–666.

Janeway CA Jr, Wigzell H, Binz H (1976): Hypothesis: Two different V_H gene products make up the T cell receptors. Scand J Immunol 5:593.

Jardetzky TS, Lane WS, Robinson RA, Madden DR, Wiley DC (1991): Identification of self peptides bound to purified HLA-B27. Nature 353:326–329.

Jenkins MK, Pardoll DM, Mizuguchi J, Quill H, Schwartz RH (1987): T cell non-responsiveness in vivo and in vitro: Fine specificity of induction and molecular characterization of the unresponsiveness state. Immunol Rev 95:113.

Lanzavecchia A (1985): Antigen-specific interaction between T and B cells. Nature 314:537.

Lehmann PV, Forsthuber T, Miller A, Sercarz EE (1992): Spreading of T-cell auto-immunity to cryptic determinants of an autoantigen. Nature 358:155–157.

Linsley PS, Brady W, Grossmair L, Aruffo A, Damle NK, Ledbetter JA (1991): Binding of the B cell activation antigen B7 to CD28 costimulates T-cell proliferation and interleukin-2 mRNA accumulation. J Exp Med 173:721.

Liu Y, Janeway CA Jr (1992): Cells that present both specific ligand and costimulatory activity are the most efficient inducers of clonal expansion of normal CD4 T cells. Proc Natl Acad Sci USA 89:3845–3849.

Liu Y and Janeway CA Jr (1991): Microbial induction of co-stimulatory activity for CD4 T-cell growth. Int Immunol 3:323–332.

Liu Y, Jones B, Aruffo A, Sullivan KM, Linsley PS, Janeway CA Jr (1992): Heat-stable antigen is a costimulatory molecule for CD4 T cell growth. J Exp Med 175:437–445.

Liu Y, Jones B, Brady W, Janeway CA Jr, Linsley PS (1993): Co-stimulation of murine CD4 T cell growth: Cooperation between B7 and heat stable antigen. Eur J Immunol 22:2855–2859.

Madden DR, Gorga JC, Strominger JL, Wiley DC (1991): The structure of HLA-B27 reveals nonamer self-peptides bound in an extended conformation. Nature 353:321.

Mamula MJ (1993): The inability to process a self-peptide allows autoreactive T cells to escape tolerance. J Exp Med 177:567–571.

Marrack P, Kappler J (1988): The T-cell repertoire for antigen and MHC. Immunol Today 9:308–315.

Matsui K, Boniface JJ, Reay PA, Schild H, Fazekas De St. Groth B, Davis MM (1991): Low affinity interaction of peptide–MHC complexes with T cell receptors. Science 254:1788–1791.

Reich E-P, Sherwin RS, Kanagawa O, Janeway CA Jr (1989): An explanation for the protective effect of the MHC class II I-E molecule in murine diabetes. Nature 341:326–328.

Rock KL, Benacerraf B, Abbas AK (1984): Antigen presentation by hapten-specific B lymphocytes. I. Role of surface immunoglobulin receptors. J Exp Med 160:1102.

Rudensky AY, Preston-Hurlburt P, Al-Ramadi B, Rothbard J, Janeway CA Jr (1992): Truncation variants of peptides isolated from MHC class II molecules suggest sequence motifs. Nature 359:429–431.

Rudensky AY, Rath S, Preston-Hurlburt P, Murphy DB, Janeway CA Jr (1991a): On the complexity of self. Nature 353:660–662.

Rudensky AY, Preston-Hurlburt P, Hong SC, Barlow A, Janeway CA Jr (1991b): Sequence analysis of peptides bound to MHC class II molecules. Nature 353:622–627.

van Seventer GA, Shimizu Y, Shaw S (1991): Roles of multiple accessory molecules in T-cell activation. Curr Biol 3:294–303.

von Boehmer H, Teh HS, Kisielow P (1989): The thymus selects the useful, neglects the useless and destroys the harmful. Immunol Today 10:57–60.

Weber S, Traunecker A, Oliveri F, Gerhard W, Karjalainen K (1992): Specific low-affinity recognition of major histocompatibility complex plus peptide by soluble T-cell receptor. Nature 356:793–796.

Zamvil S, Nelson P, Trotter J, Mitchell J, Knobler R, Fritz R, Steinman L (1985): T-cell clones specific for myelin basic protein induce chronic relapsing paralysis and demyelination. Nature 317:355–358.

5

STIMULATION OF T AND B CELLS

Jan Andersson, Yves Modigliani, and Alf Grandien

Department of Immunology, University of Uppsala Biomedical Center,
Uppsala, Sweden (J.A., A.G.); Unité d'Immunobiologie, Institut Pasteur,
Paris, France (Y.M., A.G.)

INTRODUCTION

A considerable part of our knowledge concerning activation of T and B lymphocytes arises from studies of continuous cell lines kept in vitro. Although much valuable information has been extracted from such approaches, these systems are far from ideal. What we really would like to know is how normal lymphocytes are activated in vivo. Which are the relevant mechanisms for in vivo activation, and what are the rules that govern whether activation actually will take place? An important step in this direction is represented by the possibilities of in vitro growth and differentiation of *normal lymphocytes*. If conclusions concerning the behavior of lymphocytes in vitro are to be transposed onto the in vivo situation a number of criteria have to be fulfilled, and even then the conclusions will remain preliminary, awaiting validation in vivo. One of the major obstacles with in vitro systems in general concerns the problem of representativity. Thus questions like what fraction of the normal cells becomes activated to clonal growth and differentiation in a particular in vitro system has to be answered. In addition to this, once activated, the observed in vitro responses must find their in vivo correlates at the phenotypical level. Ideally, we also

Autoimmunity: Physiology and Disease, Pages 45–56
© 1994 Wiley-Liss, Inc.

would like to use methods whereby the qualities of single cells can be revealed so as to be able to distinguish different populations within a heterogeneous sample.

Already at this early point in our discussion it becomes apparent that the study of lymphocyte activation not only encounters problems of a technical character but also concerns the definition of activation itself. Is activation an event leading to a change in the size of the cell, an increase in the number of ribosomes, or an increased expression of certain membrane or intracellular molecules? To that end, even cell death could be regarded as activation considering the fact that protein de novo synthesis is required for apoptosis.

In this chapter we argue that activation, in order to be meaningful, must result in function. We therefore focus our attention on the activation events leading normal lymphocytes to acquire their terminal differentiation stage: for B cells, antibody secretion; and for T cells, help or suppression/cytotoxicity.

RESTING AND ACTIVATED CELLS IN THE NORMAL IMMUNE SYSTEM

The normal immune system contains lymphocytes in all stages of activation. Most cells are small and resting, but a fraction of both T and B cells (around 1%) have become activated even when the experimental animals are kept under specific pathogen-free (SPF) and antigen-free conditions [Pereira et al., 1986]. Since the fraction of activated cells is small, it is generally disregarded and referred to as background activity or "noise." We see no reason why the activation of these cells should follow different rules concerning their activation compared with the activation occurring during the regular immune response. Might it not even be so that these cells would be the best candidates for the study of mechanisms underlying lymphocyte activation in vivo?

STUDYING LYMPHOCYTE ACTIVATION IN VITRO

Both T and B cells leave the site of production (thymus or fetal liver/bone marrow) as small, resting cells. In the periphery such cells then await the encounter of antigen so as to become activated into effector functions—for B cells, antibody secretion; and for T cells, helper or suppressor/cytotoxic activity. Upon activation the resting cell changes morphology and takes on the appearance of larger sized blast cells.

From in vitro studies it turns out that resting cells and in vivo activated blast cells not only display different metabolic activities but also have different activation requirements. Thus small resting T cells respond readily to mitogens and antigens presented by antigen-presenting cells (APC) but do not respond to interleukin-2 (IL-2), for example. T-cell blasts, on the other hand, respond to both, albeit the response to IL-2 is independent of APC [Coutinho et al., 1979]. Similarly, small resting B cells as well as activated B-cell blasts respond readily to mitogens like lipopolysaccharides (LPS), but only blasts respond to mitogens like purified protein derivative (PPD) [Sultzer and Nilsson, 1972] or T-cell-derived interleukins by both proliferation and differentiation into high rate antibody-producing cells [Andersson et al., 1979a,b]. As a consequence, there are agents that differ in their action on cells depending on the stage of activation, which also translates into the position of the cell within the cell cycle. This is certainly true for substances, mostly mitogens, that seemingly operate on nonclonally distributed receptors. The question is whether such rules also apply to ligand binding of clonally distributed V-region-containing receptors on T and B cells. This certainly is the case for alloreactive T cells, which cannot mount a primary proliferative in vitro response to MHC antigens presented in the form of lipid vesicles, whereas such preparations induce a vigorous secondary restimulation of already primed, isolated T-cell blasts (P. Peterson, personal communication).

Similar differences have not yet been reported for B cells at different stages of differentiation when binding of antigen or anti-Ig antibodies have been studied. In fact, we have repeatedly failed to record induction into effector cell development when resting B cells or activated B-cell blasts are subjected only to ligands binding to immunoglobulin.

For studies on cellular activation in vitro, therefore, one has to select those cells that have not previously been activated by unknown means. This can be achieved by means of size separation, for example, by sedimentation at 1g, according to Miller and Phillips [1969].

FROM IN VITRO TO IN VIVO AND BACK AGAIN

From now on, we will leave the studies on T cells and T-cell activation and instead concentrate on B cells. The reason is related to the following problems: *How can one know whether one took the right avenue if one never arrives? How can one know whether one has arrived if one does not know where one is going?* The problem in discussing T-cell activation is the absence of quantitative, single cell assays for terminally differentiated T cells. As a consequence, the bridge between in vitro and in vivo observations cannot be constructed, and one is left in a mist of phenomenology. Notions such as partial activation, abortive activation, apoptotic activation, erroneous activation, as well as anergic activation are consequences of the lack of assays for terminally differentiated T cells.

Certainly, our knowledge concerning B cells and B-cell activation is fragmentary and incomplete, but at least we have a method of scoring single cells at the stage of terminal differentiation. Therefore we can easily compare our activated cells in vitro with their in vivo counterparts, and the interplay between in vitro and in vivo observations become possible.

We here briefly describe the assays for terminal B-cell differentiation, thymus-independent antigens, and polyclonal B-cell activators; stimulation of small resting B cells; and the roles of surface IgM and surface IgD in such stimulation. Furthermore, the balance between proliferation and maturation of B cells as well as their development and turnover will be discussed. Our conclusions concern the rules governing both "background activation" and activation during regular immune responses.

QUANTITATIVE ASSAYS FOR LYMPHOCYTE FUNCTIONS

The only quantitative, single cell assay for a differentiated lymphocyte function is the plaque-forming cell (PFC) [Jerne and Nordin, 1963; Gronowicz et al., 1976] assay scoring for high rate antibody-secreting B cells. Its modern adaptation to the microtiter plate system uses enzyme-linked antibody reagents to reveal spots of chromogenic insoluble substrate products formed around B lymphocytes secreting antibodies. This assay, called ELI-Spot Assay (or ESA) [Sedgwick and Holt, 1983], will score for cells secreting specific antibody when antigen is used in the assay or will score for cells producing a particular isotype or idiotype when appropriate catching antibody reagents are used in the assay. Only B cells that have become activated and have proceeded in the differentiation pathway toward the plasma cell will score in these assays. Likewise, such cells have accumulated large enough amounts of Ig-specific mRNA to be scored by in situ hybridization with isotype- or VH-specific DNA probes [Grandien et al., 1991]. Only in the particular differentiation stage, which allows secretion of enough antibodies to be revealed by the PFC or ESA assay, will one also score positive cells with the radioactive probe technique for in situ hybridization.

THYMUS-INDEPENDENT ANTIGENS

Although much of our understanding of B-lymphocyte stimulation derives from studies on T–B-cell collaboration, when discussing B-cell induction we would like to emphasize also some other basic findings from the past. Thus it was somewhat surprising to find a large set of molecules, principally derived from bacteria, that do not require the participation of T cells in order to elicit an antibody response [Möller and Michael, 1971]. Consequently, such compounds were termed *thymus-independent (TI) antigens*. Subsequently it was shown that all TI antigens were selectively mitogenic for B cells and therefore also belong to the group of agents known as *polyclonal B-cell activators* [Coutinho and Möller, 1973]. Thus the connection was made between B-cell mitogens and TI antigens, but was regarded by some to be an "abnormal induction," [Bretscher, 1972] whereas others made it the rule that B-cell clonal growth and differentiation is driven by ligands occupying receptors not clonally distributed [Coutinho and Möller, 1974], specificity of the response being ensured by the passive focusing of mitogenic antigen by clonally distributed specific Ig molecules on the surface of antigen-sensitive B cells [Andersson et al., 1972; Coutinho and Gronowicz, 1975].

STIMULATION OF SMALL B CELLS

Only after the introduction of in vitro techniques that allowed the study of single clones of B cells could one make statements concerning the number of cells involved in a reaction. Thus quantitative assessments of B-cell stimulation is crucial for our understanding of induction.

B cells, like other eukaryotic cells, cannot grow in the absence of yet largely undefined survival and growth factors. This becomes obvious when attempting to dilute cells down to 1 cell/ml culture medium. Not only is the frequency of takes dependent on the type and batch of serum, but it is also strictly dependent on the number of cells initially plated. Thus, under optimal conditions of tissue culture, small resting B cells cannot be diluted below 5,000 cells per milliliter even to yield one cell responding to the mitogen LPS. However, by introducing thymus filler cells at high density, the number of responding B cells increases to at best one out of three [Andersson et al., 1977]. The fact that under these circumstances not every resting B cell responds has caused some arguments as to the possible existence of subpopulations of B cells responding to different stimuli. This notion became stronger since it was shown that after 18 hours of induction by LPS the separated blasts could be restimulated under the same culture conditions at 100% efficiency both by the same mitogen (LPS) and by other, heterologous B-cell mitogens [lipoprotein; Melchers et al., 1975] and [Nocardia mitogen, Bona et al., 1974] [Andersson et al., 1979a]. The reason for the inability of thymus filler cells to sustain induction by LPS of every small B cell is not understood. In fact, it is now more than 15 years since the thymus filler cell effect was described, but its molecular basis is yet to be elucidated.

We have reasons to believe that the LPS induction of only one out of three B cells is due to shortcomings of the thymus filler cell system and not an inherent property of the B cells themselves. In recent limiting dilution experiments, however, we found that, after replacing the conventional thymus filler cells by the bone marrow stromal cell line S17 [Collins and Dorshkind, 1987], the frequency of LPS-induced B cells increased to nearly 100% of plated B cells [Cumano et al., 1990; Modigliani et al., unpublished data]. Thus it seems now that every resting B cell can be induced by LPS to develop into growing clones of high rate Ig-secreting cells. Furthermore, under such conditions, small resting B cells from the IgM transgenic animals Sp6 [Rusconi and Köhler, 1985] and M54 [Grosschedl et al., 1984] are readily induced by LPS in frequencies similar to those of normal animals [Grandien et al., 1990; Modigliani et al., unpublished data]. More than 95% of the resting B cells from such transgenic animals express only the IgM transgene, and due to allelic exclusion no endogenous heavy chain Ig, including IgD, is expressed in those cells. The phenotype of the resting transgenic B cell is kept after LPS induction, when clones of growing B-cell blasts are scored for Ig secretion by the plaque assay or ESA [Grandien et al., 1990, 1992].

Resting small cells induced by LPS divide every 18 hours but require the continuous presence of the inducer. Growing clones of B cells secrete IgM so as to be scored positive by the PFC assay or by the ESA technique. Clones growing under limiting dilution conditions continue to secrete IgM during the first 5 days of culture to the extent that every cell in the clone is scored as a plaque [Andersson et al., 1977]. After some time in culture an increasing fraction of the IgM-secreting cells switch isotype so that at day 7–8 more than 10% of the cultures now contain cells secreting IgG [Andersson et al., 1978a,b].

ROLE OF SURFACE IgM IN B-CELL DEVELOPMENT AND INDUCTION

Thus the example of IgM transgenic mice demonstrates that functional B cells develop normally, although, due to allelic exclusion, they express only that isotype. It therefore becomes feasible to investigate the role of IgM, and in particular the membrane form of IgM in B cell development. To that end, the laboratory of Rajewsky produced mice, using the "knock-out" technique, that lacked a functional μ-membrane exon in the germline [Kitamura et al., 1991]. Theoretically, such animals might make B cells that produce splice forms of heavy chain messages for all isotypes including the μ-secreted form as well as the IgD-membrane form of Ig. However, this is not the case, and no B cells at all are produced under these circumstances. Thus membrane-bound IgM is a necessary component for the development of normal B cells. An interesting finding, though, is that mice transgenic for a μ gene containing both membrane and secretory exons, but truncated in the V region [Corcos et al., 1991], will produce normal levels of B cells in the periphery expressing the membrane form of μ heavy chain, but they are unable to proceed further in development to Ig-secreting plasma cells. Also, such B cells do not respond to LPS, neither by proliferation nor by differentiation to Ig-secreting cells (A. Grandien et al., unpublished observation). Thus membrane μ-chain is necessary but not sufficient for normal B-cell development and induction.

It seems possible that surface Ig is capable of mediating induction of B cells as indicated by proliferation induced by insolubilized anti-Ig monoclonal antibodies as well as experiments showing induction of both proliferation and differentiation by anti-Ig antibodies in the presence of interleukins [Phillips and Klaus, 1992]. But it is also clear that B-cell induction can take place in the absence of surface Ig involvement, as evidenced by numerous studies showing induction to proliferation and differentiation by alloreactive T-helper cells [Augustin and Coutinho, 1980] or B-cell mitogens like LPS [Andersson et al., 1972] or mycoplasma [Ruuth et al., 1985]. In the former case, it now seems likely that the class II–restricted T-helper cell–B-cell interaction, which leads to induction of B cells, is mediated by a mechanism involving the focusing of the CD40 ligand [Armitage et al., 1992] to the B-cell surface. Thus, in both Ig- and non-Ig-mediated induction, we favor the view that induction of B cells take place as a consequence of focusing inducer molecules to nonclonally distributed receptors on the B-cell surface. The cross-linking of surface Ig is likely to influence the outcome of such "mitogen"-like actions on B cells in a way that may lead to clonal growth and expansion in the presence or absence of differentiation. Also, it seems possible that, under these circumstances, Ig cross-linking may lead to reactions that render the B cells nonfunctional [Bullock and Andersson, 1973; Andersson et al., 1974, 1978b].

ROLE OF SURFACE IgD IN STIMULATION

At some time after the resting B cells have entered the immune system, surface IgD is also expressed on the cell with a V region identical to that of surface IgM already displayed. The role of surface IgD is obscure, but it has been implicated as a coreceptor able to modify the response of B cells as a consequence of antigen binding to V regions. Recently, however, it has become possible to utilize Ig transgenic animals to elucidate further the role of IgD. Animals transgenic for the membrane form of isotypes other than IgD will produce large numbers of B cells, which, due to effective allelic exclusion, only will express the transgene and not endogenous IgD on the surface [Grandien et al., 1990]. Analyses show that such B cells readily can be produced and induced by, for example, LPS, to undergo the normal steps of clonal growth and differentiation to high rate Ig (transgenic) production. Thus IgD is not mandatory for small B cells to survive in the periphery or to undergo normal reactions as a result of induction. Also, in such animals normal rates of conversion from resting cells to naturally activated background Ig-secreting cells can be observed [Grandien et al., 1990]. This is also the observation made by Roes and Rajewsky [1991] in their Delta "knock-out" mice. Thus whatever the mechanism is for driving a fraction of the small resting B cells to naturally activated plasma cells, it operates in the absence of surface IgD.

BALANCE BETWEEN PROLIFERATION AND DIFFERENTIATION

Addition of anti-heavy or anti-light chain antibodies to cells will prevent their LPS-induced differentiation but not affect the induction of proliferation [Andersson et al., 1974]. The effect is dose dependent and can be observed at any time during the growth of the clone. Recent experiments show a direct downregulation of the transcription over both the heavy and light chain loci, presumably mediated by proteins of the oct-2 family [Högbom et al., 1987]. We have recently confirmed and extended the notion that different B cells show different sensitivities to the anti-Ig-mediated inhibition [Raff et al., 1975; Nossal et al., 1979]. Thus fresh bone-marrow-derived B lymphocytes are 20–100 times more sensitive to the inhibition than splenic B cells (Y. Modigliani et al., unpublished observation). This might imply that ligand binding to bone marrow B cells will more easily prevent differentiation of these cells and allow for clonal expansion or cause negative selection by processes that lead to clonal elimination.

It is possible that small resting B cells in the periphery always have a choice to enter into proliferation only, differentiation only, or both as a result of induction [Melchers and Andersson, 1974]. But anti-Ig or anti-Id do not induce differentiation—on the contrary, in conjunction with inducing mitogens like LPS, anti-μ heavy or light chain antibodies always inhibit differentiation. This inhibition is not mediated by the Fc receptor, since F(ab)$_2$ fragments are as efficient as whole antibody molecules [Andersson et al., 1974, 1978b].

Thus B cells have an option to enter differentiation or not, and it is likely that the inhibited cells, which otherwise would both proliferate and mature to high rate antibody-secreting cells, under the influence of anti-receptor antibodies only proliferate into clones of specific cells. A remarkable fact is that after induction of small resting cells with LPS, all cells in the clone proliferate and all of them mature into high rate antibody-secreting cells [Andersson et al., 1977]. This of course would lead to exhaustion of specific clones if this is the role for any induction occurring after antigenic challenge. But the case of anti-Ig inhibition seems to operate under normal conditions of induction by antigen where frequently one finds a substantial fraction of specific cells proliferating but not maturing into terminally differentiated clones.

B-CELL DEVELOPMENT AND TURNOVER

When discussing B-cell induction we will have to describe normal B-cell physiology during development and ask the question what drives B cells under normal circumstances. B cells are made from progenitor cells in the fetal liver during embryonic life and from bone marrow during neonatal and adult life. Their development requires cellular division and concomitant rearrangements of the variable region genes in the Ig loci coding for heavy and light chain, respectively. Once a mature surface IgM molecule is formed and inserted into the membrane, B cells cease to divide and leave the site of production (fetal liver or bone marrow) to enter the periphery via the blood. Thus newly formed B cells are resting cells in the periphery and require induction for further differentiation toward high rate Ig-producing cells and plasma cells. The production of B cells is continuous throughout life, and consequently a fraction of the newly formed cells will constantly be removed from the peripheral immune system. Estimates of the fraction of B cells leaving the immune system varies, but since the production is large the number of cells destined for an early death is considerable [Freitas et al., 1986].

To this end, it is possible that selection occurs for those dying or for those B cells chosen to remain, but the evidence in favor of either alternative is scarce and a prevailing belief is that elimination occurs by chance and is a random process. Transfer experiments performed by passing resting small B cells from LPS-responder animals into the circulation of LPS-nonresponder animals reveals that also cells destined to die are responsive to LPS and may develop into clones of growing, Ig-secreting cells [Freitas et al., 1986]. Thus elimination of B cells by sudden death is not due to a failure of the B cells to respond after induction, indicating that these cells are not actively eliminated but rather lack stimulatory influences. Considering the successive diminution in numbers of various differentiation stages of B cells, we would like to address the question of background activities, like normal Ig production, whether they occur following the same rules as have been delineated using mitogens and activated T cells as B-cell inducers. To that end, we have used Ig transgenic animals so as to permit the analysis of a large fraction of the immune system expressing one particular specificity.

BACKGROUND ACTIVITY AND IMMUNE RESPONSES IN B CELLS SHOW V-REGION-DEPENDENT SELECTION

The spleen of a normal mouse contain around 1×10^5 high rate Ig-secreting cells or plasma cells. As the spleen contains some 5×10^7 B cells it is obvious that only a small fraction of these cells actually differentiate into plasma cells (a fraction of around 0.2%). Do these plasma cells, often referred to as *background* Ig-secreting cells, arise through a process of V-region-dependent selection, or are they simply the result of random differentiation events?

Empirically, the question is hard to address due to the large number of different V regions. That is why we have chosen to investigate this question by comparing the repertoire of restng splenic B cells with that of naturally secreting plasma cells in Ig transgenic mice. In such μ-transgenic mice around 95%–98% of all resting splenic B cells express the transgene, while the remaining 2%–5% have rearranged and are expressing endogenous Ig. The variability of the small fraction of B cells expressing endogenous Ig is large compared with the cells expressing only the transgene. Hypothetically, if natural Ig-secreting cells would be the result of nonspecific stimulation, the expectation would be that the repertoire of plasma cells would be similar to the repertoire of resting cells. On the other hand, if natural Ig-secreting cells would be selected and stimulated as a consequence of a V-region-mediated mechanism, one would expect the repertoire of plasma cells to be enriched for cells expressing endogenous Ig.

Indeed, the analyses of μ-transgenic mice revealed a strong over-representation of cells expressing endogenous Ig in the pool of naturally Ig-secreting cells. Out of these cells some 50% of the IgM-secreting plasma cells were synthesizing endogenous IgM. These studies were performed by using quantitative single cell assays as described above.

We can therefore conclude that V-region-dependent selection drives the differentiation of resting cells into natural Ig-secreting cells. This process seem to be similar to those observed during regular immune responses.

ACKNOWLEDGMENTS

These studies were supported by The Swedish Medical Research Council and by grants from the ANRS, DRET, INSERM, and EEC to A. Coutinho, Paris.

REFERENCES

Andersson J, Sjöberg O, Möller G (1972): Induction of immunoglobulin and antibody synthesis in vitro by lipopolysaccharides. Eur J Immunol 2:349.

Andersson J, Bullock WW, Melchers F (1974): Inhibition of mitogen stimulation of mouse lymphocytes by anti-mouse immunoglobulin antibodies. I. Mode of action. Eur J Immunol 4:715.

Andersson J, Coutinho A, Lernhardt W, Melchers F (1977): Clonal growth and maturation to immunoglobulin secretion in vitro of every growth-inducible B lymphocyte. Cell 10:27–34.

Andersson J, Coutinho A, Melchers F (1978a): The switch from IgM to IgG secretion in single mitogen-stimulated B-cell clones. J Exp Med 147:1744–1754.

Andersson J, Coutinho A, Melchers F (1978b): Stimulation of murine B lymphocytes to IgG synthesis and secretion by the mitogens lipopolysaccharide and lipoprotein and its inhibition by anti-immunoglobulin antibodies. Eur J Immunol 8:336–343.

Andersson J, Coutinho A, Melchers F (1979a): Mitogen-activated B-cell blasts reactive to more than one mitogen. J Exp Med 149:553–563.

Andersson J, Lernhardt W, Melchers F (1979b): The purified protein derivative of tuberculin: A B cell mitogen that distinguishes in its action resting, small B cells from activated B cell blasts. J Exp Med 150:1339.

Armitage RL, Fanslow WC, Strockbine L, Sato TA, Clifford KN, Macduff BM, Anderson DM, Gimpel SD, Davis-Smith T, Malisweski CR, Clark EA, Smith CA, Grabstein KH, Cosman D, Spriggs MK (1992): Molecular and biological characterization of a murine ligand for CD40. Nature 357:80–82.

Augustin AA, Coutinho A (1980): Specific T helper cells that activate B cells polyclonally. In vitro enrichment and cooperative function. J Exp Med 151:587–601.

Bona C, Damais C, Chedid L (1974): Blastic transformation of mouse spleen lymphocytes by a water-soluble mitogen extracted from *Nocardia*. Proc Natl Acad Sci USA 71:1602.

Bretscher PA (1972): The control of humoral and associative antibody synthesis. Transplant Rev 11:217.

Bullock WW, Andersson J (1973): Mitogens as probes for immunocyte regulation: specific and non-specific suppression of B cell mitogenesis. In G. Wolstenholme G, Knight S (eds): "Immunopotentiation." Amsterdam: Elsevier, Excerpta Medica, North-Holland, pp 173–188.

Collins LS, Dorshkind K (1987): A stromal cell line from myeloid long-term bone marrow cultures can support myelopoiesis and B lymphopoiesis. J Immunol 138:1082–1087.

Corcos D, Iglesias A, Dunda O, Bucchini D, Jami J (1991): Allelic exclusion in transgenic mice expressing a heavy chain disease-like human μ protein. Eur J Immunol 11:2711–2716.

Coutinho A, Möller G (1973): B-cell mitogenic properties of thymus-independent antigens. Nature [New Biol] 245:12–14.

Coutinho A, Möller G (1974): Immune activation of B cells: Evidence for "one nonspecific triggering signal" not delivered by the Ig receptors. Scand J Immunol 3:133–145.

Coutinho A, Gronowicz E (1975): Genetical control of B-cell responses. III. Requirement for functional mitogenicity of the antigen in thymus-independent specific responses. J Exp Med 141:753–760.

Coutinho A, Larsson E-L, Grönvik K, Andersson J (1979): Studies on T lymphocyte activation. II. The target cells for ConA-induced growth factors. Eur J Immunol 9:581–592.

Cumano A, Dorshkind K, Gillis S, Paige CJ (1990): The influence of S17 stromal cells and interleukin 7 on B cell development. Eur J Immunol 20:2183–2189.

Freitas AA, Rocha B, Coutinho A (1986): Lymphocyte population kinetics in the mouse. Immunol Rev 91:5.

Grandien A, Coutinho A, Andersson J (1990): Selective peripheral expansion and activation of B cells expressing endogeneous immunoglobulin in μ-transgenic mice. Eur J Immunol 20:991–998.

Grandien A, Coutinho A, Andersson J, Freitas A (1991): Endogenous VH-gene family expression in immunoglobulin-transgenic mice: Evidence for selection of antibody repertoires. Int Immunol 3:67–73.

Grandien A, Coutinho A, Freitas A, Andersson J, Marcos M (1992): On the origin of natural IgM in Ig-transgenic mice. Int Immunol 4:1153–1160.

Gronowicz E, Coutinho A, Melchers F (1976): A plaque assay for all cells secreting Ig of a given type or class. Eur J Immunol 6:588–590.

Grosschedl R, Weaver D, Baltimore D, Constantini F (1984): Introduction of a m immunoglobulin gene into the mouse germ line: Specific expression in lymphoid cells and synthesis of functional antibody. Cell 38:647.

Högbom E, Mårtensson I-L, Leanderson T (1987): Regulation of immunoglobulin transcriptional rates and mRNA processing in proliferating normal B lymphocytes by activators of protein kinase C. Proc Natl Acad Sci USA 84:9135–9139.

Jerne NK, Nordin AA (1963): An hemolytic plaque assay. Science 140:405.

Kitamura D, Roes J, Kühn R, Rajewsky K (1991): A B-cell deficient mouse by targeted disruption of the membrane exon of the immunoglobulin μ chain gene. Nature 350:423–426.

Melchers F, Andersson J (1974): The kinetics of proliferation and maturation of mitogen-activated bone marrow-derived lymphocytes. Eur J Immunol 4:687.

Melchers F, Braun V, Galanos C (1975): The lipoprotein of the outer membrane of *Escherichia coli:* A B lymphocyte mitogen J Exp Med 142:473.

Miller RG, Phillips RA (1969): Separation of cells by velocity sedimentation. J Cell Physiol 73:191.

Möller G, Michael G (1971): Frequency of antigen-sensitive cells to thymus-independent antigens. Cell Immunol 2:309.

Nossal GJV, Pike BL, Battye FL (1979): Mechanisms of clonal abortion tolerogenesis. II. Clonal behaviour of immature B cells following exposure to anti-μ chain antibody. Immunology 37:203–215.

Pereira P, Forni L, Larsson E-L, Cooper MD, Heusser C, Coutinho A (1986): Autonomous activation of B and T cells in antigen-free mice. Eur J Immunol 16:685–688.

Phillips C, Klaus GGB (1992): Soluble anti-μ monoclonal antibodies prime resting B cells to secrete immunoglobulins in response to interleukins-4 and -5. Eur J Immunol 22:1541–1545.

Raff MC, Owen JJT, Cooper MD, Lawton AR, Megson M, Gathings WE (1975): Differences in susceptibility of mature and immature mouse B lymphocytes to anti-immunoglobulin-induced immunoglobulin suppression in vitro. J Exp Med 142:1052–1064.

Roes J, Rajewsky K (1991): Cell autonomous expression of IgD is not essential for the maturation of conventional B cells. Int Immunol 12:1367.

Rusconi S, Köhler G (1985): Transmission and expression of a specific pair of rearranged immunoglobulin m and k genes in a transgenic mouse line. Nature 314:330.

Ruuth E, Ranby M, Friedrich B, Persson H, Goustin A, Leandersson T, Coutinho A, Lundgren E (1985): Mycoplasma mimicry of lymphokine activity in T cell lines. Scand J Immunol 21:593–600.

Sedgwick JD, Holt PG (1983): A solid-phase immunoenzymatic technique for the enumeration of specific antibody-secreting cells. J Immunol Methods 57:301–310.

Sultzer BM, Nilsson BS (1972): PPD-tuberculin—A B cell mitogen. Nature [New Biol] 240:198.

6

B-1 (CD5 B) CELLS

Paolo Casali, Marion T. Kasaian, and Geoffrey Haughton

Department of Pathology and Kaplan Comprehensive Cancer Center, New York University School of Medicine, New York, New York (P.C., M.T.K.); Department of Microbiology and Immunology, University of North Carolina, Chapel Hill, North Carolina (G.H.)

INTRODUCTION

$CD5^+$ B cells and their murine homologues, $Ly-1^+$ B cells are the dominant clonotypes in the early B-cell repertoire and persist throughout adult life [Antin et al., 1986; Hayakawa and Hardy, 1988; Casali and Notkins, 1989; Kasaian et al., 1991; Kasaian and Casali, 1993; Haughton et al., 1993; Herzenberg and Kantor, 1993]. The murine subset was first recognized because some of its members and the lymphomas derived from them bear the cell surface antigen Ly-1 (the equivalent of the human CD5 molecule), which had been previously thought to be expressed only by T cells [Lanier et al., 1981]. Semantic difficulties arose when it became clear that CD5 was only a low fidelity marker of the population; some cells do not express surface CD5, but resemble surface $CD5^+$ B cells in many of their features [Herzenberg et al., 1986]. The issue was addressed by a recent agreement to refer to the "CD5" B-lymphocyte population as *B-1 cells*, with its surface $CD5^+$ and $CD5^-$ components being termed *B-1a* and *B-1b* cells, respectively [Kantor, 1991]. If necessary for purposes of making a distinction, conventional B lymphocytes would be called *B-2 cells*. Although this usage may lead to some semantic difficulties of its own, it is used here.

Human and murine B-1 lymphocytes include a significant proportion of

Autoimmunity: Physiology and Disease, Pages 57–88
© *1994 Wiley-Liss, Inc.*

cells committed to the production of antibodies that bind a variety of self-antigens, including hormones, nucleic acids, phospholipids, and/or exogenous antigens, including bacterial components, viruses, protozoa, and fungi, in addition to isologous and heterologous serum proteins, erythrocytes, and tissues [Casali et al., 1987; Casali and Notkins, 1989a; Turman et al., 1991; Casali, 1992; Kasaian et al., 1992; Geller et al., 1993; Riboldi et al., 1993; Kasaian and Casali, 1993]. Antibodies with these features arise independently of known specific immunization and have been referred to as *natural antibodies* [Casali and Notkins, 1989a,b; Kasaian et al., 1991, 1992; Casali, 1992; Riboldi et al., 1993]. A considerable proportion of natural antibodies are polyreactive, i.e., they bind to two or more different antigens. Because of their ability to bind self-antigens, including other Ig, natural antibodies would provide the structural correlate for the high degree of interclonal "connectivity," i.e., high idiotypic cross-reactivity of the early B-cell repertoire. In addition, they may play an important role in the establishment of autoimmune phenomena. The polyreactivity of a major proportion of natural antibodies contrasts with the monoreactivity of others, such as antiphosphatidylcholine (PtC) antibodies, also made by B-1 cells, and that of the "specific" antibodies produced by (conventional) B-2 cells and elicited in a T-cell-dependent fashion by antigen. The phenotypic and functional features that distinguish B-1 cells and the suggestion that these lymphocytes are subject to different regulatory mechanisms than those of B-2 cells raise the possibility that B-1 lymphocytes belong to a lineage different from that of B-2 lymphocytes [Herzenberg et al., 1986; Hayakawa and Hardy, 1988; Kantor, 1991; Bhat et al., 1992]. In this report, we 1) review our current understanding of the human and murine B-1 cell populations and the antibodies produced by these cells; 2) review the evidence addressing the two hypotheses of the origin of the B-1 population—the "lineage" hypothesis and the "differentiation pathway" hypothesis; 3) discuss a model that may potentially accommodate all of the evidence in a single unifying hypothesis; and 4) discuss the role of B-1 cells in the ontogeny of the B-cell repertoire and in autoimmune diseases and malignancies.

B-1 CELL POPULATION

Although there is substantial agreement about the features that distinguish B-1 from B-2 cells, there remains a controversy regarding their origin and the possible evidence that B-1 lymphocytes belong to a lineage different from that of B-2 lymphocytes. Consistent with this hypothesis in the human are 1) the distinctive features of the antibodies produced by the two B-cell populations; 2) the striking similarity in the relative proportion of circulating B-1 cells in monozygotic twins, suggesting a genetic control of B-1 cell levels [Kipps and Vaughan, 1987]; and 3) the constancy over time of the proportions of B-1 cells in different individuals [Kipps and Vaughan, 1987; Kasaian et al., 1992;

Kasaian and Casali, 1992]. However, the findings concerning the emergence of B-1 cells following human bone marrow transplantation are controversial and inconclusive in addressing the issue of a distinct B-1 cell lineage. Because more data have been generated over a longer period of time, the debate regarding the origin of the homologous cell population in the mouse is closer to resolution. Before entering the B-1 cell lineage controversy, it would be useful to list the features of B-1 cells that most investigators in the field consider to be noncontroversial.

Phenotype

Murine B-1 cells display several distinguishing features when compared with their B-2 counterparts: 1) They express relatively high levels of surface IgM and low levels of IgD (high surface IgM/IgD ratio) [Hayakawa et al., 1984; Herzenberg et al., 1986; Hayakawa and Hardy, 1988]; 2) they express relatively low levels of the high molecular weight isoform of the leukocyte common antigen (LCA) B220 [Hayakawa et al., 1984; Herzenberg et al., 1986; Hayakawa and Hardy, 1988]; 3) in the peritoneum, they express surface Mac-1, a marker characteristic of the myelomonocytic lineage [Klinman and Holmes, 1990; McIntyre et al., 1991]; 4) they may be relatively larger and more granular than B-2 cells, as revealed by their greater ability to scatter light [Herzenberg et al., 1986]; and 5) they do not express CD23, the low affinity receptor for IgE [Waldschmidt et al., 1991]. Although human B-1 cells are not larger in size than their B-2 counterparts [Casali et al., 1987, 1989; Burastero et al., 1988; Burastero and Casali, 1989; Kasaian et al., 1992], they share at least two of the abovementioned features of mouse B-1 cells: the relatively low density surface expression of the high molecular weight isoform of the LCA CD45RA and the relatively low density of surface expression of CD11b, the equivalent of the murine Mac-1 [Kipps and Vaughan, 1987; Kasaian et al., 1992; Kasaian and Casali, 1992].

Lymphokine Production and Responsiveness

The activation and proliferation of B-1 and B-2 cells may be regulated differently. B-1 cells are much more responsive than B-2 cells to IL-5 [Wetzel, 1989; Vaux et al., 1990; Tominaga et al., 1991]. Freshly isolated mouse peritoneal B-1 cells express the receptor for interleukin-5 (IL-5R) and undergo blastogenesis, proliferation, and antibody secretion in response to this lymphokine [Wetzel, 1989]. Mice made transgenic for IL-5 develop increased numbers of splenic B-1a and B-1b cells, which express IL-5R and produce natural IgM antibodies but show no increase in B-2 cell number or activation [Tominaga et al., 1991].

In addition, B-1 cells are distinguished from B-2 cells by the ability of Ly-1[+] B cell lymphomas and normal peritoneal B-1a and B-1b cells to produce constitutively and respond to IL-10 [O'Garra et al., 1990, 1992]. Newborn mice treated with antibody to IL-10 are selectively depleted in B-1a and B-1b cells, display drastically reduced levels of circulating IgM, and fail to mount the characteristic B-1 cell-dependent antibody responses to phosphorylcholine and α1–3 dextran [Ishida et al., 1992]. In these mice, depletion of B-1 cells is mediated by increased levels of inteferon (IFN)-γ. Thus IL-10 appears to be a specific regulator of B-1-cell development, exerting its activity through modulation of IFN-γ production by lymphocytes other than B-1 cells [Ishida et al., 1992].

Influence of Mutant Genes

The concept of uniqueness of the B-1 compartment has been supported by studies of inbred mouse strains expressing mutant genes, including: 1) the me^v (viable motheaten) mutation results in most or all of the B cells being B-1 [Sidman et al., 1986]. These mice develop severe autoimmune disease; 2) athymic nude (nu/nu) mice have normal levels of B-1 cells in the peritoneum, but lack B-1 cells in the spleen [Hardy et al., 1984], and thus functional T cells are not necessary for development of these B cells but may influence their distribution; 3) mice expressing the recessive X-linked immunodeficiency genes, *Xid*, are unable to respond to T-cell-independent type 2 (TI-2) antigens and are also deficient in B-1 cells [Hayakawa et al., 1983, 1986a].

Distribution as a Function of Age

In the Normal Adult, B-1 Cells Have a Distinct Tissue Distribution. In humans, they comprise 10%–30% of peripheral blood and splenic B cells, and 5%–10% of tonsillar B cells [Gadol and Ault, 1986; Casali et al., 1987; Hardy et al., 1987; Burastero and Casali, 1989; Kasaian et al., 1991, 1992]. In the mouse, B-1 cells are very rare in peripheral blood and spleen and are virtually absent from lymph nodes, but are very frequent among free-living lymphocytes in the peritoneal and pleural cavities, comprising more than 90% of peritoneal B cells [Hayakawa et al., 1984; Herzenberg et al., 1986; Hayakawa and Hardy, 1988]. They are also highly represented among the B cells in the lamina propria of the gut [Kroese et al., 1989, 1992].

B-1 Cells Are the Predominant B Lymphocytes Found in the Late Developmental Stages of the Fetus and in the Neonate. B-1 cells account for 50%–75% of the B cells in human fetal spleen [Antin et al., 1986; Hardy et al., 1987] and for more than 90% of the B cells in cord blood [Durandy et al., 1990]. In fetal and newborn mice, B-1 cells also account for most B lymphocytes. Their proportion decreases to adult levels during the first few weeks of postnatal life and remains so from puberty throughout young adulthood.

In Aged Mice, B-1 Cells Frequently Undergo Clonal or Oligoclonal Expansion and Often Become Neoplastic. Their expansion [Haughton et al., 1986], is shown by the B-1 origin of most murine B cell lymphomas. Similarly,

B-1 cells are also prone to neoplastic transformation in aged humans, as suggested by the prominent "CD5$^+$" features of most chronic lymphocytic leukemia cells (CLL) [Kipps, 1989].

Antibody Specificity and Structure

IgM Is the Main Class of Antibody That B-1 Cells Are Committed to Produce.
Only IgM has been seen to be produced by B-1 cells in the mouse peritoneum or in blood. Gut-associated B-1 cells have been reported to produce IgA and some splenic B-1 cells to produce IgG [Kroese et al., 1992]. Certainly, B-1 cells are capable of isotype switching; some B-1 lymphoma cells maintained in tissue culture switch spontaneously to a variety of isotypes, and this intrinsic switching rate can be increased by treatment with lymphokines [Whitmore et al., 1992]. These cells show a marked predilection for switching to IgA [Kroese et al., 1992]. In the healthy human, the majority of B-1 cells produce IgM antibodies, but B-1 cells producing IgG or IgA are also found [Casali et al., 1987; Burastero and Casali, 1989; Kasaian et al., 1992]. B-1a and B-1b cells making IgG and IgA autoantibodies are frequent in patients with different autoimmune diseases, including rheumatoid arthritis and systemic lupus erythematosus [Burastero et al., 1988; Burastero and Casali, 1989; Casali et al., 1989; Harindranath et al., 1991; Ikematsu et al., 1992a; Kasaian et al., 1993; Mantovani et al., 1993].

Human and Murine Natural Antibodies Produced by B-1 Cells React With Self- and Exogenous Antigens.
A high proportion of these antibodies are polyreactive [Hayakawa et al., 1984, 1986a; Hayakawa and Hardy, 1988; Nakamura et al., 1988a,b; Casali and Notkins, 1989a,b; Kasaian et al., 1991, 1992, 1993]. In the mouse, antibodies that react with mouse erythrocytes that have been treated with the proteolytic enzyme bromelain are produced exclusively by B-1 cells [Hayakawa et al., 1984; Hayakawa and Hardy, 1988]. These antibodies all recognize the tetraethylammonium polar head group of PtC [Mercolino et al., 1988]. Anti-PtC is the single most frequent specificity of the antibodies produced by murine B-1 cells; it is produced by about 10% of normal adult peritoneal B-1 cells as well as by B-1 cells in the spleen [Mercolino et al., 1988; Hardy et al., 1989; Carmack et al., 1990]. In mice and humans, other specificities produced by B-1 cells include anti-IgG (rheumatoid factor), anti-DNA, and antithymocyte surface antigens [Hayakawa et al., 1984; Casali et al., 1987; Hardy et al., 1987; Nakamura et al., 1988a; Hayakawa et al., 1990; Kasaian et al., 1991, 1992; Kasaian and Casali, 1993].

A High Rate Somatic Mutation of Assembled Ig Genes Has Not Been Shown to Occur in B-1 Cells of Healthy Individuals.
The majority of available data state that Ig V genes are expressed in germline form, without any mutation [Sanz et al., 1989; Baccala et al., 1989; Harindranath et al., 1993]. There are a few reports that small numbers of somatic point mutations may occur, but there is no evidence of the clonal expansion, accompanied by

hierarchical accumulation of mutations, that is typical of induced secondary responses by B-2 cells and that is believed to be the mechanism responsible for the affinity maturation seen in such responses. There is no evidence yet that antibody responses by normal B-1 cells display a progressive increase in antibody affinity. This contrasts with the evidence (vide infra) that somatic hypermutation yielding high affinity antibodies may occur in B-1 cells in humans with autoimmune disease [Harindranath et al., 1991; Ikematsu et al., 1992a; Kasaian et al., 1993; Mantovani et al., 1993].

B-1b CELLS

The high surface IgM/IgD ratio of Ly-1$^+$ B-1 cells is also displayed by a small proportion of murine surface Ly-1$^-$ B cells. Similar to Ly-1$^+$ B cells, these lymphocytes display surface Mac-1 in the peritoneum and produce mainly IgM natural antibodies with multiple antigen specificities. Because they share the properties of Ly-1$^+$ (B-1a) cells but lack surface Ly-1, these lymphocytes were originally termed Ly-1 *sister* B cells [Herzenberg et al., 1986; Hayakawa and Hardy, 1988], and are now designated B-1b cells [Kantor, 1991].

In the human, the vast majority of the circulating natural antibody-producing cell precursors are surface CD5$^+$ B lymphocytes, but some surface CD5$^-$ natural antibody-producing cell precursors can also be found [Casali et al., 1987; Burastero and Casali, 1989]. Similarly, some natural antibody-producing surface CD5$^-$ B cell precursors have been identified in human cord blood [Mackenzie et al., 1991]. These observations prompted us to attempt to segregate natural antibody-producing CD5$^-$ cell precursors from the remaining CD5$^-$ B cells. Our effort led to the resolution and isolation, by three-color flow cytometry and sorting, of a discrete surface CD5$^-$ B lymphocyte subset that expresses low levels of surface CD45RA [Kasaian et al., 1992, 1993; Kasaian and Casali, 1992] (Fig. 1). This subset accounts for 2%–6% of human peripheral B lymphocytes, and, in the same individual, its proportion is constant over time [Kasaian et al., 1992]. By transformation with Epstein-Barr virus (EBV) and culture under limiting dilution conditions, we found that, similar to the CD5$^+$ B-cell subset, the CD5$^-$CD45RA^{lo} subset contains a high proportion of natural antibody-producing cells [Kasaian et al., 1992; Kasaian and Casali, 1992] (vide infra). In contrast, the CD5$^-$CD45RA^{hi} subset virtually does not contain natural antibody-producing cell precursors and is highly enriched in cells committed to the production of IgG, including some memory B lymphocytes.

To investigate further the relatedness of human CD5$^-$CD45RA^{lo} B cells to the surface CD5$^+$ B-cell subset, we analyzed the expression of CD5 mRNA by human CD5$^-$CD45RA^{lo} cells and compared it with those of CD5$^+$ and CD5$^-$CD45RA^{hi} B lymphocytes, using a CD5-specific polymerase chain reaction (PCR) amplification technique we developed [Kasaian et al., 1992, 1993]. High levels of CD5 mRNA were detected not only in sorted

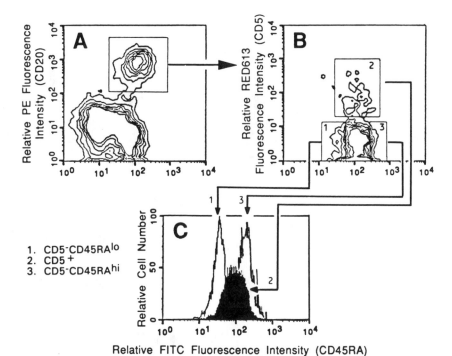

1. CD5⁻CD45RA^{lo}
2. CD5⁺
3. CD5⁻CD45RA^{hi}

FIGURE 1. Identification and sorting of human B lymphocyte subsets. Peripheral blood mononuclear cells from a healthy subject were reacted with PE-labeled monoclonal antibody (mAb) to CD20, FITC-labeled mAb to CD45RA (2H4), and biotin-labeled mAb to CD5, followed by RED613-labeled streptavidin, and then applied to the fluorescence-activated cell sorting (FACS) for analysis of their PE, FITC, and RED613 fluorescence intensities. B cells were identified by their high levels of expression of both CD20 and CD45RA and were gated as indicated by the inset in **A.** Gated B cells were analyzed for expression of surface CD5 and CD45RA and three subsets operationally identified, as shown in **B**: the cells that fell within rectangles 1, 2, and 3 were designated as B-1a (CD5⁻CD45RA^{lo}), B-1b (CD5⁺), and B-2 (CD5⁻CD45RA^{hi}), respectively. These cells could be isolated as discrete fractions by simultaneous three-color FACS. The degree of expression of the CD45RA molecule by the sorted cells is depicted in **C.**

CD5⁺ B cells, but also, and in comparable amounts, in autologous sorted CD5⁻CD45 RA^{lo} B lymphocytes (Fig. 2) [Kasaian et al., 1992, 1993; Kasaian and Casali, 1992]. In contrast, CD5⁻CD45RA^{hi} lymphocytes, tentatively defined as "conventional" (B-2) B cells, expressed very low to undetectable amounts of CD5 mRNA [Kasaian et al., 1992, 1993]. The CD5⁻CD45RA^{lo} B cells do not merely represent an "activated" phenotype of CD5⁺ cells, as they display the features of quiescent cells [Kasaian et al., 1992]. The high frequency of IgM-producing cell precursors, the prominent commitment to the production of natural antibodies, and the relatively high levels of CD5 mRNA expression of the surface CD5⁻CD45RA^{lo} B cells suggest that these lymphocytes are related to CD5⁺ B cells. This relationship may be based on

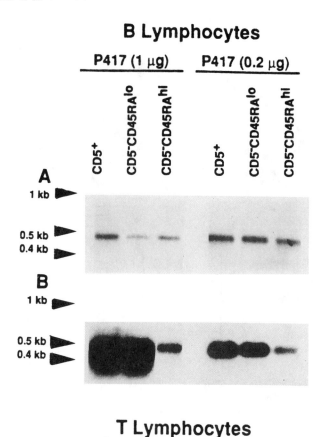

FIGURE 2. Expression of CD5 mRNA by B-1a, B-1b, and B-2 cells from a healthy subject (P417). mRNA from each B-cell subset (1 or 0.2 μg) or T lymphocytes (1.0–0.002 μg) was reverse transcribed. cDNA was amplified by PCR using β-actin-specific or CD5-specific primers and analyzed on a 1.2% agarose gel [for details, see Kasaian et al., 1992; Kasaian and Casali, 1992]. **A** shows ethidium-bromide-stained gel containing amplified β-actin (~0.6 kb) DNA from cDNA prepared using the three B cell subsets. **B** depicts the hybridization of the ^{32}P-labeled CD5-specific oligonucleotide probe to fractionated amplified CD5 DNA (~0.45 kb) from the same cDNA samples used for the amplifications in A. **C** depicts the hybridization of the ^{32}P-labeled CD5-specific oligonucleotide probe to fractionated, amplified cDNA reverse transcribed from purified T cell mRNA.

common origin, ontogeny, and/or development and suggests that the $CD5^-CD45RA^{lo}$ B cells represent the human equivalent of the mouse Ly-1 "sister" (B-1b) cell subset. In Table I the features of human B-1b cells are summarized and then compared with those of B-1a and B-2 cells, as well as with those of the equivalent murine B cell populations.

ORIGIN OF B-1 CELLS

Cell transfer experiments have suggested that the precursors of B-1 cells are distinct from those of conventional B cells. In unimmunized adult mice, B-1 cells are not generated by differentiation from precursors in bone marrow, but have arisen from cells emerging and therefore rearranging their Ig genes during fetal or early postnatal life. Studies of lethally irradiated and, more recently, of severe combined immunodeficiency (SCID) mice injected with allotype marked progenitor cells revealed that fetal liver gave rise to both B-1 and B-2 cells, but that adult bone marrow gave rise to B-2 cells and most often failed to replenish the B-1 population [Hayakawa et al., 1985; Herzenberg et al., 1986]. Experiments in which murine allotype chimeras were depleted of surface Ig^+ cells of one allotype, then monitored for replenishment of B-1 or B-2 cells, showed that in contrast to that of B-2 cells the development of B-1 cells from surface Ig^- progenitors is primarily restricted to the fetal, neonatal, and juvenile periods [Herzenberg et al., 1986; Lalor et al., 1989]. These data all are derived from studies of B-1 cells that arise spontaneously, possibly in response to self-antigens, and indicate that B-1 cells, unlike B-2 cells, usually do not arise spontaneously in the adult.

In adult life, murine B-1 cells originate from division of other surface Ig^+ cells [Herzenberg et al., 1986; Hayakawa et al., 1986b; Lalor et al., 1989]. Recently, Hardy et al. [1991] identified a surface IgM^- $B220^+$ HSA^+ (heat stable antigen) $CD43^+$ (leukosialin; sialophorin) early B-cell population present in both fetal liver and adult bone marrow and analyzed the differentiation potential of this cell type isolated from the two sources [Hardy and Hayakawa, 1991]. Fetal-liver-derived early B cells displaying the IgM^- $B220^+$ HSA^+ $CD43^+$ phenotype cultured in vitro on a stromal cell layer gave rise to progeny B cells expressing surface Ly-1. In contrast, bone-marrow-derived IgM^- $B220^+$ HSA^+ $CD43^+$ B cells cultured in vitro under identical conditions gave rise to $Ly-1^-$ progeny B cells. Furthermore, when irradiated, SCID mice were reconstituted with fetal-liver-derived surface IgM^- $B220^+$ HSA^+ $CD43^+$ cells, the majority of B cells recovered in both spleen and peritoneal cavity were B-1, and some of the IgM produced by these cells exhibited the characteristic PtC-binding activity of natural antibodies. Reconstitution of irradiated SCID mice with adult bone-marrow-derived cells of the same phenotype gave rise to B-2 cells in both spleen and peritoneum, and these cells did not produce PtC-binding antibodies [Hardy and Hayakawa, 1991]. Once generated, B-1 cells are long lived and capable of

TABLE I. Features of human and murine B lymphocyte populations

| | | Surface | | | | Expression of Ratio of IgM/IgG Frequency | | | | |
| | IgM/IgD Ratio | CD11b Mac-1 | CD5 Ly-1 | CD23 CD23 | CD45RA B220 | CD5 mRNA Ly-1 mRNA | Natural Producing Cell Precursors | Antibody-Producing Cell Precursors | Somatic Hypermutation | N-Segment Addition |
B Cells										
Human										
B-1a	?	++	Yes	?[a]	Low to intermediate	High	High	Very high	Yes	Yes
B-1b	?	++	No	?	Low	High	High	Very high	Yes	No
B-2	Low	+	No	?	High	Very low	Low	Low	Yes	Yes
Mouse										
B-1a	High	+++	Yes	No	Low	ND[b]	High	Very high	ND	No?
B-1b	High	+++	No	?	Low	ND	High	Very high	ND	ND
B-2	Low	+	No	Yes	High	ND	Low	Low	Yes	Yes

[a] Inconclusive findings.
[b] Not determined.

self renewal; i.e., B-1 cells are maintained throughout the life of the animal by virtue of their potential for continuous division [Herzenberg et al., 1986; Hayakawa et al., 1986b; Lalor et al., 1989].

Although they share many properties with B-1a cells, B-1b cells may belong to a discrete B-cell lineage stemming from precursors separate not only from those for B-2 cells but also from those for B-1a cells. B-cell precursors taken from hematopoietic tissues of different aged mice and from different locations in the 13-day-old fetus give rise to different proportions of B-1a, B-1b, and B-2 cells [Hardy and Hayakawa, 1991; Solvason et al., 1991; Kantor et al., 1992]. In transfer experiments using irradiated allotype congenic recipient mice [Kantor et al., 1992], fetal liver reconstituted both B-1a and B-1b, as well as B-2 cells, whereas adult bone marrow reconstituted B-2 and B-1b cells efficiently but B-1a cells very poorly [Kantor et al., 1992]. Thus bone marrow is a source not only of B-2, but also of B-1b cells. Recent studies by Solvason et al. [1991] identified the omentum, in addition to the liver, as a primary site of B-cell development in the murine fetus. When SCID mice were engrafted with fetal omentum obtained from normal donor mice, their peritoneal cavities were reconstituted with B lymphocytes that displayed the phenotypic features of B-1 cells: surface IgM^{hi}, IgD^{lo}, Mac-1^+, IL-5R^+. About one-half of these cells expressed Ly-1 (B-1a cells), and one-half were surface Ly-1^- (B-1b cells). When mice were engrafted with fetal liver, their peritoneal cavities contained donor B-1a, B-1b, and B-2 cells [Solvason et al., 1991]. Thus the fetal omentum is a source only of B-1a and B-1b cells, and, not "conventional" B-2 cells.

Examination of the human fetal omentum for the presence of B-cell precursors revealed pro/pre-B cells (CD24$^+$, cytoplasmic and surface IgM$^-$) and pre-B cells (CD24$^+$, cytoplasmic IgM$^+$, surface IgM$^-$), as well as mature B cells (CD24$^+$, surface IgM$^+$) [Solvason and Kearney, 1992]. These B-cell precursors are seen as early as 8 weeks of gestation, consistent with the time of appearance of B-cell precursors in the fetal liver. About 50% of the mature B cells found in the fetal omentum expressed surface CD5. The mature CD5$^-$ B cells of the human omentum likely constitute B-1b cells.

"Lineage" Hypothesis

The results of the transfer experiments outlined above have been interpreted to mean that, by the pro-B-cell stage of differentiation (before V gene rearrangement), the individual precursor is absolutely committed to produce progeny of only a single lineage, be it B-1a, B-1b, or B-2 [Herzenberg and Kantor, 1993]. The three lineages are postulated to replace one another during ontogeny, as a result of some developmental switch event. During fetal life, the B-1 lineages would predominate, with B-1b persisting into postnatal life, while the B-2 lineage arises relatively late and predominates in the mature adult. However, the fundamental evidence on which this hypothesis rests, that (at least some) fetal pro-B cells give rise only to B-1 cells whereas (at least some) adult pro-B cells yield only B-2 cells, although very substantial, may not be definitive, i.e., these differences are relative rather than absolute. For instance, it was reported that SCID mice transplanted with adult pro-B cells displayed up to 15% of $CD5^+$ B cells in their spleens and peritoneal cavities, while those given fetal pro-B cells displayed up to 10% of their B cells bearing the high levels of IgD characteristic of B-2 cells [see Fig. 4 of Hardy and Hayakawa, 1991]. Thus, although there is a clear difference in the ratio of B-1 : B-2 cells generated by similar precursors taken at different ontogenic stages, the evidence that this is due to a difference in the ratio of two types of committed precursor rather than a change in the ratio of different types of progeny from a single type of precursor is not conclusive.

The concept of distinct lineages implies that all of the features that distinguish B-1 cells are programmed prior to Ig gene rearrangement and thus, for example, that the characteristic antibody repertoire of B-1 cells is a consequence of that program. This interpretation would exclude the possibility that a single pro-B cell could yield progeny of more than one phenotype and would deny that antibody specificity plays any part in determining phenotype. The adult repertoire of B-1 cells could be a subset, selected by antigen, of a larger range of specificities generated earlier. Reactivity of B-1 cells in the adult would be entirely dependent on the spectrum of antigens encountered by these cells early in life [Vakil et al., 1986]. It would not be possible for B-1 cells de novo to generate, reactivity for an antigen first encountered in the adult.

"Differentiation Pathway" Hypothesis

A different view of the origin of B-1 cells has been proposed by Wortis and colleagues [Ying-Zi et al., 1991; Rabin et al., 1992; Haughton et al., 1993]. They reported that normal splenic B cells, lacking surface Ly-1 but expressing CD23 and a high ratio of IgD : IgM, when cultured in the presence of anti IgM and IL-6, assumed the phenotype of B-1a cells. These activated B cells expressed surface Ly-1, displayed a reduced surface IgD density, and lost surface CD23. There was no evidence that these changes were reversible. Wortis and colleagues concluded that the phenotypic change had been initiated by cross-linking of surface Ig. The similarity of these cells, generated in vitro, to B-1 cells that arise during normal development would suggest that the commitment to the B-1 phenotype may be made by a B cell after appearance of the surface IgM receptor for antigen. In the human fetal omentum, B-cell precursors acquire surface IgM and surface CD5 at the same stage of development [Solvason and Kearney, 1992]. Thus recognition of self-antigens and engagement of surface IgM at early (fetal) stages of B-cell ontogeny could result in cell activation and subsequent expression of CD5-specific mRNA resulting (B-1a cell) or not resulting (B-1b cells) in expression of surface CD5. If cross-linking of surface Ig is essential for commitment to occur, it further implies that entry into the B-1 differentiative pathway is determined by the binding specificity of surface Ig and hence that the distinctive repertoire of antibodies produced by B-1 cells is the cause rather than the consequence of their phenotype. In this case, the B-1 phenotype is better considered as the product of a differentiative pathway available to any young B cell rather than as the marker of a separate lineage.

The fundamental difference between the two hypotheses outlined above is the question of whether commitment to the B-1 phenotype occurs before or after expression of cell surface Ig. The "lineage" hypothesis envisions the occurrence of a timed developmental switch, which changes an absolute commitment to one lineage into an absolute commitment to the other. The "differentiation pathway" hypothesis considers that the determining event involves interaction between surface Ig and antigen. An initial activating interaction that leads to cross-linking of Ig, without involvement of T cells, would lead into the B-1 pathway, whereas cognate interaction with a T-helper cell, without cross-linking of Ig, leads into the B-2 pathway. The two hypotheses would apparently be irreconcilable. However, if a developmental switch occurs that does not cause a change in absolute lineage commitment, but merely reduces the probability that the surface Ig, when made, can be cross-linked by self-antigen, then it becomes possible to propose an integrated hypothesis that accommodates virtually all of the available data.

NATURAL ANTIBODIES

A key issue in integrating the differentiation pathway hypothesis into the lineage hypothesis is whether events occur in B-cell development that alter the probability that surface Ig can be cross-linked by self-antigen and promote the B-1 phenotype. To address this issue, we must consider the features of the natural antibodies, often with antiself-reactivity, produced by B-1 cells. In contrast to antigen-induced antibodies, which are monoreactive, a major proportion of natural antibodies are polyreactive, displaying different affinities for different antigens (K_d, 10^{-5} to 10^{-8} M) (Fig. 3) [Nakamura et al., 1988a,b; Casali and Notkins, 1989a,b; Casali, 1990; Ueki et al., 1990; Turman et al., 1991; Kasaian et al., 1992, Riboldi et al., 1993; Ikematsu et al., 1993b]. The antigens recognized by polyreactive antibodies are very different in nature, e.g., proteins, nucleic acids, phospholipids, or polysaccharides, and are unlikely to share identical or similar epitopes. This suggests that the multiple antigen-binding activity of natural antibodies relies on properties inherent to the antigen-binding site and implies that a polyreactive antibody binds different antigens by virtue of its ability to recognize different epitopes.

Conceivably, expression of natural antibodies on the cell surface could result in surface Ig cross-linking not only by antigens with repetitive identical epitopes but also by any antigen with more than one recognizable discrete epitope. The structures lining the antigen-binding site of an antibody molecule consist essentially of the three heavy (H) chain complementarity-

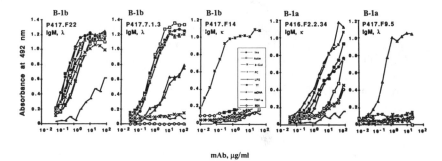

FIGURE 3. Dose-dependent binding of IgM monoclonal antibodies derived from B-1b cells and B-1a cells to solid-phase antigens, as determined by ELISA. Each antigen-binding activity is expressed as optical absorbance at 492 nm. The antigens used were ssDNA, insulin, actin, phosphorylcholine (PC), tetanus toxoid (TT), *Escherichia coli* β-galactosidase (β-gal), LPS, TNF-α, and BSA.

determining regions (CDRs) and the three light (L) chain CDRs [Colman, 1988]. In the case of relatively large antigens, such as those occurring naturally, the V_H segment, particularly its CDR3 (encoded in a nucleotide sequence consisting of the D gene flanked or not by N-segment additions and the first, variable, portion of J_H), is the major contributor to antigen binding [Amit et al., 1986; Stanfield et al., 1990]. In the mouse, two changes occur at or about the time of birth that affect the process of Ig gene expression and could alter the probability that surface Ig may be cross-linked by self-antigen: 1) the bias in favor of utilization of the most D-proximal V_H genes, which is observed in fetal life, changes to a more nearly random usage in the adult [Yancopoulos et al., 1988], a process that may result from exposure to environmental antigens [Freitas et al., 1991]; and 2) in the adult, N nucleotides are inserted at the junctions between V_H, D, and J_H genes, thereby changing the structure of H-chain CDR3 from that which can be coded by germline genes alone; this process does not occur in the fetus [Gu et al., 1990; Feeney, 1990]. If self-reactivity for cross-linking antigens is most frequently encoded by D-proximal V_H genes, or if it usually involves germline-encoded sequences at the H-chain CDR3, then one or both of these processes might have the effect of reducing the frequency of B cells expressing surface Ig that can bind to and be cross-linked by self-antigen. This would decrease the probability that the B cell would develop as B-1.

There are substantial data showing that mouse B-1 cells, producing natural antiself-antibodies, often do not employ N nucleotides and that the H-chain CDR3 is important in determining self-reactivity [Pennell et al., 1989; Martin et al., 1992]. For instance, murine antibodies that react with PtC are produced exclusively by B-1 cells [Mercolino et al., 1988], and most are encoded in either of two specific combinations of V_H and V_κ genes ($V_H11/V_\kappa9$ or $V_H12/$

$V_\kappa 4$) [Mercolino et al., 1989; Hardy et al., 1989; Carmack et al., 1990; Pennell et al., 1989]; both rearranged V_H and V_κ genes display combinatorial constraints that are characteristic of antigen-driven selection [Pennell et al., 1989], and the whole CDR3 sequence of the H-chain can be encoded by germline genes; randomly inserted N nucleotides are not needed and are frequently absent [Pennell et al., 1989]. Thus H chain V_H–D–J_H gene rearrangements suitable to encode anti-PtC antibodies are more likely to be formed during fetal life than in the adult. Anti-PtC is the most common antibody made by murine B-1 cells, being produced by about 10% of normal adult peritoneal B-1 cells as well as by B-1 cells in the spleen [Mercolino et al., 1988]. Its production is clearly antigen driven, but its function remains unknown. The $V_H 11$ and $V_H 12$ genes show strong evidence of evolutionary conservation. The expressed Ig V gene alleles contain a large excess of silent (S) over replacement (R) point mutations (Booker et al., unpublished data). This implies that the gene product (anti-PtC) is beneficial and has substantial survival value for the mouse. These findings and implications do not necessarily extrapolate to other types of antibodies produced by B-1 cells. There is no good reason to believe that antibodies reactive with nonself, polymeric antigens, or displaying polyreactivity, could not be coded by gene rearrangements including N-region nucleotides. Indeed, it is established that some B-1 cells (B-1b, vide supra) can arise either from adult bone marrow or fetal omentum.

The human B-1 cell compartment may differ in several ways from its murine equivalent: 1) Similar to that shown in the mouse, in the human, Ig genes sequenced from the fetal [Schroeder and Wang, 1990; Raaphorst et al., 1992], newborn [Mortari et al., 1992], or adult (B-1a, B-2, or unfractionated) repertoires [Harindranath et al., 1991; Yamada et al., 1991; Kasaian et al., 1992; Chai et al., in preparation; Ikematsu et al., 1993a,b; Mantovani et al., 1992] contain progressively greater amounts of N-segment additions at the V_H–D–J_H joining regions, contributing to long CDR3s. However, in contrast with their murine counterparts, the V_H genes encoding many human polyreactive natural antibodies produced by B-1a cells display relatively long CDR3s, which may provide the structural correlate for a large antigen-combining site capable of accommodating multiple ligands [Sanz et al., 1989; Harindranath et al., 1991; Kasaian et al., 1991; Ikematsu et al., 1992; Riboldi et al., 1993]. 2) Reminiscent of the murine fetal B-cell repertoire and in contrast with human adult B-1a cells, B-1b cells display a striking and highly statistically significant lack of N-segment addition [Chai et al., in preparation]. 3) Human B-1 cells can make somatically hypermutated monoreactive and polyreactive antibodies. In general, somatic mutations in the Ig V region genes contribute greatly to the specificity of the single antibody molecule. During the maturation of an antigen-driven immune response, the selective accumulation of somatic mutations in the CDRs is associated with the increase in antibody affinity and specificity. Consistent with the view that natural antibodies are generated independently of specific antigenic stimulation is the germline (unmutated) configuration of the genes encoding the V regions not only of most polyreactive, but also monoreactive natural antibodies [Sanz et al., 1989; Harindranath et al., 1991, 1993; Riboldi et al., 1993; Kasaian et al., 1992]. This, however, may not be a general rule and is certainly not a prerequisite for polyreactivity. We have found that the V genes of polyreactive IgG and IgA antibodies frequently contain somatic mutations, as defined by comparison of the expressed V gene sequence with the germline Ig gene sequences of the individual whose B cells were used for the preparation of the monoclonal antibodies [Harindranath et al., 1991; Kasaian et al., 1992; Ikematsu et al., 1993b]. The distribution of the nucleotide substitutions (clustering in the CDRs) and their high R to S mutation (R/S) ratio are consistent with antigen selection of such mutations. Thus natural antibodies produced by B-1 cells are able to participate in a selection process similar to that which gives rise to monoreactive antibodies to foreign antigens. 4) V_H gene segment utilization in the human adult repertoire does not seem to differ significantly from that in the fetal repertoire. In the mouse, members of the D,J_H-proximal gene families, V_H7183 and V_HQ52, are overrepresented in the fetal repertoire [Yancopoulos et al., 1984; Reth et al., 1986; Malynn et al., 1990], which "normalizes" in terms of V_H gene expression later in the life of the animal. A comparable skewed expression of members of the V_HV and V_HVI families, the most DJ_H-proximal of the human V_H gene families, has been suggested but not conclusively demonstrated in the fetal human B-cell repertoire [Cuisinier et al., 1989]. A large body of experimental data from our laboratory [Ikematsu et al., 1992a; Riboldi et al., 1993; Chai et al., in preparation; Kasaian et al., 1993; Harindranath et al., 1993] suggests that, among the seven human V_H gene families, members of the largest families, V_HIV and V_HIII, are utilized at a frequency higher than that expected on the basis of their representation in the haploid genome in the adult B-cell repertoire. Such an overutilization reflects what has been reported by Schroeder and collaborators [Schroeder et al., 1987; Schroeder and Wang, 1990] in the fetal B-cell repertoire. The overexpression of V_HIV genes in the adult (Casali et al., in preparation) and neonatal [Mageed et al., 1991] B-cell repertoires seems to be due to their overexpression by B-1a cells; that of V_HIII genes seems to be due to their preferential expression by B-1b and B-2 cells. Both V_HIV and V_HIII genes are overutilized to encode polyreactive natural antibodies (Casali et al., in preparation).

Thus human B-1a cells differ in their choice of V_H gene utilization form both B-1b and B-2 cells, but display degrees of N-segment addition comparable with those of B-2 cells. In contrast, human B-1b do not differ from B-2 cells in their choice of V_H genes, but differ from both B-1a and B-2 cells in their lack of N-segment addition. These findings suggest that different mechanisms of Ig gene expression and/or B-cell commitment may be operative at similar ontogenetic stages in the mouse and the human. They may also suggest that the events leading to B-1 "lineage" commitment may be only partially shared by human and murine B lymphocytes.

B-1 CELLS IN AUTOIMMUNE DISEASES AND
B-CELL MALIGNANCIES

The random processes of V_H-D-J_H and V_L-J_L recombination as well as V_H and V_L gene pairing ensure the potential for the emergence of B clonotypes recognizing self-antigens. Such potential is more frequently expressed by B-1a and B-1b cells, which are self-replenishing and provide a source of autoantibody-producing cell precursors throughout adult life. If the expression of surface Ig with antiself-specificity comprises the major developmental distinction between B-1 and B-2 cells, it is not surprising that B-1 cells participate in autoantibody production in the adult.

B-1a cells are greatly increased in number in several autoimmune diseases, including rheumatoid arthritis [Hardy et al., 1987; Burastero et al., 1988; Casali and Notkins, 1989a; Burastero and Casali, 1989; Mantovani et al., 1993], Sjögren's syndrome [Dauphinee et al., 1988], and primary antiphospholipid syndrome [Velasquillo et al., 1991]. In rheumatoid arthritis patients, B-1a cells can account for more than 50% of circulating B lymphocytes. They are large sized, actively proliferating, and produce IgM, IgG, and IgA rheumatoid factors [Burastero et al., 1988; Burastero and Casali, 1989; Harindranath et al., 1991; Mantovani et al., 1993]. Whereas most of these factors are polyreactive and display a low affinity for IgG Fc fragment, some are monoreactive and high affinity ($K_d\ 10^{-7}$ to 10^{-8} M) [Burastero et al., 1988; Harindranath et al.,1991; Williams et al., 1992; Mantovani et al., 1993]. In contrast to the germline configuration of the genes encoding the V regions of most low affinity rheumatoid factors, rheumatoid high affinity factors contain a number of somatic point mutations [Harindranath et al., 1991; Ikematsu et al., 1992a; Mantovani et al., 1993]. Consistent with antigen-driven clonal selection origin in their generation, these mutations are clustered in the CDRs and displayed a high R/S ratio [Harindranath et al., 1991; Ikematsu et al., 1992a; Mantovani et al., 1993]. Thus the same (B-1) lymphocytes that give rise to natural antibody-producing cells can in fact give rise to high affinity monoreactive autoantibody-producing cells. In most cases, this is accomplished by expression of V genes similar to those of natural antibodies, but in a somatically mutated configuration.

In systemic lupus erythematosus (SLE) patients, preliminary experiments by us and others suggest that, rather than surface CD5$^+$, surface CD5$^-$ and in particular B-1b cells are the major cell type involved in the production of the disease-characteristic autoantibodies [Casali et al., 1989; Suzuki et al., 1990; Kasaian et al., 1993]. These are IgG and IgA and, to a lesser extent, IgM to single stranded (ss)DNA and/or double-stranded (ds)DNA, often crossreacting with other nucleic acids and phospholipids. The genes encoding the V regions of these antibodies bear the imprints of an antigen-driven selection process, in that they contain extensive somatic mutations, yielding high R/S ratios in the CDRs (Fig. 4) [Dersimonian et al., 1987; Mannheimer-Lory et al., 1991; Diamond et al., 1992; Kasaian et al., 1993]. Our recent demonstra-

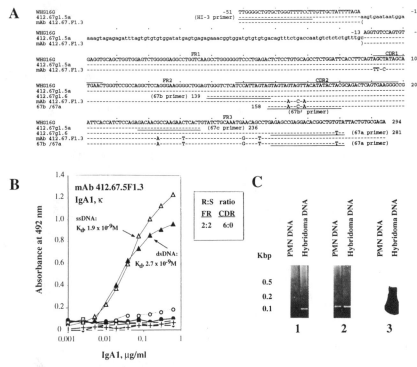

FIGURE 4. B-1 cells make somatically hypermutated high affinity antibodies. Nucleotide sequence of the V_H gene of human monoclonal antibody 412.67.5F1.3, an IgA1,κ antibody generated using B-1 cells from an SLE patient **(A)**. 412.67.5F1.3 binds to ssDNA and dsDNA with high affinity **(B)**. The sequence of the gene encoding the 412.67.5F1.3 V_H region was 96.6% homologous to that of WHG16G (Kueppers et al., unpublished), the closest known germline gene, a genomic segment belonging to the V_HIII family. An oligo-nucleotide identical to the CDR2 sequence of the 412.67.5F1.3 V_H gene and different in three nucleotides from the WHG16G CDR2 sequence was synthesized, 67b' primer. This oligonucleotide was utilized along with a 3' primer encompassing 21 residues shared by both 412.67.5F1.3 and WHG16G V_H FR3 regions (67a primer), to amplify by PCR the expressed and putative autologous genomic V_H genes. The 67b' and 67a oligonucleotide primer pair yielded a DNA product of appropriately 133 bp when used to amplify geno-mic DNA from the 412.67.5F1.3-producing hybrid cell line **(C,** panel 1, hybridoma DNA, ethidium bromine staining of amplified DNA fractionated in agarose gel electrophoresis), but not genomic DNA extracted from polymorphonuclear leukocytes (PMN) (C, panel 1, PMN DNA) obtained from the same subject whose B cells were used for generation of the monoclonal antibody-producing cell hybrid. These findings were consistent with the hy-pothesis that the expressed 412.67.F1.3 V_H CDR2 gene sequence constituted a so-matically mutated form of the WHG16G gene or a WHG16G-like gene. To determine the actual sequence of the germline gene that putatively gave rise to the 412.67.5F1.3 V_H gene, we synthesized an oligonucleotide identical with a shared stretch of the 412.67.5F1.3 V_H and WHG16G gene FR2 sequences (67b primer). Using this primer in conjunction with the 67a primer, we amplified products of identical and appropriate size (143 bp) from template DNA extracted from either 412.67.5F1.3-producing cells (C, panel 2, hybridoma DNA, ethidium bromide staining of amplified DNA fractionated in agarose gel electrophoresis) or autologous PMNs (C, panel 2, PMN DNA). Southern blot hybrid-ization of the PCR products shown in C, panel 2, with the ^{32}P-labeled 67b' oligonucleo-

tion that a significant proportion of surface CD5⁻ B cells displaying some of the phenotypic features of B-1a cells, B-1b cells, and is an important source of only natural autoantibodies in healthy subjects but also of autoantibodies in SLE patients may suggest that these lymphocytes play an important role also in other autoimmune diseases.

Further supporting the role of B-1 cells in autoimmune phenomena are the serological findings associated with chronic lymphocytic leukemia (CLL), the most frequent leukemia in Western societies, in which the malignant cell type is thought to be the neoplastic counterpart of the normal CD5⁺ B cell [Gadol and Ault, 1986; Freedman et al., 1987; Kipps, 1989]. A minority of CLL B cells, however, lack surface expression of CD5. It would be important to determine whether such surface CD5⁻ CLL B cells express CD5 mRNA, consistent with a possible B-1b origin. Self-antigen-binding activities can be frequently ascribed to the monoclonal IgM, IgG, or IgA isolated from these patients [Broker et al., 1988; Sthoeger et al., 1989]. Accordingly, a large proportion of the monoclonal IgMs produced by murine Ly-1⁺ (CH) lymphomas bind to PtC [Haughton et al., 1986; Mercolino et al., 1988; Arnold and Haughton, 1992]. Many CLL patients display autoimmune traits, including circulating antigen–antibody complexes, positive Coombs' test, cryoglobulinemia, and/or polyneuropathies. In addition to CLL, solid-tissue B-cell lymphomas may also coexpress surface CD5 and/ or CD5 mRNA and may stem from mono- or pauciclonal expansion of B-1a and/or B-1b cells, such as small lymphocytic lymphoma (SLL), Waldenstrom's macroglobulinemia, or, as we recently found, Burkitt-type lymphoma arising in patients with acquired immunodeficiency [Riboldi et al., 1993]. In spite of the putative structural similarity between some monoclonal CLL Ig and natural antibodies, and in contrast to the natural antibody-producing B-1a and B-1b cell precursors in healthy subjects, CLL B cells express at disproportionately high frequency V_H genes of the small families, such as the members of the V_HV and the single copy V_HVI families [Kipps, 1989; Kipps et al., 1992].

---

tide used as a probe, further suggested that the expressed 412.67.5F1.3 V_H segment was in mutated configuration (panel 3). This was formally proved by cloning and sequencing the V_H gene segment amplified from the PMN DNA using a 5' leader primer (not shown) and the 3' oligonucleotide 67a primer. The amplified genomic segment 412.67gl was 100% identical in sequence to WHG16G. The comparison of the expressed 412.67.5F1.3 V_H gene with the "progenitor" template (412.67gl) indicated that monoclonal antibody V_H segment accumulated 10 somatic point mutations, 3 in CDR1 and 3 in CDR2. These mutations result in six amino acid substitutions, yielding an R/S ratio of 6:0. The four nucleotide mutations in the FR3 resulted in two amino acid substitutions, yielding an R/S ratio of 1:1. The concentration of somatic point mutations in the CDRs, their high R/S ratio, and the very high affinity for antigen of the 412.67.5F1.3 V region strongly suggest that this antibody arose through a process of clonal selection and somatic point mutation driven by antigen. The nucleotide sequences of the 412.67.5F1.3 V_H and WHG16G genes are reported by Kasaian et al. [1993].

Parallel to the incidence of autoimmune traits, the frequency of B-1-related lymphoproliferative disorders increases with age. The tendency of B-1 cells to clonal outgrowth in association with an autoimmune background in aged individuals is emphasized by observations in the mouse. Autoimmune NZB-related mice develop clonal populations of self-perpetuating B-1 cells that arise in the peritoneal cavity early in life and eventually invade all lymphoid tissues. Similar spontaneous clonal B-1 lymphoproliferations occur normally in senescent healthy mice (more than 18 months old) of a variety of strains, including BALB/c, C57BL/6, and CBA [Stall et al., 1988]. In these aged animals, mono- or oligoclonal B-1 cell proliferation is often associated with serological autoimmune traits.

Taken together, these observations emphasize that a major component of autoantibody production not only in healthy adults but also in autoimmune patients segregates with B-1 cells. This conclusion is consistent with the suggestion that recruitment into this B-cell population requires expression of surface Ig with some degree of antiself-reactivity.

B-1 CELL ONTOGENY AND DEVELOPMENT: A SPECULATIVE MODEL

The requirements for maturation of B-1 lymphocytes (membrane Ig cross-linking) select for cells bearing a surface Ig receptor that is either monoreactive with a polymeric antigen or polyreactive with a variety of simultaneously present substances. In this context, the concept of polyreactivity includes the possibility that different "antigens" may bind to different sites on each antibody half-molecule. It is also implied that each "antigen" molecule bears more than one antibody-reactive site. Thus the limited spectrum of V genes expressed by murine B-1 cells is entirely a result of antigen selection and should be manipulable by immunization with appropriate forms of antigen. It follows that, in unimmunized, axenic animals, and in conventional neonates, all B-1 cells produce self-reactive (natural) antibody [Dighiero et al., 1985; Lydyard et al., 1990], since they could not have become B-1 cells unless they had already encountered a cross-linking (self)-antigen. Such antigens might well include the IgM idiotype. In normal adult mice, B-1 cells also produce antibodies reactive with environmental TI-2 antigens.

At least some of the antibodies selected for production via the B-1 pathway (e.g., anti PtC) are encoded in conserved V_H genes and have substantial survival value. Allelic forms of V_H11 and V_H12 contain a remarkably low ratio of R to S mutations $(2:11)$ as compared with the V_H genes of the S107 family $(21:11)$ that are typically expressed by B-2 cells in adaptive responses (Booker et al., unpublished data). Thus the antibodies are both constrained with respect to somatically generated $V_H–D–J_H$ diversity and conserved with respect to germline mutation. It can be speculated that such antibodies, entirely coded by conserved germline V_H, D, and J_H genes and requiring specific H-chain CDR3 sequences, are less likely to be made under conditions obtaining in adult bone marrow, where substantial N regions are generated by insertion of noncoded nucleotides, than in fetal liver, where they are not. Thus these antibodies are most frequently generated by rearrangements occurring in the fetal and neonatal periods, resulting in a greater probability that B cells made during this period will spontaneously acquire the B-1 phenotype. There is no a priori reason why such antibodies should not include N regions, but the mechanism is less likely to create the required CDR3 structure than use of preexisting germline sequences.

If this interpretation is correct, induced responses to polymeric, nonself-TI-2 antigens should be made by cells that have newly acquired the B-1 phenotype. These antibodies are probably not coded by evolutionary conserved genes; their specificity does not depend on germline-encoded H-chain CDR3 and hence is not disrupted by N-region addition. Thus the ability to produce such antibodies should not decline with age. We find that the antibody response to polyvinyl pyrrolidone (PVP) has these characteristics (Whitmore et al., unpublished data). According to this hypothesis, the B-1 population may be considered to contain cells producing three distinct, and potentially recognizable, types of antibody. Each of these types is associated with a different function. The three types of antibody are as follows:

1. *Monoreactive with multivalent self-antigens,* e.g., anti-PtC. These antibodies are beneficial, are encoded by conserved germline genes, and their antigen reactivity always involves H-chain CDR3. They are produced, predominantly, by cells whose Ig genes were rearranged early in life. This set may also include the regulatory antiidiotypes produced by murine fetal B cells [Elliott and Kearney, 1992; Coutinho, 1989] and the 7183.1 (81X) gene product [Carlsson et al., 1992] and would include the human monoreactive anti-β-galactosidase and anti-ssDNA antibodies produced by B-1b and B-1a cells, respectively, discussed above (Fig. 2).

2. *Polyreactive with a variety of self- and nonself-antigens* (see above). These include (but need not be confined to) "rogue" antibodies that would subvert the clonal selection process if the antibody-producing cell were allowed to interact with T-helper cells and develop as B-2 cells. A function of the B-1 pathway, in this instance, is to remove potentially dangerous cells from the T-dependent repertoire. N regions, of any size, may occur in these cells. Conditions that cause this set of antibody-producing cells to activate the somatic mutational mechanism might be particularly likely to lead to autoimmune disease.

3. *Monoreactive with multivalent, nonself-antigens.* These are made by the only B-1 cells responsive to deliberate immunization of the adult; they do not acquire the B-1 phenotype until after immunization and are usually generated from adult bone marrow precursors. Their function is to protect against pathogens by responding to polymeric antigens, such as carbohy-

drates, that cannot be processed for MHC-restricted recognition by T-helper cells.

The core of the model (Fig. 5) integrating the lineage hypothesis and the differentiation pathway hypothesis, i.e., that expression of surface CD5 is secondary to expression of surface Ig, is highly probable. Because Hardy and Hayakawa [1991] have unequivocally shown that similar populations of pro-B cells, whether in the fetal liver or adult bone marrow, give rise to very different proportions of B-1 and B-2 cells, it must be assumed that the inherent propensity of fetal pro-B cells to develop along the B-1 line is due to their high probability of expressing surface Ig with antiself-reactivity. By virtue of their commitment to production of natural antibodies reactive to self-antigens, B-1a and B-1b cells would be selected for differentiation and xpansion by cross-linking of surface Ig in the absence of a cognate T-

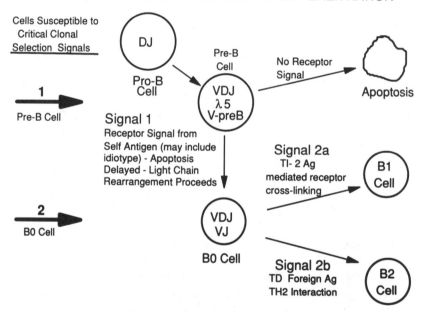

CRITICAL STEPS IN B LYMPHOCYTE DIFFERENTIATION

FIGURE 5. The "differentiation pathway" hypothesis. The alternative view of the origin of B-1 cells postulates two critical clonal selection signals occurring during the differentiation of B cells. The first, delivered to the pre-B cell, is a rescue signal that aborts preprogrammed cell death and ensures that survivors, which mature into B0 cells, all bear functional H chains. The second delivered to the B0 cell commits the cell to differentiates along either the B-1 or B-2 pathway. During fetal life, germline encoded V_H–D–J_H assemblies are expressed that have been subject to evolutionary selection. Some of these code for reactivity with polymeric self-antigens and thus lead a high proportion of cells into the B-1 pathway. In the adult, N-region insertion disrupts the germline encoded V_H–D–J_H structures and thus decreases the spontaneous generation of B-1 cells.

helper cell interaction. In contrast, B-2 cells would have to await for selection by cognate interaction with antigen and a T-helper cell. The above arguments would imply that the key to this inability is the lack of junctional N-segment addition, that is, terminal deoxynucleotidyltransferase activity in these fetal cells. This is consistent with many of the findings the murine and human fetuses and it may be reconciled with the following observations: 1) a large proportion of fetal and neonatal murine B-1a cells display consistent N-segment addition and surface Ly-1 [Gu et al., 1990]; 2) a large proportion of adult murine B-1a cells display degrees of N-segment addition comparable with those displayed by B-2 cells [Gu et al., 1990]; and 3) human B-1a cells from adults and cord blood display massive N-segment addition not different from those displayed by B-2 cells [Sanz et al., 1989; Harindranath et al., 1991; Chai et al., in preparation; Mantovani et al., 1993; Schroeder et al., 1987, 1990].

Thus, while some of the observations discussed in the above sections may make it possible to integrate the data quoted in support of the lineage hypothesis with those of the differentiation pathway model, some others are consistent with an inherent skewness to B-1 cell development from precursors, regardless of surface Ig expression. The hypothesis that phenotypically identical fetal-liver-derived and adult bone-marrow-derived B cell precursors inherently differ in developmental potential would be consistent with the recent findings by Oltz et al. [1992] that the expression of at least one gene, the precursor lymphocyte-specific regulatory myosin light chain gene, distinguishes fetal-liver- and adult bone-marrow-derived pre-B cells. Thus surface Ig cross-linking, while a necessary and, possibly, committing step, is probably not the only way or is not sufficient to induce B-1-cell development. Other characteristic features related to different developmental stages and ontogeny of B cells may play an important role in the establishment of the B-1 pathway.

SUMMARY AND CONCLUSION

The delineation of distinct subsets committed to the production of antibodies with different antigen-binding activities supports the view of a compartmentalization and specialization of function in the B-cell repertoire and is consistent with the hypothesis of a developmentally layered immune system, as originally proposed by Herzenberg and Herzenberg [1989]. It is now apparent that the B-cell repertoire includes at least three distinct B-cell subsets: B-1a cells, which develop from progenitors in the fetal splanchnic district, namely, the omentum, and are maintained in adult life by virtue of their self-replenishing nature; B-1b cells, progenitors of which can be found in the splanchnic district and, possibly, adult bone marrow; and B-2 cells, which arise in the fetal liver and are continuously replenished in adult life by progenitors in the bone marrow. The different B-cell types are distinguished by their differential expression of surface CD5, their differential expression of CD5 mRNA, and the different classes and specificities of the Ig they produce.

B-1 lymphocytes play a major role in autoimmunity and constitute the physiological equivalent of the neoplastic elements in various lymphoproliferative disorders, such as CLL and SLL, which are often associated with the production of monoclonal antibodies to self-antigens. The controversy concerning the developmental origins of the B-1a and B-1b populations centers on whether they represent B-cell lineages distinct from that which gives rise to B-2 cells or whether they are produced by alternative differentiation schemes acting on a common B-cell progenitor. In this report, we have proposed a speculative model that attempts to unify the major observations made by a number of researchers and that incorporates elements of both the lineage hypothesis and the differentiation pathway hypothesis. This model entails a number of testable features and should provide a basis for experimentation to help to resolve the issue of B-1-cell generation.

ACKNOWLEDGMENTS

This work was supported by U.S. Public Health Service grants AR-40908 and CA-16087. P.C. is a Kaplan Cancer Scholar. This is publication No. 14 from *The Jeanette Greenspan Laboratory for Cancer Research.*

REFERENCES

Amit AG, Mariuzza RA, Phillips SE, Poliak RJ (1986): Three-dimensional structure of an antigen–antibody complex at 2.8 Å resolution. Science 233:747–753.

Antin JH, Emerson SG, Martin P, Gadol N, Ault KA (1986): Leu-1$^+$ (CD5$^+$) B cells: A major lymphoid subpopulation in human fetal spleen: Phenotypic and functional studies. J Immunol 136:505–510.

Arnold LW, Haughton G (1992): Autoantibodies to phosphatidylcholine: The murine antibromelain RBC response. Ann NY Acad Sci 651:354–359.

Baccala R, Quang TV, Gilbert M, Ternynck T, Avrameas S (1989): Two murine natural polyreactive autoantibodies are encoded by nonmutated germ-line genes. Proc Natl Acad Sci USA 86:4624–4628.

Bhat NM, Kantor AB, Bieber MM, Stall AM, Herzenberg LA, Teng NNH (1992): The ontogeny and functional characteristics of human B-1 (CD5$^+$ B) cells. Int Immunol 4:243–252.

Broker BM, Klajman A, Youinou P, Jouquan J, Worman CP, Murphy J, Mackenzie L, Quartey-Papafio R, Blaschek M, Collins P, Lal S, Lydard PM (1988): Chronic lymphocytic leukemic (CLL) cells secrete multispecific autoantibodies. J Autoimmun 1:469–481.

Burastero SE, Casali P (1989): Characterization of human CD5 (Leu-1, OKT1)$^+$ B lymphocytes and the antibodies they produce. Contrib Microbiol Immunol 11:231–262.

Burastero SE, Casali P, Wilder RL, Notkins AL (1988): Monoreactive high affinity and polyreactive low affinity rheumatoid factors are produced by CD5$^+$ B cells from patients with rheumatoid arthritis. J Exp Med 168:1979–1992.

Carlsson L, Overmo C, Holmberg D (1992): Selection against N-region diversity in immunoglobulin heavy chain variable regions during the development of pre-immune B cell repertoires. Int Immunol 4:549–553.

Carmack CE, Shinton SA, Hayakawa K, Hardy RR (1990): Rearrangement and selection of V_H11 in the Ly-1 B cell lineage. J Exp Med 172:371–374.

Casali P (1990): Polyclonal B cell activation and antigen-driven antibody response as mechanisms of autoantibody production in SLE. Autoimmunity 5:147–150.

Casali P (1992): Immunoglobulin M. In Roitt IM, Delves PJ (eds): "Encyclopaedia of Immunology." London: Academic Press, pp 743–747.

Casali P, Burastero SE, Balow JE, Notkins AL (1989): High affinity antibodies to ssDNA are produced by CD5$^-$ B cells in systemic lupus erythematosus patients. J Immunol 143:3476–3483.

Casali P, Burastero SE, Nakamura M, Inghirami G, Notkins AL (1987): Human lymphocytes making rheumatoid factor and antibody to ssDNA belong to the Leu-1$^+$ B-cell subset. Science 236:77–81.

Casali P, Inghirami G, Nakamura M, Davies MT, Notkins AL (1986): Human mono-clonal antibodies generated by antigen-specific selection of B lymphocytes and transformation by EBV. Science 234:476–479.

Casali P, Nakamura M, Ginsberg-Fellner F, Notkins AL (1990): Frequency of B cells committed to the production of antibodies to insulin in newly diagnosed patients with insulin-dependent diabetes mellitus and generation of high affinity human monoclonal IgG to insulin. J Immunol 144:3741–3747.

Casali P, Notkins AL (1989a): Probing the human B-cell repertoire with EBV: Po-lyreactive antibodies and CD5$^+$ B lymphocytes. Annu Rev Immunol 7:513–535.

Casali P, Notkins AL (1989b): CD5$^+$ B cells, polyreactive antibodies and the human B cell repertoire. Immunol Today 10:364–368.

Colman PM (1988): Structure of antibody–antigen complexes: Implications for im-mune recognition. Adv Immunol 43:99–132.

Coutinho A (1989): Beyond clonal selection and network. Immunol Rev 110:63–87.

Cuisinier A-M, Guigou V, Boubli L, Fougereau M, Tonnelle C (1989): Preferential expression of V_H5 and V_H6 immunoglobulin genes in early human B-cell ontog-eny. Scand J Immunol 30:493–497.

Dauphinee M, Tovar Z, Talal N (1988): B cells expressing CD5 are increased in Sjögren's syndrome. Arthritis Rheum 31:642–647.

Dersimonian H, Schwartz RS, Barrett KJ, Stollar DB (1987): Relationship of human variable region heavy chain germ-line genes to genes encoding anti-DNA autoan-tibodies. J Immunol 139:2496–2501.

Diamond B, Katz JB, Paul E, Aranow C, Lustgarten D, Scharff MD (1992): The role of somatic mutation in the pathogenic anti-DNA response. Annu Rev Immu-nol 10:731–757.

Dighiero G, Lymberi P, Holmberg D, Lundquist I, Coutinho A, Avrameas S (1985): High frequency of natural autoantibodies in normal newborn mice. J Immunol 134:765–771.

Durandy A, Thuillier L, Forveille M, Fischer A (1990): Phenotypic and functional characteristics of human newborns' B lymphocytes. J Immunol 144:60–65.

Elliott M, Kearney JF (1992): Idiotypic regulation of development of the B-cell repertoire. Ann NY Acad Sci 651:336–345.

Feeney AJ (1990): Lack of N regions in fetal and neonatal mouse immunoglobulin V–D–J junctional sequences. J Exp Med 172:1377–1390.

Freedman AS, Boyd AW, Bieber FR, Daley J, Rosen K, Horowitz JC, Levy DN, Nadler LM (1987): Normal cellular counterparts of B cell chronic lymphocytic leukemia. Blood 70:418–427.

Freitas AA, Viale A-C, Sundblad A, Heusser C, Coutinho A (1991): Normal serum immunoglobulins participate in the selection of peripheral B-cell repertoires. Proc Natl Acad Sci USA 88:5640–5644.

Gadol N, Ault KA (1986): Phenotypic and functional characterization of human Leu 1 (CD5) B cells. Immunol Rev 93:23–34.

Geller RL, Bach FH, Turman MA, Casali P, Platt JL (1993): Natural antibodies bearing a "polyreactive" idiotype are deposited in rejected discordant xenografts. Transplantation (in press).

Gu H, Forster I, Rajewsky K (1990): Sequence homologies, N sequence insertion and J_H gene utilization in V_H D J_H joining: Implications for the joining mechanism and the ontogenic timing of Ly1 B cell and B-CLL progenitor generation. EMBO J 9:2133–2140.

Hardy RR, Carmack C, Shinton S, Kemp JD, Hayakawa K (1991): Resolution and characterization of pro-B and pre-pro-B cell stages in normal mouse bone marrow. J Exp Med 173:1213–1225.

Hardy RR, Carmack CE, Shinton SA, Riblet RJ, Hayakawa K (1989): A single V_H gene is utilized predominantly in anti-BrMRBC hybridomas derived from purified Ly-1 B cells: Definition of the V_H11 family. J Immunol 142:3642–3651.

Hardy RR, Hayakawa K (1991): A developmental switch in B lymphopoiesis. Proc Natl Acad Sci USA 88:11550–11554.

Hardy RR, Hayakawa K, Parks DR, Herzenberg LA, Herzenberg LA (1984): Murine B cell differentiation lineages. J Exp Med 159:1169–1188.

Hardy RR, Hayakawa K, Shimuzu M, Yamasaki K, Kishimoto T (1987): Rheumatoid factor secretion from human Leu-1$^+$ B cells. Science 236:81–83.

Harindranath N, Goldfarb IS, Ikematsu H, Burastero SE, Wilder RL, Notkins AL, Casali P (1991): Complete sequence of the genes encoding the V_H and V_L regions of low and high affinity monoclonal IgM and IgA1 rheumatoid factors produced by CD5$^+$ B cells from a rheumatoid arthritis patient. Int Immunol 3:865–875.

Harindranath N, Ikematsu H, Notkins AL, Casali P (1993): The V_H and V_L regions of polyreactive and monoreactive human natural antibodies to HIV-1 and E. coli galactosidase are encoded in germline genes. Submitted.

Haughton G, Arnold LW, Bishop GA, Mercolino TJ (1986): The CH series of murine B cell lymphomas: Neoplastic analogues of Ly-1$^+$ normal B cells. Immunol Rev 93:35–51.

Haughton G, Arnold LW, Whitmore AC, Clarcke SH (1993): B-1 cells are made not born. Immunol Today 14:84–87.

Hayakawa K, Carmack CE, Hyman R, Hardy RR (1990): Natural autoantibodies to thymocytes: Origin, V_H genes, fine specificities, and the role of Thy-1 glycoprotein. J Exp Med 172:869–878.

Hayakawa K, Hardy RR (1988): Normal, autoimmune, and malignant CD5[+] B cells: The Ly-1 B lineage? Annu Rev Immunol 6:197–218.

Hayakawa K, Hardy RR, Herzenberg LA (1985): Progenitors for Ly-1 B cells are distinct from progenitors for other B cells. J Exp Med 161:1554–1568.

Hayakawa K, Hardy RR, Herzenberg LA (1986a): Peritoneal Ly-1 B cells: Genetic control, autoantibody production, increased lambda light chain expression. Eur J Immunol 16:450–465.

Hayakawa K, Hardy RR, Honda M, Herzenberg LA, Steinberg AD, Herzenberg LA (1984): Ly-1 B cells: Functionally distinct lymphocytes that secrete IgM autoantibodies. Proc Natl Acad Sci USA 81:2492–2498.

Hayakawa K, Hardy RR, Parks DR, Herzenberg LA (1983): The "LY-1" B cell subpopulation in normal, immunodefective, and autoimmune mice. J Exp Med 157:202–218.

Hayakawa K, Hardy RR, Stall AM, Herzenberg LA (1986b): Immunoglobulin-bearing B cells reconstitute and maintain the murine Ly-1 B cell lineage. Eur J Immunol 16:1313–1316.

Herzenberg LA, Herzenberg LA (1989): Toward a layered immune system. Cell 59:953–954.

Herzenberg LA, Kantor AB (1993): B-cell lineages exist in the mouse. Immunol Today 14:79–83.

Herzenberg LA, Stall AM, Lalor PA, Sidman C, Moore WA, Parks DR, Herzenberg LA (1986): The LY-1 B lineage. Immunol Rev 93:81–102.

Ikematsu H, Harindranath N, Casali P (1992a): Somatic mutations in the V_H genes of high affinity antibodies to self and foreign antigens produced by human CD5[+] and CD5[−] B cells. Ann NY Acad Sci 651:319–327.

Ikematsu H, Harindranath N, Notkins AL, Ueki Y, Casali P (1993a): Clonal analysis of a human antibody response. II. Sequences of the V_H genes of human monoclonal IgM, IgG and IgA to rabies virus reveal preferential utilization of the V_HIII segments and somatic hypermutation. J Immunol 150:1325–1337.

Ikematsu H, Kasaian MT, Schettino EW, Steger TH, Casali P (1993b): Structural analysis of the $V_H–D–J_H$ segments of human polyreactive IgG: Evidence for somatic selection. J Immunol (in press).

Ikematsu H, Kasaian MT, Goldfarb IS, Harindranath N, Casali P (1992b): Generation of human monoclonal antibody-producing cell lines by Epstein-Barr virus (EBV)-transformation and somatic cell hybridization techniques. J Tissue Culture Methods 14:9–12.

Ishida H, Hastings R, Kearney J, Howard M (1992): Continuous anti-interleukin 10 antibody administration depletes mice of Ly-1 B cells but not conventional B cells. J Exp Med 175:1213–1220.

Kantor AB (1991): The development and repertoire of B-1 cells (CD5 B cells). Immunol Today 12:389–391.

Kantor AB, Stall AM, Adams S, Herzenberg LA, Herzenberg LA (1992): Differential development of progenitor activity for three B cell lineages. Proc Natl Acad Sci USA 89:3320–3324.

Kasaian MT, Casali P (1992): Analysis of the human $CD5^-CD45RA^{low}$ B cell subset. Ann NY Acad Sci 651:59–69.

Kasaian MT, Casali P (1993): Natural antibodies, self-recognition, and autoimmunity-prone B-1 (CD5 B) lymphocytes. Autoimmunity (in press).

Kasaian MT, Ikematsu H, Balow JE, Casali P (1993): Cellular origin and V_H genes of monoreactive and polyreactive IgA and IgG autoantibodies to DNA in patients with systemic lupus erythematosus. Submitted for publication.

Kasaian MT, Ikematsu H, Casali P (1991): $CD5^+$ B lymphocytes. Proc Soc Exp Biol Med 197:226–241.

Kasaian MT, Ikematsu H, Casali P (1992): Identification and analysis of a novel human surface $CD5^-$ B lymphocyte subset producing natural antibodies. J Immunol 148:2690–2702.

Kipps TJ (1989): The CD5 B cell. Adv Immunol 47:117–185.

Kipps TJ, Rassenti LZ, Duffy S, Johnson T, Kobayashi R, Carson DA (1992): Immunoglobulin V gene expression in CD5 B-cell malignancies. Ann NY Acad Sci 651:373–383.

Kipps TJ, Vaughan JH (1987): Genetic influence on the levels of circulating CD5 B lymphocytes. J Immunol 139:1060–1064.

Kitamura D, Kudo A, Schaal S, Muller W, Melchers F, Rajewsky K (1992): A critical role of λ5 protein in B cell development. Cell 69:823–831.

Klinman DM, Holmes KL (1990): Differences in the repertoire expressed by peritoneal and splenic Ly-1 $(CD5)^+$ B cells. J Immunol 144:4520–4525.

Kroese F, Butcher E, Stall A, Lalor P, Adams S, Herzenberg LA (1989): Many of the IgA producing plasma cells in murine gut are derived from self-replenishing precursors in the peritoneal cavity. Int Immunol 1:75–84.

Kroese FGM, Ammerlaan WAM, Deenen GJ (1992): Location and function of B-cell lineages. Ann NY Acad Sci 651:44–58.

Lalor PA, Stall AM, Adams S, Herzenberg LA (1989): Permanent alteration of the murine Ly-1 B repertoire due to selective depletion of Ly-1 B cells in neonatal animals. Eur J Immunol 19:501–506.

Lanier LL, Warner NL, Ledbetter JA, Herzenberg LA (1981): Expression of Lyt-1 antigen on certain murine B cell lymphomas. J Exp Med 153:998.

Lydyard PM, Quartey-Papafio R, Broker B, Mackenzie L, Jouquan J, Blascek MA, Steele J, Petrou M, Collins P, Isenberg D, Youinou PY (1990): The antibody repertoire of early human B cells. I. High frequency of autoreactivity and polyreactivity. Scand J Immunol 31:33–43.

Mackenzie LE, Youinou PY, Hicks R, Yuksel B, Mageed RA, Lydyard PM (1991): Auto- and polyreactivity of IgM from $CD5^+$ and $CD5^-$ cord blood B cells. Scand J Immunol 33:329–335.

Mageed RA, MacKenzie LE, Stevenson FK, Yuksel B, Shokri F, Maziak BR, Jefferis R, Lydyard PM (1991): Selective expression of a V_HIV subfamily of immunoglobulin genes in human $CD5^+$ B lymphocytes from cord blood. J Exp Med 174:109–113.

Malynn BA, Yancopoulos GD, Barth JE, Bona CA, Alt FW (1990): Biased expression of J_H-proximal V_H genes occurs in the newly generated repertoire of neonatal and adult mice. J Exp Med 171:843–859.

Mannheimer-Lory A, Katz JB, Pillinger M, Ghossein C, Smith A, Diamond B (1991): Molecular characteristics of antibodies bearing an anti-DNA-associated idiotype. J Exp Med 174:1639–1652.

Mantovani L, Kasaian MT, Wilder RL, Casali P (1993): Rheumatoid B-1 cells make somatically hypermutated high affinity IgM rheumatoid factors. J Immunol (in press).

Martin T, Duffy SF, Carson DA, Kipps TJ (1992): Evidence for somatic selection of natural autoantibodies. J Exp Med 175:983–991.

Mayer R, Logtenberg T, Strauchen J, Dimitriu-Bona A, Mayer L, Mechanic S, Chiorazzi N, Borche L, Dighiero G, Mannheimer-Lory A, Diamond B, Alt F, Bona C (1990): CD5 and immunoglobulin V gene expression in B-cell lymphomas and chronic lymphocytic leukemia. Blood 75:1518–1524.

McIntyre TM, Holmes KL, Steinberg AD, Kastner DL (1991): CD5$^+$ peritoneal B cells express high levels of membrane, but not secretory, Cμ mRNA. J Immunol 146:3639.

Mercolino TJ, Arnold LW, Hawkins LA, Haughton G (1988): Normal mouse peritoneum contains a large population of Ly-1$^+$ (CD5) B cells that recognize phosphatidyl choline: Relationship to cells that secrete hemolytic antibody specific for autologous erythrocytes. J Exp Med 168:687–698.

Mercolino TJ, Locke AL, Afshari A, Sasser D, Travis WW, Arnold LW, Haughton G (1989): Restricted immunoglobulin variable region gene usage by normal Ly-1 (CD5$^+$) B cells that recognize phosphatidylcholine. J Exp Med 169:1869–1877.

Mortari F, Wang J, Schroeder W (1993): Human cord blood antibody repertoire. Mixed population of V_H gene segments and CDR3 distribution on the expressed C$_\alpha$ and C$_\gamma$ repertoires. J Immunol 150:1348–1357.

Nakamura M, Burastero SE, Notkins AL, Casali P (1988a): Human monoclonal rheumatoid factor-like antibodies from CD5 (Leu-1)$^+$ B cells are polyreactive. J Immunol 140:4180–4186.

Nakamura M, Burastero SE, Ueki Y, Larrick JW, Notkins AL, Casali P (1988b): Probing the normal and autoimmune B cell repertoire with Epstein-Barr virus. Frequency of B cells producing monoreactive high affinity autoantibodies in patients with Hashimoto's disease and systemic lupus erythematosus. J Immunol 141:4165–4172.

O'Garra A, Chang R, Go N, Hastings R, Haughton G, Howard M (1992): Ly-1 B (B-1) cells are the main source of B cell-derived interleukin 10. Eur J immunol 22:711–717.

O'Garra A, Stapleton G, Dhar V, Pearce M, Schumacher J, Rugo H, Barbis D, Stall A, Cupp J, Moore K, Vieira P, Mosmann T, Whitmore A, Arnold L, Haughton G, Howard M (1990): Production of cytokines by mouse B cells: B lymphomas and normal B cells produce interleukin 10. Int Immunol 2:821–832.

Oltz EM, Yancopoulos GD, Morrow MA, Rolink A, Lee G, Wong F, Kaplan K, Gillis S, Melchers F, Alt FW (1992): A novel regulatory myosin light chain gene distinguishes pre-B cell subsets and is IL-7 inducible. EMBO J 11:2759–2767.

Pennell CA, Mercolino RJ, Grdino TA, Arnold LW, Haughton G, Clarke SH (1989): Biased immunoglobulin variable region gene expression by Ly-1 B cells due to clonal selection. Eur J Immunol 19:1289–1295.

Raaphorst FM, Timmers E, Kenter MJH, Van Tol MJD, Vossen JM, Schuurman RKB (1992): Restricted utilization of germ-line V_H3 genes and short diverse third complementarity-determining regions (CDR3) in human fetal B lymphocytes immunoglobulin heavy chain rearrangements. Eur J Immunol 22:247–251.

Rabin E, Ying-Zi C, Wortis HH (1992): Loss of CD23 is a consequence of B-cell activation. Ann NY Acad Sci 651:130–142.

Reth MG, Jackson S, Alt FW (1986): DJ_H formation and DJ_H replacement during pre-B differentiation: Non-random usage of gene segments. EMBO J 5:2131–2138.

Riboldi P, Kasaian MT, Mantovani L, Ikematsu H, Casali P (1993): Natural antibodies. In Bona CA, Siminovitch K, Zanetti M, Theofilopoulos AN (eds): "The Molecular Pathology of Autoimmune Diseases." Philadelphia: Gordon & Breach (in press).

Sanz I, Casali P, Thomas JW, Notkins AL, Capra JD (1989): Nucleotide sequences of eight human natural antibody V_H regions reveals apparent restricted use of V_H families. J Immunol 142:4054–4061.

Schroeder HW Jr, Hillson JL, Perlmutter RM (1987): Early restriction of the human antibody repertoire. Science 238:791–793.

Schroeder HW Jr, Wang JY (1990): Preferential utilization of conserved immunoglobulin heavy chain variable gene segments during human fetal life. Proc Natl Acad Sci USA 87:6146–6150.

Schutte EM, Ebeling AB, Akkermans KE, Gmelig-Meyling FHJ, Logtenberg T (1991): Antibody specificity and immunoglobulin V_H gene utilization of human monoclonal $CD5^+$ B cell lines. Eur J Immunol 21:1115–1121.

Sidman CL, Shultz LD, Hardy RR, Kayakawa K, Herzenberg LA (1986): Production of immunoglobulin isotypes by Ly-1$^+$ B cells in viable motheaten and normal mice. Science 232:1423–1425.

Solvason N, Kearney JF (1992): The human fetal omentum: A site of B cell generation. J Exp Med 175:397–404.

Solvason N, Lehuen A, Kearney JF (1991): An embryonic source of Ly1 but not conventional B cells. Int Immunol 3:543–550.

Stall AM, Farinas MC, Tarlinton DM, Lalor PA, Herzenberg LA, Strober S, Herzenberg LA (1988): Ly-1 B-cell clones similar to human chronic lymphocytic leukemias routinely develop in older normal mice and young autoimmune (New Zealand Black-related) animals. Proc Natl Acad Sci USA 85:7312–7316.

Stanfield RL, Fieser TM, Lerner RA, Wilson IA (1990): Crystal structures of an antibody to a peptide and its complex with peptide antigen at 2.8 Å. Science 248:712–719.

Sthoeger ZM, Wakai M, Tse DB, Vinviguerra VP, Allen SL, Budman DR, Lichtman SM, Schulman P, Weiselber LR, Chiorazzi N (1989): Production of autoantibodies by CD5-expressing B lymphocytes from patients with chronic lymphocytic leukemia. J Exp Med 169:255–268.

Suzuki N, Sakane T, Engleman EG (1990): Anti-DNA antibody production by CD5$^+$ and CD5$^-$ B cells of patients with systemic lupus erythematosus. J Clin Invest 85:238–247.

Tominaga A, Takaki S, Kayama N, Katoh S, Matsumoto R, Migita M, Hitoshi Y, Hosoya Y, Yamauchi S, Hanai Y, Miyazaki J-I, Usuki G, Yamamura K-I, Takatsu K (1991): Transgenic mice expressing a B cell growth and differentiation factor gene (interleukin 5) develop eosinophilia and autoantibody production. J Exp Med 173:429–437.

Turman MA, Casali P, Notkins AL, Bach FH, Platt JS (1991): Polyreactive antibodies from CD5$^+$ B cells: Antigen specificity and relationship to xenoreactive natural antibodies. Transplantation 52:710–717.

Ueki Y, Goldfarb IS, Harindranath N, Gore M, Koprowski H, Notkins AL, Casali P (1990): Clonal analysis of a human antibody response: Quantitation of precursors of antibody-producing cells and generation and characterization of monoclonal IgM, IgG and IgA to rabies virus. J Exp Med 171:19–34.

Vakil M, Sauter H, Paige C, Kearney JF (1986): In vivo suppression of perinatal multispecific B cells results in a distortion of the adult B cell repertoire. Eur J Immunol 16:1159.

Van Es JH, Gmelig-Meyling FHJ, Van De Akker WRM, Aanstoot H, Derksen RHWM, Logtenberg T (1991): Somatic mutations in the variable regions of a human IgG anti-double-stranded DNA autoantibody suggest a role for antigen in the induction of systemic lupus erythematosus. J Exp Med 173:461–470.

Vaux DL, Lalor PA, Cory S, Johnson GR (1990): In vivo expression of interleukin 5 induces eosinophilia and expanded Ly-1 B lineage populations. Int Immunol 2:965–971.

Velasquillo MC, Alcocer-Varela J, Alarcon-Segovia D, Cabiedes J, Sanchez-Guerrero J (1991): Some patients with primary antiphospholipid syndrome have increased circulating CD5$^+$ B cells that correlate with levels of IgM antiphospholipid. Clin Exp Rheum 9:1–5.

Waldschmidt TJ, Kroese FGM, Tygrett LT, Conrad DH, Lynch RG (1991): The expression of B cell surface receptors. III. The murine low-affinity IgE Fc receptor is not expressed on Ly 1 or "Ly 1-like" B cells. Int Immunol 3:305–315.

Wetzel GD (1989): IL-5 regulation of peritoneal Ly1 B lymphocyte proliferation, differentiation and autoantibody secretion. Eur J Immunol 19:1701–1707.

Whitmore AC, Haughton G, Arnold LW (1992): Isotype switching in CD5 B cells. Ann NY Acad Sci 651:143–151.

Williams RC Jr, Malone CC, Casali P (1992): Heteroclitic polyclonal and monoclonal anti-Gm(a) and anti-Gm(g) human rheumatoid factors react with epitopes induced in Gm (a-), Gm(g-) IgG by interaction with antigen or by non-specific aggregation. A possible mechanism for the in vivo generation of rheumatoid factors. J Immunol 149:1817–1824.

Yamada M, Wasserman R, Reichard BA, Shane S, Caton AJ, Rovera G (1991): Preferential utilization of specific immunoglobulin heavy chain diversity and joining segments in adult human peripheral blood B lymphocytes. J Exp Med 173:395–407.

Yancopoulos GD, Desiderio SV, Paskind M, Kearney JF, Baltimore D, Alt F (1984): Preferential utilization of the most J_H-proximal V_H gene segments in pre-B cell lines. Nature 311:727–733.

Yancopoulos GD, Malynn BA, Alt FW (1988): Developmentally regulated and strain-specific expression of murine V_H gene families. J Exp Med 168:417–435.

Ying-Zi C, Rabin E, Wortis HH (1991): Treatment of murine CD5⁻ B cells with anti-Ig, but not LPS, induces surface CD5: Two B-cell activation pathways. Int Immunol 3:467–476.

7

SELECTION OF THE B-CELL REPERTOIRE AND NATURAL AUTOANTIBODIES

Dan Holmberg and John Kearney

Institute for Cell and Molecular Biology, University of Umeå, Umeå, Sweden (D.H.); Division of Developmental and Clinical Immunology, Department of Microbiology, University of Alabama at Birmingham, Birmingham, Alabama (J.K.)

INTRODUCTION

Specificity of the vertebrate immune system (IS) is mediated by the immuno-globulin (Ig) receptor of the B lymphocyte and by the α,β- and γ,δ-receptors of T lymphocytes (TCR). These three classes of molecules have a similar structure, each of them displaying a variable region and a constant region. The genes encoding the variable (V) regions are formed by the recombination of a set of discrete gene segments during early stages of lymphocyte differen-tiation [reviewed by Tonegawa, 1983; Kronenberg et al., 1986]. In the case of Ig, the genes encoding the heavy (H) and light (L) chains are assembled in an ordered fashion during the differentiation pathway of the B cell. The Ig H-chain V region is encoded by a V_H–D–J_H segment and the Ig L-chain V region is encoded by a V_L–J_H segment.

The number of unique V regions that can potentially be generated through

Autoimmunity: Physiology and Disease, Pages 89–106

this recombination process by far exceeds the size of the repertoire of B-cell specificities available in an individual at any moment in life [Tonegawa, 1983]. The enormous potential of the immune system to generate diversity presents the possibility to select from a large number of V-region specificities those that will constitute the available immune repertoire. This selection procedure appears to be critical for some of the most fundamental characteristics of the immune system, including establishment of self–nonself-discrimination. The accumulating information about the rules and mechanisms mediating the selective processes involved in the establishment of the B-cell repertoire constitutes the scope of this review.

PROGRAMMED ESTABLISHMENT OF ANTIBODY REPERTOIRES

The establishment of B-cell-specificity repertoires during the ontogeny of the vertebrate IS is known to occur in a programmed fashion [Alt et al., 1986]. Such a programmed development of B-cell repertoires has been suggested from many observations that antibody responsiveness to distinct antigens appear at different points of ontogeny in both humans and other vertebrates [Klinman and Linton, 1988]. Molecular analyses of normal B-lymphoid populations selected at different stages of ontogeny and cell lines representative of different stages of the B-cell lineage have demonstrated that the expression of V_H gene segments occurs nonrandomly in fetal liver and neonatal spleen and shows a preference for D-proximal V_H gene families [Yancopoulos et al., 1984; Perlmutter et al., 1985; Lawler et al., 1987; Jeong and Teale, 1988]. In contrast, the expressed V_H gene repertoire of the adult spleen shows no obvious bias to family representation [Dildrop et al., 1985].

The nonrandom V gene utilization observed in the perinatal period may result from mechanisms favoring (or disfavoring) selection of certain V gene segments during the process of V(D)J assembly at the early pre-B-cell stage. Alternatively, certain V(D)J rearrangements may be intra- or intercellularly selected on the basis of specificity. Evidence has been accumulating during the last few years suggesting that mechanisms of both types contribute to the establishment of the mature B-cell repertoire [Yancopoulos et al., 1984; Malynn et al., 1990; Freitas et al., 1990; Carlsson et al., 1992; Gu et al., 1991].

Intrinsic Rates of V(D)J Rearrangements

Analyses of Abelson murine leukemia virus (A-MuLV)–transformed pre-B-cell lines, which continuously undergo V_H to DJ_H rearrangements in tissue culture, were the first to suggest that V_H genes are utilized in a nonrandom fashion [Yancopoulos et al., 1984]. These studies, together with similar analyses of fetal liver hybridomas [Perlmutter et al., 1985], suggested that the observed bias in the fetal and perinatal B-cell repertoires was a result of mechanistic constraints on the Ig gene assembly process and that chromosomal positioning and accessibility to the recombinational machinery were important parameters in mediating these constraints [Yancopoulos et al., 1984; Alt et al., 1984].

It is clear from the analysis of A-MuLV–induced pre-B-cell lines that V_H gene families positioned in the proximity of the D region of the Ig H locus tend to be preferred in the process of V_H to D–J_H rearrangements all through ontogeny [Yancopoulos et al., 1984; Lawler et al., 1987]. However, as already pointed out by Yancopoulos et al. [1984], chromosomal positioning cannot be the only factor determining the frequency with which individual V_H gene segments are rearranged. This is illustrated by the observation that the $V_H7183.8$ (V_HE4.Psi) gene rearranges at a lower frequency than the $V_H7183.1$ (V_H81X) gene segment, despite its closer position to the D region in the BALB/c genome [Yancopoulos et al., 1984].

We have recently analyzed a large set of nonfunctional V_H7183–D–J_H rearrangements and observed that the utilization of individual V_H gene segments within this family remains constant, independent of organ localization and ontogenetic stage [Carlsson et al., 1992; Huetz et al., 1993]. Thus the fraction of $V_H7183.1$ rearrangements remains constant at about 70% of the total V_H7183 rearrangements, whereas the other members of the family appear to rearrange at a distinctly lower frequency. Since nonfunctional rearrangements are not susceptible to cellular selection, these observations suggest that mechanistic constraints exist that favor the rearrangement of some gene segments, notably the $V_H7183.1$ (V_H81X) gene over the other members of the V_H7183 gene family.

The mechanistic constraints on V_H gene utilization may be imposed by several different factors. As discussed above, one such factor that has been suggested is chromosomal position, which may confer an advantage to V_H genes localized to the proximity of the D region [Alt et al., 1984]. Another possibility may involve the control rates of V_H gene rearrangements. The unique flanking region sequences of the $V_H7183.1$ gene segment [Yancopoulos et al., 1984; Schroeder et al., 1990] may also constitute possible targets for a unique V gene specific control of rearrangements. Irrespective of the mechanism responsible for the unique representation of V_H81X rearrangements, it is clear that this preference has been maintained in most strains of mice and rats, and it would appear to provide some functional consequence on the development of the B-cell repertoire.

Characteristics of the Developing B-Cell Repertoire

It is evident that the fetal and neonatal B-cell repertoire differs from that of the adult with respect to many characteristics. One of these important differences is the high degree of connectivity that is observed in panels of IgM antibodies, from perinatal but not adult B cells [Holmberg et al., 1984, 1986; Vakil and Kearney, 1986, 1988; Vakil et al., 1986]. There are difficulties in defining and measuring connectivity, but most methods have relied on the measurement of self-binding between IgM members of the same panel in a variant of a solid phase binding assay [Holmberg et al., 1984; Vakil and Kearney, 1986]. This connectivity is implied to occur through idiotypes of Ig V regions, and in some cases this can be shown formally by classic inhibition assays [Holmberg et al., 1984; Vakil and Kearney, 1986].

While it is clear that there are reasons for this connectivity such as the preferential use of D_H proximal V_H genes and the constraints on complementarity-determining region 3 (CDR3) formation, there is still the problem of how it develops. Is connectivity encoded in the germline V_H genes that are used early but not late in development, or does it occur through a "learning process" as clones of B cells developing in early liver and spleen interact with self-antigen and/or self-idiotypes in situ or after emigration to peripheral lymphoid organs resulting in an increase in the size of the early interconnected network of B cells?

Most studies have tested sets of antibodies made within a given mouse strain [Holmberg et al., 1984, 1986; Vakil and Kearney, 1986, 1988; Vakil et al., 1986]. We have attempted to illuminate these two questions by comparing connectivity between genetically different sets of antibodies generated under alternative situations. In the first case, sets of antibodies were generated from perinatal BALB/cJ (IgCH^a) or C57Bl/6 (IgCH^b) parental strains of mice. These were then tested against each other in conventional assays, i.e., analysis of connectivity *within* a given IgCH haplotype versus reactivity *between* the different IgCH^a and IgCH^b haplotypes. When this was done and connectivity was calculated by a simple measure of the frequency and intensity of individual antibody reactivities, it was clear that there was preferential connectivity between IgMs of the same haplotype. At face value these results would imply that there was a strong genetic element to the observed connectivity and that sets of V genes were expressed in genetically distinct individuals that are complementary to each other but not to others from a different strain.

In a second approach, similar sets of antibodies of either the IgCH^a or IgCH^b allotype were made from perinatal F_1 mice derived from the same parental strains and were then tested in a similar manner. This time, however, preferred reactivity between antibodies using V_H genes from the same Ig H locus was not observed, and reactivity between antibodies tended to be equal among all combinations tested. This second result suggested that connectivity was not IgCH linked and that the observed connectivity preference between antibodies of parental strains was lost in the F_1 mice.

These results suggest that connectivity develops during the perinatal period through interactions between the *available* repertoire that is generated from the genetically different heavy chain alleles. This conclusion does not take into account the role of light chain expression in this observed connectivity. There were some other trends observed in these experiments that are apparent between the C57BL/6 and BALB/c repertoires that may relate to differences discussed earlier. BALB/c IgMs appear to be more connected than C57BL/6. This was apparent not only when these antibodies were tested within the BALB/c haplotype but also in their reactivity to C57BL/6. Second, there appeared to be a comparative deficit of connectivity in IgMs from hybridomas derived from earlier (fetal liver) tissues than in later 2–3-day-old C57BL/6 hybridomas. This may relate to the increased tendency to select against functional V_H7183 rearrangements within this haplotype [Freitas et al., 1989], the extreme case being that of V_H81X [Andersson et al., 1992]. It is also worth noting that in the preliminary V_H gene analysis of the ~150 hybridomas being discussed here there does appear to be a marked expression of non-V_H7183 genes in the C57BL/6 panel, supporting at a B-cell level the genetic selection against V_H7183 expression apparent in analyses of whole liver or spleen [Wu and Paige, 1986].

How does the connectivity develop mechanistically, and what is its physiological role? Although there is only limited structural data available, there are characteristics of the gene rearrangements that occur in perinatal life that may explain connectivity. From many studies it has been shown that the perinatal V gene repertoire is marked by 1) lack of N-segment additions, 2) preferential utilization of certain V, D, and J_H segments, 3) use of a preferred reading frame, and 4) lack of somatic hypermutation. It is easy to see that these characteristics would have the potential to contribute to shared primary amino acid sequences in CDR regions and in particular the normally highly diverse CDR3 regions [Feeney, 1990; Gu et al., 1991]. Thus perinatal IgM antibodies would have a much higher probability of sharing idiotopes than would a given set of antibodies derived from adult B cells where N-segment addition would tend to give extreme diversity to CDR3 regions.

While it is easy to demonstrate that connectivity exists experimentally, it is less easy to show in a noninterventional way where and how these proposed cellular and antibody interactions occur and what the physiological sequelae of such proposed interactions may be. These will be discussed later.

V_H81X

An extreme example of the selection process involves the expression of the V_H81X gene. As stated earlier, this V_H gene is rearranged at a high frequency in B-cell generative sites all through ontogeny and appears to be positively selected in the perinatal period. In contrast, it is not found as part of a functioning B-cell or immunoglobulin product in the peripheral B-cell repertoire of the adult individual, suggesting that B cells expressing functional V_H81X rearrangements appear to be negatively selected.

Isolation of several hybridomas from fetal liver that express functional V_H81X rearrangements together with light chains permitted us to examine the specificity of immunoglobulin secreted by these rescued B cells. These were found to be highly reactive in ELISA assays and bound to ~50% of 75 other perinatal IgM immunoglobulins. Fluorescence staining showed that several of these antibodies bound to a variety of cell types, including B-cell lines and subpopulations of splenic and bone marrow cells. This characteristic was also evident when V_H81X μ-only pre-B-cell hybridomas derived from fetal liver were fused with L chain plasmacytomas or hybridomas, and in this way V_H81X IgM derived from pre-B cells could be secreted in association with light chains. These IgM molecules were also highly self-reactive, suggesting that these early functionally rearranged pre-B cells may also, if they had been forced to seek and express a light chain in vivo, have resulted in their elimination as B cells, which seems to be the fate of most functional V_H81X rearrangements in vivo, but instead were rescued by hybridoma formation.

Examination of the sequences of these V_H81X-expressing hybridoma lines shows that the V regions are highly unusual in that they contain five pairs of positively charged amino acids that may be responsible for their high degree of autoreactivity as demonstrated by reactivity to other IgM proteins and a variety of cell membrane surfaces. Alternatively, these characteristics may limit the diversity of L chains that can form a functional IgM molecule; however, preliminary modeling experiments did not show any striking differences at sites where heavy and light chains interact that may preclude interactions during the assembly of heavy and light chains into a functional molecule.

We have recently constructed transgenic mice in which a rearranged germline V_H81X gene is expressed at a protein level in B cells, not only in fetal life but throughout the life of the adult mouse. The phenotype of this mouse as revealed in preliminary analyses showed reduced levels of B lymphocytes most of which expressed the transgene in spleen, lymph nodes, and blood. Total serum IgM was much lower than normal and consisted entirely of small amounts of endogenous product whereas serum IgGH[a] derived from the transgene was totally absent despite the presence of B cells expressing the transgene. CD5[+] B cells were absent from the peritoneal cavity of these mice, a phenotype that has not been described previously in transgenic mice. It also appears that the introduced V_H81X transgene can only be expressed together with endogenous κ chains since λ chains have not been detected.

These studies show that the transgenic V_H81X can be expressed in peripheral B cells, which, however, appear to exist in a profound state of anergy since they are incapable of expressing the transgenic product. Thus it remains to be seen whether the continued expression of this highly self-reactive V_H gene has effects on or produces autoimmune phenomena later in life and also reveal a specialized function for pre-B or B cells expressing this gene early in development.

CD5 B CELLS AND CONNECTIVITY

It is obvious that most connectivity is observed between the earliest B cells as they develop during the neonatal period. This then appears to subside and provide a smaller core of connective antibodies in the adult. It is clear that mouse serum IgM is derived from the $CD5^+$ (B-1) B-cell subset [Ishida et al., 1992]. Although the lineage nature of $CD5^+$ B cells is controversial [Herzenberg et al., 1986; Cong et al., 1991], there is clear evidence that this B-cell subset is physiologically different from the major $CD5^-$ (B-2) population. There is some evidence that there may be more evolutionarily primitive precursors for B-1 cells [Hardy and Hayakawa, 1991] and that they appear to derive at least partially from extrahepatic sites during development [Solvason et al., 1991; Solvason and Kearney, 1992].

The disseminated sites of early B-cell origin and the possibility that they may come from separate precursors may be reflected in the observed differences between B-1 versus B-2 cells. Notable among these and pertinent to this discussion is the repeated inability to demonstrate any degree of somatic hypermutation in V regions of B-1 cells [Gu et al., 1991]. Certainly also, in early development these cells show little evidence for N-segment addition [Holmberg et al., 1989; Gu et al., 1990; Feeney, 1990]. The preferred use of reading frame and the use of illegitimate recombination in the forming of V–D–J joints may reflect the retention of more primitive methods of gene recombination. All of these mechanisms serve to retain the production of clones to germline-like antibodies containing the special self and autoreactivities we have observed.

Although it is clear that B-1 cells can switch isotypes under appropriate conditions, it appears to occur much less frequently and may be restricted mainly to certain isotypes, notably IgG3 and IgA [Solvason et al., 1991]. The latter propensity may be related to the ability of B-1 cells to give rise to IgA production in local mucosal sites [Kroese et al., 1988]. There are other characteristics such as IL-10, IL-4, and IL-6 production that are also exhibited by B-1 and $CD5^+$ B-cell lines, but not B-2 cells [O'Garra et al., 1992]. The ability of these cells to produce cytokines makes it feasible to propose that B-1 cells have a propensity to direct or initiate other B–B interactions or B-cell regulatory functions [O'Garra et al., 1992; O'Garra and Howard, 1991].

There have been recent findings that support previous demonstrations that the normal level of background IgM in serum is derived from CD5 cells. IL-10 suppression by chronic administration of IL-10 dramatically reduced PEC B-1 cells and simultaneously severely reduced serum IgM and ablated the ability to make antibodies to certain carbohydrate antigens [Ishida et al., 1992]. Furthermore, neonatal treatment of F1 mice with antiallotype antibodies directed to either of the parental allotypes permanently depletes the corresponding $CD5^+$ B-1 subset and simultaneously the expression of serum IgM of that allotype. These results also support the previous experiment that suggested a strong competition for a niche within the immune system by B-1 cells. Once this is established, in this case the suppressed parental type B-1 cells can no longer establish themselves in the peritoneum. A strong feedback mechanism must be occurring in this situation that may include the IgM or IgM receptor interaction between the established B-1 parental type in these treated mice.

What then is the relationship between B-1 and conventional B-2 cells in the sense of internal interconnectivity? It is clear that at least cells bearing the two different phenotypes are sequestered under normal circumstances into anatomically distinct sites. Is there a functional reason for this? It has previously been demonstrated by immunofluorescence that in the marginal zones surrounding germinal centers there exists a layer of bright IgM-producing B cells. There is some evidence that these are not B-2 type cells since they lack the Fcε receptor, and there is some evidence that these may be of B-1 origin [Waldschmidt et al., 1991]. These marginal zone areas are believed to be sites where polysaccharide antigens are accumulated and where T-independent responses occur. It is tempting to suggest that these cells may also be producing IgM molecules with high connectivity. It was postulated by Bloom et al. [1992] that the autoreactive IgM produced by B-1 cells and interaction with self-antigens is responsible for the presentation of self-peptides and induction of T-cell suppression. Perhaps the anatomical location described for these cells serves as a monitoring mechanism to limit feedback on the proliferation and differentiation of B-1 cells that is occurring in germinal centers after antigen stimulation.

There has been one recent notable example of a transgenic mouse bearing transgene-encoded anti-mRBC activity whose CD5 B cells, which have apparently escaped tolerance induction as a result of their sequestration in the peritoneal cavity, are involved in the production of autoimmune hemolytic anemia. The epitope of this antibody on mRBC has not been identified, and it is not clear whether this antibody has other specificities or to what degree it was connected with other CD5 B cells [Murakami et al., 1992].

CONNECTIVITY AND DEVELOPMENT OF THE REPERTOIRE

It is clear that in mouse and man the B-cell repertoire develops at a characteristic rate and with a chronology that is similar for different strains and in different species [Perlmutter, 1987]. One of the most notable differences between the neonatal and adult B-cell repertoire is evident in the ability to raise antibody responses to certain T-independent antigens. Characteristically in humans and in mouse the ability to respond to T-independent bacterial-associated antigens appears relatively late during development. Some of the best studies are the responses to various dextrans, phosphorylcholine (PC), and fructosans in mice and the responses to HIBS from hemophilus and pneumococcal polysaccharides, and so forth, in humans [Klinman and Press, 1975; Bona et al., 1979; Stohrer and Kearney, 1984; Barrett, 1985]. These show a broad temporal range of developmental initiation. The ability to respond to PC occurs reproducibly at about 6 days after birth in BALB/c mice, and antibody responses to $\alpha 1$–3-dextran and certain idiotypes in $\beta 2$–6-fructosan responses do not arise until much later [Klinman and Press, 1975; Bona et al., 1979; Stohrer and Kearney, 1984]. Similar delays also occur in the ability of infants to respond to bacterial-associated antigens such as pneumococcal and hemophilus polysaccharides [Barrett, 1985], with the result that this failure to respond leads to increased susceptibility to infections with these organisms to which antibodies to the polysaccharides normally provide protective immunity.

This seeming paradox may have at its roots the connectivity existing between developing germline-encoded B-cell clones in the perinatal period. It is clear that negative selection in early development can be easily induced by exogenous administration of very small amounts of anti-idiotypic antibodies. The T15 idiotype and others can be permanently suppressed by perinatal administration and also by maternal passage of artificially constructed anti-idiotypic antibodies. It is generally assumed that the ease with which this suppression is induced is due to the greater ease by which newly formed B cells are functionally inactivated and deleted compared with adult B cells by cross-linking of their IgM receptors [Stohrer and Kearney, 1984]. It is also clear from the examples we discuss later that there is intense competition between developing clones of $CD5^+$ cells for a position in the early repertoire [Lalor et al., 1989].

More subtle alterations to the B-cell repertoire have been induced by manipulation with IgM antibodies derived from hybridomas of perinatal B cells. We have been able to isolate in this way anti-idiotypic antibodies that upon reintroduction to the neonatal mouse had profound effects on the establishment of the adult repertoire. One of the striking observations made in these kinds of experiments was the appearance of critical windows during ontogeny when enhancement of the activity of a clone of B cells could be affected that differed chronologically for the antigen under study. These windows appeared to coincide with the time of normal emergence of responsive B-cell clones in nonmanipulated animals that have been described previously in a variety of functional assays [Vakil et al., 1986]. These results suggested that there are critical periods when a B-cell emerges, during which it is more highly sensitive to positive or negative selection. Our hypothesis is that engagement of the IgM receptor with IgG Fc-bearing anti-idiotype antibodies leads to a strong negative selection [Pollok et al., 1984], while engagement with an IgM Fcμ antibody may deliver an enhancing or positive signal depending on the concentration of the interacting IgM ligands. Of course, there may be a balance in that overinduction with too many individual or high-affinity IgM antibodies may lead to an overall suppression that would result in that clone being functionally silenced (anergic) and cause it to be a late-appearing clone that emerges functionally when connectivity has declined and IgM binding has decreased.

This idea that connectivity is involved in the selection of germline V_H- and V_L-encoded clones also provides an explanation for clonal dominance. The preponderant expression of one or a few clones of B cells expressing conserved germline heavy and light chain Ig genes in response to certain kinds of antigens has been repeatedly observed in mice [Claflin 1976; Hansburg et al.,

1978; Lieberman et al., 1974; Schilling et al., 1980], and there is also increasing evidence that this also occurs in man. Clonal dominance appears to be established by programmed idiotype direction interactions between B cells and their products and thus provides a mechanism for the development of useful protective clones prior to exposure to antigen [Vakil and Kearney, 1986, 1991; Vakil et al., 1986]. It is clear that clonal dominance in some cases can only occur during critical developmental periods, perhaps because of the long-lived and self-renewing capability of the CD5 B-cell lineage in which a large proportion of B cells that produce these antibodies appear to be sequestered [Förster and Rajewsky, 1987; Masmoudi et al., 1990]. These dominant responses do not appear subsequent to normal bone marrow transplantation. In this case transfer of adult stem cells and immature progenitors from bone marrow to an adult irradiated mouse or even severe combined immunodeficient (SCID) mice does not result in the restoration of clonal dominance in a number of situations [Elliot and Kearney, 1992]. However, it is possible to restore clonal dominance by transfer of adult bone marrow into neonatal SCID mice [Elliot and Kearney, 1992]. These results suggest that both the precursor status (newborn or adult) as well as the microenvironment are important in the establishment of the clones of cells responsible for the normally observed dominance.

One of the major differences in a newborn and adult is an absence of a large pool of preformed immunoglobulin. This is not removed by irradiation in the normal mouse, and would not be present in SCID mice. The V region interactions that potentially could occur between this preformed pool of immunoglobulin and the newly emerging B cells arising from the progenitor cells in transferred bone marrow may be sufficient to prevent the emergence of the dominant clones. Indeed, it has been claimed that coadministration of appropriate anti-idiotypic reagents at the time of or after administration can facilitate the emergence of the normally dominant clones. In addition, the recapitulation of the neonatal repertoire observed in the molecular analysis of V regions expressed by B cells developing from transferred bone marrow in SCID mice (lacking immunoglobulin) but not in normal mice (D. Holmberg, unpublished observations) points to the importance of these interactions. Similarly the administration of exogenous sources of immunoglobulin may cause functional changes in the repertoire [Freitas et al., 1991].

The deliberate administration of polysaccharide protein conjugate vaccines into the neonatal human is being tested as a means to hasten the normally delayed appearance of protective antibody responses to important pathogens. Similarly, acquisition of such antibodies either by passive administration or active transmission of immunized maternal immunoglobulin has been proposed as a means to booster neonatal protection in humans [Barrett, 1985]. It is clear, however, that in mice administration of particular antigens, e.g., PC, not only did not expand the appropriate protective clones of B cells but presumably, through the interconnection we have demonstrated, resulted in the ablation or down-modulation of other clones of B cells with specificities for a variety of other organisms. These results suggest that interference with this connectivity is detrimental to the normal development of repertoires [Vakil et al., 1991; Vakil and Kearney, 1991]. Similarly we have shown that passive administration of purified fluid phase immunoglobulin expressing the V regions responsible for the expression of the dominant idiotypes into neonates results in a very significant drop in the ability of adults thus treated to respond to these antigens [Vakil et al., 1991; Vakil and Kearney, 1991]. These results are interpreted to occur because of interference of B–B interactions or anti-idiotypic B-cell interactions during selection of the appropriate emerging clones.

Taking all these findings together, we have the paradox that during neonatal life interactions such as those described are necessary for the emergence of useful and sometimes dominant clones and yet at the same time may be responsible for the delay in emergence of other clones and the comcomitant inability to respond with the production of protective antibody. Is this the price paid for having a "complete" repertoire, or, as has been suggested, is it that many of these germline-encoded antibody responses also exhibit self-reactivity toward fetal and neonatal antigens expressed during development [Briles and Carroll, 1987]. The inability to respond therefore is a result of anergy induction during the period that these self-antigens are expressed and that afterwards disappears subsequent to further development. It is clear that in some cases cross-reactivity exists between self-components and bacterial products [Finne et al., 1987]. Perhaps neoantigens also share this cross-reactivity.

ANTILYMPHOCYTE ACTIVITY

It has been shown in many situations that the production of antibodies with antilymphocyte activity is characteristic of several immunopathologic diseases, including the systemic lupus erythematosus-like disease of NZB and nonobese diabetic (NOD) mice [Alpert et al., 1987, Bocchieri et al., 1982; Izui et al., 1979; Lehuen et al., 1990a,b; Raveche et al., 1981; Shirai and Mellors, 1971; van der Veen et al., 1981] as well as in graft-versus-host situations under conditions of intense lymphocyte proliferation. Antibodies produced in these conditions are characteristically of the IgM isotype and react mainly with thymocytes and to a lesser extent T cells [Shirai and Mellors, 1971; Huston et al., 1980].

Although there is a clear association of production of these antibodies with disease states, there has been no evidence that they are directly involved in the pathogenesis of these diseases. In the screening of the perinatal mouse B-cell repertoire it was found that ~11% of IgM antibodies exhibited antilymphocyte activity against thymocytes and both peripheral T and B cells. These were found in the two normal strains of perinatal C57BL/6 and BALB/c mice analyzed but were not found in adult B cells from the same strains [Lehuen et al., 1992]. At the molecular level many of these antibodies reacted with epitopes on lymphocytes that were sensitive to PI-PLC treatment associated with a predominant molecule of 100,000 MW [Lehuen and Kearney, 1992]. V-region nucleotide analysis of several of the antibodies that appeared to bind to the same epitope was revealing in that three antibodies from independent fusions had identical or very similar V_HD and J_H genes and also, of more interest, identical V_H–D_H joints. That these hybridomas were isolated independently, used similar V genes and identical joints suggest that these antibody-forming B cells arise normally as part of the developing perinatal repertoire, as a consequence of the restricted mechanisms at play in the recombination of gene segments early but not later in life. Again it was of interest that particular V_H gene segments used belonged to the newly described SM-7 family [Tutter et al., 1991], which is sufficiently distinct from the large distal J558 family to warrant a separate designation. This family is located more D proximal but would generally not be considered one of the proximal V_H gene families, which appear to be predominantly expressed early in life.

It is known that the first lymphoid cells to appear in peripheral lymphoid tissues in man and mouse are B cells [Bofill et al., 1985; J. Kearney, unpublished observations]. In man these also appear to be $CD5^+$. These B lymphocytes appear characteristically in tight clusters around the central arterioles in spleen and follicles of lymph nodes that eventually become T dependent [Bofill et al., 1985]. The neonatal generation of B cells with autoreactivity to lymphocytes appears then to be a hallmark of not only certain autoimmune diseases but also the newly generated B-cell repertoire. The interactions afforded by the specificity of B cells for non-MHC products of self-lymphocytes may be involved in the organization of lymphocytes into typical B- and T-cell areas or may provide yet another mechanism for the development of self-assertiveness. The relationship between these perinatal antibodies and the IgM antilymphocyte antibodies characteristic of autoimmune disease remain to be elucidated.

AUTOREACTIVITY AND AUTOIMMUNE DISEASE

While normal mice undergo a process of selection against the expression of D-proximal V_H genes from the perinatal period to adulthood [Jeong and Teale, 1988; Freitas et al., 1990; Malynn et al., 1990], we have recently observed that the adult NOD mouse displays an abnormal pattern of V_H gene utilization [Leijon and Holmberg, 1992; Andersson et al., 1992]. Thus in situ hybridization studies of V_H gene expression demonstrated that the neonatal pattern of V_H gene utilization, with a bias toward expression of D-proximal V_H genes, is retained in the adult NOD mouse. Whereas the vast majority of rearrangements utilizing the V_H 7183.1 gene segment were found to be nonfunctional in adult BALB/c [Carlsson et al., 1992] and in adult C57BI/6 mice, a considerable fraction of such rearrangements were scored as functional in the adult NOD mouse.

As we have argued before [Carlsson et al., 1992], the unique pattern of positive selection of this V_H gene in the perinatal period, together with an almost total selection against its expression in adult peripheral lymphoid tissue, may imply that the V_H 7183.1 gene mediates a function specific for the early development of the immune system. If so, the presence of functional V_H 7183.1 rearrangements in the adult NOD mouse could be a reflection of an aberrant development of the immune repertoire, which may be either directly or indirectly related to the development of autoimmunity in the NOD mouse. Moreover, the analysis of individual V_H gene utilization revealed that the rearrangements using the 81X gene was not selected against in the adult NOD mouse in contrast to normal mouse strains like BALB/c and C57BI/6. Most interestingly, we observed that neonatal treatment of NOD mice with a "natural" monoclonal antibody, previously reported to prevent the development of diabetes [Andersson et al., 1992], could partly restore the abnormal V_H 7183 utilization pattern in adult NOD mice.

These data demonstrate that neonatal immunoglobulin treatment can alter the development of the adult B cell repertoire. Furthermore the possibility that B cells and immunoglobulin may, directly or indirectly, influence the development of T-cell-mediated autoimmunity in the NOD mouse is also suggested. The observation that prevention of disease is paralleled by the total absence of functional 7183.1 rearrangements in the splenic B-cell population is in line with this hypothesis.

The finding that neonatal administration of a "natural," highly connected monoclonal antibody can induce changes in the repertoire of V-region specificities as well as prevent the development of diabetes suggests a possible link between the establishment of B-cell repertoires and the development of T-cell-mediated autoimmunity in the NOD mouse. In agreement with this notion, the monoclonal-antibody-induced alterations in the V-region repertoires all appear to lead to "normalization" of the adult NOD repertoire, so that it then resembles that of a normal adult C57BI/6 mouse. In view of the well-documented T-cell dependence of the disease process in the NOD mouse, it is tempting to speculate that the observed effects on B-cell repertoire development directly or indirectly induce modifications of the T-cell compartment. Examples of such B-cell/immunoglobulin-induced shaping of peripheral T-cell repertoires have been previously reported [Martinez-A et al., 1985; Sy et al., 1984], suggesting plausible mechanisms for linking B-cell repertoires to the development of T-cell-mediated autoimmunity. Further investigations addressing this point may be important for the understanding of the development of autoimmunity in the NOD mouse.

Most interestingly, neonatal monoclonal antibody treatment of NOD mice also appeared to influence the intrinsic rate of rearrangement of the V_H 7183.1 gene. Thus, whereas about 40% of the total V_H 7183 rearrangements of nontreated neonatal and adult NOD mice utilized this V_H gene segment, this frequency was increased to about 80% in animals neonatally treated with BA.N 1:1.8. These data suggest the possibility that the relative frequency of rearrangements of individual V_H gene segments may be controlled by external signals. In this context, it should be noted that the V_H 7183.1 gene has been demonstrated to display unique noncoding flanking sequences, including the recombination signal sequences [Schroeder et al., 1990] constituting potential sites for control of V–D–J recombination.

REFERENCES

Alpert SD, Turek PJ, Foung SKH, Engelman EG (1987): Human monoclonal anti-T cell antibody from a patient with juvenile rheumatoid arthritis. J Immunol 138:104–108.

Alt F, Yancopoulos GD, Blackwell TK, Wood C, Thomas E, Boss M, Coffman R, Rosenberg N, Tonegawa S, Baltimore D (1984): Ordered rearrangement of immunoglobulin heavy chain V segment. EMBO J 3:1209–1219.

Alt FW, Blackwell TK, DePinho RA, Reth MG, Yancopoulos GD (1986): Regulation of genome rearrangement events during lymphocyte differentiation. Immunol Rev 85:5–24.

Andersson Å, Leijon K, Holmberg D (1993): Neonatal treatment with monoclonal natural antibodies inhibits development of diabetes and restores a normal pattern of VH utilization in the non-obese diabetic (NOD) mouse. Submitted for publication.

Barrett DJ (1985): Human immune responses to polysaccharide antigens: An analysis of bacterial polysaccharide vaccines in infants. In Barnes LA (ed): "Advances in Pediatrics." Medical Publishers, pp 139–158.

Bloom BR, Salgame P, Diamond B (1992): Revisiting and revising suppressor T cells. Immunol Today 13:131–136.

Bocchieri MH, Cooke A, Smith JB, Weigert M, Riblet RJ (1982): Independent segregation of NZB immune abnormalities in NZB × C58 recombinant inbred mice. Eur J Immunol 12:349–354.

Bofill M, Janossy G, Burford GD, Seymour GJ, Wernet P, Kelemen E (1985): Human B cell development. II. Subpopulations in the human. J Immunol 134:1531–1538.

Bona C, Mond JJ, Stein KE, House S, Lieberman R, Paul WE (1979): Immune response to levan. III. The capacity to produce anti-inulin antibodies and cross-reactive idiotypes appears late in ontogeny. J Immunol 123:1484–1491.

Briles DE, Carroll J (1987): Natural selection and the response to polysaccharides. In Kelsoe G, Schulze DH (eds): "Evolution and Vertebrate Immunity: The Antigen Receptor and MHC Families." Austin: University of Texas Press, pp 117–133.

Carlsson L, Övermo C, Holmberg D (1992): Developmentally controlled selection of antibody genes: Characterization of individual VH 7183 genes and evidence for stage-specific somatic diversification. Eur J Immunol 22:71–78.

Claflin JL (1976): Uniformity in the clonal repertoire of the immune response to phosphorylcholine in mice. Eur J Immunol 6:669–675.

Cong Y, Rabin E, Wortis H (1991): Treatment of CD5- B cells with anti-Ig but not LPS, induces surface CD5: Two B cell activation pathways. Int Immunol 3:467–476.

Dildrop R, Krawinkel V, Winter E, Rajewsky K (1985): V_H gene expression in murine lipopolysaccharide blasts distribute over the nine known V_H gene groups and may be random. Eur J Immunol 15:1154–1156.

Elliot M, Kearney JF (1992): Idiotypic regulation of development of the B cell repertoire Ann NY Acad Sci 651:336–345.

Feeney A (1990): Lack of N regions in fetal and neonatal mouse immunoglobulin V–D–J junctional sequences. J Exp Med 172:1377–1390.

Finne J, Bitter-Suermann D, Goridis C, Finne U (1987): An IgG monoclonal antibody to group B meningococci cross-reacts with developmentally regulated polysialic acid units of glycoproteins in neural and extraneural tissues. J Immunol 138:4402–4407.

Förster I, Rajewsky K (1987): Expansion and functional activity of Ly-1$^+$ B cells upon transfer of peritoneal cells into allotype-congenic, newborn mice. Eur J Immunol 17:521–528.

Freitas AA, Andrade L, Lembezat MP, Coutinho A (1990): Selection of VH gene repertoires: differentiating B cells of adult bone marrow mimic fetal development. Int Immunol 2:15–23.

Freitas AA, Lembezat M-P, Coutinho A (1989): Expression of antibody V-regions is genetically and developmentally controlled and modulated by the B lymphocyte environment. Int Immunol 1:342–354.

Freitas AA, Viale AC, Sundblad A, Heusser C, Coutinho A (1991): Normal serum immunoglobulins participate in the selection of peripheral B cell repertoires. Proc Natl Acad Sci USA 88:5640–5644.

Gu H, Förster I, Rajewsky K (1990): Sequence homologies, N sequence insertion and JH gene utilization in VHDJH joining: Implications for the joining mechanism and the ontogenetic timing of Ly1 B cell and B-CLL progenitor generation. EMBO J 9:2133–2140.

Gu H, Tarlinton D, Müller W, Rajewsky K (1991): Most peripheral B cells in mice are ligand selected. J Exp Med 173:1357–1371.

Hansburg D, Perlmutter RM, Briles DE, Davie JM (1978): Analysis of the diversity of murine antibodies to dextran B 1355. III. Idiotypic and spectrotypic correlations. Eur J Immunol 8:352–359.

Hardy RR, Hayakawa K (1991): A developmental switch in B lymphopoiesis. Proc Natl Acad Sci USA 88:1150–1154.

Herzenberg LA, Stall AM, Lalor PA, Sidman C, Moore WA, Parks DR, Herzenberg LA (1986): The Ly-1 B cell lineage. Immunol Rev 93:81–102.

Holmberg D, Andersson Å, Carlsson L, Forsgren S (1989): Establishment and functional implications of B-cell connectivity Immunol Rev 110:89–103.

Holmberg D, Forsgren S, Ivars F, Coutinho A (1984): Reactions amongst IgM antibodies derived from normal, neonatal mice. Eur J Immunol 14:435–441.

Holmberg D, Wennerström G, Andrade L, Coutinho A (1986): The high idiotypic connectivity of "natural" newborn antibodies is not found in adult, mitogen-reactive B cell repertoires. Eur J Immunol 16:82–87.

Huetz F, Carlsson L, Tornberg U-C, Holmberg D (1993): V-region directed selection in differentiating B lymphocytes. EMBO J 12:1819–1826.

Huston DP, Raveche ES, Steinberg AD (1980): Preferential lysis of undifferentiated thymocytes by natural thymocytotoxic antibodies from New Zealand black mice. J Immunol 124:1635–1641.

Ishida H, Hastings R, Kearney J, Howard M (1992): Continuous anti-IL-10 antibody administration depletes mice of Ly1 B cells but not conventional B cells. J Exp Med 175:1213–1220.

Izui S, Kobayakawa T, Louis J, Lambert P-H (1979): Induction of thymocytotoxic autoantibodies after injection of bacterial lipopolysaccharides in mice. Eur J Immunol 9:338–341.

Jeong HD, Teale J (1988): Comparison of the foetal and adult functional B cell repertoires by analysis of V_H gene family expression. J Exp Med 168:589–603.

Klinman NR, Linton PJ (1988): The clonotype repertoire of B cell subpopulations. Adv Immunol 42:1–93.

Klinman NR, Press JL (1975): The B cell specificity repertoire: Its relationship to definable subpopulations. Transplant Rev 24:41–83.

Kroese FGM, Butcher EC, Stall AM, Lalor PA, Adams S, Herzenberg L (1988): Many of the IgA plasma cells for the murine gut are derived from self replenishing precursors in the peritoneal cavity. Int Immunol 1:75–84.

Kronenberg M, Siu G, Hood L, Shastri N (1986): The molecular genetics of the T-cell antigen receptor and the T-cell antigen recognition. Annu Rev Immunol 4:529–591.

Lalor PA, Herzenberg LA, Adams S, Stall A (1989): Feedback regulation of murine Ly1 B cell development. Eur J Immunol 19:507–513.

Lawler AM, Lin PS, Gearhart P (1987): Adult B-cell repertoire is biased toward two heavy-chain variable-region genes that rearrange frequently in fetal pre-B cells. Proc Natl Acad Sci USA 84:2454–2458.

Lehuen A, Altman J, Bach J-F, Carnaud C (1990a): Natural thymocytotoxic autoantibodies in non-obese diabetic (NOD) mice: Characterization and fine specificity. Clin Exp Immunol 81:406–411.

Lehuen A, Bartels J, Kearney JF (1992): Characterization, specificity and Ig V gene usage of anti-lymphocyte monoclonal antibodies from perinatal mice. Int Immunol 4:1073–1084.

Lehuen A, Bendelac A, Bach J-F, Carnaud C (1990b): The nonobese diabetic mouse model. Independent expression of humoral and cell-mediated autoimmune features. J Immunol 144:2147–2151.

Lehuen A, Monteiro RC, Kearney JF (1992): Identification of a 100 kD molecule associated with two PI-linked molecules: Thy-1 and the ThB. Eur J Immunol 22:2373–2380.

Leijon K, Freitas A, Holmberg D (1993): Analysis of V_H gene utilization in the non-obese diabetic mouse. Autoimmunity 15:11–18.

Lieberman R, Potter M, Mushinsky EB, Humphrey W Jr, Rudikoff S (1974): Genetics of a new IgVH (T15 idiotype) marker in the mouse regulating natural antibody to phosporylcholine. J Exp Med 139:983–998.

Malynn B, Yancopoulos G, Barth J, Bona C, Alt F (1990): Biased expression of J_H-proximal V_H genes occurs in the newly generated repertoire of neonatal and adult mice. J Exp Med 171:843–859.

Martinez-A C, Bernabé RR, De la Hera A, Pereira P, Cazenave P-A, Coutinho A (1985): Establishment of idiotypic helper T-cell repertoires early in life. Nature 317:721–723.

Masmoudi H, Mota-Santos T, Huetz F, Coutinho A, Cazenave PA (1990): All T15 Id positive antibodies (but not the majority of V_H T15$^+$ antibodies) are produced by peritoneal CD5$^+$ B lymphocytes. Int Immunol 2:515–520.

Murakami M, Tsubala T, Okamato M, Shimizu A, Kumagai S, Imura H, Honjo T (1992): Antigen induced apoptotic death of Ly1 B cells responsible for autoimmune disease in transgenic mice. Nature 357:77–81.

O'Garra A, Chang R, Go N, Hastings R, Haughton G, Howard M (1992): Ly-1 B (B-1) cells are the main source of B cell-derived interleukin 10. Eur J Immunol 22:711–717.

O'Garra A, Howard M (1991): IL-10 production by CD5 B cells. Ann NY Acad Sci 651:182–199

Perlmutter RM (1987): Programmed development of the antibody repertoire. Curr Top Microbiol Immunol 135:95–109.

Perlmutter RM, Kearney JF, Chang SP, Hood LE (1985): Developmentally controlled expression of immunoglobulin V_H genes. Science 227:1597–1601.

Pollok B, Stohrer R, Kearney J (1984): Selective alteration of the humoral immune response to α1-3 dextran and phosphoryl choline. In Köhler H, Urbain J, Cazenave P-A (eds): "Idiotypy in Biology and Medicine." New York: Academic Press, pp 187–202.

Raveche ES, Novotny EA, Hansen CT, Tjio JH, Steinberg AD (1981): Genetic studies in NZB mice. V. Recombinant inbred lines demonstrate that separate genes control autoimmune phenotype. J Exp Med 153:1187–1197.

Schilling J, Clevinger B, Davie JM, Hood L (1980): Amino acid sequence of homogeneous antibodies to dextran and DNA rearrangements in heavy chain V-region gene segments. Nature 283:35–40.

Schroeder HWJ, Hillson JL, Perlmutter RM (1990): Structure and evolution of mammalian V_H families Int Immunol 2:41–50.

Shirai R, Mellors ER (1971): Natural thymocytotoxic autoantibody and reactive antigen in New Zealand black and other mice. Proc Natl Acad Sci USA 68:1412–1416.

Solvason N, Kearney J (1992): The human fetal omentum: A site of B cell generation. J Exp Med 175:397–404.

Solvason N, Lehuen A, Kearney JF (1991): An embryonic source of Ly1 but not conventional B cells. Intern Immunol 3:543–550.

Stohrer R, Kearney JF (1984): Ontogeny of B cell precursors responding to alpha1-3 dextran in BALB/c mice. J Immunol 133:2323–2326.

Sy M-S, Lowy A, Hayglass K, Janeway CAJ, Gurish M, Greene MI, Benacerraf B

(1984): Chronic treatment with rabbit anti-mouse m-chain antibody alters the characteristic immunoglobulin heavy-chain restriction of murine suppressor T-cell factors. Proc Natl Acad Sci USA 81:3846–3850.

Tonegawa S (1983): Somatic generation of antibody diversity. Nature 302:575–581.

Tutter A, Brodeur P, Schlomchik M, Riblet R (1991): Structure, map position, and evolution of two newly diverged mouse Ig V_H gene families. J Immunol 147:3215.

Vakil M, Briles DE, Kearney JF (1991): Antigen independent selection of T15 idiotype during B cell ontogeny in mice. Dev Immunol 1:203–213.

Vakil M, Kearney JF (1986): Functional characterization of monoclonal auto-anti-idiotype antibodies isolated from the early B cell repertoire of BALB/c mice. Eur J Immunol 16:1151–1158.

Vakil M, Kearney JF (1988): Expression of idiotypes and anti-idiotypes during development: Frequencies and functional significance in the acquisition of the adult B cell repertoire. In Bona C (ed): "Elicitation and Use of Anti-Idiotype Antibodies and Their Biological Properties." Boca Raton, FL: CRC Press, pp 75–89.

Vakil M, Kearney JF (1991): Functional relationship between T15 and J558 idiotypes in BALB/c mice. Dev Immunol 1:213–224.

Vakil M, Sauter J, Paige C, Kearney JF (1986): In vivo suppression of perinatal multispecific B cells results in a distortion of the adult B cell repertoire. Eur J Immunol 16:1159–1165.

Waldschmidt TJ, Kroese FGM, Tygrett LT, Conrad DH, Lynch RG (1991): The expression of B cell surface receptors. III. The murine low affinity IgE FcεR is not expressed on Ly1 or "Ly1-like" B cells. Int Immunol 3:305–315.

Wu GE, Paige CJ (1986): V_H gene family utilization in colonies derived from B and pre-B cells detected by the RNA colony blot assay EMBO J 5:3475–3481.

Yancopoulos GD, Desiderio SV, Paskind M, Kearney JF, Baltimore D, Alt FW (1984): Preferential utilization of the most D_H-proximal V_H gene segments in pre-B cell lines. Nature 311:727–733.

8

HUMAN NATURAL SELF-REACTIVE ANTIBODIES

Gilles Dietrich and Michel D. Kazatchkine

Service d'Immunologie and INSERM U·28, Hôpital Broussais, Paris, France

INTRODUCTION

Paradigms about autoreactivity have evolved considerably since P. Ehrlich proposed "horror autotoxicus" to illustrate his notion that antibody responses may not occur against self-components. The presence of autoantibodies was first described in the serum of patients with autoimmune anemias and has long been considered only to be associated with pathological conditions. As a correlate, clonal selection theories proposed that self-reactive B-cell clones are deleted during ontogeny. Studies performed over the last 10 years have, however, established that autoreactive B cells are not eliminated upon differentiation of lymphoid precursor into B cells and that natural antibodies occur in sera of healthy individuals and of various animal species without need for external stimulation. Evidence is now accumulating that natural autoreactive antibodies, organized in a tightly regulated V-region-dependent network, are essential in establishing self-tolerance and maintaining the homeostasis of the immune system under physiological conditions. Although the concept of natural autoreactivity is now generally accepted in the mouse, it seems to be somehow more slowly recognized in humans.

Autoimmunity: Physiology and Disease, Pages 107–128
© 1994 Wiley-Liss, Inc.

AUTOANTIBODIES

The term *autoantibody* refers to antibodies that react with at least one self-antigen, whether the antibodies originate from diseased or from healthy individuals. Target self-antigens may be located on the cell surface (e.g., acetylcholine receptor and idiotypes of antigen receptors), inside the cell (e.g., DNA and ribosomal proteins), or be extracellular molecules (e.g., insulin and intrinsic factor).

AUTOREACTIVE B CELLS ARE PRESENT IN THE AVAILABLE B-CELL REPERTOIRE OF HEALTHY INDIVIDUALS

The available human B-cell repertoire has in most instances been assessed by analyzing the reactivity of monoclonal antibodies, be they malignancy-associated paraproteins, products of hybridomas, or Epstein-Barr Virus (EBV)–transformed normal B cells. EBV-transformed B lymphocytes represent a random sample of the available B-cell repertoire rather than the expressed antibody repertoire. Thus monoclonal immunoglobulins from patients with chronic lymphocytic leukemia (CLL), IgM from patients with Waldenström's macroglobulinemia, and antibodies secreted by EBV-transformed B cells have often been found to exhibit reactivity with self-antigens such as DNA, thyroglobulin, cytoskeleton proteins, and transferrin [Avrameas et al., 1981; Winger et al., 1983; Uhlig et al., 1985; Bröker et al., 1988; Seigneurin et al., 1988; Sthoeger et al., 1989; Borche et al., 1990]. Assuming that monoclonal antibodies or EBV transformants obtained from B cells of healthy individuals are representative of the normal B-cell repertoire, autoantibody producers are thus frequent within the normal human B-cell repertoire. These findings in the human are similar to those in healthy animals in which autoreactive B-cell precursors can be directly quantitated among naturally activated cells and have been found to be as frequent as 1 : 200 for precursors of antithyroglobulin-secreting cells [Portnoï et al., 1986].

NATURAL AUTOREACTIVE ANTIBODIES ARE PRESENT WITHIN THE EXPRESSED B-CELL REPERTOIRE OF HEALTHY INDIVIDUALS

Normal human serum contains autoantibodies of the IgM and IgG classes that recognize a wide range of self-antigens, including nuclear antigens, intracellular and membrane components, and circulating plasma proteins [Yadin et al., 1989; Maire et al., 1989; Hunt-Gerardo et al., 1990; Pfueller et al., 1990]. The presence of autoantibodies of the IgG isotype indicates that, under physiological conditions, T cells are involved in the regulation of the expression of the autoreactive B-cell repertoire. Natural autoantibodies were first defined using evolutionarily conserved proteins such as tubulin, actin, myoglobin, albumin, or transferrin [Avrameas et al., 1981; Guilbert et al., 1982]. Some of the antigens recognized by natural autoantibodies are also the targets of autoantibodies in autoimmune diseases, e.g., thyroglobulin, neutrophil cytoplasmic antigens, glomerular basement membrane, intrinsic factor, and Factor VIII [Rossi et al., 1989; Algiman et al., 1992; Dietrich et al., 1992a], although the fine epitopic specificity of natural antibodies may (but does not necessarily) differ from that of disease-specific autoantibodies [Piechaczyk et al., 1987; Bouanani et al., 1989, 1991; Naito et al., 1990; Bresler et al., 1990; Sabbaga et al., 1990; Dietrich et al., 1991; Ronda et al., 1993a]. As larger panels of antigens are being used for determining antibody reactivities, the frequency and the spectrum of reactivities of natural autoantibodies extend; this is best illustrated by the multiplicity of bands now observed when blotting normal human serum IgG on electrophoresed proteins from tissue extracts (Fig. 1). Some of the self-antigens that are recognized by natural IgM and IgG autoantibodies present in normal serum are idiotypes of autologous complementary antibodies of either class [Zouali and Eyquem, 1983; Muryoï et al., 1988; Dietrich et al., 1992b; Hurez et al., 1993a].

Autoantibodies are detected and quantitated by assessing their ability to bind to or to functionally interact with self-antigens. The antigens used in the assays are "true" self-antigens (e.g., autologous renal tissue for the detection of the antiglomerular basal membrane autoantibodies), heterologous, evolutionarily -conserved antigens (e.g., cytoskeleton proteins), and antigens from tissue extracts of individuals of the same species (e.g., most antigens used for the detection of autoantibodies for clinical purposes). The use of such allogeneic material may sometimes be misleading with regard to the antibody nature of some antibody activity in serum. Thus autoantibodies to Factor VIII are detected either by ELISA or by a functional assay measuring the ability of IgG to neutralize procoagulant Factor VIII activity in a pool of plasma of healthy donors. Therefore, some of the antibodies detected may be directed against allotypic determinants on a polymorphic target molecule. A caution in the definition of autoantibodies in this regard is justified by the finding that Factor VIII antibodies found in the plasma of healthy donors inhibit activity of allogeneic Factor VIII but do not neutralize autologous Factor VIII function [Algiman et al., 1992].

NATURAL AUTOANTIBODIES ARE MORE OFTEN FOUND TO BE POLYREACTIVE THAN IMMUNE ANTIBODIES

Studies employing human monoclonal immunoglobulins originating from normal B cells have shown that natural autoantibodies of both IgM and IgG isotype usually recognize several self-antigens as well as foreign antigens [Nakamura et al., 1988a; Seigneurin et al., 1988; Rossi et al., 1990]. Such polyreactivity was early recognized as a feature of naturally expressed anti-

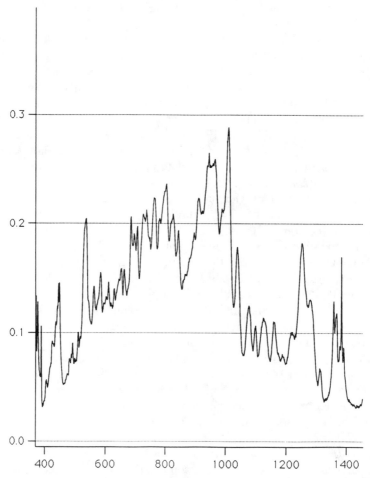

FIGURE 1. Pattern of reactivity of pooled normal human IgG (IVIg) upon Western blotting with total mouse liver extract. The ordinate indicates optical density; the abscissa indicates the relative distance of migration of protein antigens in the gel.

bodies in human and in mouse serum [Avrameas, 1991]. Polyreactivity is a general property of immunoglobulins because of the degeneracy of the antigen-combining site of the B-cell antigen receptor. Testing an antibody for polyreactivity may yield different results depending on the panel of antigens that is used and on the amount of antibody present in the assay. Polyreactivity is a frequent rather than exclusive characteristic of natural antibodies in that certain disease-specific autoantibodies or immune antibodies may exhibit high polyreactivity. Thus affinity-purified anti-DNA antibodies from patients with systemic lupus erythematosus bind to the same extent to a large panel of self-antigens as their affinity-purified counterparts from the sera of healthy individuals [Hurez et al., 1993b], and monoclonal antibodies produced by peripheral blood lymphocytes from donors deliberately immunized with mismatched red blood cells were found to be polyreactive [Thompson et al., 1992].

NATURAL AUTOANTIBODIES ARE NOT PRODUCED BY A SUBSET OF B CELLS EXPRESSING DISTINCT PHENOTYPIC MARKERS

The question of whether natural polyreactive autoantibodies in the human are exclusively produced by $CD5^+$ B cells remains in doubt (as discussed in Chapter 6). B cells bearing the CD5 antigen constitute approximately 20% of B cells in normal peripheral blood and in the spleen and 40%–60% of B cells in human fetal spleen. $CD5^+$ B cells account for a large part of activated B-cell blasts in healthy individuals. EBV-transformed $CD5^+$ peripheral blood B cells from healthy individuals secrete polyreactive antibodies [Nakamura et al., 1988b; Casali and Notkins, 1989a]. However, $CD5^-$ B cells from normal donors are also capable of producing natural polyreactive autoantibodies [Kasaian et al., 1992]. Although $CD5^+$ B cells are predominant among fetal B cells, they are more poorly represented among normal B cells in the adult. One of two hypotheses may explain these changes: (1) the existence of two independent lineages with one preceding the other or being positively selected during ontogeny or (2) the selective activation of $CD5^-$ B cells to become $CD5^+$ B cells through stimulation by environmental factors (i.e., self during ontogeny). $CD5^+$ B lymphocytes have been suggested to undergo neoplastic transformation more readily than $CD5^-$ cells [Kipps, 1989]. The number of $CD5^+$ B lymphocytes is increased in patients with rheumatoid arthritis and Sjögren's syndrome and may be associated with the production of high-affinity autoantibodies in which utilized V_H genes show a high degree of somatic mutation [Youinou et al., 1988; Burastero et al., 1988; Harindranath et al., 1991]. Thus it could be speculated that $CD5^+$ B lymphocytes that produce polyreactive natural autoantibodies under physiological conditions may be selected to produce high-affinity somatic mutants under pathological conditions. We have recently identified the presence of reactivity to CD5 in pooled normal human immunoglobulin for therapeutic use (IVIg) [Vassilev et al., 1993]. The findings suggest the presence of low amounts of anti-CD5 antibodies in healthy individuals and may be relevant to the immunoregulatory effect of IVIg in autoimmune diseases [Kaveri et al., 1991; Dietrich et al., 1992c].

AUTOREACTIVE B CELLS ARE PRESENT IN THE EARLY AVAILABLE REPERTOIRE DURING HUMAN B-CELL ONTOGENY

Autoreactive B cells account for the major part of the available B-cell repertoire in the fetus and in the neonatal period. Dominance of autoantibody-producing cells has been assessed by testing IgM secreted by EBV-transformed cord B cells for reactivity with self-antigens and may be inferred from the finding of as much as 70% and 90% of $CD5^+$ B cells in fetal spleen and cord blood, respectively [Uhlig et al., 1985; Antin et al., 1986; Lydyard et al., 1990a; Guigou et al., 1991; Casali and Notkins, 1989b; Kipps, 1989; Paavonen et al., 1990; Durandy et al., 1990; Mackenzie et al., 1991; Schutte et al., 1991]. The spontaneous production of natural polyreactive autoantibodies by cord blood B cells does not require the presence of T cells [Barbouche et al., 1992]. During early B-cell ontogeny, the recombination of individual V_H genes does not follow a probabilistic model of utilization, with preferential use of D-proximal V_H segments [Cuisinier et al., 1989; Nickerson et al., 1989; Schroeder and Wang, 1990; Berman et al., 1991; Raaphorst et al., 1992]. The biased use of V genes that is observed in the fetal liver is not found upon analysis of cord blood B cells [Mortari et al., 1992]. The sequences of the V_H genes that are preferentially expressed during early B-cell ontogeny are the same as those encoding certain natural polyreactive autoantibodies secreted by normal B cells in adults [Logtenberg et al., 1989; Schutte et al., 1991]. Recent studies, however, have indicated that the pattern of usage of V_H and V_κ families in polyreactive B-cell clones is not always restricted and may not differ in some instances from that of clones of unknown specificity [Guigou et al., 1991]. The overlap between the V gene repertoire used by fetal liver B cells and that which is associated with natural autoantibodies supports the concept of coordinated development of the immune system requiring autoreactive B cells.

IS THERE A HIGHER INCIDENCE OF NATURAL AUTOANTIBODIES IN SERUM WITH AGING?

Several studies have shown an increased frequency of occurrence of autoantibodies (e.g., antinuclear and antithyroglobulin antibodies) in the serum of aged individuals [Moulias et al., 1984; Manoussakis et al., 1987; Tomer and Shoenfeld, 1988]. The increase in IgG autoreactivity in serum and the concomitant decrease in antibody responses to vaccinal antigens with aging have been interpreted as being related to intrinsic changes in T-cell function and acquired immune dysregulation with age [Gillis et al., 1981; Bovbjerg et al., 1991]. The titers of serum IgG autoantibodies, however, have also been observed to be equivalent in aged and in young adults [Gordon and Rosenthal, 1984; Mariotti et al., 1992]. In accordance with these results, we have found no difference in autoreactivity of the purified IgG fraction from serum and of IgG in the serum between donors from various age groups, including young infants, young adults aged 20 to 30 years, and individuals between 50 and 80 years (Fig. 2) [Hurez et al., 1993a]. Published follow-up studies of healthy individuals expressing significant autoantibody titers in serum indicate that there is no relationship between occurrence of autoantibodies in aged individuals and that of overt autoimmune disease [Talor and Rose,

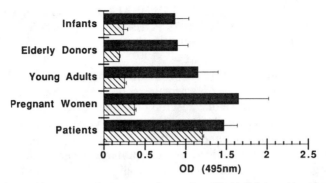

FIGURE 2. Mean binding to various autoantigens of purified IgG (closed bars) and of IgG in whole serum (hatched bars) from infants, elderly donors, young adults, pregnant women, and patients with autoimmune thyroiditis. Each column represents the mean OD ± SD of binding of IgG from 20 donors in each group. (Adapted from Hurez et al., 1993a).

1991]. As a matter of fact, the most prevalent and clinically severe autoimmune diseases occur in younger people rather than in the elderly.

NATURAL AUTOANTIBODIES ARE ENCODED BY A RESTRICTED PANEL OF GERMLINE V GENES

Analysis of human monoclonal autoantibodies derived from normal peripheral blood B cells has shown that these antibodies express germline immunoglobulin variable region genes with little or no somatic mutation [Siminovitch et al., 1989, 1990; Sanz et al., 1989a]. In most cases, some variable region genes of natural autoantibodies are identical or nearly identical with variable region genes preferentially expressed in the fetal pre-B-cell repertoire [Schroeder et al., 1987; Dersimonian et al., 1987; Zouali et al., 1988; Chen et al., 1990; Berman et al., 1991; Pascual and Capra, 1991]. Idiotypic cross-reactivity has been described among autoantibodies from healthy individuals, those from patients with autoimmune diseases, and paraproteins from patients with B-lineage malignancies [Davidson et al., 1987, 1988; Dang et al., 1988]. A high proportion of natural polyreactive antibodies express idiotypes commonly found on disease-related autoantibodies [Lydyard et al., 1990b]. The expression of cross-reactive idiotypes may reflect the use of specific V_H gene(s) and provides a structural basis for shared idiotypy between antigen receptors of natural autoreactive B cells and cells from patients with B-cell malignancies or from patients with autoimmune diseases [Newkirk et al., 1987; Chen et al., 1988; Kipps et al., 1988, 1989; Takei et al., 1988; Dersimonian et al., 1989; Sanz et al., 1989b; Davidson et al., 1990; Spatz et al., 1990; Hiraïwa et al., 1990].

DO AUTOANTIBODIES PRESENT IN HEALTHY INDIVIDUALS DIFFER FROM AUTOANTIBODIES FOUND IN PATIENTS WITH AUTOIMMUNE DISEASE?

Despite the presence of autoreactive B cells in the normal available immune repertoire, autoimmune diseases remain a relatively rare event. Since autoimmune diseases cannot be diagnosed by the mere finding of increased titers of autoantibodies in serum, the question arises of whether the fine specificity, structure, and genetics of autoantibodies in healthy subjects differ from those of autoantibodies from patients with autoimmune disease. The development of pathological autoimmunity thus results either from the abnormal expansion of natural unmutated autoreactive clones or from the emergence of somatically mutated, possibly autoantigen-driven, autoreactive clones.

There is evidence for the mutated nature of some autoantibodies associated with human autoimmune diseases: thus rheumatoid factors (RFs) from patients with rheumatoid arthritis show significant somatic mutations in contrast to natural RFs (as discussed in Chapter 17); patients with SLE generate high-affinity anti-DNA IgG autoantibodies that show no polyreactivity and extensive somatic mutation in the variable region gene sequences of heavy and light chains, whereas normal individuals make polyreactive low-affinity IgM antibodies to DNA that do not undergo significant somatic mutation [Davidson et al., 1990; Winkler et al., 1992]. The mutated nature of anti-DNA antibodies from patients with SLE suggests that autoimmune anti-DNA clones in lupus are antigen driven. It is interesting to note that at least a fraction of the high-affinity IgG anti-DNA autoantibodies from patients show mutations within V_H genes that usually encode for natural IgM antibodies and derive from the restricted V_H repertoire expressed in the fetal B-cell compartment [Winkler et al., 1992]. Indirect evidence for the restricted nature of pathological autoantibodies has also been obtained through analysis of idiotypes expressed by disease-associated autoantibodies. Thus the presence of cross-reactive idiotypes shared by disease-associated autoantibodies from different patients suggests that the antibody combining sites originate from restricted usage of V_H gene families.

Cross-reactive idiotypes have been identified on patients' autoantibodies in several autoimmune diseases [Matsuyama et al., 1983; Thomas et al., 1986; Lefvert, 1988; Ruiz-Arguelles, 1988; de la Fuente and Hoyer, 1984; Fong et al., 1986; Isenberg et al., 1984; Dang et al., 1988; Solomon et al., 1983; Zouali and Eyquem, 1984]. For example, the study of the idiotypic specificity of IgM antibodies with antimyelin-associated glycoprotein (anti-MAG) activity from patients with monoclonal IgM and peripheral neuropathy revealed that the autoantibodies exhibit restricted structural characteristics [Brouet et al., 1989].

We have shown that a cross-reactive α-idiotype (named T44) is specifically expressed by antithyroglobulin autoantibodies from patients with autoimmune thyroiditis [Dietrich and Kazatchkine, 1990] and that the expression of T44 idiotype was associated with the recognition by antithyroglobulin autoantibodies of a specific epitopic cluster on human thyroglobulin. In contrast, natural IgG antithyroglobulin autoantibodies from healthy individuals do not express the T44 idiotype or bind to the epitopes of human thyroglobulin recognized by T44 idiotype-expressing antibodies [Dietrich et al., 1991]. The disease-specific cross-reactive T44 idiotype could thus be a marker of specific V_H genes included in somatic diversity and selected by the autoantigen. Alternatively, the predominance of T44 idiotype-expressing clones among disease-associated antithyroglobulin antibodies could reflect the abnormal expansion of germline-encoded autoreactive clones that are kept silent in healthy individuals. There is indeed evidence that some disease-associated autoantibodies are germline encoded; thus sequencing of the gene encoding for the 16/6 idiotype, which is a dominant idiotype among anti-DNA antibodies in systemic lupus erythematosus, has demonstrated that it is a germline [Chen et al., 1988; Young et al., 1990]. Furthermore the 16/6 idiotype is also found on autoantibodies from healthy individuals [Madaio et al., 1986].

AVAILABLE AND EXPRESSED B-CELL AUTOREACTIVE REPERTOIRES ARE TIGHTLY REGULATED UNDER PHYSIOLOGICAL CONDITIONS

Evidence for intrinsic network regulation of the expression of the human autoreactive repertoire comes from (1) the finding of high V-region connectivity among natural autoantibodies; (2) the finding of V-region-mediated inhibition by autologous IgM of IgG autoreactivity in normal serum; and (3) the observation of reproducible patterns of spontaneous kinetic behavior of natural autoantibodies in serum of healthy individuals.

High connectivity among variable regions is a common feature of autoantibody-secreting B-cell clones that are expressed early in ontogeny in mouse [Holmberg et al., 1984] and man [Guigou et al., 1991]. The connected autoreactive subset of B cells that is predominant in the fetal repertoire is also expressed in the adult; thus we have recently observed that there exists a fraction of normal circulating human IgG that exhibits V-region complementarity associated with autoreactivity [Dietrich et al., 1992a]. Within the connected fraction of IgG are antibodies that react with their own variable region determinants. This property of self-idiotypic complementarity is associated with the expression on these antibodies of the T15 idiotype [Halpern et al., 1991]. The locus responsible for self-binding is located in the evolutionarily conserved CDR2/FR3 region encoded by the VH S107 germline gene [Kang and Kohler, 1986; Kaveri et al., 1990].

Expression of autoreactive IgG activity is largely masked in human serum under normal conditions. When tested with a large panel of self-antigens, autoantibody activity of natural IgG autoantibodies in whole serum is three-fivefold lower than in the purified IgG fraction from serum in healthy donors irrespective of age (Fig. 2) [Hurez et al., 1993a]. IgG-depleted serum and purified IgM from serum inhibit the binding of autologous IgG to autoantigens. The inhibitory effect of IgM is mediated by V-region-dependent interactions with IgG as indicated by the ability of IgM to bind to F(ab′)₂ fragments of autologous IgG and that of soluble F(ab′)₂ fragments of IgG to inhibit the binding competitively. However, no difference was found between autoreactivity of purified IgG and that of IgG in serum from patients with autoimmune disease. Taken together, these results, as well as previous observations in mice [Adib et al., 1990], indicate that V-region connectivity between IgM and IgG is involved in the regulation of expressed autoreactive repertoires under physiological conditions.

Mathematical analysis of the kinetic pattern of spontaneous fluctuations of autoantibodies in serum may be used to investigate directly the regulatory functions associated with V region connectivity in vivo. In healthy adults, the spontaneous kinetics of autoantibodies in serum follow highly reproducible patterns between individuals [Varela et al., 1991; Varela and Coutinho, 1991]. These patterns are similar to those observed in normal mice [Lundkvist et al., 1989; Varela et al., 1991] and reflect the regulation of activation and decay of autoantibody clones within a network organization that characterizes the steady-state equilibrium dynamics of the immune network under physiological conditions. In contrast, autoantibodies in the sera of patients with autoimmune disease follow random spontaneous fluctuations suggestive of an acquired loss of control of the expressed autoreactive repertoire (Fig. 3) [Varela et al., 1991; Varela and Coutinho, 1991].

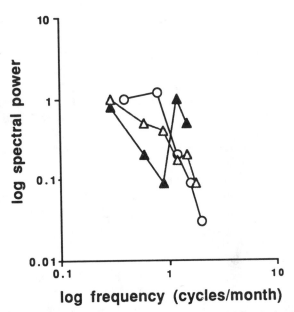

FIGURE 3. Spectral analysis of kinetics of spontaneous fluctuations of anti-TG autoantibodies in the serum of a healthy individual (○), of a patient with autoimmune thyroiditis before infusion of IVIg (▲), and following two infusions of IVIg (△). (Adapted from Dietrich et al., 1993.)

DO NATURAL AUTOANTIBODIES HAVE SPECIFIC PHYSIOLOGICAL FUNCTIONS?

Natural autoantibodies exhibit multiple homeostatic functions in normal organisms, many of which are probably unknown at this time. Natural autoantibodies play a role in first-line defense against pathogens. It has also been suggested that natural autoantibodies participate in the clearance of molecules and senescent cells [Grabar, 1983; Kay et al., 1983]. Others have speculated that natural autoantibodies prevent pathological autoimmunity by binding to microbial epitopes that are similar or identical to self [Cohen and Cooke, 1986]. As discussed above, natural autoantibodies that are found in humans and animals ensure the selection and stability of repertoires through V-region-dependent interactions with antibodies and with antigen receptors on lymphocytes [Coutinho, 1989; Stewart, 1992].

MODULATION OF PATHOLOGICAL AUTOIMMUNITY USING THERAPEUTIC POOLS OF NATURALLY EXPRESSED IgG

Intravenous immunoglobulins (IVIg) are therapeutic preparations of normal intact IgG obtained from a pool of plasma of a large number of healthy donors. IVIg thus represent the wide spectrum of the expressed normal human IgG repertoire, including antibodies to external antigens, IgG autoantibodies, and antiantibodies. IVIg were initially used for replacement therapy of antibody deficiency states. A beneficial effect of intravenous administration of IVIg has now been reported in a large number of autoimmune diseases in which there is direct or indirect evidence for a primary pathogenic role of autoantibodies or autoaggressive T cells [Dwyer, 1992; Ronda et al., 1992b]. As discussed in previous sections of this chapter, emergence of pathological autoimmunity may reflect a failure in the regulatory function of the immune network. Thus in autoimmune conditions, serum autoantibodies follow dynamic patterns indicative of random fluctuations, reflecting perturbations in network regulation that affect the expression of both disease-related autoantibodies as well as antibodies uninvolved in pathology [Varela et al., 1991]. Following this view, autoimmune diseases would be associated with disturbed network organization of autoantibodies rather than with a clonally limited escape and expansion of tissue-specific autoantibodies. Several lines of evidence have led us to propose that IVIg are effective in autoimmune disease by selecting autoimmune repertoires and restoring appropriate control mechanisms of autoreactivity in treated patients. This evidence supports a role for normal circulating IgG in selecting the expressed autoreactive repertoire under physiological conditions (Table I).

IVIg contain antibodies that interact with idiotypes expressed on autoantibodies; thus, (1) $F(ab')_2$ fragments of IVIg neutralize autoantibody activity and inhibit the binding of autoantibodies to autoantigens [Rossi et al., 1988, 1991; Rossi and Kazatchkine, 1989; Van Doorn et al., 1990; Ronda et al.,

TABLE I. Evidence for selection of autoimmune repertoires by IVIg

V-region-dependent interactions between IVIg and autoantibodies (in vitro)

Transient or long-term suppression of disease-related B-cell clones

Restricted stimulation of IVIg-reactive B-cell clones (in vivo)

Altered kinetic pattern of spontaneous fluctuations of autoantibodies in serum, indicative of induced alterations in network organization of autoantibodies (in vivo)

1993a], (2) autoantibodies are retained on affinity chromatography columns of F(ab')$_2$ fragments of IVIg coupled to Sepharose [Rossi et al., 1988, 1991; Rossi and Kazatchkine, 1989; Van Doorn et al., 1990; Ronda et al., 1993a], and (3) IVIg share anti-idiotypic reactivity toward idiotypes of autoantibodies with heterologous anti-idiotypic reagents [Dietrich and Kazatchkine, 1990; Dietrich et al., 1990; Kaveri et al., 1993]. We have also demonstrated that IVIg interact with natural polyreactive IgM antibodies through idiotypic interactions by using autoreactive monoclonal IgM antibodies secreted by EBV-transformed normal B lymphocytes [Rossi et al., 1990] (Fig. 4). The presence in IVIg of anti-idiotypes against idiotypic determinants expressed on natural IgG autoantibodies was demonstrated by using affinity chromatography of F(ab')$_2$ fragments of IVIg on Sepharose-bound F(ab')$_2$ fragments of IVIg [Dietrich et al., 1992a]. In addition, a recent study has shown that IVIg also contain antibodies directed toward complementary-determining regions and the framework constant regions of the β-chain of the T-cell receptor [Marchalonis et al., 1992]. By reacting with antigen-specific receptors and other functional membrane molecules on T and B cells, IVIg may select the available immune repertoire (Table II).

We have recently analyzed the changes that occur in the expressed antibody repertoire following infusion of IVIg in a patient with autoimmune thyroiditis [Dietrich et al., 1993]. The results indicate that changes in serum antibody concentrations after infusion of IVIg do not merely reflect passive transfer of IgG antibody activities into the patient. The two consecutive infusions of IVIg resulted in a cumulative increase in the production of IgM, indicating that B-cell clones have been stimulated in the patient. Accordingly, the concentration of IgG in the patient's serum after the second infusion of IVIg increased to higher levels than were expected from the amount of transfused IgG, suggesting the development of a secondary immune response to IVIg. The profile of antibody activity of IgG in the patient's serum after infusion of IVIg was not that expected from the passive transfer of the antibody activities present in IVIg; for example, although IVIg and the patient's preinfusion serum contain equivalent amounts of antiphosphorylcholine and antigliadin antibodies, the titer of antigliadin antibody sharply increased in the patient's serum, whereas infusion of IVIg induced no change in serum of antiphosphorylcholine titer. Furthermore, we have observed that

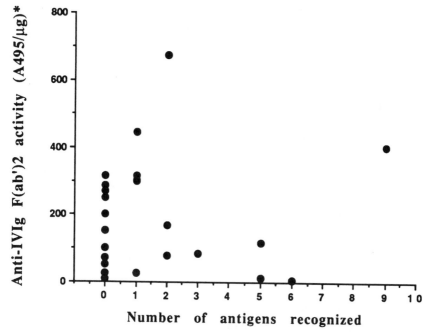

FIGURE 4. Binding of IgM antibodies from EBV-transformed human B cells to F(ab')$_2$ fragments from IVIg. The binding activity of natural IgM antibodies to F(ab')$_2$ of IVIg does not correlate with the relative degree of polyreactivity of IgM. The abscissa represents the number of antigens recognized by the IgM antibodies. Specific anti-IVIg F(ab')$_2$ activity (A495/mg) was measured by ELISA on microtiter plates coated with F(ab')$_2$ from IVIg. (Adapted from Rossi et al., 1990.)

the relative changes with time in the concentration of the fraction of serum IgG reactive with IVIg does not follow the changes in the concentration of total serum IgG [Dietrich et al., 1993]. These data indicate that infusion of IgG leads to the active recruitment of subsets of B cells reactive with IVIg. Infusion of IVIg also resulted in downregulation of the patient's B-cell clones expressing the disease-specific T44 idiotype [Dietrich and Kazatchkine, 1990] for several weeks, indicating that administration of IVIg results in transient suppression of disease-specific antibody clones. The pattern of spontaneous

TABLE II. Antilymphocyte antibodies in IVIg

Antibodies to idiotypes/variable regions of surface Ig of B cells
Antibodies to idiotype, framework, and constant regions of T-cell receptor β-chain
Antibodies to CD4
Antibodies to CD5
Antibodies to MHC class I and class II antigens

fluctuations of autoantibodies in patient's serum prior to infusion of immunoglobulin exhibits a pattern clearly distinct from normal and suggestive of disruptions of connectivity within the immune network. The kinetic pattern of serum autoantibody fluctuations following the second infusion of IVIg was similar to that seen in healthy individuals (Fig. 3) [Dietrich et al., 1992d]. Thus infusion of pooled normal immunoglobulin restored in the patient the autoregulatory functions of natural autoantibodies.

ACKNOWLEDGMENTS

This work was supported by Institut National de la Santé et de la Recherche Médicale (INSERM), France, and Baxter Healthcare Corp., Glendale, CA. G.D. is recipient of a grant from Biotransfusion, Roissy and Centre National de la Recherche Scientifique (CNRS), France.

REFERENCES

Adib M, Ragimbeau J, Avrameas S, and Ternynck T (1990): IgG autoantibody activity in normal mouse serum is controlled by IgM. J Immunol 145:3807–3813.

Algiman M, Dietrich G, Nydegger U, Boieldieu D, Sultan Y, Kazatchkine MD (1992): Antibodies to Factor VIII in healthy individuals. Proc Natl Acad Sci USA 89:3795–3799.

Antin JH, Emerson SG, Martin P, Gadol N, Ault A (1986): Leu1$^+$ (CD5$^+$) B cells: A major lymphoid subpopulation in human fetal spleen: Phenotypic and functional studies. J Immunol 136:505–510.

Avrameas S (1991): Natural autoantibodies: From "horror autotoxicus" to "gnothi seauton." Immunol Today 12:154–159.

Avrameas S, Guilbert B, Dighiero G (1981): Natural antibodies against tubulin, actin, myoglobin, thyroglobulin, fetuin, albumin and transferrin are present in normal human sera and monoclonal immunoglobulins from multiple myeloma and Waldenström's macroglobulinemia may express similar antibody specificities. Ann Immunol 132C:231–236.

Barbouche R, Forveille M, Fisher A, Avrameas S, Durandy A (1992): Spontaneous IgM autoantibody production in vitro by B lymphocytes of normal human neonates. Scand J Immunol 35:659–667.

Berman JE, Nickerson KG, Pollock RR, Barth JE, Schuurman RKB, Knowles DM, Chess L, Alt FW (1991): VH gene usage in humans: biased usage of the V_H6 gene in immature B lymphoid cells. Eur J Immunol 21:1311–1314.

Borche L, Lim A, Binet JL, Dighiero G (1990): Evidence that chronic lymphocytic leukemia B lymphocytes are frequently committed to production of natural autoantibodies. Blood 76:562–566.

Bouanani M, Bataille R, Piechaczyk M, Salhi SL, Pau B, Bastide M (1991): Respective epitopic specificity patterns of anti-human thyroglobulin autoantibodies in patients with Sjögren's syndrome and patients with Hashimoto's thyroiditis. Arthritis Rheum 34:1585–1593.

Bouanani M, Piechaczyk M, Pau B, Bastide M (1989): Significance of the recognition of certain antigenic regions on the thyroglobulin molecule by natural autoantibodies from healthy subjects. J Immunol 143:1129–1132.

Bovbjerg DH, Kim YT, Schwab R, Schmitt K, DeBlasio T, Weksler ME (1991): "Cross-wiring" of the immune response in old mice: Increased autoantibody response despite reduced antibody response to nominal antigen. Cell Immunol 135:519–525.

Bresler HS, Burek LC, Hoffman WH, Rose NR (1990): Autoantigenic determinants on human thyroglobulin: Determinants recognized by autoantibodies from patients with chronic autoimmune thyroiditis compared to auto-antibodies from healthy subjects. Clin Immunol Immunopathol 54:76–86.

Bröker BM, Klajman A, Youinou P, Jouquan J, Worman CP, Murphy J, Mackenzie L, Quartey-Papafio R, Blaschek M, Collins P, Lal S, Lydyard P (1988): Chronic lymphocytic leukemia cells (CLL) secrete multispecific autoantibodies. J Autoimmun 1:469–481.

Brouet JC, Dellagi K, Gendron MC, Chevalier A, Schmitt C, Mihaesco E (1989): Expression of a public idiotype by human monoclonal IgM directed to myelin-associated glycoprotein and characterization of the variability subgroup of their heavy and light chains. J Exp Med 170:1551–1558.

Burastero SE, Casali P, Wilder RL, Notkins AL (1988): Monoreactive high affinity and polyreactive low affinity rheumatoid factors are produced by CD5$^+$ B cells from patients with rheumatoid arthritis. J Exp Med 168:1979–1992.

Casali P, Notkins AL (1989a): CD5$^+$ B lymphocytes, polyreactive antibodies and the human B-cell repertoire. Immunol Today 10:364–368.

Casali P, Notkins AL (1989b): Probing the human B-cell repertoire with EBV: Polyreactive antibodies and CD5$^+$ B lymphocytes. Annu Rev Immunol 7:513–535.

Chen PP, Liu MF, Sinha S, Carson DA (1988): A 16/6 idiotype positive anti-DNA antibody is encoded by a conserved V_H gene with no somatic mutation. Arthritis Rheum 31:1429–1431.

Chen PP, Soto-Gil RW, Carson DA (1990): The early expression of some human autoantibody-associated heavy chain variable region genes is controlled by specific regulatory elements. Scand J Immunol 31:673–678.

Cohen IR, Cooke A (1986): Natural autoantibodies might prevent autoimmune disease. Immunol Today 7:363–364.

Coutinho A (1989): Beyond clonal selection and network. Immunol Rev 110:63–87.

Cuisiner A-M, Guigou V, Boubli L, Fougereau M, Tonnelle C (1989): Preferential expression of Vh5 and Vh6 immunoglobulin genes in early human B-cell ontogeny. Scand J Immunol 30:493–497.

Dang H, Takei M, Isenberg D, Shoenfeld Y, Backimer R, Rauch J, Talal N (1988): Expression of an interspecies idiotype in sera of SLE patients and their first-degree relatives. Clin Exp Immunol 71:445–450.

Davidson A, Livneh A, Manheimer-Lory A, Shefner R, Katz JB, Sewel KL, Diamond B (1988): Idiotypic analyses of anti-DNA antibodies in systemic lupus and monoclonal gammopathy. Ann Inst Pasteur/Immunol 139:645–650.

Davidson A, Manheimer-Lory A, Aranow C, Peterson R, Hannigan N, Diamond B (1990): Molecular characterization of a somatically mutated anti-DNA antibody bearing two systemic lupus erythematosus-related idiotypes. J Clin Invest 85:1401–1409.

Davidson A, Preud'homme JL, Solomon A, Chang M, Beede S, Diamond B (1987): Idiotypic analysis of myeloma proteins: Anti-DNA activity of monoclonal immunoglobulins bearing an SLE idiotype is more common in IgG than IgM antibodies. J Immunol 138:1515–1518.

de la Fuente B, Hoyer LW (1984): The idiotypic characteristics of human antibodies to Factor VIII. Blood 64:672–678.

Dersimonian H, Mcadam KPWJ, Mackworth-Young C, Stollar BD (1989): The recurrent expression of variable region segments in human IgM anti-DNA autoantibodies. J Immunol 142:4027–4033.

Dersimonian H, Schwartz RS, Barrett KJ, Stollar BD (1987): Relationship of human variable region heavy chain germ-line genes to genes encoding anti-DNA autoantibodies. J Immunol 139:2496–2501.

Dietrich G, Kazatchkine MD (1990): Normal immunoglobulin G (IgG) for therapeutic use (intravenous Ig) contain anti-idiotypic specificities against an immunodominant, disease-associated, cross-reactive idiotype of human anti-thyroglobulin autoantibodies. J Clin Invest 85:620–624.

Dietrich G, Piechaczyk M, Pau B, Kazatchkine MD (1991): Evidence for restricted epitopic and idiotypic specificity of anti-thyroglobulin autoantibodies. Eur J Immunol 21:811–814.

Dietrich G, Pereira P, Algiman M, Sultan Y, Kazatchkine MD (1990): A monoclonal anti-idiotypic antibody against the antigen-combining site of anti-factor VIII autoantibodies defines an idiotope that is recognized by normal human polyspecific immunoglobulins for therapeutic use (IVIg). J Autoimmun 3:547–557.

Dietrich G, Kaveri SV, Kazatchkine MD (1992a): A V-Region connected autoreactive subfraction of normal human immunoglobulins G. Eur J Immunol 22:1701–1706.

Dietrich G, Algiman M, Sultan Y, Nydegger UE, Kazatchkine MD (1992b): Origin of anti-idiotypic activity against anti-factor VIII autoantibodies in pools of normal human immunoglobulin G (IVIg). Blood 79:2946–2951.

Dietrich G, Kaveri SV, Kazatchkine MD (1992c): Modulation of autoimmunity by intravenous immunoglobulins (IVIg) through interaction with the function of the immune/idiotypic network. Clin Immunol Immunopathol 62:S73–S81.

Dietrich G, Varela F, Hurez V, Bouanani M, Kazatchkine MD (1993): Manipulating immune networks with normal immunoglobulin G. Submitted for publication.

Durandy A, Thuillier L, Forveille M, Fischer A (1990): Phenotypic and functional characteristics of human newborns' B lymphocytes. J Immunol 144:60–65.

Dwyer JM (1992): Manipulating the immune system with immune globulin. N Engl J Med 326:107–116.

Fong S, Chen PP, Gilbertson TA, Weber JR, Fox RI, Carson DA (1986): Expression of three cross-reactive idiotypes on rheumatoid factor autoantibodies from patients with autoimmune diseases and seropositive adults. J Immunol 137:122–128.

Gillis S, Kozak R, Durante M, Wecksler ME (1981): Immunological studies of aging. Decreased production of and response to T-cell growth factor by lymphocytes from aged human. J Clin Invest 67:937–942.

Gordon J, Rosenthal M (1984): Failure to detect age-related increase of nonpathological autoantibodies. Lancet 1:231–232.

Grabar P (1983): Autoantibodies and the physiological role of immunoglobulins. Immunol Today 4:337–341.

Guigou V, Guilbert B, Moinier D, Tonnelle C, Boubli L, Avrameas S, Fougereau M, Fumoux F (1991): Ig repertoire of human polyspecific antibodies and B-cell ontogeny. J Immunol 146:1368–1374.

Guilbert B, Dighiero G, Avrameas S (1982): Naturally occuring antibodies against nine common antigens in normal human sera. I. Detection, isolation, and characterization. J Immunol 128:2779–2787.

Halpern R, Kaveri SV, Kohler H (1991): Human anti-phosphorylcholine antibodies share idiotopes and are self-binding. J Clin Invest 88:476–482.

Harindranath N, Goldfarb IS, Ikematsu H, Burastero SE, Wilder RL, Notkins AL, Casali P (1991): Complete sequence of the genes encoding the Vh and Vl regions of low and high affinity monoclonal IgM and IgA1 rheumatoid factors produced by $CD5^+$ B cells from a rheumatoid arthritis patient. Int Immunol 3:865–875.

Hiraïwa A, Nugent DJ, Milner ECB (1990): Sequence analysis of monoclonal antibodies derived from a patient with idiopathic thrombocytopenic purpura. Autoimmunity 8:107–113.

Holmberg D, Forsgren S, Ivars F, Coutinho A (1984): Reactions amongst IgM antibodies derived from normal, neonatal mice. Eur J Immunol 14:435–441.

Hunt-Gerardo S, Persselin JE, Stevens RH (1990): Human IgG anti-F(ab')$_2$ antibodies possess rheumatoid factor activity. Clin Exp Immunol 81:293–300.

Hurez V, Kaveri SV, Kazatchkine MD (1993a): Expression and control of IgG autoreactivity in normal human serum. Eur J Immunol 23:783–789.

Hurez V, Dietrich G, Kaveri SV, Kazatchkine MD (1993b): Polyreactivity of natural and disease-associated anti-DNA and anti-thyroglobulin autoantibodies. Scand J Immunol (in press).

Isenberg DA, Shoenfeld Y, Madaio MP, Reichlin M, Rauch J, Stollar BD, Schwartz RS (1984): Anti-DNA antibody idiotypes in systemic lupus erythematosus. Lancet 1:417–421.

Kang C-Y, Kohler H (1986): Immunoglobulin with complementary paratope and idiotope. J Exp Med 163:787–796.

Kasaian MT, Ikematsu H, Casali P (1992): Identification and analysis of a novel human surface $CD5^-$ B lymphocyte subset producing natural antibodies. J Immunol 148:2690–2702.

Kaveri SV, Dietrich G, Hurez V, Kazatchkine MD (1991): Intravenous immunoglobulins (IVIg) in the treatment of autoimmune disease. Clin Exp Immunol 86:192–198.

Kaveri SV, Kang CY, Kohler H (1990): Natural mouse and human antibodies bind to a peptide derived from a germline variable heavy chain: Evidence for evolutionary conserved self-binding locus. J Immunol 145:4207–4213.

Kaveri SV, Rowen D, Wang H, Kohler H, Kazatchkine MD (1992): Monoclonal anti-idiotypic antibodies against anti-thyroglobulin autoantibodies define cross-reactive idiotypes recognized by normal human immunoglobulins for therapeutic use (IVIg). Submitted for publication.

Kay MMB, Goodman S, Whitfield C, Wong P, Zaki L, Rudoloff V (1983): The senescent cell antigen is immunologically related to band 3. Proc Natl Acad Sci USA 80:1631–1635.

Kipps TJ (1989): The CD5 B cell. Adv Immunol 47:117–185.

Kipps TJ, Tomhave E, Chen PP, Carson PA (1988): Autoantibody-associated kappa light chain variable region gene expressed in chronic lymphocytic leukemia with little or no somatic mutation. Implications for etiology and immunotherapy. J Exp Med 167:840–852.

Kipps TJ, Tomhave E, Pratt LF, Duffy S, Chen PP, Carson PA (1989): Developmentally restricted immunoglobulin heavy chain variable region gene expressed at high frequency in chronic lymphocytic leukemia. Proc Natl Acad Sci USA 86:5913–5917.

Lefvert AK (1988): Anti-acetylcholine receptor antibody related idiotypes in myasthenia gravis. J Autoimmun 1:63–72.

Logtenberg T, Young FM, Van Es JH, Gmelig-Meyling FHJ, Alt FW (1989): Autoantibodies encoded by the most Jh-proximal human immunoglobulin heavy chain variable region gene. J Exp Med 170:1347–1355.

Lundkvist I, Coutinho A, Varela F, Holmberg D (1989): Evidence for a functional idiotypic network among natural antibodies in normal mice. Proc Natl Acad Sci USA 86:5074–5078.

Lydyard PM, Quartey-Papafio R, Bröker B, Mackenzie L, Jouquan J, Blaschek MA, Steele J, Petrou M, Collins P, Isenberg D, Youinou PY (1990a): The antibody repertoire of early human B cells. I. High frequency of autoreactivity and polyreactivity. Scand J Immunol 31:33–43.

Lydyard PM, Quartey-Papafio RP, Bröker BM, Mackenzie L, Hay FC, Youinou PY, Jefferis R, Mageed RA (1990b): The antibody repertoire of early human B cells. III. Expression of cross-reactive idiotopes characteristic of certain Rheumatoid factors and identifying VkIII, VhI, and VhIII gene family products. Scand J Immunol 32:709–716.

Mackenzie LE, Youinou PY, Hicks R, Yuksel B, Mageed RA, Lydyard PM (1991): Auto- and polyreactivity of IgM from CD5$^+$ and CD5$^-$ cord blood B cells. Scand J Immunol 33:329–335.

Madaio MP, Schattner A, Shattner M, Schwartz RS (1986): Lupus serum and normal human serum contain anti-DNA antibodies with the same idiotypic marker. J Immunol 137:2535–2540.

Maire MA, Mittey M, Lambert PH (1989): The presence of cryoprecipitable immunoglobulins in normal human sera may reflect specific molecular interactions. Autoimmunity 2:155–164.

Manoussakis MN, Tzioufas AG, Silis MP, Pange PJE, Goudevenos J, Moutsopoulos HM (1987): High prevalence of anti-cardiolipin and other autoantibodies in a healthy elderly population. Clin Exp Immunol 69:557–565.

Marchalonis JJ, Kaymaz H, Dedeoglu F, Schlutter SF, Yocum DE, Edmundson AB (1992): Human autoantibodies reactive with synthetic autoantigens from T-cell receptor β chain. Proc Natl Acad Sci USA 89:3325–3329.

Mariotti S, Sansoni P, Barbesino G, Caturegli P, Monti D, Cossarizza A, Giacomelli T, Passeri G, Fagiolo U, Pinchera A, Franceschi C (1992): Thyroid and other organ-specific autoantibodies in healthy centenarians. Lancet 339:1506–1508.

Matsuyama T, Fukumori J, Tanaka H (1983): Evidence of unique idiotypic determinants and similar idiotypic determinants on human anti-thyroglobulin antibodies. Clin Exp Immunol 51:381–386.

Mortari F, Newton JA, Wang JY, Schroeder HW (1992): The human cord blood antibody repertoire. Frequent usage of the Vh7 gene repertoire. Eur J Immunol 22:241–245.

Moulias R, Proust J, Wang A, Congy F, Marescot MR, Deville-Chabrolle A, Paris-Hamelin A, Lesourd B (1984): Age-related increase in autoantibodies. Lancet 1:1128–1129.

Muryoï T, Sasaki T, Harata N, Takai O, Tamate E, Yoshinaga K (1988): Heterogeneity of anti-idiotypic antibodies to anti-DNA antibodies in humans. Clin Exp Immunol 71:67–72.

Naito N, Saito K, Hosoya T, Tarutani O, Sakata S, Nishikawa T, Niimi H, Nakajima H, Kohno Y (1990): Anti-thyroglobulin autoantibodies in sera from patients with chronic thyroiditis and from healthy subjects: Differences in cross-reactivity with thyroid peroxidase. Clin Exp Immunol 80:4–10.

Nakamura M, Burastero SE, Ueki Y, Larrick JW, Notkins AL, Casali P (1988a): Probing the normal and autoimmune B cell repertoire with Epstein-Barr virus: Frequency of B cells producing monoreactive high affinity autoantibodies in patients with Hashimoto's disease and systemic lupus erythematosus. J Immunol 141:4165–4172.

Nakamura M, Burastero SE, Notkins AL, Casali P (1988b): Human monoclonal rheumatoid factor-like antibodies from CD5 (Leu-1)$^+$ B cells are polyreactive. J Immunol 140:4180–4186.

Newkirk MM, Mageed RA, Jefferis R, Chen PP, Capra JD (1987): Complete amino acid sequences of variable regions of two human IgM rheumatoid factors, BOR and KAS of the Wa idiotypic family, reveal restricted use of heavy and light chain variable and joining region gene segments. J Exp Med 166:550–564.

Nickerson KG, Berman J, Glickman E, Chess L, Alt FW (1989): Early human IgH gene assembly in Epstein-Barr virus transformed fetal B cell lines. Preferential utilization of the most J_H-proximal D segment (DQ52) and two unusual V_H-related rearrangements. J Exp Med 169:1391–1403.

Paavonen T, Quartey-Papafio RP, Delves PJ, Mackenzie L, Lund T, Youinou PY, Lydyard PM (1990): CD5 mRNA expression and autoantibody production in early human B cells immortalized by EBV. Scand J Immunol 31:269–274.

Pascual V, Capra JD (1991): Human immunoglobulin heavy-chain variable region genes: Organization, polymorphism and expression. Adv Immunol 49:1–74.

Pfueller SL, Logan D, Tran TT, Bilston RA (1990): Naturally occurring human IgG antibodies to intracellular and cytoskeletal components of human platelets. Clin Exp Immunol 79:367–373.

Piechaczyk M, Bouanani M, Salhi SL, Baldet L, Bastide M, Pau B, Bastide JM (1987): Antigenic domains on the human thyroglobulin molecule recognized by autoantibodies in patients' sera and by natural autoantibodies isolated from sera of healthy subjects. Clin Immunol Immunopathol 45:114–121.

Portnoï D, Freitas A, Holmberg D, Bandeira A, Coutinho A, (1986): Immunocompetent autoreactive B lymphocytes are activated cycling cells in normal mice. J Exp Med 164:25–35.

Raaphorst FM, Timmers E, Kenter MJH, Van Tol MJD, Vossen JM, Schuurman RKB (1992): Restricted utilization of germ-line Vh3 genes and short diverse third complementarity-determining regions (CDR3) in human fetal B lymphocyte immunoglobulin heavy chain rearrangements. Eur J Immunol 22:247–251.

Ronda N, Haury M, Nobrega A, Coutinho A, Kazatchkine MD (1993a): A comparative study of natural and SLE associated anti-endothelial cell autoantibodies (AECA). Submitted for publication.

Ronda N, Hurez V, Kazatchkine MD (1993b): Intravenous immunoglobulin (IVIG) therapy of autoimmune and inflammatory diseases. Vox Sang 64:65–72.

Rossi F, Dietrich G, Kazatchkine MD (1989): Anti-idiotypes against autoantibodies in normal immunoglobulins: Evidence for network regulation of human autoimmune responses. Immunol Rev 110:135–149.

Rossi F, Guilbert B, Tonnelle C, Ternynck T, Fumoux F, Avrameas S, Kazatchkine MD (1990): Idiotypic interactions between normal human polyspecific IgG and natural IgM antibodies. Eur J Immunol 20:2089–2094.

Rossi F, Jayne DRW, Lockwood CM, Kazatchkine MD (1991): Antiidiotypes against anti-neutrophil cytoplasmic antigen autoantibodies in normal human polyspecific IgG for therapeutic use and in the remission serum of patients with systemic vasculitis. Clin Exp Immunol 83:298–303.

Rossi F, Kazatchkine MD (1989): Antiidiotypes against autoantibodies in pooled normal human polyspecific Ig. J Immunol 143:4104–4109.

Rossi F, Sultan Y, Kazatchkine MD (1988): Anti-idiotypes against autoantibodies and alloantibodies to Factor VIIIc (anti-hemophilic factor) are present in therapeutic polyspecific normal immunoglobulins. Clin Exp Immunol 74:311–316.

Ruiz-Arguelles A (1988): Spontaneous reversal of acquired autoimmune dysfibrinogenemia probably due to an anti-idiotypic antibody directed to an interspecies cross-reactive idiotype expressed on antifibrinogen antibodies. J Clin Invest 82:958–963.

Sabbaga J, Pankewycz OG, Lufft V, Schwartz RS, Madaio MP (1990): cross-reactivity distinguishes serum and nephritigenic anti-DNA antibodies in human lupus from their natural counterparts in normal serum. J Autoimmun 3:215–235.

Sanz I, Casali P, Thomas JW, Notkins AL, Capra JD (1989a): Nucleotide sequences of eight human natural autoantibodies V_H regions reveals apparent restricted use of VH families. J Immunol 142:4054–4061.

Sanz I, Dang H, Takei M, Talal N, Capra JD (1989b): Vh sequence of a human anti-Sm autoantibody: Evidence that autoantibodies can be unmutated copies of germline genes. J Immunol 142:883–887.

Schroeder HW, Hillson JL, Perlmutter PM (1987): Early restriction of the human antibody repertoire. Science 238:791–793.

Schroeder HW, Wang JY (1990): Preferential utilization of conserved immunoglobulin heavy chain variable gene segments during human fetal life. Proc Natl Acad Sci USA 87:6146–6150.

Schutte MEM, Ebeling SB, Akkermans KE, Gmelig-Meyling FHJ, Logtenberg T (1991): Antibody specificity and immunoglobulin Vh gene utilization of human monoclonal $CD5^+$ B cell lines. Eur J Immunol 21:1115–1121.

Seigneurin J-M, Guilbert B, Bourgeat MJ, Avrameas S (1988): Polyspecific natural antibodies and autoantibodies secreted by human lymphocytes immortalized with Epstein-Barr virus. Blood 71:581–585.

Siminovitch KA, Misener V, Kwong PC, Song QL, Chen PP (1989): A natural autoantibody is encoded by germline heavy and lambda light chain variable region genes without somatic mutation. J Clin Invest 84:1675–1678.

Siminovitch KA, Misener V, Kwong PC, Yang PM, Laskin CA, Cairns E, Bell D, Rubin LA, Chen PP (1990): A human anti-cardiolipin autoantibody is encoded by developmentally restricted heavy and light chain variable region genes. Autoimmunity 8:97–105.

Solomon G, Schiffenbauer J, Keiser HD, Diamond B (1983): Use of monoclonal antibodies to identify shared idiotypes on human antibodies to native DNA from patients with systemic lupus erythematosus. Proc Natl Acad Sci USA 80:850–854.

Spatz LA, Wong KK, Williams M, Desal R, Golier J, Berman JE, Alt FW, Latov N (1990): Cloning and sequence analysis of the V_H and V_L regions of an anti-myelin/DNA antibody from a patient with peripheral neuropathy and chronic lymphocytic leukemia. J Immunol 144:2821–2828.

Stewart J (1992): Immunoglobulins did not arise in evolution to fight infection. Immunol Today 13:396–399.

Sthoeger ZM, Wakai M, Tse DB, Vinciguerra VP, Allen SL, Budman DR, Lichtman SM, Schulman P, Weiselberg LR, Chiorazzi N (1989): Production of autoantibodies by CD5-expressing B lymphocytes from patients with chronic lymphocytic leukemia. J Exp Med 169:255–268.

Takei M, Dang H, Wang RJ, Talal N (1988): Characteristics of a human monoclonal anti-Sm autoantibody expressing an interspecies idiotype. J Immunol 140:3108–3113.

Talor E, Rose NR (1991): Hypothesis: The aging paradox and autoimmune disease. Autoimmunity 8:245–249.

Thomas JW, Virta VJ, Nell LJ (1986): Idiotypic determinants on human anti-insulin antibodies are cyclically expressed. J Immunol 137:1610–1615.

Thompson KM, Sutherland J, Barden G, Melamed MD, Wright MG, Bailey S (1992): Human monoclonal antibodies specific for blood group antigens demonstrate multispecific properties characteristic of natural autoantibodies. Immunology 76:146–157.

Tomer Y, Shoenfeld Y (1988): Aging and autoantibodies. Autoimmunity 1:141–149.

Uhlig H, Rutter G, Dernick R (1985): Self-reactive B lymphocytes detected in young adults, children and newborns after in vitro infection with Epstein-Barr virus. Clin Exp Immunol 62:75–84.

Van Doorn PA, Rossi F, Brand A, Lint MV, Vermeulen M, Kazatchkine M (1990): On the mechanism of high dose intravenous immunoglobulin treatment of patients with chronic inflammatory demyelinating polyneuropathy with high-dose intravenous immunoglobulins. J Neuroimmunol 29:57–64.

Varela F, Anderson A, Dietrich G, Sundblad A, Holmberg D, Kazatchkine MD, Coutinho A (1991): The population dynamics of antibodies in normal and autoimmune individuals. Proc Natl Acad Sci USA 88:5917–5921.

Varela F, Coutinho A (1991): Second generation immune networks. Immunol Today 12:159–166.

Vassilev T, Gelin C, Kaveri SV, Zilber MT, Boumsell L, Kazatchkine MD (1993): Anti-CD5 antibodies in pooled normal immunoglobulins for therapeutic use (intravenous immunoglobulins, IVIg). Clin Exp Immunol 92:369–372.

Winger L, Winger C, Shastry P, Russel A, Longenecker M (1983): Efficient generation in vitro, from human peripheral blood cells, of monoclonal Epstein-Barr virus transformants producing specific antibody to a variety of antigens without prior deliberate immunization. Proc Natl Acad Sci USA 80:4484–4488.

Winkler TH, Fehr H, Kalden JR (1992): Analysis of immunoglobulin variable region genes from human IgG anti-DNA hybridomas. Eur J Immunol 22:1719–1728.

Yadin O, Sarov B, Naggan L, Slor H, Shoenfeld Y (1989): Natural autoantibodies in the serum of healthy women—a five year follow-up. Clin Exp Immunol 75:402–406.

Youinou PY, Mackenzie L, Masson GL, Papadopoulos NM, Jouquan J, Pennec YL, Angelidis P, Katsikis P, Moutsopoulos HM, Lydyard PM (1988): CD5-Expressing B lymphocytes in the blood and salivery glands of patients with primary Sjögren's syndrome. J Autoimmun 1:185–194.

Young F, Tucker L, Rubinstein D, Guillaume T, Andre-Schwartz J, Barrett KJ, Schwartz RS, Logtenberg T (1990): Molecular analysis of a germ-line-encoded idiotypic marker of pathogenic human lupus autoantibodies. J Immunol 145:2545–2553.

Zouali M, Eyquem A (1983): Expression of anti-idiotypic clones against auto-anti-DNA antibodies in normal individuals. Cell Immunol 76:137–147.

Zouali M, Eyquem A (1984): Idiotype restriction in human autoantibodies to DNA in systemic lupus erythematosus. Immunol Lett 7:187–190.

Zouali M, Stollar BD, Schwartz RS (1988): Origin and diversification of anti-DNA antibodies. Immunol Rev 105:137–159.

9

AUTOANTIBODIES AND AUTOIMMUNE NETWORK: THE EVOLVING PARADIGM

Maurizio Zanetti

Department of Medicine and Cancer Center, University of California, San Diego, La Jolla, California

I see things differently, with more meanings, as I look for the dynamic asymmetrical binary relationship that is reflected in all the phenomena that leap into and out of my field of perception. . . . This concept of pairing manifests itself in dynamic asymmetrical binary systems and their internal and external interactions. It may well define the characteristics of all living systems which have in common a similar basic functional pattern, i.e., an interacting, dynamic, asymmetrical binary plan. This suggests that this pattern must also exist in other natural phenomena. Then it becomes possible to recognize the underlying unity in all the diversity of the phenomena of life, i.e., in biological and metabiological phenomena. . . .

—Jonas Salk [1983]

INTRODUCTION

The pathogenesis of autoimmune diseases remains one of the main unresolved issues in immunology. Although knowledge has steadily increased for the last 30 years, the origin and the nature of the basic mechanisms of

Autoimmunity: Physiology and Disease, Pages 129–141
© 1994 Wiley-Liss, Inc.

autoaggression still elude our understanding. In the past decades, some immunologists investigated model systems that are not harmful to understand better the mechanisms of immunity. Others identified and studied animal models of disease that could help elucidate the phenomenon of autoimmunity. No doubt progress has been made. The questions have been better defined and patterns among autoimmune diseases identified. Tools have been developed to analyze both the humoral and cellular arm of the immune response, determine whether a given disease is prevalently mediated by autoantibodies or cells, and assess their fine antigen reactivity (Table I). Formidable progress has also been made in identifying new lymphokines and their putative role in amplifying autoreactivity or causing tissue injury. It has also become clear that in human as well as animal autoimmune diseases genetic factors play an important role as single gene defects (e.g., autoimmune diseases that spontaneously occur in mutant murine strains), multifactorial gene defects (e.g., autoimmune diseases in which several genes controlling different autoimmune manifestations are involved), and disease-susceptibility genes (e.g., HLA genes that determine the susceptibility to disease). Because in spite of all these discoveries autoimmunity remains a mystery, it may be time to reassess our views about it by asking a few fundamental questions. Is our perception of what immunity is correct? What precisely are autoantibodies? Are current theories of immunity adequate to explain both physiology and pathology? What is the function of the immune system as a whole?

SELF-RECOGNITION: A PARADOX WITHOUT EXPLANATION

Traditionally, we regard the immune system, and its capacity to develop specific immunity, as the most important means of defense of the animal against the myriads of pathogens continuously threatening its existence. At the same time the immune system recognizes self-antigens without developing an autoimmune disease in every instance. It is almost imperative therefore that it be able to distinguish a substance as foreign and avoid reactions against its own body components to prevent the harmful consequences, that is, self–nonself-discrimination.

This apparent dichotomy of function has intrigued immunologists since the beginning of modern immunology. Here is how Burnet [1956] viewed the lack of antigenicity of self components:

> We still regard the absence of antigenicity of the body's own components as the most important feature to be interpreted. . . . In one way or another there must be a means of recognizing the difference between "self" and "nonself" material. There appears to be no limit to the number of molecular patterns that can act as antigenic determinants. On the other hand, there are hints that only a relatively small number of configurations are concerned in

TABLE I. The most common human autoimmune diseases and equivalent experimental models and their effector mechanism

Disease	Effector	Experimental Model
Myasthenia gravis	Anti-ACh receptor antibody	ACh receptor-induced muscle weakness in animals
Graves' disease	Anti-TSHR antibody	—
Hashimoto's disease	Anti-thyroglobulin and thyroid peroxidase antibodies	Thyroglobulin-induced throiditis in mice, spontaneous thyroiditis in Buffalo rats
Insulin-resistant diabetes associated with *Acanthosis nigricans* or ataxia telangectasia	Anti-insulin receptor antibodies	—
Type I diabetes (Juvenile insulin-dependent diabetes)	Anti-islet cell antibodies and T cells	Spontaneous disease in NOD mice and BB rats
Pernicious anemia	Antibodies against gastric parietal cells and intrinsic factor	—
Addison's disease	Antibodies against adrenal cells	—
Idiopathic hypoparathyroidism	Antibodies against parathyroid cells	—
Azoospermia	Antibodies to sperm	Antigen-induced orchitis in animals; postvasectomy orchitis
Premature ovarian failure	Antibodies to interstitial cells and corpus luteum	
Uveoretinitis	Antibodies and T cells specific for S-antigen	Antigen-induced uveoretinitis in animals
Vitiligo	Antimelanocyte antibodies	
Pemphigus	Antibodies against intercellular substance in the skin	
Pemphigus foliaceus	Antibodies against desmoglein I	
Primary biliary cirrhosis	Dihydrolipoyl acetyltransferase and protein X	
Multiple sclerosis	MBP specific T cells	Experimental allergic encephalomyelitis (EAE)
Autoimmune hemolytic anemia	Coombs' antibodies or cold agglutinin specific for I and i antigens	NZB mice

(Continued)

TABLE I. The most common human autoimmune diseases and equivalent experimental models and their effector mechanism (Continued)

Disease	Effector	Experimental Model
Idiopathic thrombocytopenic purpura	Antiplatelets antibodies	(BXSB × NZB) F$_1$ mice
Goodpasture's syndrome	Antibasement membrane antibodies	Masugi nephritis
Rheumatoid arthritis and Sjögren's syndrome	Rheumatoid factor, T cells	Collagen-induced arthritis in mice and rats, spontaneous arthritis and Sjögren's syndrome in MRL/lpr gld mice
SLE	Antinuclear antibodies (DNA, RNA, RNA RNA polymerase Sm, ribonucleoproteins)	Spontaneous disease in NZB × NZW F$_1$, BXSB, MRL/lpr gld mice, dogs
Scleroderma	Antitopoisomerase I, antinuclear antibodies, anticollagen I and III, anticentromere antibodies	Spontaneous disease in TSK mice
Polymiositis	Antibodies anti t-RNA synthetase	

"self-recognition." It is clearly economical of hypothesis to assume that there is a positive function of self-recognition that is followed by what can be called an "instruction" that the antibody-producing function be inhibited. Without such a positive instruction the intrusion of organic material into scavenger cells is followed by antibody production to some degree.

In recent years it has become increasingly evident that neither B nor T lymphocytes reactive with self-antigens are eliminated from the immune repertoire of normal individuals. Autoreactive B cells have been demonstrated in normal newborns and adult individuals, and the serum of normal adults has been found to contain a variety of antibodies reactive with endogenous (self) antigens [Guilbert et al., 1982; Ternynck and Avrameas, 1986; Glotz et al., 1988]. Similarly, autoreactive T cells exist in peripheral lymphoid organs and can be easily expanded by self-antigen or corresponding peptides [LaSalle et al., 1991]. Most likely, these T cells are usually silenced by the presence of antigen, lack of costimulatory factors (anergy), or active peripheral suppressive mechanisms (T-cell and anti-idiotype suppression). There have been numerous reviews on this subject, and more detailed information can be found there. What is important, however, is to realize that the dogma that has been for a long time propagated on clonal elimination of self-reactive clones is not completely correct.

Why then does the immune system recognize self at all if this is a potentially lethal process? Before directly addressing this issue, it may be helpful to discuss briefly a more general aspect, that of semiology[1] of immunology. We may find that some of the existing, conceptual obstacles may be attributable to the way we look at things rather than to things themselves.

BINARISM IN THE IMMUNE SYSTEM

Possibly, the most astonishing aspect of the immune system is the way we usually refer to it. By far, the prevalent way is duality both in its architecture as well as function. This binarism is the practice of identifying an element through its opposite or complementary. Table II lists a few paradigmatic examples of binarism in contemporary immunology.

It is common among immunologists as well as among nonimmunologists to define an antigen by the antibody that binds to it and vice versa. The same holds true for receptors and ligands. The binary relation between idiotype and anti-idiotype will be discussed in the subsequent pages. (An idiotype is defined by an anti-idiotype and the latter is the product of immunization against a reference antibody idiotype.) The distinction between B and T cells and their different and sometimes independent function in the immune system was reiterated just recently by one of the most insightful immunologists [Mitchison, 1990]. Moving to a level of greater complexity, one finds positive and negative selection, a prototype binary concept. Whereas positive selection allows for the development of lymphocytes with genetically programmed receptors recognizing foreign antigens, negative selection eliminates lymphocytes genetically programmed toward recognition of self-antigens. Last comes self–nonself discrimination, the summation of positive and negative selection of lymphocytes in central lymphoid organs for some and active regulation for others. Thus it is easy to conclude that a binary view of the immune system serves a great purpose, that of looking at its function with the idea that normal is symmetrical and pathological is loss of symmetry.

What concerns me is that in spite of such a clear dual organization, all

TABLE II. Binarism in immunology

Antigen	Antibody
Receptor	Ligand
Idiotype	Anti-idiotype
B cell	T cell
Positive selection	Negative selection
Self	Nonself

[1] *Semiology* is used in the accepted meaning of Michel Foucault [1966].

individuals possess, and continuously deal with, autoreactive B and T cells, albeit to a different degree. Therefore, I argue that immunology, like our culture in general, is embedded with an unavoidable sense of duality. I see this as a dominant sign of the Occidental culture that essentially reflects the transposition of the duality of the human brain into philosophy, religion, and science. The origin of this phenomenon is easily traceable to the early seventeenth century, the post-Renaissance and post-Galilean era dominated by Descartes' dualism of "res cogitans" and "res extensa," spirit and matter. Although a century later Kant laid the ground for radical revision of this binary view, his proposal to use the dialectic process to reconcile the reductionist–synthetic approach of experimentalists and the cognition a priori of methaphysicians had unfortunately little influence on eradicating the use of binary logic in the scientific thoughts of the last two hundred years. Embracing the dialectic process and recognizing the complexity of the system will be the next necessary step in understanding how immunity and autoimmunity work.

AUTOANTIBODIES VERSUS AUTOANTIBODIES

An issue frequently discussed among immunologists is the nature of autoantibodies, their origin, their role in disease, and how we can control them. There are in my opinion several misconceptions at this level. Based on the current, available data, I will define four categories of autoantibodies and provide a few arguments in favor of the hypothesis that autoantibodies causative of pathology are rare. As a consequence, we need stringent criteria to distinguish those that are pathogenetic from those that are not. I will also argue that autoantibodies may in selected instances serve a regulatory function.

It has now become apparent that the process of differentiation and subsequent development of pre-B and B cells—the rearrangement of immunoglobulin genes and the acquisition of cell surface characteristics—is utilized differently during late fetal and early extrauterine life and adult life. Thus, while an initial repertoire of approximately 10^4 specificities develops stochastically (i.e., independent of antigen), the repertoire of adult individuals is viewed as primarily driven by antigen, albeit a remnant of the original neonatal repertoire can be identified throughout life [Feeney, 1992].

A finding of considerable importance that is being discussed in detail elsewhere in this volume is the presence of antibodies reacting with conventional endogenous antigens in the serum of apparently normal individuals, as it will be abundantly reviewed in this volume. First in rodents [Ternynck and Avrameas, 1986; Glotz et al., 1988] and more recently in humans (see Chapter 6), it has been easy to immortalize self-reactive cells and better characterize the fine reactivity of their product at the clonal level. Because of their existence during the normal state one needs to question the role of ontogeny in shaping the B-cell repertoire and pinpoint the differences between pathogenetic and nonpathogenetic autoantibodies.

It is now clear that most of those referred to as autoantibodies are natural or innate antibodies with little if any noxious capacity. Natural autoantibodies often exhibit multiple binding characteristics and can interact with both endogenous and exogenous antigens [Avrameas, 1991]. Their affinity for antigens is generally low, and there exists no proof that these antibodies can cause pathology in animals or in humans. What could their function be? It has been proposed that innate antibodies form a web of high connectivity, e.g., multiple interactions involving mostly, but not exclusively, the variable region of the molecule. In other words, an archetypal idiotype network that may be relevant to shape the repertoire during ontogeny [Coutinho et al., 1984; Varela and Coutinho, 1991].

Related to connected, innate antibodies are self-reactive antibodies that bind with high affinity to one or several antigens. Their concentration increases significantly in autoimmune diseases, but again they do not cause disease. Possible functions could be to eliminate breakdown products and metabolites (scavenger effect) or to be the sentinel of emerging autoimmune diseases and play a role in immunoregulation by favoring, for instance, repertoire shift and/or idiotype regulation [Zanetti et al., 1987].

Pathogenic autoantibodies, on the other hand, are responsible for pathology during the course of a disease, be this an organ-specific or a systemic disease. Studies aimed at defining pathogenic autoantibodies based on affinity, epitope specificity, or mutation in variable (V)-region genes encoding for such antibodies have failed thus far to provide us with clear criteria to base a distinction. The analysis of autoantibody V-region genes demonstrated that the repertoire is random with respect to gene usage, and somatic mutation and germline gene utilization are both involved in the make-up of autoreactive antibodies.

What is striking is that the number of autoimmune diseases for which the causative role of autoantibodies has been clearly demonstrated is still very limited. Among these are myasthenia gravis, Graves' disease, Goopasture syndrome, pemphigus bullosus, autoimmune hemolytic anemia, insulin-resistant diabetes associated with *Acanthosis nigricans,* and coagulopathy by anti-Factor VIII antibodies. To this list, one may want to add the reported association with pathology of anti-SS-A/Ro antibodies (congenital heart block), anti-β_2-adrenergic receptor antibodies in Chagas' disease, and the anticoagulant effect of anticardiolipin and antiphospholipid antibodies in lupus. This clearly contrasts with the large number of known autoantibodies. In other words, a reactivity with a self-antigen is not sufficient for determining the pathogenetic potential of an autoantibody. I will illustrate this point with an example.

A decade ago, C.B. Wilson and I at the Scripps Research Institute studied a model of experimental nephritis in rats [Zanetti and Wilson, 1983; Zanetti et al., 1983]. The objective was to characterize the autoantibody response in susceptible and resistant strains and determine parameters necessary and sufficient for pathology to occur. Autoimmune diseases in laboratory animals are often induced by immunization across species barriers to terminate self-tolerance. Thus we used a semipurified antigen of heterologous kidney to incite the formation of autoantibodies and autoimmune disease in the susceptible strain. The same immunization in the resistant strain induced kidney-reactive autoantibodies but not disease. Interestingly, in the susceptible strain pathogenetic antibodies directed at the autologous nephritogenic antigen represented a minute fraction of the total antikidney antibody response. Pathogenetic autoantibodies were by and large in the diseased tissue, as their relative concentration was 500 times that in the serum. By contrast, the resistant strain failed to make antibodies to the autologous nephritogenic antigen and displayed a quantitative deficiency of the relevant nephritogenic antigen. Collectively, two important messages came from this study. One is that serum autoantibodies do not always contain and express the pathogenetic potential of an autoantibody response. The second is that both the fine specificity of the autoantibody response (quality) and the content or accessibility of the antigenic determinant required for pathology (quantity) determine whether or not a humoral autoantibody response will cause disease.

In light of these considerations it appears that simply binding to, or reacting with, an autoantigen reveals per se little about the pathogenetic potential of autoantibodies. It would certainly help to adopt stringent criteria to define pathogenetic autoantibodies (Table III), hence uniforming our understanding of autoimmunity and disease.

Finally, there exists a fourth category of autoantibodies, antibodies to self-idiotypes. Possibly they are the most faithful representation of the inner activity of lymphocytes as an ensemble of individual units that seek functional interconnection and interdependence in a higher organizational structure within the immune system.

NETWORK REGULATION: A DIALECTIC OF SELF–ANTISELF

Idiotype-based regulation still remains the most dynamic and specific mechanism available to the immune system to modulate induced and natural

TABLE III. Criteria for the definition of pathogenetic autoantibodies

Autoantibodies isolated from an affected organ or tissue must react in vitro with the same tissue antigen

Autoantibodies isolated from the diseased tissue, or produced in vitro with similar characteristics, should transfer an identical lesion in animals

Upon transfer it should be possible to reproduce the histopathological, functional, and biochemical abnormalities present in the original disease responses. Numerous experiments exist to validate what a priori seem the most essential properties of the idiotype network: regulation and homeostasis. Protection of the individual from the development and/or progression of autoimmunity is a third function of the network, but this has not been firmly established (see below).

The fact that network dynamics can occur without the involvement of antigen is an attractive feature for two reasons. First is the notion that once self-reactivity has began, the identification of the triggering antigens proves very difficult, almost implying that it may not be necessary for the perpetuation (i.e., chronicity) of the disease. Thus other forms of autoactivation need to be sought. Second is the fact that the V regions of antibodies and T-cell receptors are themselves antigenic and immunogenic and form an extended array of structures that constitute the architecture of a functional network. Thus self–nonself-discrimination and self-tolerance can both be realized using a system and a mechanism that are both endogenous and active. Although a portion of the self-reactive repertoire is deleted during ontogeny in the central lymphoid organs, one cannot discount the fact that autoreactivity arises later in life in most individuals at an astonishing rate. This makes it likely that the immune system and the organism possess ways to counterbalance autoreactivity and/or limit its potentially noxious effects.

The origin of these views dates to Jerne's first proposal [1974] that self-reactivity is a normal component of the immune system whose major function would then be to look inside and maintain the macromolecular homeostasis rather than being projected toward the outside and protect the host against invading macromolecules. This rapidly propounded view was based on the prediction that the immune system consists in a web of V regions mutually interacting via their antigenic determinants, hence constituting the major link between clones of lymphocytes. His view gained immediate popularity.

Several years later the need arose for integrating Jerne's network ideas with the phenomenology of autoimmune diseases. In the mid-1980s I proposed the concept of an *autoimmune network* [Zanetti, 1985] as the fundamental, comprehensive framework of self-recognition/reactivity events to encompass responsiveness to self-antigens and its modulation through the positive and negative influence of humoral or cellular interactions based on domain–domain interactions between antibody and T-cell receptor V regions. The question that now needs to be asked is: Have we learned what was to be learned about the autoimmune network? Did we collect sufficient evidence to explain the phenomenology of autoimmune diseases based on the structure–function of the autoimmune network?

Based on experimental results accumulated over the past 15 years, one can, no doubt, make a strong case for the existence of an autoimmune network (Table IV). What emerged is that regulation of the response to a self-antigen and modulation of disease are both possible through the direct

TABLE IV. Evidence for the existence of an autoimmune network

The humoral response to self-antigens can be suppressed by passive administration of anti-idiotypic antibodies

The humoral response to self-antigens can be suppressed by active immunization with idiotype

The humoral response to self can be suppressed in vivo by passive transfer of idiotype-primed T cells

Humoral and cellular responses to self-antigens can be suppressed in vivo by active immunization with antigen- or idiotype-reactive T cells

Active immunity using synthetic peptides of disease-inducing T-cell receptors prevent the induction of experimental disease

Self-reactive antibodies can be induced in naive animals by active immunization with idiotypic and anti-idiotypic antibodies

Immunization with a self-antigen may induce antireceptor autoantibodies via an idiotypic mechanism

Spontaneously occurring anti-idiotypes have been identified for a number of autoantibodies

manipulation of the autoimmune network. This implies that (1) the immune response to self-antigens is by and large regulated similarly to that to exogenous antigens (albeit some difference may exist) and (2) regulation within the autoimmune network may in fact be very important in physiology and physiopathology [Zanetti, 1986, 1992; Zanetti et al., 1992].

Another aspect became evident, that is, a self-centered immune system (i.e., the autoimmune network) must oscillate within a spectrum of possible dynamic outcomes (Table V). In other words, under normal circumstances (i.e., a state in which the immune system is not deliberately perturbed by antigens or mitogens) the autoimmune network must continually be confronted with the choice between physiological (nonpathogenetic) and pathogenetic (disease-causing) events. What determines whether a given set of interactions will end up in activating or silencing autoreactive clones? This is what still escapes our understanding.

TABLE V. Possible outcomes for idiotype and anti-idiotype interactions in the autoimmune network

Physiology
   Idiotype regulation
   Suppression of self-reactive idiotypic clones
   De novo activation of self-reactive clones via anti-idiotype
   Idiotype–anti-idiotype complexes and inflammation
Pathology

IMMUNE SYSTEM: UNITY OVERALL

To recognize and counteract pathogens the immune system uses ancestral nonspecific defense mechanisms (e.g., phagocytosis) and highly specific mechanisms (e.g., antibody formation and generation of antigen-reactive T cells). In vertebrates lymphoid cells, and the immune system as a whole, clearly utilize the same mechanisms to (1) respond to foreign antigens (defense mechanisms) and (2) silence the response to self-antigens (tolerance). This mere consideration necessitates that we approach the problem from a new and different perspective. For sake of simplicity I will call this the *integrated approach*. This requires consideration of the complexity of the system and identification of common patterns to its function. I will illustrate this concept by borrowing from Capra [1982]:

> The essence of life is the replication of specific pattern. We are concerned with an attempt to understand the significance of this, to point out the difficulties of considering, even at a purely theoretical level, the application of the standard physico-chemical approach to biological matters at this level and to try to develop a series of concepts in terms of macromolecular pattern which may make such matters more amenable to an effective scientific approach.

From the foregoing, a strict binary approach to immunology is a fortiori self-limiting. What is needed is to put ourselves outside a conventional, cartesian way of thinking and reconsider the enormous complexity upon which systems in living organisms, including the immune system, have and continue to operate.

> The system view looks at the world in terms of relationships and integration. Systems are integrated wholes whose properties cannot be reduced to those of smaller units. Instead of concentrating on basic building blocks or basic substances, the systems approach emphasizes basic principles of organization. Examples of systems abound in nature. Every organism from the smallest bacterium through the wide range of plants and animals to humans is an integrated whole and thus a living system. Cells are living systems, and so are the various tissues and organs of the body, the human brain being the most complex example. But systems are not confined to individual organisms and their parts. The same aspects of wholeness are exhibited by social systems such as an anthill, a beehive, or a human family and by ecosystems that consist of a variety of organisms and inanimate matter in mutual interaction. What is preserved in a wilderness area is not individual trees or organisms but the complex web of relationships between them. [Capra, 1982]

A tentative conclusion from all this is that the immune system is a self-organizing system, which means that its order in structure and function is not imposed by the environment, but is established by the system itself according to an internal principle of organization, independent of environmental influences. Precisely, the autoimmune network is an internal principle of organization [Zanetti, 1988]. Although not isolated from the environment its interaction with the outside world is not what determines its raison d'être.

Modern tools of cellular, chemical, and molecular analysis continuously refine our ability to understand the immune phenomenon. The identification of specific patterns of organization may make it possible to understand what determines the immune system as both a defense and an autoaggressive system. The challenge that lies ahead requires the change in approach mentioned above.

It seems to be of the nature of the relation between the human mind and the events which make up the universe that the approach to control and understanding is a process in which success leads always to the envisaging of more problems than it solves. At every stage in the past and at every stage in the future, the advancing edge of knowledge in every field has been and will be in a state of confusion. There are phases when the emergence of a new technique or, more rarely, of a fertile generalization allows a swift development of a new area in which ignorance and confusion can be replaced by understanding and the possibility of control and utilization for the satisfaction of human desires. But the edge where ignorance lies beyond the zone of ad hoc hypothesis and inadequate experimental technique is always there. Speculation and tentative generalization, as well as the search for and development of new technical approaches, are the legitimate weapons to take us further toward the always receding periphery. [Capra, 1982]

ACKNOWLEDGMENTS

This work was supported by grants NIH HD25787 and Council for Tobacco Research No. 2124.

REFERENCES

Avrameas S (1991): Natural antibodies: from "horror autotoxicus" to "gnothi seauton." Immunol Today 12:154–159.

Burnet FM (1956): "Enzyme Antigen and Virus." London: Cambridge University Press.

Capra F (1982): "The Turning Point." New York: Simon & Shuster.

Coutinho A, Forni L, Holmberg D, Ivars F, Vaz N (1984): From an antigen-centered, clonal perspective of the immune response to an organism-centered, network perspective of autonomous activity in a self-referential system. Immunol Rev 79:151–168.

Feeney AJ (1992): Comparison of junctional diversity in neonatal and adult immunoglobulin repertoires. Int Rev Immunol 8:113–122.

Foucault M (1966): "Les mots et les choses." Paris: Gallimard.

Glotz D, Sollazzo M, Riley S, Zanetti M (1988): Isotype, V_H genes, and antigen-binding analysis of hybridomas from newborn BALB/c mice. J Immunol 141: 383–390.

Guilbert B, Dighiero G, Avrameas S (1982): Naturally occurring antibodies against nine common antigens in humans—Detection, isolation and characterization. J Immunol 128:2779–2787.

Jerne NK (1974): Towards the network theory of the immune system. Ann Immunol Inst Pasteur (Paris) 125:373–389.

LaSalle J, Ota K, Hafler D (1991): Presentation of autoantigen by human T cells. J Immunol 147:774–780.

Mitchison A (1990): Unique features of the immune system: Their logical ordering and likely evolution. In Burger M, Sordat B, Zinkernagel R (eds): "Cell to Cell Interaction." Basel: Karger, pp 201–214.

Salk J (1983): "Anatomy of Reality: Merging of Intuition and Reason." New York: Columbia University Press.

Ternynck T, Avrameas S (1986): Murine natural monoclonal antibodies: a study of their polyspecificity and their affinities. Immunol Rev 94:99–112.

Varela F, Coutinho A (1991): Second generation immune networks. Immunol Today 12:159–166.

Zanetti M (1985): The idiotypic network in autoimmune processes. Immunol Today 6:299–302.

Zanetti M (1986): Idiotypic regulation of autoantibody production. CRC Crit Rev Immunol 6:151–183.

Zanetti M (1988): Self immunity and the autoimmune network: A molecular perspective to ontogeny and regulation of the immune system. Ann Immunol Inst Pasteur (Paris) 139:619–631.

Zanetti M (1992): Ontogeny of the immune system and the invisible frontier to immune regulation. Int Rev Immunol 8:209–218.

Zanetti M, Glotz D, Sollazzo M (1987): Idiotype regulation of self responses, autoantibody V regions and neonatal B cell repertoire. Immunol Lett 16:277–282.

Zanetti M, Mampaso F, Wilson CB (1983): Anti-idiotype as a probe in the analysis of autoimmune tubulointerstitial nephritis in the Brown Norway rat. J Immunol 131:1268–1273.

Zanetti M, Sollazzo M, Billetta R (1992): Functions and structures in a regulatory network for self-reactivity. In Bona C, Kaushik A (eds): "Molecular Immunobiology of Self-Reactivity." New York: Marcel Dekker, pp 221–238.

Zanetti M, Wilson C (1983): Characterization of anti-tubular basement membrane antibodies in rats. J Immunol 130:2173–2179.

10

LYMPHOCYTE POPULATION KINETICS: A CELLULAR COMPETITION MODEL

António A. Freitas and Benedita B. Rocha

*Unité d'Immunobiologie, Institut Pasteur (A.A.F.); INSERM U.345,
CHU Necker (B.B.R.), Paris, France*

O mundo dá tanta volta
Que a gente nem sabe já
Se, um terço do que hoje pensa
amanhã pensá-lo-á
—Ângelo de Lima

INTRODUCTION

As for any other organ or tissue of a multicellular organism the immune system is under a strict homeostatic control of cell numbers. From early development up to the adult age, lymphocyte populations increase in size. In the adult the total number of immunocompetent B and T cells remains constant in all lymphoid organs. A major question on population dynamics of the immune system is therefore related to the control of total lymphocyte numbers.

Autoimmunity: Physiology and Disease, Pages 143–160
© *1994 Wiley-Liss, Inc.*

HOMEOSTATIC CONTROL OF CELL NUMBERS

In the adult mice the size of the T- and B-lymphocyte compartments are maintained independently. The number of B cells is similar in either normal, thymectomized, athymic mice or in mice that lack T cells due to the deletion of TcR genes by homologous recombination (TcR KO) (S. Tonegawa, personal communication). In mice that lack B cells (mIgM KO) the number of T cells is similar to that in normal mice [Kitamura et al., 1991]. The numbers of TcR-gd and ab T cells is also independently kept. The TcR-gd compartment is of similar size in normal and in TcR-ab KO mice. Conversely, TcR-ab cells are present in similar numbers in TcR-gd KO mice (S. Tonegawa, personal communication).

The size of the peripheral T-cell pool is kept independently of the input of T cells into this compartment. In mice transplanted with up to 50 thymus lobes, the total T-cell pool does not increase significantly in size [Wallis et al., 1979]. Athymic nude mice injected with different numbers of T cells (ranging from 10^3 to 10^8) reconstitute their peripheral T cell compartment to a similar level [Rocha et al., 1989]. The total number of T cells in an adult mouse is independent of the input of CD4 or CD8 lymphocytes. Reconstitution of athymic nude mice with purified T-cell populations followed by anti-CD4 or anti-CD8 treatment [Rocha et al., 1989], and the analysis of β_2-microglobulin KO [Zijlstra et al., 1990], classII KO [Cosgrove et al., 1991], and CD4 KO mice [Rahemtulla et al., 1991] shows that in the absence of either of the two T-cell subsets, cell loss can be compensated by the remaining cellular subset and the total number of T cells remains similar to that of normal mice. Although dominance of one T-cell subset can occur in transgenic models [Hanaham, 1990], the ratio between CD4 and CD8 T lymphocytes is also under homeostatic control. Athymic mice reconstituted with peripheral T cells maintain a strain-specific CD4/CD8 ratio independently of the initial inoculum of each cell type [Rocha et al., 1989]. Female mice transgenic for the anti H-Y TcR show inverted CD4/CD8 ratios in the thymus, but have normal ratios in the periphery [von Boehmer, 1990].

The factors controling lymphocyte numbers may act independently of cell specificity. In mice with restricted repertoires, transgenic for complete immunoglobulin molecules, the number of mature peripheral lymphocytes, the vast majority (>95%) bearing transgenic molecules, does not differ very significantly from the number of B cells in normal mice [Weaver et al., 1985; Rusconi and Kohler, 1985; Grandien et al., 1990]. In TcR transgenic mice [von Boehmer, 1990; Weaver et al., 1985] or in athymic mice reconstituted with cells expressing a single Vβ specificity [Pereira and Rocha 1992], peripheral T-cell pools can be replenished with a restricted set of specificities.

Circulating steroids, growth factors, and interferon are likely to play an important role in regulating the total number of lymphoid cells. Steroid levels correlate with seasonal transient regression of lymphoid tissues in lower vertebrates [Rosenberg, 1978; Zapala et al., 1992]. Stress causes lymphocyte depletion [Rocha, 1985]. Adrenalectomy, ovariectomy, and castration induce the increase in the size of lymphocyte pools [Ishidate and Metcalf 1963; Eidinger and Garret, 1972], while pregnancy is associated with thymic atrophy and reduction of the number of lymphocytes in secondary lymphoid organs [Le Hoang Puc et al., 1981]. The aberrant expression of interferon regulatory factor 1 gene in transgenic mice leads to the reduction in the number of B cells [Yamada et al., 1991]. In contrast, the constitutive expression of the protooncogene bcl-2 in transgenic mice induces a four- to fivefold increase in the total numbers of lymphocytes [McDonnel et al., 1990].

The size of the lymphocyte pools can also be modulated by the environment. Germ-free mice have lower cell numbers than conventional mice [Pereira et al., 1986], and animals immunized with particulate ligands or parasites accommodate transiently higher lymphocyte numbers [Rosenberg, 1978].

LYMPHOCYTE POPULATION KINETICS

The homeostatic control of cell numbers implies, in the adult mouse, a kinetic steady state in which lymphocyte populations maintain a constant size, i.e., cell production equals cell death. The immune system must, however, adapt to changes in the environment through selection of appropriate clonal specificities. In the adult mouse, in which the total number of cells remains constant, selection of new specificities in all lymphoid compartments depends on the renewal rate of cells in that compartment. Renewal rate of cell populations depends on cell production and death within, as well as cell input and output from/to, other cellular compartments. All these parameters are reflected in the time that a cell survives inside a certain compartment, i.e., lymphocyte lifespan. Studies on population dynamics of lymphocytes evaluate all these parameters. They also study lymphocyte lifespans.

Production of Mature B- and T-Cell Populations in Precursor Pools

The total number, production, and flux of cells through the defined compartments of the percursor lymphocyte pools in the bone marrow and thymus have been determined with statmokinetic techniques [Opstelten and Osmond, 1983; Deenen et al., 1990] by following the incorporation of DNA precursors, such as BrdU and ^{3}H-thymidine [Landreth et al., 1981; Forster et al., 1989; Rocha et al., 1990] and by killing cycling cells [Freitas et al., 1982]. Most studies agree on the rates of lymphocyte production in central lymphoid organs, i.e., bone marrow and thymus.

In adult mice, the whole bone marrow organ produces 40–60 $\times$ 10^6 pre-B cells. Only part of these cells will complete maturation, and approximately 15–20 $\times$ 10^6 B cells are generated daily. The majority of newly produced B cells migrate to the peripheral lymphocyte pools [Rocha et al., 1990; Brahim and Osmond, 1970]. The bone marrow production is therefore sufficient to renew the peripheral pool of B lymphocytes every 4 days.

The thymus generates an average of 40×10^6 immature cells daily, but the number of mature single positive CD4$^+$ thymocytes produced every day is on the order of 3×10^6 [Rocha et al., 1990]. The number of mature cells reported to exit the thymus whithin the same time period is approximately 1×10^6 cells [Scollay et al., 1980].

The relative importance of de novo cell production in central lymphoid organs on the renewal of the mature peripheral lymphocyte pools will depend on the lifespan of mature B- and T-cell populations.

Lifespan of Mature Lymphocytes

Definitions of lymphocyte lifespans are complex and vary according to different conceptual and experimental systems. These differences can be summarized by the question: By *lifespan* do we mean that a cell dies at the end of its lifespan, or that it becomes two cells after its lifespan? These two definitions have different physiological significance, as well as limitations. The first does not consider that a clonal specificity may persist in vivo through continuous short-lived dividing cells. It does not distinguish clonal elimination from clonal expansion. The second does not consider that a clone may change after cell division. These changes may modify the behavior of a lymphocyte in response to the same stimulation. Different experimental approachs have been employed to define lifespans.

Rate of Cell Division. The concept that a cell becomes two cells has been the most commonly used approach to study lifespan of lymphocytes. The incorporation of labeled DNA precursors is taken as the index of cell division and the in vivo rate of accumulation (or clearing) of labeled cells is used to quantify the fraction of short- and long-lived cells in a population [Caffrey et al., 1962; Robinson et al., 1965; Everett and Tyler, 1967; Howard, 1972; Sprent and Basten, 1973; Ropke and Everett, 1975; Press et al., 1977; Rosse et al., 1978; Gray, 1988; Forster and Rajewsky, 1990; Crippen and Jones, 1989; Forster et al., 1989; Rocha et al., 1990]. Using these experimental approachs current lifespan estimates for peripheral mature lymphocytes vary according to different authors [Caffrey et al., 1962; Robinson et al., 1965; Everett and Tyler, 1967; Howard, 1972; Sprent and Basten, 1973; Ropke and Everett, 1975; Press et al., 1977; Rosse et al., 1978; Gray, 1988; Forster and Rajewsky, 1990; Crippen and Jones, 1989; Forster et al., 1989; Rocha et al., 1990]. These variations are in part due to the different cell types analyzed (e.g., total lymphoid populations or small lymphocytes) and the different protocols of administration of DNA precursors employed.

In summary, considering only studies on the accumulation or clearance of labeled cells in the spleen, and excluding those that involve surgical manipulation, which may induce nonspecific cell depletion due to stress [Rocha,

1985], two different views have emerged. One view, based on reports that show that 30%–60% of peripheral lymphocytes were labeled after 3–7 days [Everett and Tyler, 1967; Press et al., 1977; Rosse et al., 1978; Rocha et al., 1990; Crippen and Jones, 1989], claims that most peripheral lymphocytes have a relatively short lifespan [Rocha et al., 1990]. The second view, based on the findings that only 20%–30% of splenocytes were labeled after a time period of 2–3 weeks considers that the majority (70%) of mature lymphocytes are stable cellular populations with a lifespan longer than 2–4 weeks [Sprent and Basten, 1973; Gray, 1988; Forster et al., 1989; Forster and Rajewsky, 1990]. These results were obtained using different protocols of administration of DNA precursors and reflect the limitations of the experimental approach.

Lymphoid organs are mixtures of cells with different cycling times, dividing asynchronously. Studies on the accumulation of labeled cells require that, at any time point a lymphocyte is in the S phase of the cell cycle in vivo, the concentration of DNA precursors (that are rapidly cleared in vivo) present in circulation is sufficient to label it. The amount of DNA precursors incorporated by dividing cells must also be sufficient to discriminate the progeny of such cells, as the amount of incorporated DNA precursor diminishes with cell division. The mechanisms involved in the incorporation and processing of exogenous nucleotides are complex, imply competition with endogenous precursor pools, and vary according to cell type [Reichard, 1988; Cohen et al., 1983]. Exogenous nucleotides are incorporated through the salvage pathway, a process mediated by the tk enzyme, which competes with thymidylate monophosphatase of the de novo pathway of DNA synthesis [Haaskjold et al., 1988]. Lymphocytes differ in their relative usage of the salvage pathway [Cohen et al., 1983]. Exogenous nucleotides may label immature cells, which use predominantly the salvage pathway and fail to label mature lymphocytes in which the utilization of the de novo pathway predominates. Moreover, progressive incorporation of exogenous nucleotides induce cytotoxic effects due to changes in the intracellular pools of endogenous nucleotides, mimic the effects of cytostatic agents, and lead to the selective elimination of cycling cells and their progeny [Bianchi et al., 1986; Martin and Gelfand, 1981].

We conclude that these methods provide no more than minimal estimates of cell turnover. It is, however, of interest to report that only values of high turnover rates for peripheral mature B cells account for the rates of bone marrow B-cell production and export.

Persistence After Arrest of Cell Production. Cycling cells can be selectively eliminated in vivo by administration of cytostatic drugs. Cell production is blocked, and resting cells persist after treatment. The time of cell persistence has been used as a definition of lifespan [Freitas et al., 1982; Strober, 1972; Rozing et al., 1976; Rocha et al., 1983; Levy, 1985; Heyman, 1989].

Hydroxyurea, a cytostatic drug with a transient effect in vivo, which selectively eliminates all dividing cells, has been commonly used in this type of approach. This treatment leads to the depletion of approximately 40%–50% peripheral mature lymphocytes, 3 days after drug administration [Freitas et al., 1982; Rocha et al., 1983]. Similar results were obtained by treating mice transgenic for the *HSV-1 thymidine kinase* (*tk*) gene with the antiherpetic drug gancyclovir, a nucleoside analogue that is incorporated by cells in the S phase of the cell cycle [Heyman et al., 1989]. The *HSV-1 tk* transgene is under the control of the immunoglobulin k chain promoter and μ enhancer elements, which ensures its exclusive expression in B and T cells. This treatment obliterates lymphocyte prodution by selectively killing all dividing lymphoid cells and induces the disappearance of 65% T and 90% B lymphocytes within 7 days [Heyman et al., 1989].

Studies following cell persistence after cytostatic treatment are thus consistent with the view that most lymphoid cells have a short lifespan (i.e., have been recently produced). In contrast with methods employing the incorporation of DNA precursors, which label cycling cells exclusively through the salvage pathway, the use of cytostatic drugs leads to the elimination of cycling cells whatever the use of metabolic pathways of DNA synthesis. Nevertheless, cell deletion following cytostatic agents may be due to nonselective toxic effects. Although we have not detected toxicity to noncycling cells in the short schedules of hydroxyurea administration employed, this drug eliminates proliferating nonlymphoid cells and thus may induce general effects that could affect cell survival. The recent finding that gancyclovir affects solely lymphoid populations in the bone marrow without altering the numbers of nonlymphoid precursors [Heyman et al., 1989], together with the observation that its action can be fully reversed in vitro by thymidine [Oliver et al., 1985], seems to exclude possible nonselective effects of this treatment.

In general, these approachs suggest that continuous cell production is required to maintain the stable size of mature B- and T-cell populations. These methods do not allow us to discriminate if this cell production, required to maintain population sizes, takes place in the precursor pools of the bone marrow and thymus, or in the mature B- and T-cell compartments, in the periphery.

Persistence After Cell Transfer. Persistence of cells after transfer into histocompatible hosts can be used as a parameter to define lifespan of a population. The transferred cell population must bear a specific marker, absent in the new host, to allow its identification in the recipient. The cell input from precursor compartments into the transfered population is absent in the new host. Adoptive transfers thus are useful to establish the role of precursor populations in the turnover of more mature cells.

In contrast to the previous methods, cell transfers permit us to evaluate clonal persistence in vivo. They do not allow us to discriminate if clones are maintained in the periphery (because they are capable of self-renewal and divide continuously) or if they persist as long-lived, nondividing cells.

In adult mice, the fate of transferred mature B cells differs from that of mature T cells. In intact or irradiated hosts, and independently of the detection method used, donor B cells decay rapidly. By 7–10 days after transfer, approximately 60%–80% of the cells recovered initially at day 1 have disappeared from the host tissues [Park et al., 1985; Freitas and Coutinho, 1981; Freitas et al., 1986a,b; Udhayakumar et al., 1988; Goroff et al., 1989]. The remaining persisting 20%–40% B cells are able to persist with no decay upon a secondary transfer into normal host mice [Freitas et al., 1986a]. These results suggest that maintainence of peripheral B-cell pools in adult nonimmunized mice requires the continuous production and export from the bone marrow.

Transfer of peripheral mature T cells into either B-mice (thymectomized, lethally irradiated, bone marrow reconstituted) or athymic nude mice leads to the expansion and persistence of the donor T-cell populations in the adoptive hosts [Miller and Stutman, 1984; Rocha, 1987]. These results, together with studies on the effects of adult or neonatal thymectomy and studies on the kinetics of recovery of peripheral T-cell numbers in thymectomized mice following hydroxyurea treatment show that stable peripheral T-cell numbers can be maintained in the absence of the thymic precursor pool by continuous cell division at the periphery.

Cell transfer experiments have also shown that lymphocyte survival varies with environmental influences. Thus, while in intact or irradiated adult hosts most of the transferred B cells are lost shortly after transfer, in newborn hosts B cells transferred from adult donor mice can expand (at the same rate as host cells) and persist for 3–4 weeks, i.e., until these mice become adults [Thomas-Vaslin and Freitas, 1989]. Similarly, in severe combined immunodeficient (SCID) adult hosts a fraction of donor B cells can persist and increase in numbers up to 6 months after transfer [Sprent et al., 1991].

The extent of T-cell expansion, as well as the size of the peripheral T-cell pool after reconstitution with peripheral T cells, varies in different host mice. Thus purified $CD8^+$ cells do not expand after transfer into SCID hosts, even when these mice have also been injected with donor B lymphocytes [Rudolphi et al., 1991]. The extent of $CD4^+$ T-cell reconstitution in SCID mice is also inferior to that observed in other hosts [Rudolphi et al., 1991]. The total amount of T cells recovered from T-cell-reconstituted athymic nude recipients is half of that obtained after transfer into thymectomized, lethally irradiated, bone-marrow-reconstituted hosts (Rocha, unpublished observations). This may be due to the overall hormonal deficiency of nude mice [Pierpaoli and Sorkin, 1972] that conditions a smaller size of the T-cell pool.

Lymphocyte Renewal Rates

We conclude that reliable evaluations of the renewal rate of peripheral mature lymphocyte populations cannot be based solely on a single experimental strategy. It must involve a consensus of the several different definitions and take into consideration current estimates on the production and export of cells from the central lymphoid organs: the bone marrow and the thymus. Based on our own studies, using different strategies, and supported by other observations, we have suggested that about 30%–40% of peripheral immuno-competent B and T cells are renewed every 3 days and that 10 days will suffice for the renewal of most B (90%) and T (65%) lymphocytes.

The mechanisms of cell renewal differ for B and T cells. While B cells are renewed through continuous production and export from the precursor pool, T cells are mainly renewed by cell generation at the periphery. We speculate that the differential renewal of peripheral T and B cells is related to the properties of their differentiation sites. B cells develop in the open reticular frames of the bone marrow, and T cells mature in the closed environment of the thymus cortex where contact with extrathymic ligands is restricted, suggesting that newly formed T cells require further peripheral selection before fully adapted to the host. It is interesting to note that in birds, in which diversification of B cells occurs mainly in the closed environment of the bursa, peripheral mature B cells maintain self-renewal capabilities.

"Lifespan" Is Not a Predetermined Property of the Cell: At the Clonal Level, Lymphocyte Survival Is Determined By Selection

The relative sizes of the potential ($>10^9$), available ($<10^8$), and actual ($\sim 10^6$) lymphocyte repertoires and the dynamic properties of lymphocyte popula-tions (the high numbers of cells are continuously being produced in precursor pools, and the high turnover rates ensure the rapid substitution of the immu-nocompetent cell pool) suggest that (1) the immune system only uses a minor fraction of its potential diversity and (2) repertoires can be subject to continu-ous qualitative changes throughout life.

Studies on V_H gene family usage have shown that selection of immuno-globulin specificities occurs at multiple steps of B-cell differentiation: in the bone marrow at the pre-B cell stage, when a significant fraction of cells bearing 7183 V_H genes fails to complete maturation [Freitas et al., 1990], and at the periphery, where it is determined by cellular localization and interac-tions [Freitas et al., 1989a,b]. Studies using double transgenic mouse models also show B-cell selection in the bone marrow and peripheral compartments [Nemazee and Burki, 1989; Russel et al., 1991; Harley et al., 1991].

Cell transfer studies show that mature B-cell survival is influenced by selection. The disappearance of donor B cells transferred from immunoglob-ulin transgenic donor mice into major histocompatibility complex (MHC) host mice is more rapid than the disappearence of a heterogeneous population of B cells from normal donors (A.-C. Viale et al., in preparation). Studies on the differential decay of small and large activated LPS reactive cells, derived from either small resting or large activated donor B cells, have led us to suggest that B-cell longevity is an acquired property of lymphocytes that requires a preactivation step [Freitas et al., 1986a]. Transfer of mature B cells from immunized mice into irradiated hosts, if followed immediatly after transfer by appropriate challenge, results in the expansion and survival of donor cells [Moller, 1968]. The finding of a modified V_H gene family expression among long-lived B cells further demonstrates that the lifespan of B cells is determined by selection (A.-C. Viale et al., in press). Selection for persistence is likely to occur in the germinal centers [MacLennan et al., 1990] and may involve activation steps that prevent apoptosis through the induction of genes such as bcl-2 [Yamada et al., 1991; Strasser et al., 1991].

Selection of T-cell specificities also occurs at multiple steps of T-cell differentiation. The T-cell repertoire is shaped in the thymus, through negative and positive selection events [Huesman et al., 1991], which may involve differential kinetics. Further selection of T-cell repertoires occurs at the periphery. Selection of T-cell specificities in the peripheral pools involves the expansion of peripheral mature T cells, which is related to the presence of TcR specific ligands [Rocha and von Boehmer, 1991; Rocha, 1992], and also activation and expansion of mature T cells, which modifies considerably the representation of the T-cell specificities, initially selected in the thymus [Rocha and von Boehmer, 1991; Rocha, 1992].

The role of the thymus out-put in the turnover of mature T-cell populations in adult mice has yet to be established. Kinetic studies and sequential T-cell transfers into athymic hosts (Rocha, unpublished observations) show that in adult mice the peripheral T cell pool is permeable [Rocha et al., 1983, 1990]. Up to 50% of peripheral T cells can be substituted by new incoming cells.

These observations show that persistence of B and T lymphocytes is influenced by environmental selection. Thus it is not appropriate to define lymphocyte lifespan as a predetermined property of the cell, but rather to consider that lymphocytes, at different stages of differentiation, have a probability rate of survival that is continuously modulated by their interactions with the environment.

Immune System Shows a Competitive Selective Behavior That Has Been Described for Other Systems

In ecological systems the survival of different populations follows the rules of a selective competitive behavior [Eigen and Winkler, 1975; May, 1976]. The premises of such behavior have been defined. Adapted for the immune system, they postulate:

1. Each lymphocyte subclass may exist independently of the others. In other words, for the existence of a lymphocyte subclass, other lymphocyte subclasses are not necessary. This has been amply demonstrated in KO mice that lack different lymphocyte subclasses.

2. The size of each lymphocyte population is stable. The total number of lymphocytes is constant.

3. Lymphocytes of each subclass follow the same rules of recognition and activation and depend on the same growth and differentiation factors.

4. In each lymphocyte population there is continuous production of new elements.

5. New elements produced in precursor pools may integrate the mature T- and B-cell pool. Mature T- and B-cell pools are permeable and allow the incorporation of newly formed elements.

6. Cell survival in the precursor or mature pools is influenced by selection events.

CELLULAR COMPETITION

In an immune system in which there is a continuous renewal of immunocompetent cells and the total number of cells is under strict control, peripheral B- and T-cell repertoires will be shaped by the differential ability of lymphocytes to survive. Considering that the total number of cells is limited, each newly produced lymphocyte has to compete with other newly produced or resident cells for survival and/or differentiation. Selection is mediated by clonal distributed receptors and will depend on both the affinity and concentration of existing ligands and the presence of growth and differentiation factors. The relative role of each cell specie in the final repertoire will be determined not only by its relative number but also by its differential kinetics. In this context, each newly produced lymphocyte can only establish itself upon the loss or reduction of other cells. New cells may replace a less efficient variant provided that it has a selective advantage.

One of the consequences of competitive selective behavior is that it excludes a priori a pivotal role of stabilizing interactions among the different elements of the system. According to the above postulates, each lymphocyte specificity may also exist independently of the others. Network interactions exist and shape repertoires, as mutualistic interactions and exploitation (predator–prey) relationships do, but are not essential for the establishment of the system.

AUTOIMMUNITY

A model of competitive selective behavior for the immune system changes current concepts of autoimmunity. Let us consider two concrete examples: Sakagushi's experiments and the lpr mutant mouse.

In the case of Sakagushi's experiments, neonatal thymectomy in mice results in organ-specific autoimmune diseases that can be corrected by the transfer of lymphocytes from normal donors [Sakaguchi et al., 1982a,b]. A clonal competition model suggests the following interpretation: In normal mice accumulation of newly formed T-cell specificities occurs for the first 3–4 weeks of life [Kelly and Scollay, 1992] and evolves thereafter with the permanent renewal of peripheral T-cell populations. In the adult, the T-cell repertoire consists of 10^7 or more different clones competing with each other to a total of $1-2 \times 10^8$ T cells. In this case, the homeostatic control of cell numbers and the continuous influx of newly formed cells abrogates large clonal expansions. In contrast, neonatal thymectomized mice develop a T-cell repertoire that is restricted and fixed by the initial number of cells present at birth [Smith et al., 1989], i.e., a maximum of 10^3 different clones.

These mature T cells are further selected in the periphery by their reactivity toward environmental ligands, self or other, and expand to form a total of 5×10^7 T cells in the adult. Thus in the case of neonatal thymectomized mice each T-cell clone present at birth may, in the absence of competition by other newly formed cells, reach a size of 10^5 or more cells in the adult. This pauciclonality, which varies according to the different mouse strains depending on the number of T cells present in the periphery at birth, increases the probability of the dominance and fixation of clones that can induce pathology, even upon transfer into appropriate recipient mice. Transfer of disease, however, will only occur if the cells are transferred into mice where they can keep their selective advantage, i.e., noenatal or athymic hosts with restricted T-cell repertoires and bearing the appropriate ligand, but not into intact adult hosts [Sakaguchi et al., 1982a]. The immune system is permeable, and autoimmunity can be prevented or reverted upon transfer of T cells from normal adult mice. Donor T cells, however, can only prevent disease and compete successfuly with host T cells if they are transferred in large numbers [Sakaguchi et al., 1982b]. The diversity of clones reacting with the variety of ligands present in the same tissue provides control against clonal dominance and pathology. Pauciclonality may favor, but is not sufficient for, establishment of disease. Conversely autoimmunity is not solely related to oligoclonality.

The lpr mutant mouse shows an "lupus-like" autoimmune process that can be mapped to a single gene, located on chromosome 19, which codes for the Fas cell surface antigen [Watanabe-Fukunaga et al., 1992]. These mice develop lymphadenopathy with accumulation of a nonmalignant population of double-negative T cells. This is accompanied by hypergammaglobulinemia and increased serum levels of rheumathoid factors and antibodies directed against single-stranded DNA [Cohen and Eisenberg, 1991]. We suggest the following chain of events to explain pathology: Lack of expression of the Fas antigen modifies T-cell differentiation and selection in the thymus, changes the adhesion properties of thymocytes, and allows the exit of a population of $CD4^-CD8^-$ lymphocytes. These immature $CD4^-CD8^-TcR^+$ cells have been shown to express preferentially Vβ 8.2 genes [Fowlkes et al., 1987]. The TcR-expressing immature cells are selected in the periphery by ligands, self or other, and in the absence of competing mature T cells accumulate progressively by escaping normal homeostatic control of cell numbers that may involve apoptosis [Watanabe-Fukunaga et al., 1992]. Although with an immature cell surface phenotype these cells show helper functions [Sobel et al.,

1991] and induce polyclonal activation of B cells and hypergammaglobulinemia, B-cell activation is, however, selective for lymphocytes with the lpr phenotype [Sobel et al., 1991], suggesting that the altered cellular phenotype either gives a survival advantage to activated lpr B cells or facilitates a homophilic interaction with T cells of the same lpr phenotype. Increased serum immunoglobulin levels diminish B cell production in the bone marrow [Sundblad et al., 1991; Freitas et al., 1991], decrease peripheral B-cell renewal, and confer a definite selective advantage to a restricted set of peripheral B-cell clones, leading to the observed oligoclonality [Shlomchik et al., 1987a,b]. Since B cells are selected by environmental ligands and considering both the hypergammaglobulinemia and the increased cell numbers, the preferential increase in both rheumathoid factors and anti-DNA hypermutated antibodies is not surprising [Shlomchik et al., 1987a,b]. Methods of immunostimulation that induce polyclonal activation of T cells can reestablish normal cell competition by mature single positive cells, abrogate dominance of the $CD4^-CD8^-TcR^+$ cells, and prevent disease [Gutierrez-Ramos et al., 1990]. Based on the cellular competition model, two predictions can be made:

1. Autoimmunity correlates with immunodeficiency. In fact, restricted lymphocyte repertoires determine higher fluctuations in clonal frequencies that may increase the probability for the expansion and fixation of clones which in the absence of competition will become irreversibily dominant and induce pathology.

2. Immunostimulation should often offer a better prognosis for therapeutics than immunosuppression. In fact, the nonspecific polyclonal activation of lymphocytes is more likely capable of disrupting the pathological equilibrium established by favoring the growth and competition by underrepresented specificities rather than by immunodepression, which by suppressing all cells can only reinforce the already established clonal drift.

It should be noted that immunopathology will depend not only on the number and size of dominant clones, but also on the amount and distribution of the antigen and on the target tissue susceptibility, which will vary according to individuals and within the same individual with time and previous experience.

ACKNOWLEDGMENTS

We thank Drs. Alf Grandien, Delphine Guy-Grand, Alberto Nobrega, Anne Sundblad, and Caroline Tucek for discussions, suggestions, and reviews of the manuscript. We particularly thank Anne-Claire Viale for suggestions and for letting us quote her unpublished results.

REFERENCES

Bianchi V, Pontis E, Reichard P (1986): Interrelations between substrate cycles and de novo synthesis of pyrimidine deoxyribonucleoside triphosphates in 3T6 cells. Proc Natl Acad Sci USA 83:986.

Brahim F, Osmond D (1970): Migration of bone marrow lymphocytes demonstrated by selective bone marrow labelling with ^{3}H-thymidine. Anat Rec 168:139.

Caffrey RW, Rieke WO, Everett NB (1962): Radioautographic studies of small lymphocytes in the thoracic duct of the rat. Acta Haematol 28:145–154.

Cohen A, Barankiewicz J, Lederman HM, Gelfand EW (1983): Purine and pyrimidine metabolism in human T lymphocytes. J Biol Chem 258:12334.

Cohen PL, Eisenberg RA (1991): *lpr* and *gld:* single gene models of systemic autoimmunity and lymphoproliferative disease. Annu Rev Immunol 9:243.

Cosgrove D, Gray D, Dierich A, Kaufman J, Lemeur M, Benoist C, Mathis D (1991): Mice lacking MHC Class II molecules. Cell 66:1051–1066.

Crippen TL, Jones IM (1989): Cell proliferation in the bone marrow, thymus and spleen of mice studied by continuous, in vivo bromedeoxycycydine labelling and flow cytometric analysis. Cell Tissue Kinet 22:203.

Deenen GJ, van Balen I, Opstelten D (1990): In rat B lymphocyte genesis sixty percent is lost from the bone marrow at the transition of nondividing pre-B cell to sIgM+ B lymphocyte, the stage of Ig light chain expression. Eur J Immunol 20:557.

Eidinger D, Garret TJ (1972): Studies of the regulatory effects of the sex hormones on antibody formation and stem cell differentiation. J Exp Med 136:1098.

Eigen M, Winkler R (1975): "Das Spiel. Naturgesetze Steuern den Zufall." Munchen: R. Piper & Co, Verlag.

Everett NB, Tyler RW (1967): Lymphopoiesis in the thymus and other tissues: functional implications. Int Rev Cytol 22:205.

Förster I, Rajewsky K (1990): The bulk of the peripheral B-cell pool in mice is stable and not rapidly renewed from the bone marrow. Proc Natl Acad Sci USA 87:4781.

Förster I, Vieira P, Rajewsky K (1989): Flow cytometric analysis of cell proliferation dynamics in the B cell compartment of the mouse. Int Immunol 1:321.

Fowlkes BJ, Kruisbeek AM, Ton-That H, Weston MA, Coligan JE, Schwartz RH, Pardoll DM (1987): A novel population of T-cell receptor ab-bearing thymocytes which predominantly express a single Vb family. Nature 329:251.

Freitas AA, Andrade L, Lembezat MP, Coutinho A (1990): Selection of VH gene repertoires: differentiating B cells of adult bone marrow mimic fetal development. Int Immunol 2:15–23.

Freitas AA, Coutinho A (1981): Very rapid decay of mature B lymphocytes in the spleen. J Exp Med 154:994.

Freitas AA, Lembezat MP, Coutinho A (1989a): Expression of antibody V-regions is genetically and developmentally controled and modulated by the B lymphocyte environment. Int Immunol 1:342–354.

Freitas AA, Lembezat MP, Rocha B (1989b): Selection of antibody repertoires. Transfer of mature T lymphocytes modifies VH gene family usage in the actual and available B cell repertoires of athymic nude mice. Int Immunol 1:398–408.

Freitas AA, Rocha B, Coutinho A (1986a): Lymphocyte population kinetics in the mouse. Immunol Rev 91:5.

Freitas AA, Rocha B, Coutinho A (1986b): Two major classes of mitogen-reactive B lymphocytes defined by life-span. J Immunol 136:466.

Freitas AA, Rocha B, Forni L, Coutinho A (1982): Population dynamics of B lymphocytes and their precursors: demonstration of high turnover in the central and peripheral lymphoid organs. J Immunol 128:54.

Freitas AA, Viale A-C, Sundblad A, Heusser C, Coutinho A (1991): Normal serum immunoglobulins participate in the selection of peripheral B cell repertoires. Proc Natl Acad Sci USA 88:5640.

Goroff DK, Finkelman FD (1989): Life span of mature BALB/c B cells in allotype congenic CB20 mice. 7th Int Cong Immunol, Gustav Fisher Verlag, p 262.

Grandien A, Coutinho A (1990): Andersson, J. Selective peripheral expansion and activation of B cells expressing endogenous immunoglobulin in mu-transgenic mice. Eur J Immunol 20:991.

Gray D (1988): Population kinetics of rat peripheral B cells. J Exp Med 167:805.

Gutierrez-Ramos JC, Andreu JL, Revila Y, Vinuela E, Martinez AC (1990): Recovery from autoimmunity of MRL/lpr mice after infection with an interleukin-2/vaccinia recombinant virus. Nature 271:346.

Haaskjold E, Refsum SB, Bjerknes R, Paulsen TO (1988): The labelling index is not always reliable. Discrepancies between the labelling index and the mitotic rate in the rat corneal epithelium after intraperitoneal and topical administration of tritiated thymidine and colcemid. Cell Tissue Kinet 21:389.

Hanaham D (1990): Transgenic mouse models of self-tolerance and autoreactivity by the immune system. Annu Rev Cell Biol 6:493.

Hartley SB, Crosbie J, Brink R, Kantor AB, Basten A, Goodnow CC (1991): Elimination from peripheral lymphoid tissues of self-reactive B lymphocytes recognizing membrane-bound antigens. Nature 353:765–769.

Heyman RA, Borreli E, Lesley J, Anderson D, Richman DD, Baird SM, Hyman R, Evans RM (1989): Thymidine kinase obliteration: creation of transgenic mice with controlled immune deficiency. Proc Nat Acad Sci USA 86:2698.

Howard J (1972): The lifespan and recirculation of marrow derived small lymphocytes from the rat thoracic duct. J Exp Med 135:185.

Huesman M, Scott B, Kisielow P, von Boehmer H (1991): Kinetics and efficacy of positive selection in the thymus of normal and T cell receptor transgenic mice. Cell 66:533.

Ishidate M, Metcalf D (1963): The pattern of lymphopoiesis in the mouse thymus after cortisone treatment or adrenalectomy. Austral J Exp Biol 41:637.

Kelly KA, Scollay R (1992): Seeding of neonatal lymph nodes by T cells and identification of a novel population of $CD3^-CD4^+$ cells. Eur J Immunol 22:329.

Kitamura D, Roes J, Kuhn P, Rajewsky K (1991): A B-cell deficient mouse by targeted disruption of the membrane exon of the immunoglobulin mu chain gene. Nature 350:423–426.

Landreth KS, Rosse C, Clagett J (1981): Myelogeneous production and maturation of B lymphocytes in the mouse. J Immunol 127:2027.

Le Hoang Phuc, Papiernik M, Dardenne M (1981): Thymic involution in pregnant mice. II. Functional aspects of the remaining thymocytes. Clin Exp Immunol 44:253.

Levy M (1985): Long-lived lymphocytes include lipopolysaccharide-reactive B cells. Cell Immunol 96:290.

MacLennan ICM, Liu Y-J, Oldfield S, Zhang J, Lane PJL (1990): The evolution of B-cell clones. Curr Top Microbiol Immunol 159:37.

Martin DW, Gelfand EW (1981): Biochemistry of diseases of immunodevelopment. Annu Rev Biochem 50:845.

May RM (1976): Simple mathematical models with very complicated dynamics. Nature 261:459–467.

McDonnel TJ, Nunez G, Platt FM, Hockenberry D, London L, McKearn JP, Korsmeyer SJ (1990): Mol Cell Biol 10:1901–1907.

Miller RA, Stutman O (1984): T cell repopulation from functionally restricted splenic progenitors: 10,000 fold expansion documented by using limiting dilution analysis. J Immunol 133:2925.

Möller G (1968): Regulation of cellular antibody synthesis. Cellular 7S production and longevity of 7S antigen-sensitive cells in the absence of antibody feedback. J Exp Med 127:291.

Nemazee D, Burki K (1989): Clonal deletion of B lymphocytes in a transgenic mouse bearing anti-MHC Class I antibody gene. Proc Nat Acad Sci USA 86:8039–8043.

Oliver S, Bubley G, Crumpacker C (1985): Inhibition of HSV-transformed murine cells by nucleoside analogs, 2'-NDG and 2'-nor-cGMP: mechasnisms of inhibition and reversal by exogenous nucleosides. Virology 145:84–93.

Opstelten D, Osmond D (1983): Pre-B cells in mouse bone marrow: immunofluorescence stathmokinetic studies of the proliferation of cytoplasmic mu-chain-bearing cells in normal mice. J Immunol 131:2635.

Park Y-H, Yoshida Y, Uchino H, Inaba MM, Masuda T (1985): Migration and differentiation of bone marrow lymphocytes: development of surface immunoglobulin, Fc receptor, complement receptor and functional responsiveness as studied with anti-allotype serum. Cell Immunol 93:58.

Pereira P, Rocha B (1992): Post-thymic in vivo expression of mature $\alpha\beta$ T cells. Int Immunol 3:1077–1080.

Pereira P, Forni L, Larsson E-L, Cooper M, Heusser C, Coutinho A (1986): Autonomous activation of B and T cells in antigen-free mice. Eur J Immunol 16:685–691.

Pierpaoli W, Sorkin E (1972): Alterations of adrenal cortex and thyroid in mice with congenital absence of the thymus. Nature [New Biol] 238:282.

Press OW, Rosse C, Clagett J (1977): The distribution of rapidly and slowly renewed T, B, and "null" lymphocytes in the mouse bone marrow, thymus, lymph nodes and spleen. Cell Immunol 33:114.

Rahemtulla A, Fung-Leung WP, Schilham MW, Kundig TM, Sambhara SR, Narendram A, Arabian A, Wakeman A, Paige CJ, Zinkernagel RM, Miler RG, Mak TW (1991): Normal development and function of CD8$^+$ cells but markedly decreased helper cell activity in mice lacking CD4. Nature 353:180–184.

Reichard P (1988): Interactions between deoxyribonucleotide and DNA synthesis. Annu Rev Biochem 57:349.

Robinson SH, Brecher G, Lourie IS, Haley JE (1965): Leucocyte labelling in rats during and after continuous infusion of tritiated thymidine: implications for leucocyte longevity and DNA reutilization. Blood 26:281.

Rocha B, Freitas AA, Coutinho A (1983): Population dynamics of T lymphocytes. Renewal rate and expansion in the peripheral lymphoid organs. J Immunol 131:2158.

Rocha B (1985): The effects of stress in normal and adrenalectomized mice. Eur J Immunol 15:1131.

Rocha B (1987): Population kinetics of precursors of Il-2 producing T lymphocytes: evidence for short life expectancy, continuous renewal and post-thymic expansion. J Immunol 139:365.

Rocha B, Dautigny N, Pereira P (1989): Peripheral T lymphocytes: expansion potential and homeostatic regulation of pool sizes and CD4/CD8 ratios "in vivo". Eur J Immunol 19:905.

Rocha B, Penit C, Baron C, Vasseur F, Dautigny N, Freitas AA (1990): Accumulation of bromodeixyuridine-labeled cells in central and peripheral lymphoid organs: minimal estimates of production and turnover rates of mature lymphocytes. Eur J Immunol 20:1697–1708.

Rocha B, von Boehmer H (1991): Peripheral selection of the T cell repertoire. Science 251:1225.

Rocha B (1992): Peripheral tolerance. Res Immunol 143:299.

Ropke C, Everett NB (1975): Life span of small lymphocytes in the thymolymphatic tissues of normal and thymus-deprived BALB/c mice. Anat Rec 183:83.

Rosenberg YF (1978): Autoimmune and polyclonal B cell responses during murine malaria. Nature 274:170.

Rosse C, Cole SB, Appleton C, Press OW, Clagett J (1978): The relative importance of the bone marrow and spleen in the production and dissemination of B lymphocytes. Cell Immunol 37:254.

Rozing J, Buurman WA, Benner R (1976): B lymphocyte differentiation in lethally irradiated and reconstituted mice. I. Effect of strontium-89 induced bone marrow aplasia on the recovery of the B cell compartment in the spleen. Cell Immunol 24:79.

Rudolphi A, Spiess S, Conradt P, Claesson MH, Reiman J (1991): CD3[+] T cells in severe combined immunodeficiency (scid) mice. II. Transplantation of dm2 lymphoid cells into semi-allogenic scid mice. Eur J Immunol 21:1591.

Rusconi S, Kohler G (1985): Transmission and expression of a specific pair of rearranged immunoglobulin m and k genes in a transgenic mouse line. Nature 314:330.

Russel DM, Dembic Z, Morahan G, Miller JAFP, Burki K, Nemazee D (1991): Peripheral deletion of self-reactive B cells. Nature 354:308–311.

Sakaguchi S, Takahashi T, Nishizuka Y (1982a): Study on cellular events in postthymectomy autoimmune oophoritis in mice. I. Requirement of lyt-1 effector cells for oocytes damage after adoptive transfer. J Exp Med 156:1565.

Sakaguchi S, Takahashi T, Nishizuka Y (1982b): Study on the cellular events in postthymectomy autoimmune oophoritis. II. Requirement of Lyt-1 cells in normal female mice for the prevention of oophoritis. J Exp Med 156:1577.

Scollay RG, Butcher EC, Weissman I (1980): Thymus cell migration. Quantitative aspects of cellular traffic from the thymus to the periphery in mice. Eur J Immunol 10:210.

Shlomchik MJ, Aucoin AH, Pisetsky DS, Weigert M (1987a): Structure and function of anti-DNA autoantibodies derived from a single autoimmune mouse. Proc Nat Acad Sci USA 84:9150.

Shlomchik MJ, Marshak-Rothstein A, Wolfowicz CB, Rothstein TL, Weigert M (1987b): The role of clonal selection and somatic mutation in autoimmunity. Nature 328:805.

Smith H, Chen I-M, Kubo R, Tung KSK (1989): Neonatal thymectomy results in a repertoire enriched in T cells deleted in adult thymus. Science 245:749.

Sobel ES, Katagiri T, Katagiri K, Morris SC, Cohen PL, Eisenberg RA (1991): An intrinsic B cell defect is required for the production of autoantibodies in the *lpr* model of murine systemic autoimmunity. J Exp Med 173:1441.

Sprent J, Basten A (1973): Circulating T and B lymphocytes of the mouse. II. Life-span. Cell Immunol 7:40.

Sprent J, Schaefer M, Hurd M, Surh D, Ron Y (1991): Mature murine B and T cells transferred to SCID mide can survive indefinitely and may maintain a virgin phenotype. J Exp Med 174:717–728.

Strasser A, Harris A, Cory S (1991): bcl-2 Transgene inhibits T cell death and perturbs thymic self-censorship. Cell 67:889–899.

Strober S (1972): Initiation of antibody responses by different classes of lymphocytes. V fundamental changes in the physiological characteristics of virgin thymus-independent (''B'') lymphocytes and ''B'' memory cells. J Exp Med 136:851–861.

Sundblad A, Marcos M, Huetz F, Freitas AA, Heusser C, Portnoi D, Coutinho A (1991): Normal serum immunoglobulins regulates the numbers of bone marrow pre-B and B cells. Eur J Immunol 21:1155.

Thomas-Vaslin V, Freitas AA (1989): Lymphocyte population kinetics during the development of the immune system. B cell persistence and life span can be determined by the host environment. Int Immunol 1:237–246.

Udhayakumar V, Goud SN, Subarao B (1988): Physiology of murine B lymphocytes. I. Life-spans of anti-mu and hapteneted Ficoll (thymus-independent antigen)-reactive B cells. Eur J Immunol 18:1593

Von Boehmer H (1990): Developmental biology of T cells in T cell-receptor transgenic mice. Annu Rev Immunol 8:531.

Wallis VJ, Leuchars E, Chauduri H, Davies AJS (1979): Studies on hyperlymphoid mice. Immunology 38:163.

Watanabe-Fukunaga R, Brannan CI, Copeland NG, Jenkins NA, Nagata S (1992): Lymphoproliferation disorder in mice explained by defects in Fas antigen that mediates apoptosis. Nature 356:314.

Weaver D, Costantini F, Imanishi-Kari T, Baltimore D (1985): A transgenic immuno-globulin μ gene prevents rearrangement of endogenous genes. Cell 42:117.

Yamada G, Ogawa M, Akagi K, Miyamoto H, Nakano N, Itoh S, Miyazaki J-I, Nishikawa S-I, Yamamura K-I, Tanaguchi T (1991): Specific depletion of the B-cell population induced by aberrant expression of human interferon regulatory factor 1 gene in transgenic mice. Proc Nat Acad Sci USA 88:532–536.

Zapata AG, Varas A, Torroba M (1992): Seasonal variations in the immune system of lower vertebrates. Immunol Today 13:142–144.

Zijlstra M, Bix M, Simister NE, Loring JM, Raulet D, Jaenisch R (1990): β2-microglobulin deficient mice lack CD4$^-$8$^+$ cytolytic T cells. Nature 344:742–746.

11

POSTTHYMIC
T-LYMPHOCYTE
POPULATION DYNAMICS
IN MOUSE AND MAN

Lisa J. Glickstein and Osias Stutman

*Immunology Program, Memorial Sloan-Kettering Cancer Center,
New York, New York*

INTRODUCTION

Since our last review on the subject of T-cell population dynamics [Stutman, 1986a], it may be argued that the mechanisms concerning T-cell development and especially maintenance of the T-cell pool remain undefined. Only limited aspects of these issues have been addressed experimentally in mice, and, although our knowledge about the behavior of individual or cloned T cells has progressed significantly at both the biological and biochemical levels, the sociology of the interactions between T cells remains elusive. Furthermore, as will be discussed briefly at the end of this chapter, our understanding of the homeostatic T-cell population dynamics in humans is even more fragmentary.

In the present text, *T cells* means predominantly cells that utilize α–β-chains of the T receptor for antigen (TCR), and *periphery* means spleen and lymph nodes (and to a lesser extent blood and thoracic duct lymph), thus excluding the T cells that utilize γ–δ TCR chains, as well as

Autoimmunity: Physiology and Disease, Pages 161–172
© *1994 Wiley-Liss, Inc.*

the mucosa or skin-associated T cells. There is agreement that T cells develop mainly by the intrathymic processing of prethymic hemopoietic precursors that migrate to the thymus and act as direct precursors of the postthymic compartment of exported T cells in periphery [Stutman, 1977, 1978]. The inefficient extrathymic generation of T cells, as is the case in nude mice and other models, probably has a limited impact under normal physiological conditions [Stutman, 1986a].

In the most general terms, it may be stated that the mechanisms for development and maintenance of the peripheral T-cell pool in mice include three main components [Stutman, 1977, 1978, 1985, 1986a]: 1) thymus import and export, 2) postthymic expansion (of recent thymic migrants), and 3) thymus-independent postthymic renewal [Stutman, 1986a,b; Miller and Stutman, 1982, 1984]. Even at the peak of thymic export and with the most conservative estimates of T-cell loss, thymic export alone seems to be incapable of maintaining homeostatic levels of T cells in periphery [Stutman, 1986a]. These three components participate differently during ontogeny, adult life, and aging. During ontogeny, thymus export is predominant during the first 3–6 perinatal weeks [Stutman 1986a,b; Ishizaka and Stutman, 1983; Scollay et al., 1980, 1986], with important thymus-dependent postthymic expansion [Stutman 1986a; Miller and Stutman, 1982, 1984]. During most of adult life, thymus export is reduced to a minimal but detectable component [Scollay et al., 1980; Stutman, 1986a,b], and T-cell homeostasis is mediated by a predominantly thymus-independent postthymic expansion in periphery [Stutman 1986a,b; Miller and Stutman 1982, 1984; Freitas et al., 1986; Rocha, 1987, 1990; Bell et al., 1987; Rocha et al., 1989; Pereira and Rocha, 1991].

One paradox of the T-cell system is that at the time that Dante calls the "highest point of this arch" (*Convivio* IV, 23, 9) or "midway in the journey of our life" (*Divina Comedia* I.1), which is between the 30th and 40th years, the human thymus contains only about 20% of its original cortex-medulla; the rest is fat [Boyd, 1932]. Similarly, at 1 year of age, a bit less than the midway point in the life span of a CBA/H mouse [Stutman, 1974], the thymus exports about 40,000 cells per day, as opposed to the 1–2 million cells per day at 1 month of age [Stutman, 1986a,b]. However, neither this thymic atrophy nor the decline in thymic export seem to affect the overall function of the T-cell system at those ages nor produce important changes in the size and composition of the peripheral T-cell pool in humans or mice [summarized by Thoman and Weigle, 1989]. One may add that neither the 35–40-year-old normal human nor the 1-year-old normal CBA/H mouse can be considered "old" and certainly will score as immunologically normal in all tests. Thus one may conclude that, once it has been formed by thymus processing, the postthymic peripheral T-cell pool behaves in an autonomous, thymus-independent fashion and seems to require limited (if any) input of new thymus-exported T cells. However, it is worth noting that the fraction of exported thymocytes at the 1 month peak of export is about 1% [Scollay et al., 1980; Stutman, 1986b], while at 1 year of age, when the thymus is exporting about 10^4 cells per day, that fraction represents actually 7%–8% of the total thymocyte population [Stutman, 1986b]. In other words, during the export trickle of the young adult age the thymus is exporting a higher fraction of its available thymocytes than at the peak of export.

PERIPHERAL T-CELL HOMEOSTASIS IN MICE

Thymus-Independent Peripheral Renewal

Maintenance of homeostasis in the peripheral T-cell pool in adult mice has been shown to be a thymus-independent process [Stutman, 1986a]. Direct evidence that peripheral T cells could expand and be maintained in the absence of thymic input came from experiments using postthymic adult peripheral T cells from normal mice injected into T-deficient syngeneic hosts. These studies showed that the postthymic T cells could expand in B mice (thymectomized, lethally irradiated, and reconstituted with T-depleted marrow) [Miller and Stutman, 1982, 1984; Stutman, 1986a], syngeneic nude mice [Rocha, 1987], syngeneic nude rats [Bell et al., 1987], and C.B.17 *scid/scid* mice [Rudolphi et al., 1991a] in the absence of thymic input. These type of results were also predicted from studies using hydroxyurea (HU), which selectively kills all cycling cells during DNA replication and is rapidly eliminated from the circulation [Hodgson et al., 1975], which showed that thymectomized mice treated with HU exhibited a T-cell recovery comparable with that seen in normal or sham-thymectomized controls [Rocha et al., 1983].

After initial seeding from the thymus, maintenance of homeostasis in the periphery could be due to either of two mechanisms: 1) the majority of peripheral T cells could be long-lived or 2) there could be constant renewal of cells at the periphery. Much early work labeling T cells with tritiated thymidine or BrdUrd as DNA precursors gave highly variable estimates of percentages of short-lived (the number of cells labeling after a single pulse or a short series of injections) and long-lived cells (the number of labeled cells remaining some time after label removal). This variability was later accounted for by toxicity of the substances used, reutilization of label, and inefficiency of labeling cycling peripheral lymphoid cells [Rocha et al., 1990]. Of particular significance, mature lymphoid cells utilize a de novo pathway to synthesize DNA precursors to a larger extent than the salvage pathway and therefore exhibit an unusually low labeling efficiency. Also, many experimental protocols involved administering BrdUrd orally. This was shown to increase the rate of debromination in the liver, which in turn prevented visualization by the anti-BrdUrd reagents. All of these factors have contributed to low estimates of the number of cycling T cells in the periphery. Experiments maximizing labeling efficiency [Rocha et al., 1990] and those utilizing HU to remove cycling cells [Rocha et al., 1983] result in renewal rates of 30%–40% of the peripheral T-cell pool every 24–48 hours.

The balance of evidence weighs in favor of the second hypothesis of considerable peripheral expansion. The earliest experiments using B mice demonstrated that engraftment of syngeneic T cells was possible with limiting numbers of donor cells [Miller and Stutman, 1982, 1984] as tested by the presence of allospecific cytotoxic T lymphocyte (CTL) precursors, that the frequency of the CTL progenitors for a given haplotype was about 1 per 10^5 T cells, and that these postthymic cells could increase 10,000-fold in the recipients in the absence of allogeneic antigenic stimulation. Furthermore, as predicted from the CTL progenitor frequencies, in mice injected with $1–5 \times 10^5$ T cells, some were repopulated clonally with single progenitor for a given allogeneic specificity, in other words, could be sensitized to generate CTL to only one allogeneic specificity [Miller and Stutman, 1984]. These limiting dilution in vivo experiments gave strong evidence against equal division of all injected cells and led to the proposal of the existence of progenitor cells responsible for maintenance of normal cell numbers [Stutman, 1986a] and also suggested that expansion was independent of conventional antigenic stimulation [Miller and Stutman, 1984].

T cells were also shown to have great expansion potential (probably close to a factor of 10^{-8}) in syngeneic nude mice, even after serial passages into new hosts [Rocha, 1987]. Markers used to examine the expansion at a subset level include alloresponsiveness [Miller and Stutman, 1984], interleukin-2p or CTLp frequency [Rocha, 1987], or staining for surface proteins such as CD4 and CD8 [Rocha et al., 1989; Rudolphi et al., 1991a,b]. Only limiting dilution experiments [Miller and Stutman, 1984; Rocha et al., 1989] allow determination of anything other than maximum or minimum numbers of divisions following adoptive transfer of T cells. The signal for peripheral expansion also remains unknown. Antigen-driven expansion can be shown to occur [Rocha and von Boehmer, 1991], and some therefore conclude that cells with a virgin phenotype have not divided recently [Sprent et al., 1991]. However, T cells possess many other surface proteins in addition to the T-cell receptor, and the postulation of a ligand internal to the immune system driving expansion of T cells in periphery in a T-cell-receptor-independent manner is certainly plausible. Surface proteins that, based on gene structure, show cytoplasmic domains with the capacity to activate T cells and for which internal ligands expressed on non-T cells are defined, such as CD2 and CD28, have been described in mice and humans. Thus the possibility of selected but polyclonal T-cell proliferation triggered by nonconventional signals that are independent of the conventional T-cell antigen receptor are certainly a possibility.

Expansion Kinetics

Expansion of T cells in the periphery has been studied in four different systems: 1) recovery from treatment with HU [Rocha et al., 1983], 2) adoptive transfer into B-mice [Miller and Stutman 1982, 1984], 3) adoptive transfer into nude mice [Rocha, 1987, 1990; Rocha et al., 1989; Rocha and von Boehmer, 1991], and 4) adoptive transfer into SCID mice [Rudolphi et al., 1991a,b; Reimann et al., 1991a; Sprent et al., 1991; Sunshine et al., 1991; Claesson et al., 1991; Tschnerning et al., 1991; reviewed by Reimann et al., 1991b]. Although the donor cells in all cases were from normal adult mice, engraftment differed in terms of rate of expansion, the eventual plateau number of cells reached, and the behavior of the CD4 and CD8 single positive (SP) subsets.

Plating efficiency determines the number of T-cell progenitors in adoptive transfer systems that home to a location favoring engraftment. By definition, plating efficiency is 100% in the HU experiments. Plating efficiency may be affected by the condition of the recipient organs (i.e., possibly damaged by irradiation in the B-mice; possible temporary refractoriness to engraftment in nude mice), the treatment of the cells before injection, and the route of administration (i.p. vs. i.v.). For example, a commonly made assumption is that the lymphoid organs of the host are permanently receptive to the injected cells, although the lack of expansion of injected cells into some individual nude hosts within most experiments is usually the case [Rocha et al., 1989; Freitas and Rocha, unpublished results]. Cells injected i.p. have been shown to home primarily to lymph nodes and those injected i.v. to spleen. Since all adoptive transfer experiments involved transfer of cells i.v. after similar preparative protocols, these factors are minimized. Transfer into unmanipulated nude and SCID hosts probably minimizes differences in plating efficiency still further.

A plateau of T-cell engraftment was observed in all experimental protocols. This plateau was dose dependent at higher (10^7) than very low (10^4) doses of cells, but at narrower ranges was not. A stable plateau was reached at various rates (discussed below) but was virtually never equal to the numbers of T cells in a normal mouse. Cells taken from one nude recipient mouse after reaching plateau would expand further after transfer into a second recipient [Rocha et al., 1987], indicating that the potential to expand was not lost at the plateau level. The plateaus were highest in the HU mice (normal numbers of cells) and lowest in the SCID recipients. These differences in plateau were a function of the recipients, not the donors; host environment therefore determines the plateau.

Rate of expansion (defined as the time to reach a stable plateau or the peak number of cells) is the fastest after treatment with HU and slowest after adoptive transfer into B-mice. In the adoptive transfer systems rate was shown to be dependent on the dose of cells injected until a maximum rate was reached at which time increasing the dose had no effect. The slow rate of expansion in the B-mice may also be due to the slow recovery of the rest of the hematopoietic system; if this is the case then presumably cells have engrafted, but some stimulus for expansion is initially lacking. The rate of expansion is independent of the plateau reached; thus nude and SCID recipients have different plateau levels but reach them at the same rate for a given cell dose.

The above findings regarding the relationship of dose, host environment, plateau, and rate lead to a model for T-cell expansion in periphery and peripheral homeostasis. The non-T portion of the immune system (epithelial, B cell, or myeloid) contains the signal required for T cells to expand when present in limited quantities. T cells contain cells able to engraft and expand and cells in limiting quantities able to provide accessory function necessary for optimal expansion [Stutman, 1986a]. The amounts of signal (non-T) and accessory function (T) determine the plateau. Therefore the plateau is dose dependent only at low doses when accessory function is limiting [Stutman, 1986a]. The rate of expansion is dependent on intrinsic properties of T cells (such as cell cycle length) and the delivery of optimal amounts of signal and accessory function. Maximal rate of expansion is independent of plateau reached because the ratio of signal and accessory function to progenitors is determinate, not the absolute amount of either. If signal and accessory function are in excess, the rate will be dose dependent. If these factors are limiting, the rate will be maximal and not dose dependent. Finally, a gradually increasing amount of signal will cause the plateau to rise gradually as well until the signal reaches maximal levels. This would appear as a slower rate to plateau levels and in fact is exactly what is observed in the T expansion of the B-mice [Miller and Stutman, 1982, 1984].

CD4 and CD8 Subset Ratios

In all experiments in which CD4 and CD8 SP subsets were examined, the normal ratio (2–3 : 1) was maintained during the homeostatic plateau. In fact even skewing the SP subset ratio in the donor cell inoculum failed to affect a change in the recovery to a normal ratio [Rocha, 1989]. CD4 SP cells were shown to have a greater expansion potential than CD8 SP cells in SCID mice, which required continuous interleukin-2 replacement therapy in the host mice for successful engraftment on their own [Rudolphi et al., 1991b]. In the nude recipients CD4 and CD8 SP cells could engraft and expand independently, and in fact the CD8 SP cells expanded to a greater extent in the absence of the CD4 SP subset. The cause of the discrepancy in the engraftment of the CD8 SP cells in SCID and nude recipients is unknown. Despite varying plateaus in the different systems the ratio of CD4 to CD8 SP cells is maintained, indicating tight regulatory mechanisms operating between these subsets that do not depend on extrinsic stimuli to operate. These regulatory mechanisms may also be the source of the accessory function discussed above.

Antigen-Driven Selection of Repertoire

The question of the affect of antigenic stimulation on the peripheral T-cell repertoire has been addressed by injecting transgenic T cells specific for the male HY antigen into male and female nude recipients [Rocha and von

Boehmer, 1991] or allogeneic or semiallogeneic donor spleen cells into SCID recipients [Rudolphi et al., 1991b; Tschnerning et al., 1991; Claesson et al., 1991].

Transgenic HY-Specific T Cells in Male and Female Nude Mice. The majority of peripheral T cells in female mice transgenic for the α- and β-chains of a TCR specific for the male HY antigen express the β-transgene, with a minority expressing the α-transgene as well. The remaining peripheral T cells express endogenous α-chains and do not react with HY. The finding that thymectomy in these mice reduced the percentage of T cells expressing the transgenic heterodimer led to the hypothesis that these cells were failing to expand in periphery due to lack of antigen and thus required continuous thymic output to maintain their numbers. T cells from female transgenic mice transferred into male and female nude recipients expanded in the periphery in both sexes [Rocha and von Boehmer, 1991]. However, the α–β-transgene expressing T cells expanded in an antigen-driven manner in male but not female mice. This initial expansion was followed by an equally rapid decline, and the remaining α–β-transgene-expressing cells were shown to be tolerant to male cells. The final level of these cells was still higher in the male than the female mice.

Cells expressing endogenous α-chains expanded to a similar extent in both sex recipients. Although this was taken to reflect a need for antigen-driven expansion (or, more precisely, TCR-mediated expansion) in the periphery, the effect of the great overproduction of transgene-positive cells in the donor mice was not addressed. The overproduction of cells with a TCR that binds preferentially to class I MHC leads to an overproduction in the thymus of CD8+ cells. The tight regulatory mechanisms detailed above are insufficient to control this overproduction completely in the periphery, as the ratio of CD4 to CD8 SP cells in the donor mice was nearly 1 : 1. In fact, in the nude recipients the CD8 SP subset comprises more cells than the CD4 SP subset.

Allogeneic Lymphoid Cells in SCID Mice. Semiallogeneic and allogeneic cells do not induce graft-vs. host disease (GVHD) when injected i.v. into SCID recipients [Tschnerning et al., 1991; Rudolphi et al., 1991b]. The route of administration was shown to be important, as the same dose of cells injected i.p. did induce GVHD. The allogeneic cells required a higher dose (i.v.) to provide successful engraftment and expansion than syngeneic cells, indicating a rejection mechanism in the SCID recipients. T cells that engrafted were shown to be tolerant to host in vivo and in vitro, although a proliferative response could be shown. This tolerance was not dependent on host-derived T or B cells, and no suppressor or veto activity could be shown by SCID spleen cells against a third-party, MLR.

General Remarks on Antigen-Driven Expansion. Although antigen-driven expansion or deletion may be demonstrated in the periphery [Rocha and von Bohemer, 1991], and although this indicates that the repertoire after thymic selection is flexible to change, the extent to which antigen-driven expansion is responsible for normal T-cell peripheral expansion cannot be concluded from these experiments. However, two points are worth mentioning: 1) The peripheral expansion of postthymic T cells is polyclonal [hypothesized by Stutman 1986a; demonstrated by Pereira and Rocha, 1991], and 2) even in the constant presence of the appropriate antigen the clonal expansion of the antigen-specific transgenic T cells is transient and self-limited [Rocha and von Boehmer, 1991].

Conclusions From Murine Experiments

Certainly all of the above-detailed experiments have contributed greatly to our knowledge of T-cell expansion and homeostasis. The canonic dogma of the long-lived T-cell population waiting for conventional exogenous antigen to ever divide has given way to a new view of a constantly renewing population with great potential for change. Many mechanisms that are operating during T-cell expansion must also be flexible enough to allow decreases in T-cell numbers, such as after resolution of antigenic challenge (when greater than 60% of T cells may reflect a limited number of specificities as reflected by V-β usage). The constant tension between the need for non-T stimuli to drive the T cells to expand and intrinsic limits to such expansion (such as cell cycle length or T–T subset controls) is reflected in the observed variations in plateaus that can be achieved in different systems.

Although certainly it has now been demonstrated that the system is flexible enough to allow changes in repertoire, it is difficult to support the view that expansion is exclusively antigen driven (or mediated through specificity of the TCR) while still assuming a large heterogeneous repertoire. More likely, there is a general mechanism for cellular expansion that requires interaction between T cells and other cells of the immune system and still undefined ligands; whether a certain subset of T cells possesses this ability to expand or it is a function of limited numbers of cells at any given point in time is still unknown.

HUMAN STUDIES

As mentioned in the Introduction, our knowledge of T-cell population dynamics in humans is very limited. T-cell lifespans are still undefined. The studies showing that patients irradiated in infancy had chromosome breaks in their blood lymphoid cells, detected with phytohemagglutinin stimulation, when studied 23–40 years later [Goh et al., 1976] were usually interpreted as indicating T cells that have never divided within that period of time and generated views on T-cell lifespans that are identical to the lifespan of the individual [Jerne, 1984]. However, even the radiobiologists who made the original observation could not be sure whether the high incidence of chromosome breaks was due to the irradiation received in childhood or to other reasons, such as the primary diseases of the patients [Goh et al., 1976].

The notion of an eternal postthymic T cell was used to explain the fact that adult thymectomy in humans (usually performed as treatment for myasthenia gravis) produced only very marginal immunological defects when studied 10–20 years later [Glenis et al., 1979; Van de Griend et al., 1982; Berrih et al., 1983; Haynes et al., 1983]. The alternative interpretation could be derived from the postthymic but thymus-independent T-cell renewal discussed above.

The studies on reconstitution of humans with SCID with bone marrow transplantation, although related to the murine studies discussed above, are essentially different. Rather than injecting postthymic T cells, the treatments inject stem cells and carefully deplete for any T cells to avoid GVHD reactions, since most of the cases have to use non-MHC-matched donors (summarized by Johnson and Pochedly [1990] in a multiauthored book on bone marrow transplantation). Thus the marrow-treated SCID patients would be examples in which a peripheral T-cell compartment develops as a consequence of the seeding of the patient's thymus with normal stem cells from the donor and the subsequent export and expansion in periphery (as well as a similar development of a B-cell compartment by seeding of the patient's marrow with the normal donor stem cells and subsequent export to the peripheral lymphoid organs). Although these are complex cases, the general picture that emerges is that T-cell restoration after successful engraftment takes time (usually about 3 months), that commonly the first T cells to appear are CD4, and that in general B cell reconstitution follows a similar time pattern.

Finally, and probably the most important potential derivation of the murine T cell population studies is that the proposed model of T cell maintenance based on the antigen-independent but internal-signal-driven expansion of CD4 or CD8 peripheral T cells, which uses extensive expansion of a generative compartment that probably contains a small number of progenitors, may explain the paradox of the severe CD4 depletion in HIV-infected patients in spite of relative low levels of actual virus-infected T cells [Fauci, 1988].

CONCLUSION

Many unknowns of peripheral T-cell expansion and homeostasis remain, including the internal signals driving expansion and the intrinsic properties of T cells that limit expansion or control subset ratios, among others. Experiments in nude and SCID mice have demonstrated that periphery is not inert and can have important effects on T-cell numbers. For example, it was shown that CD8 SP T cells could expand independently in nude [Rocha et al., 1989] but not in SCID [Rudolphi et al., 1991a] mice. Although periphery may be demonstrated to affect changes in repertoire by expanding certain clones [Rocha and von Boehmer, 1991] or removing self-reactive clones [Claesson et al., 1991], the effects of periphery on T-cell repertoire under normal conditions are probably quite limited.

Concerning self-tolerance, however, periphery may in fact be important as a site for induction of anergy [Schwartz, 1990], and peripheral anergy to self may play a role in preventing autoimmunity. Regardless of the importance of anergy induction in vivo under normal conditions, the existence of such a mechanism may eventually be exploited for therapeutic ends. Finally, although the model discussed here considers "periphery" as a single compartment, it is highly possible that important regional and local events may be critical in determining the maintenance and functional behavior of T cells.

REFERENCES

Bell EB, Sparshott SM, Drayson MT, Ford WL (1987): The stable and permanent expansion of functional T lymphocytes in athymic nude rats after a single injection of mature T cells. J Immunol 139:1379–1384.

Berrih S, Le Brigand H, Levasseur P, Gaud C, Bach JF (1983): Depletion of helper/inducer T cells after thymectomy in myasthenic patients. Clin Immunol Immunopathol 28:272–281.

Boyd E (1932): The weight of the thymus gland in health and disease. Am J Dis Child 43:1162–1214.

Claesson MH, Rudolphi A, Tscherning T, Reimann J (1991): $CD3^+$ T cells in severe combined immunodeficiency (scid) mice IV. Graft-vs.-host resistance of $H-2^d$ scid mice to intravenous injection of allogeneic $H-2^b$ (C57BL/6) spleen cells. Eur J Immunol 21:2057–2062.

Fauci AS (1988): The human immunodeficiency virus: Infectivity and mechanisms of pathogenesis. Science 239:617–622.

Freitas AA, Rocha B, Coutinho AA (1986): Lymphocyte population kinetics in the mouse. Immunol Rev 91:5–37.

Glenis K, Scadding HC, Havard CWH (1979): The immunological effects of thymectomy in myasthenia gravis. Clin Exp Immunol 36:205–213.

Goh K, Reddy MM, Hemperlmann, LH (1976): Chromosomal aberrations in lymphocytes of normal adults long after thymus irradiation. Radiol Res 67:82–85.

Haynes BF, Harden EA, Olanov CW, Eisenbarth GS, Wechsler AS, Hensley LL, Roses AD (1983): Effect of thymectomy on peripheral lymphocyte subsets in myasthenia gravis: Selective effect on T cells in patients with thymic atrophy. J Immunol 131:773–777.

Hodgson GS, Bradley TR, Martin RF, Sumner M, Fry P (1975): Recovery of proliferating haemopoietic progenitor cells after killing by hydroxyurea. Cell Tissue Kinet 8:51–60.

Ishizaka ST, Stutman O (1983): Analysis by limiting dilution of interleukin 2-producing T cells in murine ontogeny. Eur J Immunol 13:936–942.

Jerne NK (1984): Idiotypic networks and other preconceived ideas. Immunol Rev 79:5–24.

Johnson FL, Pochedly C (eds) (1990): "Bone Marrow Transplantation in Children." New York: Raven Press.

Miller RA, Stutman O (1982): Generation of functionally distinct T cell subsets from post-thymic T cell progenitors in vivo. Behring Inst Mitt 70:101–105.

Miller RA, Stutman O (1984): T cell repopulation from functionally restricted splenic progenitors: 10,000-fold expansion documented by using limiting dilution analyses. J Immunol 133:2925–2932.

Pereira P, Rocha B (1991): Post-thymic in vivo expansion of mature alpha-beta T cells. Int Immunol 3:1077–1080.

Reimann J, Rudolphi A, Claesson MH (1991a): $CD3^+$ T-cells in severe combined immunodeficiency (scid) mice III: Transferred congenic, selfreactive $CD4^+$ T cell clones rescue IgM-producing, scid-derived B cells. Int Immunol 3:657–663.

Reimann J, Rudolphi A, Claesson MH (1991b): Selective reconstitution of T lymphocyte subsets in scid mice. Immunol Rev 124:75–95.

Rocha B (1987): Population kinetics of precursors of IL 2-producing peripheral T lymphocytes: Evidence for short life expectancy, continuous renewal, and post-thymic expansion. J Immunol 139:365–372.

Rocha B (1990): Characterization of $V\beta$-bearing cells in athymic (nu/nu) mice suggest an extrathymic pathway for T cell differentiation. Eur J Immunol 29:919–925.

Rocha B, Dautigny N, Pereira P (1989): Peripheral T lymphocytes: Expansion potential and homeostatic regulation of pool sizes and CD4/CD8 ratios in vivo. Eur J Immunol 19:905–911.

Rocha B, Freitas AA, Coutinho AA (1983): Population dynamics of T lymphocytes, renewal rate and expansion in the peripheral lymphoid organs. J Immunol 131:2158–2164.

Rocha B, Penit C, Baron C, Vasseur F, Dautigny N, Freitas AA (1990): Accumulation of bromodeoxyuridine-labeled cells in central and peripheral lymphoid organs: Minimal estimates of production and turnover rates of mature lymphocytes. Eur J Immunol 20:1697–1708.

Rocha B, von Boehmer H (1991): Peripheral selection of the T cell repertoire. Science 251:1225–1228.

Rudolphi A, Spiess S, Conradt P, Claesson MH, Reimann J (1991a): $CD3^+$ T cells in severe combined immune deficiency (scid) mice I. Transferred purified $CD4^+$ T cells, but not $CD8^+$ T cells are engrafted in the spleen of congenic scid mice. Eur J Immunol 21:523–533.

Rudolphi A, Speiss S, Conradt P, Claesson MH, Reimann J (1991b): $CD3^+$ T cells in severe combined immunodeficiency (scid) mice II. Transplantation of dm2 lymphoid cells into semi-allogeneic scid mice. Eur J Immunol 21:1591–1600.

Schwartz RH (1990): A cell culture model for T lymphocyte clonal anergy. Science 248:1349–1356.

Scollay R, Butcher EC, Weissman I (1980): Thymus cell migration: Quantitative aspects of cellular traffic from the thymus to the periphery in mice. Eur J Immunol 10:210–218.

Scollay R, Smith J, Stauffer V (1986): Dynamics of early T cells: Prothymocyte migration and proliferation in the adult mouse thymus. Immunol Rev 91:129–157.

Sprent J, Schaefer M, Hurd M, Surh CD, Ron Y (1991): Mature murine B and T cells transferred to SCID mice can survive indefinitely and may maintain a virgin phenotype. J Exp Med 174:717–728.

Stutman O (1974): Cell-mediated immunity and aging. Fed Proc 33:2028–2032.

Stutman O (1977): Two main features of T-cell development. Contemp Top Immunobiol 7:1–46.

Stutman O (1978): Intrathymic and extrathymic T cell maturation. Immunol Rev 42:138–184.

Stutman O (1985): Ontogeny of T cells. Clin Immunol Allergy 5:191–234.

Stutman O (1986a): Postthymic T-cell development. Immunol Rev 91:159–194.

Stutman O (1986b): Ontogeny, maintenance and ageing of T cell function in mice. In Facchini A, Haaijman JJ, Labo G (eds): "Immunoregulation in Aging. Topics in Aging Research in Europe." Vol. 9. Rijswijk, the Netherlands: EURAGE, pp 3–8.

Sunshine GH, Jimmo BL, Ianelli C, Jarvis L (1991): Strong priming of T cells adoptively transferred into scid mice. J Exp Med 174:1653–1656.

Thoman ML, Weigle WO (1989): The cellular and subcellular bases of immunosenescence. Adv Immunol 46:221–261.

Tscherning T, Rudolphi A, Reimann J, Claesson MH (1991): CD3$^+$ T cells in severe combined immunodeficiency (SCID) mice V. Allogeneic T cells engrafted into SCID mice do not induce graft-versus-host disease in spite of the absence of host veto and natural suppressor cell activity. Scand J Immunol 34:795–801.

Van de Griend RJ, Carreno M, Van Doorn R, Leupers CJM, Van den Ende A, Wijermans P, Oosterhuis HJGH, Astaldi A (1982): Changes in human T lymphocytes after thymectomy and during senescence. J Clin Immunol 2:289–295.

12

QUANTIFICATION OF AUTOREACTIVE LYMPHOCYTES IN HEALTH AND DISEASE

Rudolf H. Zubler, Alessandra Tucci, Robert Rieben, Thomas Matthes, and Urs E. Nydegger

Division of Hematology, Hôpital Cantonal Universitaire, Genève, Switzerland (R.H.Z., A.T., T.M.); Central Laboratory of Hematology, University of Bern, Bern, Switzerland (R.R., U.E.N.)

INTRODUCTION

Although autoimmunity plays an important role in many human diseases, most of the time the immune system performs rather well in avoiding pathologic self-reactivity. A priori it seems impossible that the immune system of complex organisms, on the one hand, eliminates all self-reactive lymphocytes and, on the other, is able to develop an extensively diverse, preformed antigen receptor repertoire for defense against foreign pathogens. However, solutions to this dilemma have been found by adaptive evolution, and significant progress has been made during recent years with regard to our understanding of the strategies involved. Most important in this context is that T and B lymphocytes (in spite of similar generation of diversity of B- and T-cell antigen receptors) recognize antigens in fundamentally different manners and use complementary strategies to deal with self-reactivity. The focus of this

Autoimmunity: Physiology and Disease, Pages 173–190
© 1994 Wiley-Liss, Inc.

chapter is on the results obtained by limiting dilution analysis (LDA), which suggested the frequent occurrence of autoreactive lymphocytes (in fact, the available data primarily concern the B cells) in normal individuals, mice, and humans. These findings are critically discussed in view of the recent observations on the molecular differences between natural versus disease-associated autoantibodies, on self-tolerance in transgeneic mice, and on human B-cell tolerance to ABO histoblood group self-antigens as found in our own studies.

AUTOREACTIVE T CELLS

It has been shown that self-molecules such as murine hemoglobin are normally processed by specialized antigen-presenting cells (APC) and their peptides presented by major histocompatibility complex (MHC) class II molecules [Lorenz and Allen, 1988]. To find out which antigens autologous APC "naturally" present, peptides can now be eluted from the MHC molecules and chemically characterized [Hunt et al., 1992]. This sophisticated approach has shown that many self-peptides are present on autologous MHC molecules, including signal peptide domains of normal cellular proteins [Henderson et al., 1992], and it has also indicated that many of the peptides may occur at a too low density on the APC either to tolerize or to activate T cells [Schild et al., 1990]. Thus experimental in vitro loading of APC with self-peptides could give an unnaturally high antigen density.

Liver membrane antigen-reactive T clones were established from patients with autoimmune chronic active hepatitis [Wen et al., 1990]. T clones responding to collagen and/or proteoglycans could be derived not only from joint tissue of patients with rheumatoid arthritis [Londei et al., 1989] but also from T cells of normal individuals [Ofusu-Appiah et al., 1989]. T clones with apparent autoreactivity were frequently obtained by culturing T cells from normal individuals in the presence of irradiated autologous non-T cells and autologous serum [Strober and James, 1990]. T-cell clones were also found to recognize heat shock protein sequences that are shared between bacteria and humans [Munk et al., 1989; Haregewoin et al., 1991]. These and other clonal studies indicate the existence of autoreactive T cells in health and disease. However, LDA data on the actual frequencies of T cells responding to molecularly defined self-epitopes (as exist for various antigen-specific B cells) are presently not available. One of the main problems is that APC always present many different antigen–MHC complexes.

AUTOREACTIVE B CELLS

B-Cell Assays

The basic principle for investigating the B-cell specificity repertoire by LDA is to titrate down the number of B cells in a polyclonal culture system until a certain specificity (as detected by antibody assay) becomes limiting. The fraction of antibody-nonproducing cultures/total number of cultures tested (F0) is then considered the zero term of the Poisson distribution; the formula $F0 = e^{-\mu}$ or $-\ln(F0) = \mu$ gives the mean number (μ) of antibody-producing cell precursors per culture [Lefkovits, 1979; Taswell, 1981]. The B-cell mitogen LPS (lipopolysaccharide of gram-negative bacteria such as *Escherichia coli*) together with filler cells, such as thymocytes, was most frequently used for murine B-cell LDA; about one-third of all murine B cells respond [Andersson et al., 1977]. In contrast, human B cells do not directly respond to LPS [Zubler et al., 1987]. Protein A–rich *Staphylococcus aureus*, strain Cowan I (SAC) is a human B-cell mitogen that leads to immunoglobulin secretion by about 1% of all B cells. The lectin pokeweed mitogen (PWM) gives polyclonal human B-cell activation of a similar proportion to SAC through leading to macrophage–T cell–B cell interactions.

Three types of high efficiency culture systems have been reported for human B cells: 1) The EL-4 assay uses a subclone of the mouse thymoma EL-4 that stimulates B cells through direct cell contact in conjunction with phorbol ester (PMA) or culture supernatant of activated human T cells (T-SUP) [Zubler et al., 1987; Wen et al., 1987]. More than 90% of all B cells can respond by generating clones of antibody-secreting cells, and the mean cloning frequency in different experiments is 50% (see below). 2) A similarly efficient B-cell stimulation can be obtained by coculturing B cells with mitomycin C–treated $CD4^+$ T cells, which are activated by adding insolubilized anti-CD3 antibody and thus react polyclonally with B cells; interleukin (IL)-2 and accessory cells are also added (anti-CD3 T cell system) [Amoroso and Lipsky, 1990]. 3) Stimulation of B cells by anti-CD40 antibody-coated fibroblasts in conjunction with IL-4 alone or with other cytokines also gives potent B-cell responses; this is the only nonviral system for which long-term growth of B cells was reported [Banchereau et al., 1991]. As yet no LDA data obtained with this system have been reported. Epstein-Barr virus (EBV) has two types of effect [Aman et al., 1984; Straub and Zubler, 1989]: EBV binding to complement receptor-2 (CD21) activates about 30% of human B cells to proliferate and secrete antibodies during a limited period of time (about 10 days, as for the other short-term culture systems); in addition, about 1%–10% of B cells become immortalized by EBV infection and continue to grow and secrete antibodies. Activation of apparently different B-cell subpopulations occurs in some culture systems (see below). Finally, B-cell immortalization via hybridoma formation with plasmocytoma cells [Köhler and Milstein, 1975] can be used to probe the murine and human B-cell-specificity repertoires.

LDA of the Murine B Cell-Specificity Repertoire

Rheumatoid factor (RF)–producing B cells were frequently detected in many studies; sometimes it appeared that the majority of all B cells make IgM RF [Dziarski, 1982]. RF react with the constant (Fc) portion of autologous immunoglobulins and bind aggregated immunoglobulin with higher avidity than monomeric immunoglobulin. They occur so frequently that a physiologic role, e.g., enhanced clearance of circulating immune complexes, has to be considered. Anti-denatured DNA (single-stranded DNA [ssDNA])–specific B cells also occur frequently; they represent 1%–5% of all murine B cells in the LPS assay [Conger, 1984]. It is now known that many different germline V genes encode natural RF [Duchosal et al., 1989] and anti-ssDNA antibodies [Panosian-Sahakian et al., 1989] and that the corresponding antibodies in autoimmune mice arise by somatic mutations that are typical for affinity maturation [Marion et al., 1989; Schlomchik et al., 1990].

Other autoantibody-producing B cells were detected in normal mice. Their investigation was stimulated by a report showing the frequent presence of natural autoantibodies against a variety of self-antigens in normal human sera [Guilbert et al., 1982]. Dighiero et al. [1985] found that 6% of 384 hybridomas derived from B cells of normal newborn mice produced antibodies reacting with mouse actin, tubulin, myosin, peroxidase, renin, and ssDNA. These authors noted the frequent cross-reactivities with various antigens, the "polyreactivity" of natural autoantibodies. In another study one-third of such hybridoma antibodies reacted with a panel of 17 autoantigens (including red blood cells, thyroglobulin, T-cell surface antigens, and the antigens mentioned above); about one-half of the autoantibodies were pluri- or polyreactive, and this was not correlated with the usage of particular V_H gene families [Glotz et al., 1988]. The latter point was confirmed by others [Souroujon et al., 1988]. The findings with newborn mice showed that the preimmune B-cell repertoire is particularly rich in autoreactive B cells. Moreover, Portnoi et al. [1986] showed that autoreactive B cells are more frequent among the large, activated B cells than among the small, resting B cells obtained by Percoll gradient before the stimulation with LPS; the frequencies were 1/200 large versus 1/1,900 small B cells for mouse thyroglobulin-reactive B cells and 1/150 large versus 1/1,400 small B cells for B cells reactive with bromealin-treated mouse red blood cells (BrMRBC). These authors thus proposed that self-reactivity could play a role in shaping the preimmune B-cell repertoire. However, an age-dependent increase of autoreactivity was also found in that old mice had 3–10 times more anti-BrMRBC and antithyroglobulin B cells than young mice [Weksler et al., 1990].

Polyreactive antibodies are nevertheless specific with respect to different epitopes on a single molecule. Kuppers [1991] observed that 80% of antithyroglobulin antibody-producing B cells (1/3,900 B cells in the LPS assay) reacted only with mouse and not with human thyroglobulin. Hybridoma studies showed that natural antitubulin antibodies recognize the same or very overlapping epitopes, whereas immune antibodies to this molecule recognize a variety of epitopes [Matthes et al., 1988]. It seems that polyreactive IgM antibodies are generally encoded by nonmutated germline V genes [Baccala et al., 1989]. Among monoclonal anti-MRBC antibodies from the autoimmune disease-prone NZB mice, those capable of producing hemolytic anemia after transfer to normal mice were specific for MRBC only, whereas nonpathogenic antibodies cross-reacted with RBC from other species [Shibata et al., 1990].

LDA of the Human B-Cell Specificity Repertoire

As in mice, one frequently finds RF– and anti-ssDNA–producing B cells in normal humans. In one study, 1%–4% of human B cells made IgM RF in the anti-CD3 T cell assay, and as much as 30%–60% of those B cells that responded in the SAC assay [Hirohata et al., 1990]. Thus, as noted in other studies, SAC preferentially stimulates the RF-producing cells; perhaps this is related to RF binding to SAC–immunoglobulin complexes. The relative frequencies of EBV-inducible IgM RF– (and antithyroglobulin antibody)–producing B cells increase with age according to Fong et al. [1981], whereas Levinson et al. [1987] found that only 3% of adult compared with 17% of neonatal (cord blood) SAC-responsive B cells make IgM RF. The frequency. of RF B cells increases after immunization with tetanus toxoid [Welch et al., 1983]. Up to 15% of EBV-immortalized B cells were found to produce RF; the frequency was higher in patients with rheumatoid arthritis (RA) than in normal individuals, and synovial fluid was enriched with such B cells [Burastero et al., 1990]. For comparison, B cells specific for *Haemophilus influenzae* type b capsular polysaccharide were found with a frequency of 0.1%–0.2% of immunoglobulin-secreting cells induced by polyclonal stimulation with EBV [Munoz and Insel, 1987]. Fifty percent of plasma cells in the diseased joints of patients with RA generate RF [Natvig et al., 1989]. RF activity was produced by 8 of 15 heterohybridomas derived from human B chronic lymphocytic leukemia B cells [Borche et al., 1990]. The other protagonist autoantibody, anti-ssDNA, is also produced in large amounts by EBV-transformed human B cells from normal individuals [Hoch et al., 1983] and by normal adult and cord blood B cells responding in bulk cultures in the anti-CD3 T-cell assay [Splawski et al., 1991].

Properties of Natural Versus Disease-Associated Autoantibodies

Polyreactivity of human antibodies was studied by LDA of EBV-transformed B cells in conjunction with antigen-competition for ELISA assays. Nakamura et al. [1988] found B cells with reactivity for ssDNA, thyroglobulin, thyroid microsomal antigen, insulin, and tetanus toxoid, each with a frequency of 3%–6% of all EBV-transformed B cells from normal humans. The antibodies were almost exclusively IgM, with frequent polyreactivity and sometimes very low affinity (10^{-3} to 10^{-7} mol/liter). By the same approach, natural RF were found to exhibit polyreactivity and low affinity for all tested antigens ($k_d \pm 10^{-5}$ mol/liter), while RF from patients with RA included monospecific IgG with 100-fold higher affinity [Burastero et al., 1988]. Similarly, naturally occurring anti-DNA antibodies are polyreactive and of low affinity, while their counterparts in patients with systemic lupus erythematosus (SLE) are specific and of 10- to 100-fold higher affinity [Casali et al., 1989]. Anti-insulin IgG antibody-producing B cells are more frequent in patients with newly diagnosed, untreated, insulin-dependent diabetes mellitus (IDDM) (0.2% of EBV-transformed B cells) than in normal controls (0.03%), are more monoreactive, and of higher affinity [Casali et al., 1990]. About 2% of the normal circulating B cells immortalized by EBV make antirabies virus antibodies (polyreactive IgM), while after rabies immunization the frequency apparently increases to 10%, with antirabies immune B cells producing mostly IgG, monospecific, higher affinity antibody [Ueki et al., 1990].

Anti-DNA antibodies produced by hybridomas derived from the B cells of patients with SLE still show various patterns of cross-reactivity, in this case particularly with platelet and/or phospholipid antigens [Rauch et al., 1987]. Such anti-DNA antibodies can cross-react with cell surface proteins [Jacob et al., 1987]. Serum antibodies to different lupus autoantigens have different IgG subclass patterns, suggesting an influence of the antigens on isotype switch [Rubin et al., 1986]. As in mice, the natural IgM autoantibodies are mostly derived from germline V genes, while the IgG antibodies in autoimmune disease show nonrandom mutations indicating clonal selection [Carson, 1991; Pascual and Capra, 1991]. Although certain V genes may be present or absent in some individuals, this does not appear to play an important role in whether the individual develops autoimmune disease or not [Pascual and Capra, 1991]. The actual antigens responsible for driving the autoimmune response in diseases such as SLE or RA are not known.

CD5[+] B Cells

The natural, polyreactive IgM autoantibodies in humans and mice are frequently produced by CD5-expressing B cells [Hardy and Hayakawa, 1986; Casali et al., 1987; Kantor, 1991]. This cell surface molecule is present on a subset of B cells, on all T cells, and also on endothelial cells [Gogolin-Ewens et al., 1989]. In mice, the highest concentration of CD5[+] B cells is found in the peritoneal cavity, and cell transfer experiments have shown that CD5[+] B cells are self-regenerating in syngeneic hosts, while CD5[−] B cells do not expand and remain CD5[−]; it has thus been proposed that there exist two separate B-cell lineages [Herzenberg et al., 1986].

However, CD5 expression can be induced in human CD5[−] B cells by phorbol ester (PMA) [Miller and Gralow, 1984], while CD5[+] human B cells become CD5[−] when incubated with IL-2 [Caligaris-Cappio et al., 1989]. Our own studies demonstrated transient expression of CD5 on most B cells during the first few days of culture of FACS-sorted CD5[−] B cells in the EL-4 B-cell assay [Werner-Favre et al., 1989]. This has been confirmed in the anti-CD3 T-cell system [Vernino et al., 1992]. CD5 expression was also shown to be inducible in murine CD5[−] B cells by stimulation with anti-immunoglobulin antibody [Ying-zi et al., 1991]. The straightforward (but not generally accepted) conclusion is that CD5 is a marker of activated B cells and that polyreactive B cells are frequently activated in vivo and thus self-regenerating in cell transfers between syngeneic mice [Werner-Favre et al., 1989]. CD5 expression by chronic lymphocytic leukemia B cells most likely reflects their stage of maturation arrest rather than the participation of only one of two B-cell lineages in this disease, and the frequency with which such tumor cells express V genes for autoreactive (polyreactive) receptors could simply mirror the germline repertoire. In addition, the recent finding of an accumulation of nonrandom V gene mutations during the progression of a B-cell lymphoma suggests that self-reactivity provides a growth advantage to tumor cells [Friedman et al., 1991].

The finding that only anti-immunoglobulin but not LPS induces CD5 expression on murine B cells [Ying-zi et al., 1991] is similar to the observation that anti-immunoglobulin is also required (in addition to LPS) for the IL-2 receptor expression on murine B cells [Zubler et al., 1987]. Clearly, different pathways of B-cell activation lead to different B-cell phenotypes. It will be important to study why most of the B cells producing polyreactive IgM antibodies express CD5 and are in the peritoneum, in contrast to the B cells producing high-affinity IgG autoantibodies [Casali et al., 1989].

LDA of Human B Cells With the EL-4 B-Cell Assay

Clonal expansion of B cells in the EL-4 assay stops after 10 days, leading to a mean of 400 plasma cells that secrete a mean of 80 μg of immunoglobulins per clone in cultures set up with a single B cell per 200 μl well [Wen et al., 1987; Zhang et al., 1991]. With higher numbers of starting B cells the clonal expansion becomes reduced. Of 11 cytokines tested, the most efficient cytokines in replacing T-cell supernatant were IL-1 together with TNFα [Tucci et al., 1992]. Most of the B clones derived from membrane IgM-positive B cells produce IgG and/or IgA in addition to IgM (and 10% of the clones produce IgE in the presence of IL-4) [Zhang et al., 1991]. Therefore, the analysis of the immunoglobulin isotypes does not help in distinguishing primary versus memory B cells. However, since adult and cord blood B cells [Tucci et al., 1991], CD5$^+$ and CD5$^-$ B cells (see above), and membrane IgM$^+$, IgG$^+$, or IgA$^+$ B cells [Zhang et al., 1991] respond in this system, it seems that all types of B cells become stimulated.

The LDA results obtained with this assay are summarized in Table I. B cells generating RF [Werner-Favre et al., 1989] or anti-ssDNA antibodies (Zubler and Doucet, unpublished data) were detected at similar frequencies in normal individuals and in patients with RA or SLE, respectively. However, their affinity could not be tested with the amounts of antibodies available. The frequency of RF-producing B cells among the FACS-sorted responder B cells was, however, nine times higher in the synovial fluid than in the peripheral blood of patients with RA. Native DNA (dsDNA)–specific B cells were detected in patients with SLE by a specific ELISA that did not reveal such B cells in normal individuals. For comparison, it is also shown

TABLE I. Human B-cell frequencies detected in the EL-4 assay

B-cell specificity	B-cell donors (Nos. of donors)	Mean frequency[a]
Tetanus toxoid	Normal individuals (10)	1/1,900
BSA	Normal individuals (10)	1/2,200
P. falciparum (total parasite)	Normal individuals (9)	1/1,890
P. falciparum (total parasite)	Recent malaria (6)	1/160
HIV	HIV-seronegative individuals (9)	1/25,400
HIV	HIV-seropositive individuals (12)	1/4,350
RF activity (human IgG Fc)	Normal individuals (10)	1/1,400 (IgM)
RF activity (human IgG Fc)	Seropositive RA (8)	1/860 (IgM)
RF activity (human IgG Fc)	Seropositive RA, synovial fluid (5)	1/100 (IgM)
Denatured (ss) DNA	Normal individuals (10)	1/60
Denatured (ss) DNA	SLE patients (8)	1/50
Native (ds) DNA	Normal individuals (6)	<1/200,000
Native (ds) DNA	SLE patients (5)	1/12,500
Self-ABO histoblood group antigens	Blood groups A, B, AB (11)	1/11,600 (IgM)
Allo-ABO histoblood group antigens	Blood groups A, B, O (10)	1/104,000 (IgM)

[a] LDA data from the indicated individuals were pooled for Poisson Statistics and corrected for a mean B-cell cloning efficiency of 50% in the EL-4 assay. Total immunoglobulin (IgM and IgG together) was measured except where IgM is indicated.

that malaria parasite-reactive (immune fluorescence assay with *Plasmodium falciparum* [Wen et al., 1987]) or HIV-reactive (ELISA and Western blot [Zubler et al., 1992]) B cells could be detected in normal individuals. The mean frequency of the corresponding B cells was about 10 times higher in individuals who had recently recovered from malaria or in HIV-seropositive individuals. Two new findings, which were recently made with the EL-4 assay, will be briefly discussed.

Selective Activation of dsDNA-Specific B Cells in Human SLE. It is well known that in autoimmune diseases such as SLE, increased spontaneous immunoglobulin secretion occurs in cultures of total peripheral blood mononuclear cells (PBMC). The spontaneous immunoglobulin is mostly derived from in vivo activated B cells. In contrast, as mentioned above, the EL-4 assay seems to probe the total, activated and nonactivated, B-cell specificity repertoire. We found that the relative proportion of anti-dsDNA antibodies among the total spontaneously secreted immunoglobulin in PBMC cultures from patients with active SLE was 960 times higher than the corresponding anti-dsDNA/total immunoglobulin ratio that was found in the EL-4 assay (Fig. 1). PWM-stimulated PBMC cultures produced a similar ratio of anti-dsDNA antibodies/total immunoglobulin as spontaneous PBMC cultures in SLE, while neither type of culture with PBMC from normal individuals produced anti-dsDNA antibodies.

This finding suggests that highly selective activation of dsDNA-specific B cells occurs in SLE, which could hardly result from antigen-independent, polyclonal B-cell activation in this disease. A very similar enrichment factor (800 times) was recently found by comparing the anti-HIV antibody/total immunoglobulin ratios in spontaneous PBMC cultures versus in EL-4 B cell cultures from HIV-seropositive individuals [Zubler et al., 1992]. In this case, the selective B-cell activation is expected to reflect the anti-HIV immune response. However, although potent helper T-cell activation could be detected in SLE [Huang et al., 1988], neither the T epitopes (DNA-binding proteins, virus?) nor in fact the B epitopes (DNA itself or an antigen with which lupus anti-DNA antibodies crossreact?) that trigger the B cell autoimmune response are known for this disease.

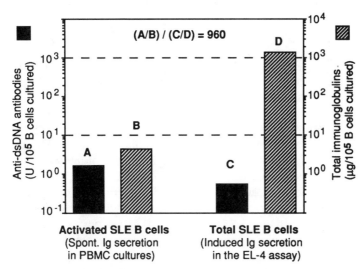

FIGURE 1. Relative ratio of anti-dsDNA antibodies/total immunoglobulin is increased in spontaneous PBMC cultures as compared with EL-4 B-cell cultures in SLE. These are mean data from five patients with active SLE. PBMC cultures were performed with 2×10^5 total mononuclear cells (containing a mean of 10^4 B cells according to flow cytometry)/200 μl culture, in triplicates; EL-4 B-cell cultures were performed with 1,000 B cells/200 μl culture, mean of 50 cultures per patient. The anti-dsDNA antibody levels (ELISA units representing absorbance) and the total immunoglobulin levels (μg) are expressed per 10^5 starting B cells cultured.

B-Cell Tolerance in the ABO Histoblood Group System. In another study we used the EL-4 assay to address the question of whether the normal B-cell specificity repertoire contains B cells that recognize autologous determinants of the ABO histoblood group system [Rieben et al., 1992]. A key feature of this system is that all normal individuals have natural serum antibodies against those A or B carbohydrate determinants that are not present in their organism. The natural antibodies result from bacterial infections; the A and B carbohydrate antigens occur frequently in the natural environment. We used a sensitive ELISA assay for the quantitation of IgM and IgG antibodies against A and B antigens [Rieben et al., 1991]. In the EL-4 assay, B clones from all individuals frequently generated IgM (but not IgG) antibodies with apparent double-specificity for A and B antigens. These were polyreactive antibodies in that they also frequently reacted with BSA, bee venom phospholipase A_2, and sometimes uncoated plastic plates. However, the patterns of A or B antigen-specific B-cell responses were in agreement with classic blood group serology: allo A/B-specific IgM-producing B cells occurred 10 times more frequently (1/11,600 B cells) than apparently self-A/B-specific IgM-producing B cells (1/104,000 B cells) in 2,600 B-cell cultures from 14 individuals with different blood group phenotypes (A, B, AB, or O); for IgG-producing B cells the corresponding frequencies were 1/26,000 B cells for anti-allo A/B and 1/350,000 B cells for anti-self-A/B determinants. These results show self-tolerance at the B-cell level.

Comparison With Transgenic Mice

In transgenic mice in which most B cells express the same immunoglobulin, the fate of autoreactive B cells can be directly visualized. In a model of autoimmune hemolytic anemia, a certain erythrocyte self-antigen induced both clonal deletion and functional inactivation (anergy) of B cells with variable contributions to self-tolerance in individual mice [Okamoto et al., 1992]. From other models it appeared that cell-bound autoantigens induce clonal deletion [Nemazee and Bürki, 1989], while soluble autoantigens such as lysozyme [Goodnow et al., 1991] or ssDNA [Erikson et al., 1991] cause anergy. Usually, anergy can be overcome to various extents by stimuli that bypass the B-cell antigen receptor; anergic B cells from antilysozyme immunoglobulin and lysozyme double-transgenic mice generated potent antilysozyme antibody responses after 6 days of coculture with LPS [Goodnow et al., 1991]. In our study on B-cell tolerance in the ABO system, the B-cell assay lasted 10 days and led to very potent, antigen receptor-independent, polyclonal B-cell activation, clonal expansion, and antibody secretion. The results mentioned above suggest therefore that either a highly resistant state of anergy or—more likely—clonal deletion is responsible for B cell tolerance to human A and B histoblood group self-antigens.

Problems With In Vitro Assays

The affinity of the antibody reactivity that can be detected in antigen-coated ELISA plates can be so low, in particular, in the case of the multivalent IgM antibodies, that it may be irrelevant under in vivo conditions [Friguet et al., 1985; Conger et al., 1988]. In mice that are transgenic for a polyreactive IgM, the B cells expressing this immunoglobulin are not much downregulated and are apparently quite well tolerated [Zöller and Achtnich, 1991]. An analogous problem exists with regard to T-cell assays. As mentioned above, the density of self-peptide–MHC complexes on APC may be much lower under physiologic conditions than after in vitro feeding of large amounts of such antigen. Finally, anergy of either T or B cells, such as has been demonstrated in transgenic mice, can be broken by potent activation in vitro; the information on the functional state of the cells in vivo is thus lost. These caveats must be taken into consideration for the interpretation of the in vitro findings about self-reactive lymphocytes.

INTERPRETATION OF STUDIES DEMONSTRATING AUTOREACTIVE LYMPHOCYTES IN NORMAL INDIVIDUALS

Clonal deletion of immature autoreactive lymphocytes, and functional inactivation (anergy) of mature cells due to antigen encounter in the absence of appropriate accessory signals, have been demonstrated for T cells [Kisielow et al., 1988; Schwartz, 1989] and for B cells (see above). T and B cells interact in immune responses and in tolerance. Regarding the latter, autoantigen-presenting, anergic B cells may help in maintaining the anergy of autoreactive T cells [Eynon and Parker, 1992]; the breaking of anergy in such B cells may in turn lead to stimulation of the T cells [Lin et al., 1991]. Nevertheless, important differences exist regarding the control of autoreactivity of the two classes of lymphocytes (Fig. 2).

Most fundamentally, control of T-cell autoreactivity is facilitated by 1) MHC presentation of antigens, which limits the number of possible T epitopes and the number of APC (for MHC class II); and 2) the absence of affinity maturation during the immune responses of mature T cells, which precludes further changes of the antigen receptor repertoire after the clonal deletion/positive selection time point in T-cell ontogeny. In contrast, because there are no constraints on the B-cell antigen recognition of the kind due to the MHC antigen presentation for T cells, clonal elimination of autoreactive B cells is expected to be less complete. High-affinity self-reactive B cells and/or those reacting with high-density membrane antigens that strongly cross-link the B-cell antigen receptors (see ABO Histoblood Group Determinants, above) are most likely deleted as immature cells, but the elimination of all (including the very-low-affinity) self-reactive B cells would certainly re-

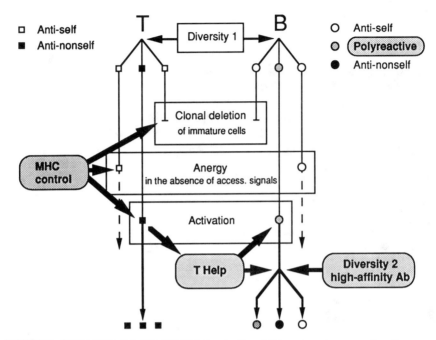

FIGURE 2. Similarities and differences between T and B lymphocytes regarding the control of autoreactivity (see text).

strict too much the B-cell specificity repertoire available for responses to foreign pathogens. Idiotypic interactions, in which antigen receptors recognize the variable regions of other antigen receptors, belong to the latter type of reactivity, which simply cannot be avoided. Idiotypic interactions may in fact contribute to the control of harmful autoreactivity, as is suggested, for example, by the existence in healthy human individuals of both autoantibodies to clotting Factor VIII and corresponding anti-idiotypic antibodies [Algiman et al., 1992; Dietrich et al., 1992].

Darwinian evolutionary constraints may have selected for a primary (germline) B-cell repertoire in which many receptors are of the polyreactive, "low affinity for everything" type. During immune responses, these B cells are then driven by antigenic selection/antibody feedback regulation to undergo mutations in the complementarity-determining regions of their V genes in order to become specific for toxins, bacteria, and viruses. This is in fact "adaptation" of receptors to antigens rather than "preformation." The helper T-cell dependence of affinity maturation indirectly confers MHC control upon B-cell responses. However, high affinity antibodies can also sometimes cross-react among foreign and self-antigens; self-reactivity can suddenly appear by somatic mutation.

It is not within the scope of this chapter to discuss the pathogenesis of autoimmune disease: lack of tolerance to "cryptic antigens," escape of

CD4/8 double-negative cells from clonal deletion [Reimann et al., 1988; von Boehmer et al., 1991], altered MHC expression due to virus infection [Maudsley and Pound, 1991], and so forth. Some chaos-type unpredictability also applies to immunology. This appears clearly in a transgenic mouse model of autoimmune hemolytic anemia: in mice from the same strain with the same immunoglobulin transgene for a certain erythrocyte self-antigen—which should thus all be genetically identical—B-cell clonal deletion, anergy, and sometimes hemolytic anemia occurred to various degrees in different individual mice [Okamoto et al., 1992]. Interestingly, the nontolerant B cells in the mice with anemia were $CD5^+$ and resided in the peritoneum; possibly the B cells were not much in contact with antigen at this anatomical site [Murakami et al., 1992]. An other possibility is that some particular kind of B-cell activation (see above, $CD5^+$ B Cells), which breaks the anergy of B cells and leads to CD5 expression, occurs in the peritoneum.

ACKNOWLEDGMENTS

Our experimental work mentioned in this chapter was supported in part by the Swiss National Science Foundation (grant 31-26502.89), the Fondation pour la recherche hématologique Geneva, and the Fondation Dubois-Ferrière/Dinu Lipatti, Geneva.

REFERENCES

Algiman M, Dietrich G, Nydegger UE, Boieldieu P, Sultan Y, Kazatchkine MD (1992): Antibodies to FVIII (anti-hemophilic factor) in healthy individuals. Proc Natl Acad Sci USA 89:3795–3799.

Aman P, Ehlin-Henriksson B, Klein G (1984): Epstein-Barr virus susceptibility of normal human B lymphocyte populations. J Exp Med 159:208–220.

Amoroso K, Lipsky PE (1990): Frequency of human B cells that differentite in response to anti-CD3–activated T cells. J Immunol 145:3155–3161.

Andersson J, Coutinho A, Lernhardt W, Melchers F (1977): Clonal growth and maturation to immunoglobulin secretion in vitro of every growth inducible B lymphocyte. Cell 10:27–34.

Baccala R, Quant TV, Gilbert M, Ternynck, Avrameas S (1989): Two murine natural polyreactive autoantibodies are encoded by nonmutated germ-line genes. Proc Natl Acad Sci USA 86:4624–4628.

Banchereau J, de Paoli P, Alle A, Garcia E, Rousset F (1991): Long term human B cell lines dependent on interleukin 4 and antibody to CD40. Science 251:70–72.

Borche L, Lim A, Binet J-L, Dighiero G (1990): Evidence that chronic lymphocytic leukemia B lymphocytes are frequently committed to production of natural autoantibodies. Blood 76:562–569.

Burastero SE, Casali P, Wilder RL, Notkins AL (1988): Monoreactive high affinity and polyreactive low affinity rheumatoid factors are produced by $CD5^+$ B cells from patients with rheumatoid arthritis. J Exp Med 168:1979–1992.

Burastero SE, Cutolo M, Dessi V, Celada F (1990): Monoreactive and polyreactive rheumatoid factors produced by in vitro Epstein-Barr virus–transformed peripheral blood and synovial B lymphocytes from rheumatoid arthritis patients. Scand J Immunol 32:347–357.

Caligaris-Cappio F, Riva M, Tesio L, Schena M, Gaidano G, Bergui L (1989): Human normal CD5$^+$ B lymphocytes can be induced to differentiate to CD5$^-$ B lymphocytes with germinal center cell features. Blood 73:1259–1263.

Carson DA (1991): The specificity of anti-DNA antibodies in systemic lupus erythematosus. J Immunol 146:1–2.

Casali P, Burastero SE, Balow JE, Notkins AL (1989): High-affinity antibodies to ssDNA are produced by CD$^-$ B cells in systemic lupus erythematosus patients. J Immunol 143:3476–3483.

Casali P, Burastero SE, Nakamura M, Inghirami G, Notkins AL (1987): Human lymphocytes making rheumatoid factor and antibody to ssDNA belong to Leu-1$^+$ B-cell subset. Science 236:77–80.

Casali P, Nakamura M, Ginsberg-Fellner F, Notkins AL (1990): Frequency of B cells committed to the production of antibodies to insulin in newly diagnosed patients with insulin-dependent diabetes mellitus and generation of high affinity human monoclonal IgG to insulin. J Immunol 144:3741–3747.

Conger JD, Pike BL, Nossal GJV (1984): Clonal analysis of the anti-DNA repertoire of murine B lymphocytes. Proc Natl Acad Sci USA 84:2931–2935.

Conger JD, Pike BL, Nossal GJV (1988): Analysis of the B lymphocyte repertoire by polyclonal activation. Hindrance by clones yielding antibodies which bind promiscuously to plastic. J Immunol Methods 106:181–189.

Dietrich G, Algiman M, Sultan Y, Nydegger UE, Kazatchkine MD (1992): Origin of anti-idiotypic activity against anti-factor VIII autoantibodies in pols of normal human immunoglobulin G (IVIg). Blood 79:2946–2951.

Dighiero G, Lymberi P, Holmberg D, Lundquist I, Coutinho A, Avrameas S (1985): High frequency of natural autoantibodies in normal newborn mice. J Immunol 134:765–771.

Duchosal MA, Kofler R, Balderas RS, Aguado MT, Dixon FJ, Theofilopoulos AN (1989): Genetic diversity of murine rheumatoid factors. J Immunol 142:1737–1742.

Dziarski R (1982): Preferential induction of autoantibody secretion in polyclonal activation by peptidoglycan and lipopolysaccharide. I. In vitro studies. J Immunol 128:1018–1025.

Erikson J, Radic MZ, Camper SA, Hardy RR, Carmack C, Weigert M (1991): Expression of anti-DNA immunoglobulin transgenes in non-autoimmune mice. Nature 349:331–334.

Eynon EE, Parker DC (1992): Small B cells as antigen-presenting cells in the induction of tolerance to soluble protein antigens. J Exp Med 175:131–138.

Fong S, Tsoukas CD, Frincke LA, Lawrance SK, Holbrook TL, Vaughan JH, Carson DA (1981): Age-associated changes in Epstein-Barr virus–induced human lymphocyte autoantibody responses. J Immunol 126:910–914.

Friedman DF, Cho EA, Goldman J, Carmack CE, Besa EC, Hardy RR, Silberstein LE (1991): The role of clonal selection in the pathogenesis of an autoreactive human B cell lymphoma. J Exp Med 174:525–537.

Friguet B, Chaffott AF, Djavadi-Ohaniance L, Goldberg M (1985): Measurements of the true affinity constant in solution of antigen–antibody complexes by enzyme-linked immunoabsorbent assays. J Immunol Methods 77:305–319.

Glotz D, Sollazzo M, Riley S, Zanetti M (1988): Isotype, V_H genes, and antigen-binding analysis of hybridomas from newborn normal Balb/c mice. J Immunol 141:383–390.

Gogolin-Ewens K, Meeusen E, Lee C-S, Brandon M (1989): Expression of CD5, a lymphocyte surface antigen, on the endothelium of blood vessels. Eur J Immunol 19:935–938.

Goodnow CC, Brink R, Adams E (1991): Breakdown of self-tolerance in anergic B lymphocytes. Nature 352:532–536.

Guilbert G, Dighiero G, Avrameas S (1982): Naturally occurring antibodies against nine common antigens in human sera. I. Detection, isolation and characterization. J Immunol 128:2779–2785.

Hardy RR, Hayakawa K (1986): Development and physiology of LY-1 B and its human homologue, LEU-1 B. Immunol Rev 93:53–79.

Haregewoin A, Singh B, Gupta RS, Finberg RW (1991): A mycobacterial heat-shock protein-responsive $\gamma\delta$ T cell clone also responds to the homologous human heat-shock protein: A possible link between infection and autoimmunity. J Infect Dis 163:156–160.

Henderson RA, Michel H, Sakaguchi K, Shabanowity J, Appella E, Hunt DF, Engelhard VH (1992): HLA-A2.1-associated peptides from a mutant cell line: A second pathway of antigen presentation. Science 255:1264–1266.

Herzenberg LA, Stall AM, Lalor PA, Sidman C, Moore WA, Parks DR, Herzenberg LA (1986): The LY-1 B cell lineage. Immunol Rev 93:81–102.

Hirohata S, Inoue T, Miyamoto T (1990): Frequency analysis of human peripheral blood B cells producing IgM-rheumatoid factor. Differential effects of stimulation with monoclonal antibodies to CD3 and *Staphylococcus aureus*. J Immunol 145:1681–1686.

Hoch S, Schur PH, Schwaber J (1983): Frequency of anti-DNA antibody producing cells from normals and patients with systemic lupus erythematosus. Clin Immunol Immunopathol 27:28–37.

Huang Y-P, Perrin LH, Miescher PA, Zubler RH (1988): Correlation of T and B cell activities in vitro and serum IL-2 levels in systemic lupus erythematosus. J Immunol 141:827–833.

Hunt DF, Henderson RA, Shabanowitz J, Sakaguchi K, Michel H, Sevilir N, Cox AL, Appella E, Engelhard VH (1992): Characterization of peptides bound to the class I MHC molecule HLA-A2.1 by mass spectrometry. Science 255:1261–1263.

Jacob L, Lety M-A, Choquette D, Viard J-P, Jacob F, Louvard D, Bach J-F (1987): Presence of antibodies against a cell-surface protein, cross-reactive with DNA, in systemic lupus erythematosus: A marker of the disease. Proc Natl Acad Sci USA 84:2956–2959.

Kantor AB (1991): The development and repertoire of B-1 cells (CD5 B cells). Immunol Today 12:389–391.

Kisielow P, Blüthmann H, Staerz UD, Steinmetz M, von Boehmer H (1988): Tolerance in T-cell-receptor transgenic mice involves deletion of nonmature $CD4^+8^+$ thymocytes. Nature 333:741–746.

Köhler G, Milstein C (1975): Continuous cultures of fused cells secreting antibody of predefined specificity. Nature 256:495–498.

Kuppers RC (1991): The frequency of LPS-responsive B cells to autologous and heterologous thyroglobulin. Cell Immunol 132:94–101.

Lefkovits I (1979): Limiting dilution analysis. In Lefkovits I, Pernis B (eds): "Immunological Methods." New York: Academic Press, pp 355–370.

Levinson AI, Dalal NF, Haidar M, Tar L, Orlow M (1987): Prominent IgM rheumatoid factor production by human cord blood lymphocytes stimulated in vitro with *Staphylococcus aureus* Cowan 1. J Immunol 139:2237–2241.

Lin R-H, Mamula MJ, Hardin JA, Janeway CA (1991): Induction of autoreactive B cells allows priming of autoreactive T cells. J Exp Med 173:1433–1439.

Londei M, Savill C, Verhoef A, Brennan F, Leech ZE, Duance V, Maini RN, Feldmann M (1989): Persistence of collagen type II–specific T cell clones in the synovial fluid of a patient with rheumatoid arthritis. Proc Natl Acad Sci USA 86:636–640.

Lorenz RG, Allen PM (1988): Direct evidence for functional self protein/Ia molecule complexes in vivo. Proc Natl Acad Sci USA 85:5220–5223.

Marion TN, Bothwell ALM, Briles DE, Janeway CA Jr (1989): IgG anti-DNA autoantibodies within an individual autoimmune mouse are the products of clonal selection. J Immunol 142:4269–4274.

Matthes T, Wolff A, Soubiran P, Gros F, Dighiero G (1988): Antitubulin antibodies. II. Natural autoantibodies and induced antibodies recognize different epitopes on the tubulin molecule. J Immunol 141:3135–3141.

Maudsley DJ, Pound JD (1991): Modulation of MHC antigen expression by viruses and oncogenes. Immunol Today 12:429–431.

Miller RA, Gralow J (1984): The induction of Leu-1 antigen expression in human malignant and normal B cells by phorbol myristic acetate (PMA). J Immunol 133:3408–3414.

Munk ME, Shoel B, Modrow S, Karr RW, Young RA, Kaufman SHE (1989): T lymphocytes from healthy individuals with specificity to self-epitopes shared by mycobacterial and human 65-kilodalton heat shock protein. J Immunol 143:2844–2849.

Munoz JL, Insel RA (1987): In vitro human antibody production to the *Haemophilus influenzae* type b capsular polysaccharide. J Immunol 139:2026–2031.

Murakami M, Tsubata T, Okamoto M, Shimizu A, Kumagai S, Imura H, Honjo T (1992): Antigen-induced apoptotic death of Ly-1 B cells responsible for autoimmune disease in transgenic mice. Nature 357:77–79.

Nakamura M, Burastero SE, Ueki Y, Larrick JW, Notkins AL, Casali P (1988): Probing the normal and autoimmune B cell repertoire with Epstein-Barr virus. Frequency of B cells producing monoreactive high affinity autoantibodies in patients with Hashimoto's disease and systemic lupus erythematosus. J Immunol 141:4165–4172.

Natvig JB, Randen I, Thompson K, Forre O (1989): The B cell system in the rheumatoid inflammation. New insights into the pathogenesis of rheumatoid arthritis using synovial B cell heterohybridoma clones. Springer Semin Immunopathol 11:301–313.

Nemazee DA, Bürki K (1989): Clonal deletion of B lymphocytes in a transgenic mouse bearing anti-MHC class I antibody genes. Nature 337:562–566.

Ofusu-Appiah WA, Warrington RJ, Wilkins JA (1989): Interleukin 2-responsive T cell clones from rheumatoid and normal subjects: Proliferative responses to connective tissue elements. Clin Immunol Immunopathol 50:264–271.

Okamoto M, Murakami M, Shimizu A, Ozaki S, Tsubata T, Kumagai S, Honjo T (1992): A transgenic model of autoimmune hemolytic anemia. J Exp Med 175: 71–79.

Panosian-Sahakian N, Klotz JL, Ebling F, Kronenberg M, Hahn B (1989): Diversity of Ig V gene segments found in anti-DNA autoantibodies from a single (NZB × NZW)F$_1$ mouse. J Immunol 142:4500–4506.

Pascual V, Capra JD (1991): Human immunoglobulin heavy-chain variable region genes: Organization, polymorphism, and expression. Adv Immunol 49:1–74.

Portnoi D, Freitas A, Holmberg D, Bandeira A, Coutinho A (1986): Immunocompetent autoreactive B lymphocytes are activated cycling cells in normal mice. J Exp Med 164:25–35.

Rauch J, Meng Q-H, Tannenbaum H (1987): Lupus anticoagulant and antiplatelet properties of human hybridoma autoantibodies. J Immunol 139:2598–2604.

Reimann J, Bellan A, Conradt P (1988): Development of autoreactive L3T4 + T cells from double-negative (L3T4-Ly-2) Thy-1 + spleen cells of normal mice. Eur J Immunol 18:989–1000.

Rieben R, Buchs JP, Flückiger E, Nydegger UE (1991): Antibodies to histo-blood group substances A and B: Agglutination titers, Ig class, and IgG subclasses in healthy persons of different age categories. Transfusion 31:607–615.

Rieben R, Tucci A, Nydegger UE, Zubler RH (1992): Self tolerance to human A and B histo-blood group antigens exists at the B cell level and can not be broken by potent polyclonal B cell activation in vitro. Eur J Immunol 22:2713–2717.

Rubin RL, Tang F-L, Chan EKL, Pollard KM, Tsay G, Tan EM (1986): IgG subclasses of autoantibodies in systemic lupus erythematosus, Sjögren's syndrome, and drug-induced autoimmunity. J Immunol 137:2528–2534.

Schild H, Rötzschke O, Kalbacher H, Rammensee H-G (1990): Limit of T cell tolerance to self proteins by peptide presentation. Science 247:1587–1589.

Schlomchik M, Mascelli M, Shaw H, Radic MZ, Pisetsky D, Marshak-Rothstein A, Weigert M (1990): Anti-DNA antibodies from autoimmune mice arise by clonal expansion and somatic mutation. J Exp Med 171:265–297.

Schwartz RH (1989): Acquisition of immunologic self-tolerance. Cell 57:1073–1081.

Shibata T, Berney T, Reininger L, Chicheportiche Y, Ozaki S, Shirai T, Izui S (1990): Monoclonal anti-erythrocyte autoantibodies derived from NZB mice cause autoimmune hemolytic anemia by two distinct pathogenic mechanisms. Int Immunol 2:1133–1141.

Souroujon M, White-Scharf ME, Andre-Schwartz J, Gefter ML, Schwartz RS (1988): Preferential autoantibody reactivity of the preimmune B cell repertoire in normal mice. J Immunol 140:4173–4179.

Splawski JD, Jelinek DF, Lipsky PE (1991): Delineation of the functional capacity of neonatal human lymphocytes. J Clin Invest 87:54–61.

Straub C, Zubler RH (1989): Immortalization of EBV-infected B cells is not influenced by exogenous signals acting on B cell proliferation. Effects of mutant EL-4 thymoma cells and transforming growth factor-β. J Immunol 142:87–93.

Strober W, James SP (1990): Immunoregulatory function of human autoreactive T cell lines and clones. In "Immunological Reviews." Copenhagen, Denmark: Munksgaard, pp 133–138.

Taswell C (1980): Limiting dilution assays for the determination of immunocompetent cell frequencies. I. Data analysis. J Immunol 126:1614–1620.

Tucci A, James H, Chicheportiche R, Bonnefoy J-Y, Dayer J-M, Zubler RH (1992): Effects of eleven cytokines, and of IL-1 and TNF inhibitors, in a human B cell assay. J Immunol 148:2778–2784.

Tucci A, Mouzaki A, James H, Bonnefoy J-Y, Zubler RH (1991): Are cord blood B cells functionally mature? Clin Exp Immunol 84:389–394.

Ueki Y, Goldlfarb IS, Harindranath N, Gore M, Koprowski H, Notkins AL, Casali P (1990): Clonal analysis of a human antibody response. Quantitation of precursors of antibody-producing cells and generation and characterization of monoclonal IgM, IgG, and IgA to rabies virus. J Exp Med 171:19–34.

Vernino LA, Pisetsky DS, Lipsky PE (1992): Analysis of the expression of CD5 by human B cells and correlation with functional activity. Cell Immunol 139:185–197.

von Boehmer H, Kirberg J, Rocha B (1991): An unusual lineage of α/β T cells that contains autoreactive cells. J Exp Med 174:1001–1008.

Weksler ME, Schwab R, Huetz F, Kim YT, Coutinho A (1990): Cellular basis for the age-associated increase in autoimmune reactions. Int Immunol 2:329–335.

Welch MJ, Fong S, Vaughan J, Carson D (1983): Increased frequency of rheumatoid factor precursor B lymphocytes after immunization of normal adults with tetanus toxoid. Clin Exp Immunol 51:299–304.

Wen L, Hanvanich M, Werner-Favre C, Brouwers N, Perrin LH, Zubler RH (1987): Limiting dilution assay for human B cells based on their activation by mutant EL-4 thymoma cells: Total and anti-malaria responder B cell frequencies. Eur J Immunol 17:887–892.

Wen L, Peakman M, Lobo-Yeo A, McFarlane BM, Mowat AP, Mieli-Vergani G, Vergani D (1990): T-cell-directed hepatocyte damage in autoimmune chronic active hepatitis. Lancet 336:1527–1530.

Werner-Favre C, Vischer TL, Wohlwend D, Zubler RH (1989): Cell surface antigen CD5 is a marker for activated huma B cells. Eur J Immunol 19:1209–1213.

Ying-zi C, Rabin E, Wortis HH (1990): Treatment of murine CD5 B cells with anti-Ig, but not LPS, induces surface CD5: Two B-cell activation pathways. Int Immunol 3:467–476.

Zhang X, Werner-Favre C, Tang H, Brouwers N, Bonnefoy J-Y, Zubler RH (1991): Interleukin-4 dependent IgE switch in membrane IgA-positive human B cells. J Immunol 174:3001–3004.

Zöller M, Achtnich M (1991): Evidence for regulation of naturally activated autoreactive B cells. Eur J Immunol 21:305–312.

Zubler RH, Perrin LH, Doucet A, Zhang X, Huang Y-P, Miescher PA (1992): Frequencies of HIV-reactive B cells in seropositive and seronegative individuals. Clin Exp Immunol 87:31–36.

Zubler RH, Werner-Favre C, Wen LI, Sekita K, Straub C (1987): Theoretical and practical aspects of B cell activation: Murine and human systems. Immunol Rev 99:281–299.

13

TOLERANCE AND AUTOIMMUNITY IN THE PERIPHERAL T-CELL REPERTOIRE

J.F.A.P. Miller

The Walter and Eliza Hall Institute of Medical Research, Post Office Royal Melbourne Hospital, Victoria, Australia

INTRODUCTION

The immune system must not only resist infections but also ensure that it does not react against the body's own tissues. Since individual clones of lymphocytes have predetermined reactivities, some will be self-reactive and have the potential to cause damage. They should therefore be eliminated or neutralized in some way. It may be expected that in a system as complex and important as that governing self-tolerance many mechanisms should exist to neutralize autoaggressive lymphocytes.

Various explanations for the imposition and maintenance of tolerance have been suggested. They can be classified under two main categories. In one the tolerant state arises from the physical or functional silencing of potentially reactive lymphocytes after antigen encounter. This may involve clonal deletion, clonal abortion, or clonal anergy [Nossal, 1986]. In the second, regulatory mechanisms of the immune system itself hold the reac-

Autoimmunity: Physiology and Disease, Pages 191–202
© *1994 Wiley-Liss, Inc.*

tive lymphocytes in check, for example, through the operation of idiotypic network interactions and the action of specialized suppressor cells.

In many experimental studies designed to investigate the processes responsible for inducing immunological tolerance, the immune system has been confronted, not with *self*-constituents, but with *exogenous* antigens introduced systemically. There are several reasons why this may not mimic the natural situation. The most important is that an immune response does not result from a simple interaction of antigen and lymphocyte, but from the activation of a complex network of interacting cells and molecules. Each response is an amplified reaction and is thus subjected to appropriate control mechanisms. Hence unresponsiveness following the introduction of exogenous antigen may result from normal control processes that limit the immune response rather than from events that actually occur during the induction of immunological tolerance to a *self*-constituent. It is therefore important to bear this in mind when considering mechanisms of self-tolerance in light of results obtained from work done in vitro or in vivo using exogenous antigens.

In this discussion, I deal with some aspects of tolerance in T cells to exogenous antigens and to antigens synthesized by the body's own cells, i.e., self-tolerance. I first consider what pertains to lymphocytes differentiating within the thymus and then what might be relevant to mature peripheral T cells.

INTRATHYMIC NEGATIVE SELECTION

The intrathymic negative selection of differentiating T cells with antiself-reactivity is clearly one way in which self-tolerance can be achieved. This has been proven experimentally by using models in which the frequency of T cells specific for a given self-antigen was unusually high. One such model exploited the naturally high frequency of T cells reactive to superantigens. In mice with such antigens, T cells with superantigen-specific T-cell receptors (TCR) were found in the immature population of thymus lymphocytes but not in the mature intrathymic or peripheral T-cell pools [Kappler et al., 1987, MacDonald et al., 1988]. Differentiating T cells were thus deleted within the thymus. In another model, transgenic technology was used to introduce, into the germline of mice, rearranged TCR genes encoding a specificity directed to the male (H-Y) antigen in the context of the class I H-2D^b molecule. Tolerance to H-Y could be demonstrated in male H-2^b mice but not in female mice, H-Y-autospecific T cells being deleted at the CD4$^+$CD8$^+$ stage in the former [Kisielow et al., 1988]. Self-epitopes existing intrathymically may thus be presented to maturing T cells in a manner that leads to what I had referred to as a *selective immunological thymectomy* 30 years ago [Miller, 1962].

If we consider that self-tolerance in T cells is imposed solely within the thymus, two questions arise. Are all autoantigens expressed intrathymically? If not, what happens to T cells that have the potential to respond to antigens not represented within the thymus but unique to extrathymic tissues? Conceivably extrathymic autoantigens could be shed and ferried to the thymus either as such or via circulating monocytes or macrophages. These incoming cells might then tolerize potentially reactive T cells as they differentiate within the thymus. This may be so for $CD4^+$ T cells that usually recognize exogenous peptides [Braciale et al., 1987]. The situation with $CD8^+$ T cells is clearly different as these cells generally perceive endogenously synthesized peptides. As hypothesized by Boon and van Pel [1989], antigenic peptides derived from the cellular genome may not be degradation products of the cellular proteins but may be generated directly by autonomous transcription and translation of short subgenic regions that they termed *peptons*. Key cells in the thymus might thus be able to transcribe peptons very efficiently and present the entire pepton repertoire within the thymus. If that is so, tolerance to self-constituents would occur only by the intrathymic deletion of potentially autoaggressive T cells.

As there is, at the time of writing, no direct evidence for the pepton hypothesis, and no evidence to show that all genes are transcribed and translated in the thymus, the fate of autoreactive T cells outside the thymus must be investigated. It is in fact very important to determine whether such T cells may be silenced extrathymically, because an insight into the mechanism of silencing may shed light on the pathogenesis of some autoimmune conditions. In addition, it may give us hints as to how we might proceed to switch off those specific T cells responsible for rejecting transplants of tissues and organs.

It is, however, quite possible that extrathymic autoantigens need not induce tolerance simply because they could elude the immune system and hence not provoke an immune response. This may be the case if they are sequestered in an immunologically privileged site, or exposed on cell types not expressing MHC molecules, and thus unable to present peptides to T cells. It may also be so if the cell surface concentration of autoantigens is too low to be detected by T cells or if the avidity of the combined TCR and CD4 or CD8 molecules is not high enough for T cells to make effective contact. If these conditions are not met, however, do postthymic T-cell toleragenic mechanisms exist?

TOLERANCE OF PERIPHERAL T CELLS TO EXOGENOUS ANTIGENS

It is a fact that tolerance to *exogenous* antigens can be induced in adult thymectomized mice. It has been achieved both with deaggregated protein antigens [Mitchison, 1968] and, more recently, with skin grafts [Qin et al., 1992]. In the latter case, life-long tolerance to skin allografts was established by using a short course of nondepleting anti-CD4 and anti-CD8 monoclonal antibodies. Tolerance could not be broken by infusing normal lymphocytes from genetically identical donors, this phenomenon being termed *resistance*. The cells responsible for resistance were shown to be the host's own T cells. By infusing genetically marked but otherwise syngeneic lymphocytes, it could also be shown that the donor T cells became tolerant of graft antigens within 2 weeks. Hence tolerance could "spread" from a tolerant T-cell population to a nontolerant one, provided the two coexisted for at least 2 weeks. While the mechanism responsible for this "pervasive" tolerance is not clear, the results show that tolerance can indeed be induced in mature peripheral T cells.

As shown by several investigators [Rocha and von Boehmer, 1991; Webb et al., 1990], tolerance can be imposed on a population of injected mature T cells as the end result of a powerful immune response to an antigen that is not eliminated but that persists. For example, following the injection of syngeneic spleen cells into irradiated transgenic mice expressing the class I molecule, K^b, on liver cells, activated lymphocytes infiltrated the liver lobules and proliferated. Most were confined to the portal tracts where they inflicted piecemeal necrosis of the adjacent hepatocytes. With increasing time after inoculation, the response became more subdued, and by 12 weeks the few portal tracts that were still infiltrated showed no accompanying necrosis and the lymphocytes were small and apparently inactive [Morahan et al., 1989a]. In a similar model, but in one using appropriate strain combinations, it was shown that adult thymectomized transgenic recipients of syngeneic spleen cells could reject K^b skin grafts at 3 weeks but were tolerant at 12 weeks (Morahan et al., unpublished data). Hence even mature T cells can be silenced after a powerful immune response to a persisting antigen.

In vitro work has also provided excellent evidence for tolerance induction in mature peripheral T cells. Using a clone of human T cells specific for a defined peptide of influenza hemagglutinin, some investigators were able to induce a form of immunological tolerance by incubating the clone for several hours at 37°C with a high concentration of peptide in the absence of antigen-presenting cells (APC). The T cells remained alive and were therefore "anergic." Since APC reduced the degree of tolerance induced at any single peptide concentration, a costimulator signal derived from these APC seemed to be essential for immune induction [Lamb et al., 1983]. Furthermore, interleukin-2 (IL-2), but not interferon-γ or IL-1, inhibited the induction of tolerance, and the addition of IL-2 reversed established tolerance [Essery et al., 1988]. Similar in vitro experiments with T-cell clones performed by Schwartz [1990] also showed that the anergic T cells were unable to produce their own growth factor, IL-2, on restimulation.

Attempts to elucidate the nature of the costimulator signal have not been successful [Weaver and Unanue, 1990]. It could be mediated through a cytokine such as IL-1 or through some ligand for the T-cell surface molecule CD28 [Gross et al., 1990; Harding et al., 1992]. In general, it would appear that, at least in vitro, antigen receptor occupancy in the absence of costimulator activity renders mature T cells anergic and unable to respond to a subsequent appropriate presentation of the same antigen.

One may be tempted to extrapolate these results to explain extrathymic tolerance to self-constituents in vivo by simply invoking the absence of any costimulating activity by cells expressing unique self-epitopes. The evidence summarized above for peripheral tolerance has, however, been obtained only in models in which the antigens were not self-components but exogenous with respect to the potentially autoreactive T cells. The case for peripheral tolerance to self-constituents must therefore be examined in models in which both the self-antigen and the corresponding reactive T cells can readily be identified.

DO SELF-ANTIGENS TOLERIZE PERIPHERAL T CELLS?

Whether tolerance can be induced to extrathymic self-antigens has been investigated in transgenic mouse models. For example, by linking a class I MHC gene to a tissue-specific promoter and introducing the construct into fertilized mouse eggs of a given strain, expression can be directed to specific cell types outside the thymus. The effect of these molecules on the peripheral T-cell repertoire can thus be studied.

We linked the gene coding for the class I molecule, K^b, to the rat insulin promoter and microinjected the construct into fertilized eggs derived from mice of non-B haplotypes, i.e., from strains that do not normally produce this molecule. The aim was to create transgenic mice expressing the K^b gene in the insulin-producing β-cells of the islets of the pancreas, but not in the thymus. Immunochemical techniques revealed abundant expression of K^b in the β-cells. None was detected in the thymus. No lymphocytic infiltration was seen in the islets, even if we attempted to immunize the mice. Interestingly, β-cell dysfunction and therefore diabetes became evident after 3–4 weeks of age. This resulted not from any autoimmune reaction as happens in classic diabetes, but from the toxic effects of the accumulation of the transgenic class I molecules being overexpressed [Allison et al., 1988]. The absence of lymphocyte infiltration hinted at the possibility that the mice were tolerant of K^b. Indeed, K^b-bearing skin was not rejected by young transgenic mice, designated RIP-K^b, but third-party skin was, indicating specific tolerance [Morahan et al., 1989b]. Tolerance, however, waned by about 17 weeks of age, and this was originally attributed to loss of β-cells and therefore to a fall in antigen concentration [Miller et al., 1991]. It thus became necessary to determine what happened to the K^b-specific CD8$^+$ T cells in these tolerant mice: Were they deleted or functionally silenced, and did this occur in the periphery?

Tracking these cells in the RIP-K^b mice could not, however, be done, because the frequency of K^b-specific T cells is too low to be detected directly and there is no dominant clonotype in the K^b-specific T-cell response. The problem was overcome by crossing RIP-K^b mice to mice transgenic for genes encoding a K^b-specific TCR so that a large proportion of the T cells of the double transgenic offspring were K^b-specific and of a single clonotype. In addition, the TCR of the K^b-specific T cells could be identified by a clonotypic antibody called *Désiré* or *Des,* which we gratefully received from colleagues in Marseille and Heidelberg [Schönrich et al., 1991].

When peripheral CD8 T cells in single TCR (Des) transgenic mice and double, RIP-K^b × Des, transgenic mice were compared by flow cytometry, the cells expressing the highest density of TCR were lacking in the double transgenic mice. Would these have been deleted peripherally or intrathymically? Flow cytometry showed a 50% reduction in the percentage of $CD8^+$ cells in the thymus of the double transgenic mice as compared to that of the Des mice [Heath et al., 1992]. A few molecules of K^b must therefore have been present intrathymically and able to delete T cells with the highest density of TCR and presumably with the highest avidity for K^b. Although various molecular techniques, including Northern blots and S1 nuclease mapping, failed to reveal thymus expression, the highly sensitive polymerase chain reaction did detect transgene mRNA as a slim band in the thymus of RIP-K^b mice [Miller et al., 1989].

It was necessary to determine whether the lower avidity cells (that is, the CD8 cells expressing a lower density of DES TCR), still present in the periphery of double transgenic mice, were either indifferent to the K^b molecules expressed on the β-cells or functionally silenced in some way. Young transgenic mice were therefore grafted with K^b-bearing skin: Both Des and RIP-K^b × Des mice rejected these grafts [Heath et al., 1992]. The lack of tolerance in the double transgenic mice could not be accounted for by the response of newly derived T cells that had not yet encountered β-cell antigens, because similar results were obtained in mice that had been thymectomized at 6 weeks of age. How can we reconcile the fact that tolerance was observed in the young RIP-K^b mice but not in the double transgenic mice? Possibly, the number of low avidity cells that escaped thymus censorship in the former have had to build up to a certain level before they could cause skin graft rejection. This period of time would of course be reduced in the RIP-K^b × Des transgenic mice in which the majority of the T cells in the peripheral pool are K^b-specific.

It seems therefore that in these transgenic models the β-cell antigen is ignored by antigen-specific T cells. This is in line with studies using transgenic mice expressing the lymphocytic choriomeningitis virus (LCMV) glycoprotein (GP) or nucleoprotein (NP) in the β-cells of the pancreas. The T cells in these mice did not appear to be influenced by the GP or NP antigens, but, after infection with LCMV, $CD8^+$ T cells were activated and produced selective and progressive β-cell damage leading to diabetes

[Ohashi et al., 1991; Oldstone et al., 1991]. In our RIP-K^b × Des mice, however, no lymphocytic infiltration was observed in or around the islets whether or not the mice had been primed by skin grafting. One interpretation of this result is that "low-avidity" K^b-specific T cells that escaped thymus censorship in the double transgenic mice had insufficient avidity to cause a destructive response in the islets, even after cross-stimulation with skin graft antigens.

When single transgenic RIP-K^b mice were thymectomized, irradiated, and reconstituted with bone marrow from Des transgenic mice and thymus grafts from nontransgenic mice so that the thymus could not express K^b, they showed no deletion of high avidity K^b-specific T cells in the periphery and could reject K^b skin graft as rapidly as control nontransgenic mice (Heath et al., unpublished data). Hence in this model T cells had not been silenced but had remained indifferent to antigens expressed on β-cells.

The lack of tolerance in this particular model contrasts with several other reports in which tolerance to extrathymically expressed K^b was observed. This may be due to the K^b antigen being expressed in different sites [Schönrich et al., 1991, 1992] and perhaps in different amounts or to the inability to detect the α-chain of the transgenic TCR in one of our previous models [Morahan et al., 1991].

INTERLEUKIN-2 AND AUTOIMMUNITY

In some experimental situations in vitro and in vivo, IL-2 has interfered with immunological tolerance [Kroemer et al., 1989; Morahan et al., 1989b; Dallman et al., 1991]. For example, in the rat model of tolerance induced by blood transfusion [Dallman et al., 1991], T cells did infiltrate the tolerated kidney allografts, but were unable to make biologically active IL-2, and tolerance was abrogated by the administration of IL-2 at the time of transplantation. The failure of the cells to make IL-2 was not reflected at the mRNA level, as the IL-2 gene was transcribed to similar levels in both tolerant and treated rats. There was a reduced expression of the p55 IL-2 receptor (IL-2R) chain on the T-cell surface and a lower level of transcription of both IL-2R α- and β-chain mRNA. This resulted in a reduced ability of the cells to proliferate in response to IL-2. Altered regulation of the IL-2 pathway is thus clearly an intracellular lesion of the induction of tolerance in this model.

Another in vivo situation in which IL-2 appears to have reversed tolerance was that following thymectomy of infant mice. A variety of organ-specific autoimmune diseases have developed in these mice, the particular syndrome being determined by the genetic background [Taguchi and Nishizuka, 1980; Kojima and Prehn, 1981]. Autoreactive T cells released from the neonatal thymus, which normally would have been deleted or diluted [Smith et al., 1989], were responsible for mediating the disease [Taguchi and Nishizuka, 1980]. In some cases, however, these cells behaved as anergic cells [Jones et al., 1990; Andreu-Sánchez et al., 1991], although they could be reactivated in vivo by high levels of IL-2 [Andreu-Sánchez et al., 1991].

The fact that IL-2 reversed tolerance in vitro and in some in vivo models suggests the possibility that the onset of an autoimmune response might result from the inappropriate delivery of IL-2 to T cells that had not undergone negative selection, because their antigen was not encountered in the thymus. To determine whether local IL-2 production in the pancreas of RIP-K^b transgenic mice would activate K^b-specific T cells, we created "RIP-IL-2" transgenic mice expressing IL-2 in the β cells [Allison et al., 1992]. Triple transgenic mice were then produced by mating the RIP-K^b × Des mice to homozygous RIP-IL-2 mice. These developed severe diabetes as early as 1 week after birth and died within a few weeks [Heath et al., 1992]. This contrasts with the RIP-IL-2 and the RIP-IL-2 × Des mice, which did not develop the disease, and with the RIP-IL-2 × RIP-K^b mice, which became diabetic at about 3 weeks of age following the accumulation of toxic levels of class I molecules within the β cells [Allison et al., 1988]. The severe diabetes occurring in the triple transgenic mice indicates that those K^b-specific T cells, still present in the periphery, could destroy K^b-expressing β cells provided IL-2 was also expressed by these cells. As the expression of IL-2 by β cells induces a large lymphocytic infiltrate [Allison et al., 1992], flow cytometry was used to analyze the phenotype of the T cells and their expression of IL-2 receptors (IL-2R). A large proportion of the infiltrating cells in the triple transgenic mice were Des$^+$CD8$^+$, and many of these expressed IL-2R. By contrast, age-matched RIP-IL-2 × Des had only few of these cells. It is not clear whether IL-2R expression on the infiltrating K^b-specific cells was induced by the K^b molecules on the β cells, by cross-priming on environmental antigens, by local exposure to IL-2, or by nonspecific stimulation. What is clear is that locally produced IL-2 did lead to the stimulation of an antigen-specific autoimmune response.

SUMMARY AND CONCLUSIONS

The major mechanism responsible for tolerance to self-components in the T-cell repertoire is undoubtedly intrathymic clonal deletion. The point of contention is whether peripheral tolerance mechanisms exist to neutralize potentially autoaggressive T cells, which escape thymus censorship because the corresponding autoantigen may not have been expressed intrathymically, at least in sufficient amounts. That such mechanisms exist has been clearly demonstrated in the case of tolerance to exogenous antigens as referred to above. But these mechanisms may be operating as part of the normal feedback processes limiting any immune response, and there is no proof that they operate for the induction of tolerance to *self* constituents in peripheral T cells.

Anergy in T-cell clones has readily been demonstrated in vitro and is thought to result from the presentation of antigen by "nonprofessional" antigen-presenting cells that lack costimulatory activity. If such APC do exist in vivo and are able to present antigen to T cells in the absence of costimulation, a case could be made for tolerance induction in mature peripheral T cells in vivo.

The autoimmune manifestations observed in mice in which T cell development was abnormal [e.g., Taguchi and Nishizuka, 1980] might reflect a disturbance of the balance that normally exists between different T-cell subsets with distinct lymphokine profiles [Mosmann and Coffman, 1989; Fiorentino et al., 1989; Fowell et al., 1991]. Presumably, some mature extrathymic T cells might prevent autoimmunity by producing lymphokines that antagonize the responsiveness of other T cells that have not undergone negative selection in the thymus because their receptors were specific for autoantigens not expressed intrathymically. Another possibility would be that disturbed T-cell development predisposes to infection. The ensuing inflammatory response would lead to the release of antigens normally sequestered from the immune system. Alternatively, a cross-reactive virus-encoded antigen presented on professional antigen-presenting cells would activate specific T cells that otherwise would have ignored the autoantigen. An autoimmune reaction would then ensue.

Transgenic technology has allowed a different approach to the investigation of peripheral T-cell tolerance to self-components. While some models have suggested that extrathymic tolerance has indeed been imposed and may be associated with downregulation of the TCR [Morahan et al., 1991; Schönrich et al., 1991, 1992], other models clearly indicate that potentially autoaggressive T cells can ignore extrathymic antigens [Ohashi et al., 1991; Oldstone et al., 1991; Heath et al., 1992]. If such autoimmune T cells are not normally stimulated by autoantigens, cross-reactive stimulation on environmental antigens, perhaps following virus infection, would produce an autoimmune response. In the RIP-K^b × Des model described above, the low avidity K^b-specific T cells that escaped thymus censorship were not able to cause islet cell damage even after priming by skin grafting. However, the rapid onset of islet destruction and diabetes in the triple transgenic RIP-IL-2 × RIP-K^b × Des mice indicates that these low avidity cells can be stimulated to aggression provided sufficient "help" is available in the form of IL-2. Hence the occurrence and progression of an autoimmune response may critically depend on the avidity of the self-reactive T cells and may be influenced by exogenous IL-2 that could be provided during the course of a chronic infection.

ACKNOWLEDGMENTS

The work performed by the author and his colleagues was supported by grants from the National Health and Medical Research Council of Australia, the US Cancer Research Institute, and National Institutes of Health grant 1 R01 AI29385.

REFERENCES

Andreu-Sánchez J, de Alborán IM, Marcos MAR, Sánchez-Movilla A, Martinez-AC, Kroemer G (1991): Interleukin 2 abrogates the nonresponsive state of T cells expressing a forbidden T cell receptor repertoire and induces autoimmune disease in neonatally thymectomized mice. J Exp Med 173:1323–1329.

Allison J, Campbell IL, Morahan G, Mandel TE, Harrison L, Miller JFAP (1988): Diabetes in transgenic mice resulting from over-expression of class I histocompatibility molecules in pancreatic β cells. Nature 333:529–533.

Allison J, Malcolm L, Chosich N, Miller JFAP (1992): Inflammation but not autoimmunity occurs in transgenic mice expressing constitutive levels of interleukin-2 in islet β cells. Eur J Immunol 22:1115–1121.

Boon T, van Pel A (1989): T cell-recognized antigenic peptides derived from the cellular genome are not protein degradation products but can be generated directly by transcription and translation of short subgenic regions. A hypothesis. Immunogenetics 29:75–79.

Braciale TJ, Morrison LA, Sweetser MT, Sambrook J, Gething M-J, Braciale VL (1987): Antigen presentation pathways to class I and class II MHC-restricted T lymphocytes. Immunol Rev 98:95–114.

Dallman MJ, Shiho O, Page TH, Wood K, Morris PJ (1991): Peripheral tolerance to alloantigen results from altered regulation of the interleukin pathway. J Exp Med 173:79–87.

Essery G, Feldmann M, Lamb JR (1988): Interleukin-2 can prevent and reverse antigen-induced unresponsiveness in cloned human T lymphocytes. Immunology 64:413–417.

Fiorentino DF, Bond MW, Mosmann TR (1989): Two types of mouse T helper cells. IV. Th2 clones secrete a factor that inhibits cytokine production by Th1 clones. J Exp Med 170:2081–2095.

Fowell D, McKnight AJ, Powrie F, Dyke R, Mason D (1991): Subsets of CD4[+] T cells and their roles in the induction and prevention of autoimmunity. Immunol Rev 123:37–64.

Gross JA, St John T, Allison JP (1990): The murine homologue of the T lymphocyte antigen CD28. Molecular cloning and cell surface expression. J Immunol 144:3201–3210.

Harding FA, McArthur JG, Gross JA, Raulet DH, Allison JP (1992): CD28-mediated signalling co-stimulates murine T cells and prevents induction of anergy in T-cell clones. Nature 356:607–609.

Heath WR, Allison J, Hoffmann MW, Schönrich G, Hämmerling G, Arnold B, Miller JFAP (1992): Autoimmune diabetes as a consequence of locally produced interleukin-2. Nature 359:547–549.

Jones LA, Chin LT, Merriam GR, Nelson LM, Kruisbeek AM (1990): Failure of clonal deletion in neonatally thymectomized mice: Tolerance is preserved through clonal anergy. J Exp Med 172:1277–1285.

Kappler JW, Roehm M, Marrack P (1987): T cell tolerance by clonal elimination in the thymus. Cell 49:273–280.

Kisielow P, Blüthmann H, Staerz UD, Steinmetz M, von Boehmer H (1988): Tolerance in T-cell-receptor transgenic mice involves deletion of nonmature CD4$^+$8$^+$ thymocytes. Nature 333:742–746.

Kojima A, Prehn RT (1981): Genetic susceptibility to post-thymectomy autoimmune disease in mice. Immunogenetics 14:15–27.

Kroemer G, Wick G (1989): The role of interleukin 2 in autoimmunity. Immunol Today 7:246–251.

Lamb JR, Skidmore BJ, Green N, Chiller JM, Feldmann M (1983): Induction of tolerance in influenza virus-immune T lymphocyte clones with syngeneic peptides of influenza hemagglutinin. J Exp Med 157:1434–1447.

MacDonald HR, Sneider R, Lees RK, Howe RC, Acha-Orbea H, Fetenstein H, Zinkernagel RM, Hengartner H (1988): T cell receptor V use predicts reactivity and tolerance to Mls^a-encoded antigens. Nature 332:40–45.

Miller JFAP (1962): Effect of neonatal thymectomy on the immunological responsiveness of the mouse. Proc R Soc [Biol] 156:410–428.

Miller JFAP, Morahan G, Allison J (1989): Extra-thymic acquisition of tolerance by T lymphocytes. Cold Spring Harbor Symp Quant Biol 54:807–813.

Miller JFAP, Morahan G, Hoffmann M, Allison J (1991): A transgenic approach to the study of peripheral T cell tolerance. Immunol Rev 122:103–116.

Mitchison NA (1968): The dosage requirements for immunological paralysis by soluble proteins. Immunology 15:509–530.

Morahan G, Brennan F, Bhathal PS, Allison J, Cox KO, Miller JFAP (1989a): Expression in transgenic mice of class I histocompatibility antigens controlled by the metallothionein promoter. Proc Natl Acad Sci USA 86:3782–3786.

Morahan G, Allison J, Miller JFAP (1989b): Tolerance of class I histocompatibility antigens expressed extra-thymically. Nature 339:622–624.

Morahan G, Hoffman M, Miller JFAP (1991): A non-deletional mechanism of peripheral tolerance in T cell receptor transgenic mice. Proc Natl Acad Sci USA 88:11421–11425.

Mosmann TR, Coffman RL (1989): TH1 and TH2 cells: different patterns of lymphokine secretion lead to different functional properties. Annu Rev Immunol 7:145–173.

Nossal GJV (1986): The regulatory biology of antibody formation. Proc R Soc [Biol] 228:225–240.

Ohashi PS, Oehen S, Buerki K, Pircher H, Ohashi CT, Odermatt B, Malissen B, Zinkernagel RM, Hengartner H (1991): Ablation of "tolerance" and induction of diabetes by virus infection in viral antigen transgenic mice. Cell 65:305–317.

Oldstone MBA, Nerenberg M, Southern P, Price J, Lewicki H (1991): Virus infection triggers insulin-dependent diabetes mellitus in a transgenic model: Role of anti-self (virus) immune response. Cell 65:319–331.

Qin S, Cobbold SP, Pope H, Elliott J, Kioussis D, Davies J, Waldmann H (1993): "Infectious" transplantation tolerance. Science 259:974–977.

Rocha R, von Boehmer H (1991): Peripheral selection of the T cell repertoire. Science 251:1225–1228.

Schönrich G, Kalinke U, Momburg F, Malissen M, Schmitt-Verhulst A-M, Malissen B, Hämmerling GJ, Arnold B (1991): Downregulation of T cell receptors on self-reactive T cells as a novel mechanism for extrathymic tolerance induction. Cell 65:293–304.

Schönrich G, Momburg F, Malissen M, Schmitt-Verhulst A-M, Malissen B, Hämmerling GJ, Arnold B (1992): Distinct mechanisms of extrathymic T cell tolerance due to differential expression of self antigen. Int Immunol 4:581–590.

Schwartz RH (1990): A cell culture model for T lymphocyte clonal anergy. Science 248:1349–1356.

Smith H, Chen I-M, Kubo R, Tung KSK (1989): Neonatal thymectomy results in a repertoire enriched in T cells deleted in adult thymus. Science 245:749–752.

Taguchi O, Nishizuka Y (1980): Autoimmune oophoritis in thymectomized mice: T cell requirement in adoptive cell transfer. Clin Exp Immunol 42:324–331.

Weaver CT, Unanue ER (1990): The costimulatory function of antigen-presenting cells. Immunol Today 11:49–55.

Webb SR, Morris C, Sprent J (1990): Extrathymic tolerance of mature T cells: Clonal elimination as a consequence of immunity. Cell 63:1249–1256.

14

THYMUS, T CELLS, AND AUTOIMMUNITY: VARIOUS CAUSES BUT A COMMON MECHANISM OF AUTOIMMUNE DISEASE

Shimon Sakaguchi and Noriko Sakaguchi

The Institute of Physical and Chemical Research (RIKEN), Tsukuba Life Science Center, Tsukuba, Ibaraki, Japan

The cause of the phenomenon is single, though the means for making it appear may be multiple and apparently very various.

—Claude Bernard [1865]

INTRODUCTION

Accumulating evidence indicates that T cells play a pivotal role in generating various autoimmune diseases in humans and animals [Good et al., 1957; Like et al., 1981; De Calvalho et al., 1981; Londei et al., 1985; Wofsy and Seaman; 1985; Shizuru et al., 1988]. Unlike B cells, in which somatic hypermutation of immunoglobulin genes significantly contributes to the formation of self-reactive specificities, the repertoire of T cells is solely determined in the

Autoimmunity: Physiology and Disease, Pages 203–227
© *1994 Wiley-Liss, Inc.*

thymus by rearrangement of the T-cell receptor (TCR) genes with nucleotide insertion at the junctions of gene segments and by subsequent positive–negative selections [Marrack and Kappler, 1987; Davis and Bjorkman, 1988; Sprent et al., 1988]. T cells bearing TCRs with high affinity for self-antigens expressed in the thymus are clonally deleted [Kappler et al., 1987; Kisielow et al., 1988]. It is controversial, however, how those T cells specific for self-antigens expressed outside the thymus are dealt with in the normal immune system [Schwartz, 1989].

Antigen-presenting cells are seemingly capable of presenting self-peptides to self-reactive T cells in vitro [Winchester et al., 1984; Lorenz and Allen, 1988]. Furthermore, potentially harmful T cells reactive with peripheral self-antigens are apparently present in the normal healthy individuals since T-cell-mediated organ-specific autoimmune diseases can be easily elicited by immunizing animals with self-constituents and a suitable adjuvant. For example, thyroiditis and encephalomyelitis can be easily produced by immunizing animals with thyroglobulins or myelin basic proteins, respectively, emulsified in Freund's adjuvant; T cells mediate these diseases [Weigle, 1981]. Hence critical issues in studying the pathogenetic mechanism of autoimmune disease would be to characterize the self-reactive T cells in a dormant as well as an activated state to elucidate the mechanism by which they are controlled in the normal immune system and to determine the immunological conditions required for their expansion and activation to cause autoimmune disease.

Autoimmune diseases are divided into "organ specific" (e.g., Hashimoto's thyroiditis, autoimmune gastritis with pernicious anemia, and insulitis with insulin-dependent diabetes mellitus) or "nonorgan specific" ("systemic"; e.g., systemic lupus erythematosus [SLE] and rheumatoid arthritis), depending on whether autoimmune responses are directed to antigen(s) confined to a particular organ or widely distributed in the body [Roitt, 1989; Schwartz and Datta, 1989]. In humans and animals, one organ-specific autoimmune disease is frequently associated with another, e.g., insulin-dependent diabetes mellitus, thyroiditis, and gastritis [Irvine et al., 1970; Sternthal et al., 1981; Elder et al., 1982; Doniach et al., 1982; Khoury et al., 1982; Riley et al., 1983]. Likewise, SLE and rheumatoid arthritis share many clinical features and frequently coexist in humans and animals [Andrews et al., 1978; Quimby and Schwartz, 1982; Schwartz and Datta, 1989]. These facts suggest a common pathogenetic basis for each spectrum of autoimmune disease, although it is contentious whether systemic autoimmune diseases and organ-specific ones share a common mechanism [Schwartz and Datta, 1989]. It has been documented that immunologic, genetic, and environmental factors contribute to the development of these autoimmune diseases. Assuming that T cells are key mediators of organ-specific autoimmune diseases and presumably systemic ones, it must be determined how immunologic, environmental, and genetic factors can be linked in the causal chain of autoimmune pathogenesis, especially in connection with the control of generation, expansion, and activation of self-reactive T cells.

In this chapter, we first review the experiments demonstrating that various autoimmune diseases, especially organ-specific ones, can be produced in normal rodents by manipulating the thymus or T-cell subsets and discuss the possible mechanism of a T-cell-dependent control of pathogenic self-reactived T cells in the normal immune system. We then discuss the immunological conditions required for expansion–activation of the self-reactive T cells to induce autoimmune disease and demonstrate that the environmental agents or genetical abnormalities that affect the thymus and T cells and fulfill those conditions can elicit autoimmune disease in normal animals. It is shown that the phenotype of autoimmune disease thus triggered is largely determined by the genetic background of the host, not the T-cell abnormality itself caused by environmental agents or genetic defects. Implications of these findings to the etiology and pathogenetic mechanism of human autoimmune disease is then discussed.

CELLULAR INTERACTIONS WITHIN CD4+ T-CELL SUBSET IN MAINTAINING PERIPHERAL TOLERANCE TO ORGAN-SPECIFIC SELF-ANTIGENS

Several studies have shown that expansion–activation of self-reactive T cells and induction of autoimmune disease can be achieved without manipulating target self-antigens or using potent adjuvants. Neonatal thymectomy of selected strains of mice, for example, produces various organ-specific autoimmune diseases, such as thyroiditis, gastritis, oophoritis, or orchitis [Kojima et al., 1976, 1980; Taguchi et al., 1980; Taguchi and Nishizuka, 1981]. Thymectomy of young adult rats and subsequent doses of low dose x-ray irradiations elicit thyroiditis and insulin-dependent diabetes mellitus [Penhale et al., 1973, 1990]. The development of autoimmune disease in these models can be prevented by inoculating T-cell suspensions prepared from syngeneic normal animals when the inoculation was performed within a limited period after the autoimmune-inducing treatments [Penhale et al., 1976; Sakaguchi et al., 1982b]. The T cells bearing the autoimmune-preventive activity were revealed to be CD4+ [Sakaguchi et al., 1982b; Fowell et al., 1991]. In spontaneous autoimmune models, such as insulin-dependent diabetes mellitus in BB rats or NOD mice, inoculation of CD4+ cell suspensions prepared from histocompatible nonautoimmune animals prevented the autoimmune disease as well when the cell inoculation was performed before clinical onset of autoimmune disease [Mordes et al., 1987; Boitard et al., 1989].

A number of studies on effector T cells mediating organ-specific autoimmune disease in spontaneous or induced models have documented that the key effector cells are CD4+ T cells, which mediate autoimmune disease as helper T cells for autoantibody-forming B cells, as amplifiers for cytotoxic T cells, or as mediators of cell-mediated immune responses akin to delayed-type hypersensitivity [Sakaguchi et al., 1982a; Like et al., 1985; Londei et al., 1985; Koike et al., 1987; Shizuru et al., 1988; Fukuma et al., 1988].

These findings, when taken together, suggest that there may exist two functionally distinct populations of CD4$^+$ T cells in terms of maintaining self-tolerance and induction of autoimmune disease, one mediating autoimmune disease and the other inhibiting it. They further lead to the hypothesis that one aspect of self-tolerance may be maintained by the cellular interactions between these two CD4$^+$ populations, the autoimmune-inhibitory CD4$^+$ T cells being dominant in the physiological state.

To demonstrate more directly that the cellular interactions within the CD4$^+$ subset is a key mechanism, not an epiphenomenon, of self-tolerance, attempts have been made to dissect the CD4$^+$ population by expression of cell surface differentiation antigens and to examine correlation of the dissection with autoimmune induction or inhibition. We used congenitally T-cell-deficient athymic nude mice of BALB/c background and reconstituted them with a particular T-cell subpopulation prepared from spleens of syngeneic euthymic BALB/c mice; the nude mice were histologically and serologically examined 3 months later [Sakaguchi et al., 1985] (Table I). The BALB/c nude mice spontaneously developed thyroiditis (20%), gastritis (30%), oophoritis (50%), or orchitis (50%) when they were transferrred with CD4$^+$ CD5^{lo} spleen cell suspensions prepared by in vitro treatment with mixed antisera of anti-CD8 plus anti-CD5 antibodies and complement. CD4$^+$ peripheral T cells express the CD5 antigen in various degrees from high to low, and the CD4$^+$ CD5^{lo} population prepared by the complement-dependent cytotoxic treatment comprised 10%–15% of the splenic CD4$^+$ population. Transfer of an

TABLE I. Induction of autoimmune disease in nude mice by the transfer of syngeneic T-cell subsets[a]

Cells Inoculated Into Nude Mice	Development of Autoimmune Disease in Nude Mice
Unseparated	−
CD4$^+$	−
CD8$^+$	−
CD5^{lo}	+
CD4$^+$CD5^{lo}	+
CD8$^+$CD5^{lo}	−
CD4$^+$CD5^{lo} plus CD4$^+$ cells	−
CD4$^+$CD5^{lo} plus CD8$^+$ cells	+

[a] BALB/c athymic nude mice are transferred with various T-cell subpopulations prepared from the spleens of euthymic BALB/c mice. When the mice were examined 3 months after the cell transfer, those transferred with CD4$^+$CD5^{lo} cells developed various organ-specific autoimmune disease, such as thyroiditis, gastritis, oophoritis, or orchitis. This autoimmune development was prevented by the cotransfer of unseparated CD4$^+$ cells with CD4$^+$CD5^{lo} cells, suggesting that CD4$^+$CD5^{hi} cells bear downregulatory activity on the autoimmune-inducing CD4$^+$CD5^{lo} cells.

unseparated CD4$^+$ population could not induce autoimmune disease. Furthermore, the autoimmune induction by a CD4$^+$CD5^{lo} population was completely inhibited by cotransfer of a small number of unseparated CD4$^+$ cell population. Thus these results, taken together, indicate that certain, if not all, CD4$^+$ self-reactive T cells capable of causing organ-specific autoimmune diseases can be characterized in a dormant state as expressing a low amount of CD5 molecules on the cell surface; and CD4$^+$CD5^{hi} cells in the normal immune system appear to downregulate such autoimmune-inducing CD4$^+$CD5^{lo} cells in the physiological state [Sakaguchi et al., 1985; Sakaguchi et al., manuscript in preparation] (Fig. 1).

Similar findings were made by T-cell transfer into syngeneic T-cell-depleted mice [Sugihara et al., 1988]. The C3H strain of mice were T-cell depleted by adult thymectomy, x-irradiation, and bone marrow transplantation and then inoculated with syngeneic CD4$^+$CD5^{lo} spleen cells. The majority of the mice thus treated spontaneously developed autoimmune thyroiditis with high titers of antithyroglobulin autoantibodies. Coinoculation of unseparated CD4$^+$ cells with CD4$^+$CD5^{lo} cells prevented the thyroiditis.

Autoimmune disease was also produced in rats by a similar procedure. Insulitis/insulin-dependent diabetes mellitus and thyroiditis developed in athymic PVG rats transferred with CD4$^+$RT6.1$^-$ spleen cells from syngeneic euthymic rats [McKeever et al., 1990]. PVG nude rats transferred with CD4$^+$CD45RC^{hi} spleen cells also developed various autoimmune diseases, including gastritis and thyroiditis [Powrie and Mason, 1990]. Cotransfer of CD4$^+$CD45RC^{hi} cells and CD4$^+$CD45RC^{lo} cells prevented the autoimmune disease. Common elements in these experiments suggest the following modes of cellular interactions within the CD4$^+$ T-cell subset in maintaining self-tolerance.

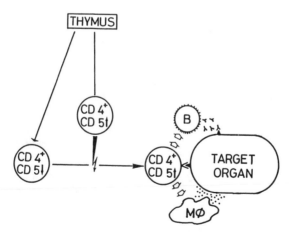

FIGURE 1. Scheme of cellular interactions within CD4$^+$ subset in maintaining self-tolerance and induction of autoimmune disease. B, B cells, Mϕ, macrophages.

Expression of CD5, CD45, and RT6.1 antigens is not specific for the autoimmune-inducing or autoimmune-inhibitory T cells, but for stages of T-cell differentiation or activation. Although precise immunological functions of the CD5, RT6.1, CD45RC molecules remain to be studied, high or low expressions of these molecules on T cells appear to correlate with a particular differentiation or activation stage of T cells rather than a functionally distinct T-cell subset or lineage [Mojcik et al., 1988; Sparshoff et al., 1991; Fowell et al., 1991]. Indeed, the final effector T cells mediating destruction of the target organs in the murine organ-specific autoimmune diseases described above were largely CD4$^+$CD5^{hi}, the same phenotype as the autoimmune-supressing T cells, and appear to help autoantibody-forming B cells and/or conduct cell-mediated immune reactions akin to delayed-type hypersensitivity toward the target self-antigens [Sakaguchi et al., 1982a; Fukuma et al., 1988] (Fig. 1).

Normal CD4$^+$ T cells control proliferation–differentiation of self-reactive T cells from a dormant state, not their autoimmune-effector functions. Our recent study using congenic strains different at Thy-1 alleles showed that the presence of CD4$^+$CD5^{hi} cells in the normal immune system inhibits the proliferation–differentiation of CD4$^+$CD5^{lo} cells (including the self-reactive T cells) to CD4$^+$CD5^{hi} cells, not the effector functions of fully differentiated CD4$^+$CD5^{hi} autoimmune effector T cells (Sakaguchi and Sakaguchi, manuscript in preparation). This explains the critical window period for autoimmune prevention by inoculating normal CD4$^+$ cells; i.e., organ-specific autoimmune disease can be prevented by the cell inoculation within a limited period after the autoimmune-inducing treatment, but the prevention is inefficient or impossible by similar cell inoculation later [Sakaguchi et al., 1982b, 1992a,b; Sakaguchi and Sakaguchi, 1989]. In this regard, the CD4$^+$CD5^{hi} cells with autoimmune-suppressive activity contrasts wtih those antigen-specific suppressor T cells that are antigen-induced and in many cases suppress functions of effector T cells in immune responses [Hodes, 1989].

There is accumulating evidence that the CD4$^+$ T-cell population consists of subpopulations distinct in profiles of lymphokine secretion or sensitivity [Mosmann and Coffman, 1989]. It is likely that the cellular interactions within CD4$^+$ subset in maintaining self-tolerance are also mediated by certain lymphokines enhancing or inhibiting proliferation–differentiation of T cells; the autoimmune-inducing CD4$^+$ cells and the autoimmune-inhibitory CD4$^+$ cells might be different in the profile of lymphokine formation or sensitivity. For example, CD4$^+$CD5^{hi} T cells might constitutively secrete certain lymphokine(s) inhibitory to the proliferation–differentiation of CD4$^+$CD5^{lo} T cells or consume lymphokine(s) necessary for their proliferation–differentiation; conversely, self-reactived CD4$^+$ T cells in the CD5^{lo} state might be especially sensitive to the inhibitory lymphokines or to the deprivation of the proliferatory lymphokines.

T-cell-dependent downregulation is not specific for self-antigens. To determine whether the autoimmune-inhibitory activity of CD4$^+$ cells is specific for self-antigens, the oophoritis-preventive activities of CD4$^+$ cells were compared among male mice, neonatally oophorectomized (NOx) mice, and female mice on the assumption that the presence of self-antigens might sensitize the CD4$^+$ T cells to acquire antigen-specific autoimmune-preventive activity (Sakaguchi and Sakaguchi, manuscript in preparation). Indeed, two to four times more undissected CD4$^+$ spleen cells from male or NOx mice than CD4$^+$ spleen cells from female mice were required for preventing oophoritis when these CD4$^+$ spleen cells were cotransferred with male-derived CD4$^+$CD5^{lo} spleen cells; the spleen cell doses required for the prevention of gastritis and thyroiditis were equivalent among female, NOx, and male mice. However, this apparently oophoritis-specific difference in the preventive activity cannot be attributed to the difference in antigen-specific suppressive activity. It is presumably due to different oophoritis-inducing activities of CD4$^+$CD5^{lo} cells included in the undissected CD4$^+$ cell inocula, since CD4$^+$CD5^{lo} cells prepared from male or NOx mice induced oophoritis at 100% incidence in nude mice while the incidence of oophoritis by inoculation of the equivalent dose of female-derived CD4$^+$CD5^{lo} cells was ~40%, the incidences of gastritis and thyroiditis being comparable irrespective of the cell donors. These results suggest that female mice may possess less potent or less numbers of ovary-specific self-reactive T cells presumably as a result of clonal deletion of T cells with high affinity for ovarian antigens rather than having T cells with more potent oophoritis-specific suppressive activity. The suppressive activity of CD4$^+$ cells on other autoimmune diseases, such as gastritis and thyroiditis, would be also antigen nonspecific, although the experiment described above did not formally exclude the role of antigen-specific suppressor T cells in this type of self-tolerance.

CD4$^+$ cell-dependent downregulation on self-reactive T cells may not hinder normal immune responses to foreign antigens. It is an absolute prerequisite that the T-cell-dependent downregulation on self-reactive T cells should not suppress or hinder the expansion and activation of nonautoimmune T cells responding to invading nonself-antigens. Based on the findings described above, it is likely that, when extrathymic self-antigens, even if at a quite low concentration in the circulation, are picked up and presented by the thymic stromal cells, T cells with high affinity TCRs for the self-antigens are clonally deleted in the thymus, but those with low affinity are released from the thymus to the periphery. Such self-reactive T cells are dormant in the normal periphery and might be different from nonself-reactive T cells not only in their low TCR affinity to the relevant self-antigens, but also in their immunological state (as illustrated as low cell surface expression of CD5 molecules) and presumably in the conditions required for their expansion–activation. These differences may form the basis for less or no sensitivity of nonself-reactive T cells to the suppressive signals in the CD4$^+$-cell-dependent regulation and will guarantee normal immune responses to foreign antigens while inhibiting autoimmune responses.

THYMIC PRODUCTION OF PATHOGENIC SELF-REACTIVE T CELLS AND A T CELL-DEPENDENT CONTROL OF THEIR EXPANSION IN THE PERIPHERY

Assuming that self-reactive T cells can be controlled in ther periphery by $CD4^+$ T-cell-dependent downregulation, autoimmune disease may develop when the pathogenic self-reactive T cells are released from the thymus to the periphery where no or few T cells are present. To address this possibility, normal thymi were engrafted into syngeneic athymic nude mice [Sakaguchi and Sakaguchi, 1990]. The BALB/c nude mice transplanted with fetal or newborn BALB/c thymi spontaneously developed various organ-specific autoimmune diseases (such as gastritis [60%], thyroiditis [10%], oophoritis [40%], or orchitis [10%]), as well as systemic ones (such as arthritis [10%], immune complex-mediated glomerulonephritis [20%], and arteritis [30%]). Engrafting of adult thymi was less efficient in inducing the autoimmunity in nude mice, but transplantation of adult thymi x-irradiated at a T-cell-depleting dose prior to engrafting produced histologically demonstrable organ-specific autoimmune diseases at high incidences.

Engrafting of newborn thymi also successfully induced organ-specific autoimmune diseases in T-cell-depleted BALB/c mice prepared by thymectomy x-irradiation, and bone marrow transplantation [Sakaguchi and Sakaguchi, 1990]. However, the thymus engrafting into T-cell-nondepleted mice (e.g., thymectomized in adult but not x-irradiated] was unable to induce serological or histological organ-specific autoimmunity despite the fact that transplanted thymi grew well in these mice. These results collectively indicate that the normal thymus is capable of producing various pathogenic self-reactive T cells, which can easily expand and cause autoimmune disease when released to a T-cell-deficient or -depleted periphery; however, the self-reactive T cells cannot expand when released to the normal T-cell nondepleted periphery. Easier autoimmune induction by engrafting newborn or x-irradiated thymi compared with engrafting normal adult thymi might result if the former contain less number of mature $CD4^+$ T cells with the auto-immune-preventive activity. It is likely that the self-reactive T cells immediately after leaving the thymus grafts (which first degenerate upon transplantation and then regenerate T cells) may bear $CD4^+CD5^{lo}$ phenotype and be quite susceptible to downregulation by $CD4^+CD5^{hi}$ peripheral T cells, as discussed above (Fig. 1).

Neonatal thymectomy (NTx) (between days 2 and 4 after birth) of selected strains of mice produces various organ-specific autoimmune diseases similar to those induced in T-cell-deficient mice by thymus engrafting or inoculation of a peripheral T-cell subset; thymectomy on day 0 or 7 is less efficient to induce the autoimmunity [Kojima et al., 1976, 1980; Taguchi et al., 1980; Taguchi and Nishizuka, 1981; Kojima and Prehn, 1981]. The development of autoimmune disease was prevented by neonatal inoculation of peripheral T-cell suspensions prepared from syngeneic adult mice, but not by those from newborns, which bear a small number of peripheral T cells [Sakaguchi et al., 1982b]. $CD4^+$ cells had this preventive activity, but $CD8^+$ cells did not [Sakaguchi et al., 1982b; Sakaguchi et al., unpublished data]. These findings, taken together, suggest that the in situ normal thymus physiologically produces pathogenic self-reactive T cells; the production may begin shortly after birth in normal mice, and NTx may abrogate the peripheralization of mature (e.g., $CD4^+CD5^{hi}$) T cells with the autoimmune-preventive activity, thereby producing relative dominance of the self-reactive T cells that have peripheralized before NTx [Sakaguchi et al., 1982b]. It was recently suggested that the neonatal thymus may be defective in clonal deletion of some self-reactive T cells [Schneider et al., 1989]. For example, the number and percentage composition of TCR $V\beta11^+$ cells increased after NTx in the strains that normally delete $V\beta11^+$ cells [Smith et al., 1989]. The nondeleted $V\beta11^+$ cells were anergic in vitro to the relevant I–E antigens [Jones et al., 1990]. However, there is thus far no evidence that the pathogenic self-reactive T cells causing organ-specific autoimmune disease utilize such "forbidden" TCR $V\beta$ segments. Furthermore, those T cells expressing the "forbidden" TCR $V\beta$ segments are mainly $CD8^+$ cells; however, main autoimmune effector T cells in NTx-induced autoimmune disease are $CD4^+$ [Sakaguchi et al., 1982a; Sakaguchi and Sakaguchi, unpublished data] (Fig. 1). Further study is needed to determine the significance of the $V\beta$ deviation in the autoimmune pathogenesis after NTx.

ENVIRONMENTAL AGENTS CAN CAUSE AUTOIMMUNE DISEASE BY AFFECTING THYMUS/T CELLS

The successful induction of autoimmune disease by simple manipulation of the thymus/T cells, not the target self-antigens, suggests that certain environmental agents may cause organ-specific autoimmune disease by affecting the thymus/T cells. For example, 1) environmental agents may eliminate or reduce $CD4^+$ T cells with autoimmune-preventive activity from the periphery and tip the balance toward the dominance of autoimmune-inducing $CD4^+$ cells; or 2) they may eliminate mature $CD4^+$ T cells from the thymus as well as periphery so that self-reactive T cells produced by the thymus may easily expand in the periphery and cause autoimmune disease. In this context, the immune system early in life might be especially vulnerable to such environmental insults because relatively small numbers of mature T cells are present in the periphery and it might be easier for the insult to deplete them for a certain length of time sufficient for pathogenic self-reactive T cells produced by the thymus to expand. As shown here, there are several examples of the environmental (chemical, physical, or biological) agents that affect the thymus/T cells and thereby cause autoimmune disease apparently by a common mechanism.

Cyclosporin A

Cyclosporin A (CsA), a fungal metabolite, is a potent immunosuppressive agent widely used in various clinical fields [Borel, 1989]. The drug abrogates mature CD4$^+$CD8$^-$ and CD4$^-$CD8$^+$ thymocytes [Sakaguchi and Sakaguchi, 1988, 1989; Gao et al., 1988; Jenkins et al., 1988; Kosugi et al., 1989]. Consequently, these populations are substantially depleted from the peripheral lymphoid organs, especially when the drug is administered from the day of birth. When BALB/c mice were daily administered with CsA at 10 mg/kg body weight/day for 1 week from the day of birth, ~60% of the treated mice later developed autoantibodies specific for gastric parietal cells and ~20% sufferred from histologically demonstrable gastritis with inflammatory damage to the parietal cells; ~10% of the treated mice developed oophoritis with antioocyte autoantibodies [Sakaguchi and Sakaguchi, 1989]. CsA administration of the equivalent dose per body weight for 1 week from day 7 after birth was less effective; and the administration to adult mice failed to induce the autoimmunity even with a higher dose for a prolonged period.

Inoculation of normal syngeneic splenic T cells immediately after the neonatal CsA treatment histologically and serologically prevented the occurrence of autoimmunity. On the other hand, removal of the thymus after the neonatal CsA treatment to sustain the CsA-induced T-cell immunodeficiency enhanced the autoimmune development; i.e., gastritis and oophoritis developed in 100% and 60% of mice, respectively. Other autoimmune diseases developed as well: thyroiditis (~30%), insulitis (~15%), adrenalitis (~15%), sialoadenitis (~25%), and orchitis (~40%). These autoimmune diseases were accompanied by the appearance of serum autoantibodies specific for thyroglobulins, cell surface antigens on Langerhans islet cells, adrenocortical cells, acinar cells of the salivary glands, and sperm.

CsA does not appear to induce de novo production of the "forbidden" clones by interfering with a thymic clonal deletion mechanism, since even the normal thymus can produce T cells capable of causing similar organ-specific autoimmune diseases (see above). It is, however, possible that the drug might affect clonal deletion and enhance the thymic production of qualitatively or quantitatively more pathogenic self-reactive T cells [Gao et al., 1988; Jenkins et al., 1988]. Indeed, a proportion of CD5^{lo} thymocytes increased in the CsA-treated thymus; and the thymic production/release of self-reactive T cells with CD4$^+$CD5^{lo} phenotype may well be increased. Together with effective prevention–ameriolation of autoimmune disease by inoculating normal T cells and aggravation of disease by thymectomy, these findings suggest that the neonatal CsA treatment abrogates from the immune system mature CD4$^+$ thymocytes/T cells with inhibitory activity on the proliferation–differentiation of self-reactive clones, thereby enhancing expansion of the latter. Successful induction of autoimmune disease by neonatal CsA treatment, but not by CsA treatment of adult mice, is presumably because CsA cannot efficiently eliminate mature peripheral T cells in adult mice, in contrast to the presence of few mature T cells in the newborn periphery and the easier elimination of them [Sakaguchi and Sakaguchi, 1989]. Indeed, organ-specific autoimmune diseases can be produced by CsA treatment of adult mice that are depleted of peripheral T cells by x-irradiation or anti-T cell serum treatment prior to CsA administration (Sakaguchi and Sakaguchi, unpublished data).

Similar findings on CsA-induced autoimmunity was made in chickens. In the Obese Strain chickens, which spontaneously develop autoimmune thyroiditis, the incidence and severity of thyroiditis was enhanced by in ovo treatment with CsA [Wick et al., 1982]. Furthermore, neonatal CsA treatment and subsequent thymectomy of a nonautoimmune strain of chickens produced various organ-specific autoimmune diseases similar to those produced in mice [Cooper et al., 1991].

Ionizing Radiation

We have recently shown that high dose fractionated irradiation of the lymphoid organs, called *total lymphoid irradiation* (TLI), can elicit organ-specific autoimmune diseases, such as thyroiditis and gastritis, in rodents. TLI consists of irradiating major lymphoid organs including the thymus and spleen, while shielding radiosensitive nonlymphoid organs (e.g., long bones, lung, and skull) with lead. By this irradiation protocol, a high dose (3,000–4,000 rads) is achieved within 4–5 weeks by multiple small fractions of 200–250 rads each [Strober et al., 1979]. TLI has been routinely used for treatment of malignant lymphomas during the past 25 years [Kaplan, 1980].

BALB/c mice subjected to TLI predominantly developed gastritis with antiparietal cell autoantibodies, as in CsA treatment of BALB/c mice, and at lesser incidences orchitis and thyroiditis; the autoimmune disease could be adoptively transferred to syngeneic athymic nude mice by CD4$^+$ cells [Sakaguchi et al., 1992a]. Irradiation of the target organs alone (e.g., stomach) did not elicit autoimmunity. TLI depletes mature T cells from the thymus and periphery for 4–6 weeks after completion of TLI. Shielding of the target organs from irradiation did not prevent the organ-specific autoimmune diseases. Autoimmune disease was, however, successfully prevented by inoculation immediately after TLI of normal peripheral CD4$^+$ T cells prepared from syngeneic nonirradiated mice.

There was a strain-dependent difference in susceptibility to this TLI-induced organ-specific autoimmune disease. BALB/c, A, and SWR strains were susceptible, while B10 and C3H strains were resistant. In contrast to gastritis in mice, TLI predominantly produced thyroiditis in rats [Sakaguchi et al., 1992a].

Mouse T-Lymphotropic Virus

Viruses have been suspected to be causative agents of various autoimmune diseases [Schwartz and Datta, 1989; Mims, 1987]. There are many viruses that affect the thymus/T cells in humans, e.g., measles, rubella, and cytomegalovirus [McChesney and Oldstone, 1987; Mims, 1987]. An intriguing question is whether such a virus that affects the thymus/T cells can cause organ-specific autoimmune disease. We employed the mouse T-lymphotropic virus (MTLV; thymic necrosis virus, murid herpesvirus 3), which causes massive necrosis of the thymus when it infects newborn mice [Morse and Valinsky, 1989]. BALB/c mice infected with MTLV immediately after birth showed thymic necrosis and depletion of CD4$^+$ thymocytes between 1 and 3 weeks after birth. They developed autoimmune gastritis with antiparietal autoantibodies when assessed at 3 months of age (Morse et al., manuscript in preparation). Furthermore, thymectomy at the time of thymus regeneration (around 3 weeks after birth) enhanced autoimmune development; i.e., not only high incidence of gastritis but also other autoimmune diseases, such as thyroiditis, developed in these mice, in a similar manner as shown in the neonatally CsA-treated and subsequently thymectomized mice.

AUTOIMMUNE DISEASE INDUCED BY GERMLINE ALTERATION OF THE T-CELL RECEPTOR GENE EXPRESSION

As discussed above, autoimmune T cells may be able to expand in the periphery if they leave the thymus earlier than the physiological time course, much earlier than the peripheralization of mature T cells with the autoimmune preventive activity or, alternatively, if ontogeny of the latter is delayed for a sufficient length of time during which the self-reactive T cells physiologically produced can expand in the periphery. With reduction of mature thymocytes, as in CsA, as a clue to such an autoimmune-causing T-cell abnormality, we have examined TCR transgenic mice for autoimmunity since the TCR is a key molecule for proliferation–differentiation of T cells in the thymus [von Boemer, 1990]. We found that a strain of transgenic mice expressing a rearranged TCR α-chain gene under the immunoglobulin heavy chain (IgH) enhancer bore organ-specific autoimmunity [Sakaguchi et al., 1992b]. After several backcrossings to inbred strains, including BALB/c, A, SWR, C3H, and B10 strains, ~60% of BALB/c-backcrossed transgenic mice histologically developed gastritis with high titers of antiparietal cell autoantibodies; ~80% of A-backcrossed mice developed oophoritis with antioocyte autoantibodies; ~60% of SWR-backcrossed mice succumbed to orchitis with antisperm autoantibodies; and ~10% of A- or SWR-backcrossed mice also developed sialoadenitis, thyroiditis, and/or insulitis. In contrast to these three strains, C3H- and B10-backcrossed mice did not show histologically evident autoimmunity. Once autoimmune disease developed, disease could be adoptively transferred to syngeneic nude mice by CD4$^+$ cells with resulting histological damage of the target organ and development of organ-specific autoantibodies.

This transgenic autoimmunity is not due to insertional inactivation or activation of host genes, since the disease was dominantly inherited and since other transgenic lines independently produced with the same transgene developed the same autoimmune disease when backcrossed to the relevant strains; e.g., BALB/c-backcrossed mice predominantly developed autoimmune gastritis. Furthermore, the antigen specificity of the original TCR from which the α-chain transgene was constructed or its usage of particular $V\alpha$–$J\alpha$ gene segments was not critical for contstructing the autoimmune-inducing TCR α-chain transgene since the mice introduced with the α-chain transgenes that were constructed of different $V\alpha$–$J\alpha$ gene segments and expressed under the same IgH enhancer also developed the same autoimmune disease.

In the TCR α-chain–IgH enhancer transgenic mice, the number of T cells decreased in the periphery to two-thirds of the nontransgenic littermates; the percentage composition of $CD4^+$ cells was about half of the normal, and $CD4^-CD8^-$ T cells increased to 10%–20% of total peripheral T cells. Approximately 80%–90% of the peripheral T cells expressed the transgenic α-chains, which paired with endogenous β-chains, and 10%–20% of T cells expressed endogenous α-chains (i.e., endogenous α-chains only or endogenous α-chains in addition to the transgenic α-chains) on the cell surface, suggesting incomplete allelic exclusion of the α-chain gene in these T cells. Transfer of T cells expressing or not expressing the transgenic α-chains into syngeneic nude mice revealed that T cells expressing endogenous α-chains (with or without the transgenic α-chains) mediate the autoimmune disease. When rearranged α-chain transgenes are expressed under the IgH enhancer, the time of cell surface α-chain expression was earlier than the physiological time course and almost at the same time as the expression of other TCR chains. Thymocyte expression of various markers including CD5 antigen indicated increase of immature thymocytes, such as $CD5^{lo}$ cells, in the transgenic mice. Furthermore, inoculation of normal $CD4^+$ T cells prepared from syngeneic nontransgenic mice completely prevented the autoimmune development when the inoculation was performed in the neonatal period (Sakaguchi et al., manuscript in preparation). Thus these results, taken together, indicate that the early expression of rearranged TCR α-chains might disrupt the normal T-cell ontogeny, including the ontogeny of self-reactive T cells and/or T cells with the autoimmune preventive activity, thereby preparing the immunologic conditions favorable for expansion of the former.

CONTRIBUTION OF THE HOST GENETIC BACKGROUND TO AUTOIMMUNE PATHOGENESIS

In the organ-specific autoimmune disease described above, there were strain-dependent differences in the spectrum of affected organs, the incidence of individual autoimmune diseases, and their pathological and clinical severities [Kojima and Prehn, 1981; Sakaguchi and Sakaguchi, 1989; Sakaguchi et al., 1992a,b]. For example, BALB/c ($H-2^d$) predominantly develop autoimmune gastritis whether affected by CsA, TLI, or MTLV or introduced with the

TCR α-chain–IgH enhancer transgenes. Likewise, the A (H-2^a) and SWR (H-2^q) strains predominantly develop autoimmune disease in the reproductive organs, such as oophoritis or orchitis. In contrast, the DBA/2 (H-2^d), C3H (H-2^k), and C57BL/6 (H-2^b) strains are resistant to these autoimmune diseases. Difference in the incidence and severity of autoimmune disease between BALB/c and DBA/2 (which share the d haplotype of MHC [Hansen and Sachs, 1989]) or between A and C3H (which share the k haplotype of class II MHC [Hansen and Sachs, 1989]) indicates that the host class II MHC gene by itself is unable or insufficient, at least in these strains, to determine susceptibility and resistance. In the genetic study with congeneic strains, BALB/c (H-2^d), BALB.B (H-2^b), and BALB.K (H-2^k) were all susceptible to gastritis, but B10.D2 (H-2^d) was resistant, indicating the predominant role of non-MHC gene(s) in determining the resistance to autoimmune gastritis. Interestingly, however, the A strain (H-2^a) was susceptible to oophoritis but the congenic A.By strain (H-2^b) and the B10.A (H-2^a) strain was resistant, suggesting that either the MHC or the non-MHC gene(s) alone can dominantly contribute to the resistance to oophoritis (Sakaguchi and Sakaguchi, manuscript in preparation). Thus MHC genes may play a significant role in determining susceptibility and resistance to some autoimmune diseases, while non-MHC genes may exert a more dominant effect in others.

The result that MHC genes alone can determine the resistance to oophoritis is similar to the finding made in NOD mice that introduction of particular class II MHC transgenes could prevent insulin-dependent diabetes mellitus [Lund et al., 1990; Miyazaki et al., 1990; Slattery et al., 1990]. It is obscure, however, how a particular class II MHC haplotype determines the resistance or susceptibility to a particular autoimmune disease. It is also little known what kind of non-MHC genes contribute to autoimmune pathogenesis [Kojima and Prehn, 1981; Prochazka et al., 1987; Todd, et al., 1991].

DEVELOPMENT OF AUTOIMMUNE DISEASE IS DETERMINED BY THE PRIMARY IMMUNOLOGICAL ABNORMALITY OF THE THYMUS/T CELLS IN THE CONTROL OF SELF-REACTIVE T CELLS AND THE HOST GENES DETERMINING THE AUTOIMMUNE PHENOTYPE

The findings on the autoimmune-inducing abnormalities of the thymus/T cells and the roles of host genetic elements in autoimmune pathogenesis lead to the hypothesis that the development of autoimmune disease is determined by two elements; one is the immunological abnormality of the thymus/T cells in the control of self-reactive T cells, and the other is the host genes, including MHC as well as non-MHC gene(s), which determine the autoimmune phenotype including the specificity and intensity of the autoimmune responses (Fig. 2). Unless the primary immunological abnormality is present, the host genes are unable to induce autoimmune disease. On the other hand, certain individuals are quite resistant, like B10 mice, to every autoimmune disease whatever

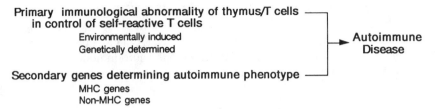

FIGURE 2. Two factors required for the development of autoimmune disease.

the autoimmune-inducing insults are. Severity of the immunological abnormality may also contribute to the autoimmune phenotype by influencing the manifestation of the genotype; in general, the longer and the more severe the immunological abnormality is, autoimmune disease develops at the higher incidence in the susceptible organ, with the more severe form, and in the wider spectrum of organs [Sakaguchi and Sakaguchi, 1989].

A similar "dual gene hypothesis" on autoimmune pathogenesis has been proposed from the study on other species. In humans, Bias et al. [1986] showed that autoimmunity is inherited as an autosomal dominant trait in familial occurrences of various systemic as well as organ-specific autoimmune diseases; this primary autoimmune gene appeared to be epistatic to other secondary genes, which confer specificity of the autoimmune phenotype. Quimby and Schwartz [1982] formulated a similar hypothesis from their study on canine colonies that spontaneously developed multiple autoimmune diseases including SLE, arthritis, thyroiditis, gastritis, insulitis, and sialoadenitis when the dogs were selectively bred for SLE. Both groups suggested that the "primary autoimmune gene" might be concerned with a defect in lymphocyte function or immunoregulation. Our findings suggest that such an immunological abnormality might be expressed in the T-cell compartment; furthermore, not only genetically determined abnormalities of the immune system but also environmentally induced immunological abnormalities play the same primary role in triggering autoimmune disease.

As discussed above, organ-specific autoimmune disease tends to occur in a particular spectrum of organs in various species. For example, Obese strain chickens spontaneously develop chronic thyroiditis and other organ-specific autoimmunities (e.g., against stomach, adrenal glands, and endocrine pancreas) [Khoury et al., 1982; Wick et al., 1990]. Neonatal CsA treatment and subsequent thymectomy of nonautoimmune-prone strains of chickens also elicit similar organ-specific autoimmune diseases [Cooper et al., 1991]. BB rats succumb to insulin-dependent diabetes mellitus, thyroiditis, and gastric autoimmunity [Sternthal et al., 1981; Elder et al., 1982; Rossini et al., 1985]. A colony of dogs spontaneously develop thyroiditis, gastritis with pernicious anemia, insulitis, and other systemic autoimmune diseases [Quimby and Schwartz, 1982]. Humans are also prone to develop autoimmune diseases in a similar spectrum of organs, e.g., thyroiditis, gastritis, and insulin-dependent diabetes mellitus [Irvine et al., 1970; Riley et al., 1983; Schwartz and Datta, 1989]. It is likely that some of the genes concerned with determining the autoimmune phenotype might have been retained from chicken to humans in the course of evolution. The genes determining the autoimmune phenotype in one species may well play a similar role in another species.

POSSIBLE CAUSES AND MECHANISM OF ORGAN-SPECIFIC AUTOIMMUNE DISEASE IN HUMANS

The prevailing notion on the etiology of autoimmune disease is that there should be a causative agent specific for a particular autoimmune disease and that the agent must affect the target self-antigens to cause autoimmune disease (Fig. 3A) [Bottazzo et al., 1983; Oldstone, 1988]. In contrast to this paradigm, we here propose another mechanism of organ-specific autoimmune disease: Environmental agents or genetic abnormalities affect the thymus/T cells, not the target self-antigens, thereby eliciting autoimmune disease; and the phenotype of the autoimmune disease thus triggered is determined by the genetic make-up of the individuals, as shown in Figures 2 and 3B. In this possible mechanism of autoimmune disease, 1) a single causative agent or a single genetic abnormality can lead to the occurrence of autoimmune disease in various organs, frequently more than one organ; 2) the same autoimmune disease can be produced in a particular individual by different causative agents through a common mechanism; and, 3) exposure to the autoimmune-inducing environmental agents or the resulting abnormality in the thymus/T cells need not be permanent to elicit chronic autoimmune

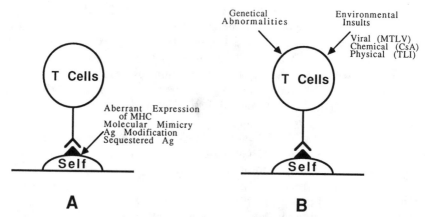

FIGURE 3. Two paradigms (**A, B**) of autoimmune pathogenesis. One postulates that the cause of autoimmune disease is in the abnormality of the target self-antigens; the other postulates that the cause is in the control of self-reactive T cells, not the target self-antigens.

disease later in life, as shown for CsA, TLI, and MTLV in mice. This suggests that, even if a specific etiologic agent is not detected at the time of disease onset, it does not exclude the possibility that the autoimmune disease was triggered in the past by an environmental agent affecting the T-cell immune system for a limited length of time.

One of the characteristics of human organ-specific autoimmune disease is that it affects many young and middle aged people. It contrasts with degenerative diseases or cancer, which increase with aging. This epidemiological pattern suggests that environmental insults early in life might have triggered the expansion–activation of self-reactive T cells, which have insidiously mediated the autoimmune disease to the clinical onset some years later. In this regard, viruses might be the most common etiological agents for the following reasons. First, people ordinarily experience the majority of virus infections before school age, and the first infection with a particular virus may well exert a serious effect on the immune system because of nonimmunity to it [Burnet and White, 1972]. Second, there are a number of common viruses (e.g., measles, rubella, mumps, and cytomegalovirus) that infect and destroy T cells or affect functions of T cells. For example, measles virus is well known to impair immunological functions of T cells severely over a fair length of time [McChesney and Oldstone, 1987].

Although etiology of the majority of human autoimmune diseases is unknown at present, there are two autoimmune syndromes whose causes are epidemiologically evident. One is organ-specific autoimmune disease associated with congenital rubella virus infection. The other is so-called polyglandular autoimmune syndrome or immunoendocrinopathy syndrome, which shows a mendelian inheritance pattern, indicating an abnormality of a single gene as the primary cause of the autoimmune disease. These two diseases, one caused by an environmental agent and the other by a genetic abnormality, are accompanied by similar organ-specific autoimmune diseases, such as insulin-dependent diabetes mellitus, gastritis with pernicious anemia, thyroiditis, or Addison's adrenalitis. They are the two touchstones on which any theory of autoimmune pathogenesis should be tested.

Autoimmune Disease Associated With In Utero Infection With Rubella Virus

In Australia and the United States, about 20% of patients with congenital rubella syndrome later developed type 1 diabetes mellitus [Forrest et al., 1971; Rubinstein et al., 1982; Ginsberg-Feller et al., 1985]. Incidences of other organ-specific autoimmunities, such as against thyroid, were also significantly high in these patients [Ginsberg-Feller et al., 1985]. Rubella virus is known to induce chromosome breakage and to reduce cell division, leading to maldevelopment or malformation of various organs and tissues that result in cardiac anomalies, cataract, deafness, and mental retardation [Cooper, 1985]. It also infects T lymphocytes and suppresses their immunological functions [Olson et al., 1967]. As a mechanism of this autoimmune syndrome, hypotheses have been proposed, e.g., molecular mimicry between a viral component and MHC molecules [Horn et al., 1988] or virus-induced destruction of the β-cells [Menser et al., 1978]. Based on our hypothesis described above, it is also likely that rubella infection early in life may affect the thymus/T cells for a certain length of time, preparing an immunological state favorable for production and expansion of pathogenic self-reactive T cells, which may cause organ-specific autoimmune diseases later in life in genetically susceptible people, as neonatal MTLV infection does in mice.

Polyglandular Autoimmune Syndrome

Two types of polyglandular autoimmune syndromes (PGA) are known [Eisenbarth, 1985; MacLaren and Riley, 1986]. PGA I, also called *autoimmune polyendocrinopathy–candidiasis–ectodermal dystrophy* (APECED), has its predominant age of onset in childhood or early adulthood and is frequently accompanied by abnormalities of the thymus/T cells [Arulanantham et al., 1979; Ahonen et al., 1990]. It shows autosomal recessive inheritance and is not associated with particular HLA haplotypes [Ahonen 1985]. PGA II is, in contrast, characterized by its onset in middle age, association with the HLA DR3/4 haplotype, and autosomal dominant inheritance [Eisenbarth, 1985]. The successful establishment of an autoimmune TCR transgenic mouse suggests that genetic abnormality in PGA, especially PGA I, might be in the T-cell compartment and related to the regulation of TCR gene expression. People with this genetic abnormality may develop various organ-specific autoimmune diseases, depending on other genes determining the autoimmune phenotype.

CsA and TLI

We showed that CsA and TLI can cause organ-specific autoimmune diseases in rodents. It remains to be determined in humans whether TLI and CsA, both of which are widely used for treatment of malignancies or immunosuppression in organ transplantation, will later elicit organ-specific autoimmune disease depending on the genetic make-up of the patients [Hancock et al., 1991].

SUMMARY

In this chapter, we have mainly discussed the causes and mechanism of organ-specific autoimmune diseases. We showed that systemic autoimmune disease, like SLE or rheumatoid arthritis, can also be produced in normal mice by manipulating the T-cell immune system [Sakaguchi and Sakaguchi, 1990]. Systemic and organ-specific autoimmune diseases occur in association in a colony of dogs and familial cases of human autoimmune diseases [Quinby and Schwartz, 1982; Bias et al., 1986]. It remains to be determined, however, whether both systemic and organ-specific autoimmunities are mediated by T cells with a similar self-reactivity. We also do not assert that every organ-localized autoimmune disease has a common pathogenetic mechanism; some of them might well be caused by molecular mimicry between self-constituents and exogenous agents, e.g., rheumatic heart or renal disease after streptococcal infection [Zabriskie, 1986; Oldstone, 1988].

We have shown that self-reactive T cells sufficiently pathogenic to cause clinical autoimmune disease are not totally deleted in apparently normal healthy animals; these self-reactive T cells are not rendered anergic after periperalization and upon contact with the target self-antigens, but their proliferation and differentiation to autoimmune effector T cells are controlled by a T-cell-dependent mechanism. This cellular interaction, which maintains one aspect of self-tolerance, appears to be within the $CD4^+$ subset, since the T cells mediating autoimmune disease and the T cells with autoimmune-preventive activity are both $CD4^+$. Environmental agents or genetic defects that affect the thymus/T cells, not the target self-antigens, and tip the balance toward the dominance of the self-reactive T cells can cause autoimmune disease. In the presence of such an autoimmune-causing T-cell abnormality, the phenotype of autoimmune disease is mainly determined by the host genes, not by the character of the T-cell abnormality. Further elucidation of the T-cell-dependent mechanism controlling self-reactive T cells and the host genes determining the autoimmune phenotype will contribute to our understanding of the pathogenetic mechanism of human autoimmune disease and designing of new ways for prevention and treatment.

ACKNOWLEDGMENTS

We thank Dr. K. Miyai for continuous encouragement; and Drs. T. Masuda, S.M. Morse, T.H. Ermak, and M.M. Davis for fruitful collaborations on the works reviewed here. Part of this work was supported by a grant from the Lucille P. Markey Charitable Trust. S.S. is a Lucille P. Markey Scholar for Biomedical Science and a Researcher of the JRDC "Sakigake 21" project (PRESTO) of the Science and Technology Agency, Japan.

REFERENCES

Ahonen P (1985): Autoimmune polyendocrinopathy–candidiasis–ectodermal dystrophy (APECED): Autosomal recessive inheritance. Clin Genet 27:535.

Ahonen P, Myllarniemi S, Sipila I, Perheentupa J (1990): Clinical variation of autoimmune polyendocrinopathy–candidiasis–ectodermal dystrophy (APECED) in a series of 68 patients. N Engl J Med 322:1829.

Andrews BA, Eisenberg RA, Theofilopoulos AN, Izui S, Wilson CB, McConahey PJ, Murphy ED, Roths JB, Dixon FJ (1978): Spontaneous murine lupus-like syndromes: Clinical and immunopathological manifestations in several strains. J Exp Med 148:1198.

Arulanantham K, Dwyer JM, Genel M (1979): Evidence for defective immunoregulation in the syndrome of familial candidiasis endocrinopathy. N Engl J Med 300:164.

Bernard C (1865): "An Introduction to the Study of Experimental Medicine." New York: Dover.

Bias WB, Reveille JD, Beaty TH, Meyers DA, Arnett FC (1986): Evidence that autoimmunity in man is a mendelian dominant trait. Am J Hum Genet 39:584–602.

Boitard C, Yasunami R, Dardenne M, Bach JF (1989): T cell-mediated inhibition of the transfer of autoimmune diabetes in NOD mice. J Exp Med 169:1669.

Bottazzo GF, Pujol-Borrell R, Hanafusa T, Feldman M (1983): Role of aberrant HLA-DR expression and antigen presentation in induction of endocrine autoimmunity. Lancet 2:1115–1119.

Borel JF (1989): Pharmacology of cyclosporin (Sandimmune). IV. Pharmacological properties in vivo. Pharmacol Rev 41:259.

Burnet M, White DO (1972): "Natural History of Infectious Disease," 4th ed. Cambridge: Cambridge University Press.

Cooper LZ (1985): The history and medical consequences of rubella. Rev Infect Dis 7(Suppl):S2.

Cooper MD, Chen C-LH, Bucy RP, Thompson CB (1991): Avian T cell ontogeny. Adv Immunol 50:87.

Davis MM, Bjorkman PJ (1988): T-cell receptor genes and T-cell recognition. Nature 334:395.

De Calvalho LC, Wick G, Roitt IM (1981): Requirement of T cells for the development of spontaneous autoimmune thyroiditis in Obese strain (OS) chickens. J Immunol 126:750.

Doniach D, Bottazo GF, Drexhage HA (1982): The autoimmune endocrinopathies. In Lachmann PJ, Peters DK (eds): "Clinical Aspects of Immunology," 4th ed. Oxford: Blackwell, pp 903–937.

Eisenbarth GS (1985): The immunoendocrinopathy syndrome. In Wilson JD, Forster DW (eds): "Williams' Textbook of Endocrinology," 7th ed. Philadelphia:WB Saunders, pp 1290–1300.

Elder M, Maclaren N, Riley W, McConnel T (1982): Gastric parietal cell and other autoantibodies in the BB rat. Diabetes 31:313.

Forrest JM, Menser MA, Burgess JA (1971): High frequency of diabetes mellitus in young adults with congenital rubella. Lancet 2:332–334.

Fowell D, McKnight AJ, Powrie F, Dyke R, Mason D (1991): Subsets of CD4$^+$ T cells and their roles in the induction and prevention of autoimmunity. Immunol Rev 123:37.

Fukuma K, Sakaguchi S, Chen W-L, Morishita R, Masuda T, Uchino H (1988): Immunological and clinical studies on murine experimental autoimmune gastritis induced by neonatal thymectomy. Gastroenterology 94:274.

Gao EK, Lo D, Cheney R, Kanagawa O, Sprent J (1988): Abnormal differentiation of thymocytes in mice treated with cyclosporin A. Nature 336:176.

Ginsberg-Fellner F, Witt ME, Fedun B, Taub F, Doberson MJ, McEvoy RC, Cooper LZ, Notkins AL, Rubinstein P (1985): Diabetes mellitus and autoimmunity in patients with the congenital rubella syndrome. Rev Infect Dis 7(Suppl):S170–176.

Good RA, Roetstein J, Mazzitello WF (1957): The simultaneous occurrence of rheumatoid arthritis and agammaglobulinemia. J Lab Clin Med 49:343.

Hancock S, Cox RS, McDougall IR (1991): Thyroid disease after treatment of Hodgkins's disease. N Engl J Med 325:599.

Hansen TH, Sachs DH (1989): The major histocompatibility complex. In Paul W (ed): "Fundamental Immunology," 2nd Ed. New York: Raven Press, pp 445–487.

Hodes RJ (1989): T-cell-mediated regulation: Help and suppression. In Paul W (ed): "Fundamental Immunology." 2nd Ed. New York: Raven Press, pp 587–620.

Horn GT, Bugawan TL, Long CM, Erlich HA (1988): Allelic sequence variation of the HLA-DQ loci: Relationship to serology and insulin-dependent diabetes susceptibility. Proc Natl Acad Sci USA 85:6012.

Irvine WJ, Clarke BF, Scarth L, Cullen DR, Duncan LJP (1970): Thyroid and gastric autoimmunity in patients with diabetes mellitus. Lancet 2:163.

Jenkins MK, Schwartz RN, Pardoll DM (1988): Effects of cyclosporin A on T cell development and clonal deletion. Science 241:1655.

Jones LA, Chin LT, Merriam GR, Nelson LM, Kruisbeek AM (1990): Failure of clonal deletion in neonatally thymectomized mice: Tolerance is preserved through clonal anergy. J Exp Med 172:1277.

Kaplan HS (1980): "Hodgkin's Disease." 2nd Ed. Cambridge, MA: Harvard University Press.

Kappler JW, Roehm N, Marrack P (1987): T cell tolerance by clonal elimination in the thymus. Cell 49:273.

Khoury EL, Bottazzo GF, Pontes de Carvalho LC, Wick G, Roitt IM (1982): Predisposition to organ-specific autoimmunity in obese strain (OS) chickens: Reactivity to thyroid, gastric, adrenal and pancreatic cytoplasmic antigens. Clin Exp Immunol 49:273.

Kisielow P, Bluethmann H, Staerz U, Steinmetz M, von Boemer H (1988): Tolerance in T-cell receptor transgenic mice involves deletion of nonmature $CD4^+8^+$ thymocytes. Nature 333:742.

Koike T, Itoh Y, Ishii T, Ito I, Takabayashi K, Maruyama N, Tomioka H, Yoshida S (1987): Preventive effect of monoclonal anti-L3T4 antibody on development of diabetes in NOD mice. Diabetes 36:539.

Kojima A, Tanaka-Kojima Y, Sakakura T, Nishizuka Y (1976): Spontaneous development of autoimmune thyroiditis in neonatally thymectomized mice. Lab Invest 34:550.

Kojima A, Taguchi O, Nishizuka Y (1980): Experimental production of possible autoimmune gastritis followed by macrocytic anemia in athymic nude mice. Lab Invest 42:387.

Kojima A, Prehn RT (1981): Genetic susceptibility of postthymectomy autoimmune disease in mice. Immunogenetics 14:15.

Kosugi A, Sharrow SO, Shearer GM (1989): Effect of cyclosporin A on lymphopoiesis: absence of mature T cells in thymus and periphery of bone marrow transplanted mice treated with cyclosporin A. J Immunol 142:3026.

Like AA, Rossini AA, Guberski DL, Appel MC, Williams RM (1981): Spontaneous diabetes mellitus: Reversal and prevention in the BB/W rat with antiserum to rat lymphocytes. Science 206:1421.

Like AA, Weringer EJ, Holdash A, McGill P, Atkinson D, Rossini AA (1985): Adoptive transfer of autoimmune diabetes mellitus in Biobreeding/Worcester (BB/W) inbred and hybrid rats. J Immunol 134:1583.

Londei M, Bottazzo GF, Feldman M (1985): Human T cell clones from autoimmune thyroid glands: Specific recognition of autologous thyroid cells. Science 228:85.

Lorenz RG, Allen PM (1988): Direct evidence for functional self protein/Ia-molecule complexes in vivo. Proc Natl Acad Sci USA 85:5220.

Lund T, O'Reilly L, Hutchings P, Kanagawa O, Simpson E, Gravery R, Chandler P, Dyson J, Picard JK, Edwards A, Kioussis D, Cooke A (1990): Prevention of insulin-dependent diabetes mellitus in non-obese diabetic mice by transgenes encoding modified I-A β-chain or normal I-E α-chain. Nature 345:727.

MacLaren NK, Riley WJ (1986): Autoimmune polyendocrinopathies. In Samter M, Talmage DW, Frank MM, Austen KF, Claman HN (eds): "Immunological Diseases." 4th Ed. Boston: Little, Brown, pp 1737–1746.

Marrack P, Kappler JW (1987): The T-cell receptor. Science 238:1073.

McChesney MB, Oldstone MBA (1987): Viruses perturb lymphocyte functions: Selected principles characterizing virus-induced immunosuppression. Annu Rev Immunol 5:279.

McKeever U, Mordes JP, Greiner DL, Appel MC, Rozing J, Handler ES, Rossini AA (1990): Adoptive transfer of autoimmune diabetes and thyroiditis to athymic rats. Proc Natl Acad Sci USA 87:7618.

Menser M, Forrest JM, Bransby RD (1978): Rubella infection and diabetes mellitus. Lancet 1:57.

Mims CA (1987): "The Pathogenesis of Infectious Disease." 3rd. Ed. London: Academic Press, pp 152–178.

Miyazaki T, Uno M, Uehira M, Kikutani H, Kishimoto T, Kimoto M, Nishimoto H, Miyazaki J, Yamamura K (1990): Direct evidence for the contribution of the unique I-A^{nod} to the development of insulitis in non-obese diabetic mice. Nature 345:722.

Mojcik CF, Greiner DL, Medlock ES, Komschlies KL, Goldschneider I (1988): Characterization of RT6 bearing rat lymphocytes. I. Ontogeny of the RT6$^+$ subset. Cell Immunol 114:336.

Mordes JP, Gallina DL, Handler ES, Greiner DL, Nakamura N, Pelletier A, Rossini AA (1987): Transfusions enriched for W3/25$^+$ helper/inducer T lymphocytes prevent spontaneous diabetes in the BB/W rat. Diabetologia 30:22.

Morse SS, Valinsky JE (1989): Mouse thymic virus (MTLV). A mammalian herpesvirus cytolytic for CD4$^+$ (L3T4$^+$) T lymphocytes. J Exp Med 169:591–597.

Mosmann T, Coffman RL (1989): Heterogeneity of cytokine secretion patterns and functions of helper T cells. Adv Immunol 46:111.

Oldstone MBA (1987): Molecular mimicry and autoimmune disease. Cell 50:819.

Olson GB, South MA, Good RA (1967). Phytohemagglutinin unresponsiveness of lymphocytes from babies with congenital rubella. Nature 214:695.

Penhale WJ, Farmer A, McKenna RP, Irvine WJ (1973): Spontaneous thyroiditis in thymectomized and irradiated Wister rats. Clin Exp Immunol 15:225.

Penhale WJ, Stumbles PA, Huxtable CR, Sutherland RJ, Pethick DW (1990): Induction of diabetes in PVG/c strain rats by manipulation of the immune system. Autoimmunity 7:169.

Penhale WJ, Irvine WJ, Ingris JR, Farmer A (1976): Thyroiditis in T cell-depleted rats: Suppression of the autoallergic response by reconstitution with normal lymphoid cells. Clin Exp Immunol 25:6.

Powrie F, Mason D (1990): Ox-22^{high} CD4$^+$ T cells induce wasting disease with multiple organ pathology: Prevention by the OX-22^{low} subset. J Exp Med 172:1701.

Powrie F, Mason D (1988): Phenotypic and functional heterogeneity of CD4$^+$ T cells. Immunol Today 9:274.

Prochazka M, Leiter EH, Serreze DV, et al. (1987): Three recessive loci required for insulin dependent diabetes in nonobese diabetic mice. Science 237:286.

Quimby FW, Schwartz RS (1982): Systemic lupus erythematosus in mice and dogs. In Lachmann PJ, Peters DK (eds): "Clinical Aspects of Immunology." 4th Ed. Oxford: Blackwell Scientific, pp 1217–1230.

Riley WJ, Winter A, Goldstein D (1983): Coincident presence of thyrogastric autoimmunity at onset of type 1 (insulin-dependent) diabetes. Diabetologia 24:418.

Roitt IM (1988): "Essential Immunology." 6th Ed. Oxford: Blackwell Scientific, pp 238–273.

Rossini AA, Mordes JP, Like AA (1985): Immunology of insulin-dependent diabetes mellitus. Annu Rev Immunol 3:291.

Rubinstein P, Walker ME, Fedun B, Witt ME, Cooper LZ, Ginsberg-Fellner F (1982): The HLA system in congenital rubella patients with and without diabetes. Diabetes 31:1088.

Sakaguchi S, Takahashi T, Nishizuka Y (1982a): Study on cellular events in postthymectomy autoimmune oophoritis in mice. I. Requirement of Lyt-1 effector T cells for oocytes damage after adoptive transfer. J Exp Med 156:1565.

Sakaguchi S, Takahashi T, Nishizuka Y (1982b): Study on cellular events in postthymectomy autoimmune oophoritis in mice. II. Requirement of Lyt-1 cells in normal female mice for the prevention of oophoritis. J Exp Med 156:1577.

Sakaguchi S, Fukuma K, Kuribayashi K, Masuda T (1985): Organ-specific autoimmune diseases induced in mice by elimination of T cell subset. I. Evidence for the active participation of T cells in natural self-tolerance: Deficit of a T cell subset as a possible cause of autoimmune disease. J Exp Med 161:72.

Sakaguchi S, Sakaguchi N (1988): Thymus and autoimmunity: Transplantation of the thymus from cyclosporin A–treated mice causes organ-specific autoimmune disease in athymic nude mice. J Exp Med 167:1479.

Sakaguchi S, Sakaguchi N (1989): Organ-specific autoimmune disease induced in mice by elimination of T-cell subsets. V. Neonatal administration of cyclosporin A causes autoimmune disease. J Immunol 142:471.

Sakaguchi S, Sakaguchi N (1990): Thymus and autoimmunity: Capacity of the normal thymus to produce pathogenic self-reactive T cells and conditions required for their induction of autoimmune disease. J Exp Med 172:537.

Sakaguchi N, Miyai K, Sakaguchi S (1992a): Ionizing radiation and autoimmunity: Induction of autoimmune disease in mice by high dose fractionated total lymphoid irradiation and its prevention by inoculating normal T cells. Manuscript submitted.

Sakaguchi S, Ermak TH, Berg LJ, Ho W, Fazekas de St. Groth B, Peterson PA, Sakaguchi N, Davis MM (1992b): Induction of autoimmune disease by germline alteration of the T cell receptor gene expression. Manuscript submitted.

Schneider R, Lees RK, Pedrazzini T, Zinkernagel RM, Hengartner H, MacDonald HR (1989): Postnatal disappearance of self-reactive (Vβ6$^+$) cells from the thymus of Mls^a mice: Implication for T cell development and autoimmunity. J Exp Med 169:2149.

Schwartz RH (1989): Acquisition of immunologic self-tolerance. Cell 57:1073.

Schwartz RS, Datta SK (1989): Autoimmunity and autoimmune disease. In Paul W (ed): "Fundamental Immunology." 2nd Ed. New York: Raven Press, pp 819–866.

Shizuru JA, Taylor-Edwards C, Banks BA, Gregory AK, Fathman CG (1988): Immunotherapy of the nonobese diabetic mouse: Treatment with an antibody to T-helper lymphocytes. Science 240:659.

Slattery RM, Kjer-Nielsen L, Allison J, Charlton B, Mandel TE, Miller JFAP (1990): Prevention of diabetes in non-obese diabetic I-A^k transgenic mice. Nature 345:724.

Smith H, Chin IM, Kubo R, Tung KSK (1989): Neonatal thymectomy results in a repertoire enriched in T cells deleted in adult thymus. Science 246:1041.

Sparshoff SM, Bell EB, Sarawar SR (1991): CD45R CD4 T cell subset reconstituted nude rats: Subset-dependent survival of recipients and bi-directional isoform switching. Eur J Immunol 21:993.

Sprent J, Lo D, Gao E-K, Ron Y (1988): T cell selection in the thymus. Immunol Rev 101:173.

Sternthal E, Like AA, Sarantis K, Braverman LE (1981): Lymphocytic thyroiditis and diabetes in the BB/W rat: A new model of autoimmune endocrinopathy. Diabetes 30:1058.

Strober S, Slavin S, Gottlieb M, Zan-Bar I, King DP, Hoppe RT, Fucks Z, Grumet FC, Kaplan HS (1979): Allograft tolerance after total lymphoid irradiation (TLI). Immunol Rev 46:87.

Sugihara S, Izumi Y, Yoshioka T, Yagi H, Tsujimura T, Tarutani O, Kohno Y, Murakami S, Hamaoka T, Fujiwara H (1988): Autoimmune thyroiditis induced in mice depleted of particular T-cell subsets. I. Requirement of Lyt-1^{dull} L3T4^{bright} normal T cells for the induction of thyroiditis. J Immunol 141:105.

Taguchi O, Nishizuka Y, Sakakura T, Kojima A (1980): Autoimmune oophoritis in thymectomized mice: Detection of circulating antibodies against oocytes. Clin Exp Immunol 40:540.

Taguchi O, Nishizuka Y (1981): Experimental autoimmune orchitis after neonatal thymectomy in the mouse. Clin Exp Immunol 46:425.

Todd JA, Aitman TJ, Cornall RJ, Ghosh S, Hall JRS, Earne M, Knight AM, Love JM, McAleer M, Prins J-B, Rodrigues N, Lathrop M, Pressey A, DeLarato NH, Peterson LB, Wicker LS (1991): Genetic analysis of autoimmune type 1 diabetes mellitus in mice. Nature 351:542.

von Boehmer H (1990): Developmental biology of T cells in T cell–receptor transgenic mice. Annu Rev Immunol 8:531.

Weigle WO (1980): Analysis of autoimmunity through experimental models of thyroiditis and allergic encephalomyelitis. Adv Immunol 30:159.

Wick G, Mueller PU, Schwarz S (1982): Effect of cyclosporin A on spontaneous autoimmune thyroiditis of obese strain (OS) chickens. Eur J Immunol 12:877.

Wick G, Brezinschek HP, Hala K, Dietrich H, Wolf H, Kroemer H (1990): The obese strain chickens: An animal model with spontaneous autoimmune thyroiditis. Adv Immunol 47:433.

Winchester G, Sunshine GH, Nardi N, Mitchison NA (1984): Antigen-presenting cells do not discriminate between self and nonself. Immunogenetics 19:487.

Wofsy D, Seaman WE (1985): Successful treatment of autoimmunity in NZB/NZW F_1 mice with monoclonal antibody to L3T4. J Exp Med 161:378.

Zabriskie JB (1986): Rheumatic fever: A model for the pathological consequences of microbial-host mimicry. Clin Exp Rheumatol 4:65.

15

AUTOIMMUNITY AND IDIOTYPIC NETWORKS

John Stewart

Unité d'Immunobiologie, Institut Pasteur, Paris, France

INTRODUCTION

In classic immunology, attention is focused on immune responses to foreign antigens. Such responses are attributed to Burnetian clonal selection; in this scheme, each clone is activated individually through its own direct interaction with the antigen, with the corollary that the B-cell clones that proliferate and secrete immunoglobulin do not interact with each other. The major problem in this schema is to account for the fact that antigens belonging to the somatic self do not generally provoke strong immune responses, which would of course lead to autoimmunity and thus be highly dysteleological. The classic answer to this problem is to postulate that self-reactive clones are eliminated or inactivated (by clonal deletion or clonal anergy) during a special period during early ontogeny. This solution to the problem of autoimmunity is, however, invalidated by the rapidly accumulating evidence showing that normal individuals produce autoreactive antibodies (albeit in relatively low concentrations), not only in early ontogeny but also in the mature immune system [Avrameus, 1991].

The aim of this chapter is to summarize the theoretical work, based largely on computer simulations, that examines the possibility that network interactions between lymphocyte clones may make a decisive contribution to self-tolerance, i.e., to the avoidance of autoimmunity. The focus will be

Autoimmunity: Physiology and Disease, Pages 229–240
© *1994 Wiley-Liss, Inc.*

on our own work in this area; we shall refer to the work of other groups primarily in so far as it supports, complements, or contrasts with our work. Thus far, we have concentrated on the role of B cells and idiotypic interactions between the variable regions of immunoglobulins; the possible role of major histocompatibility complex (MHC) and T cells, notably the differentiation between Th1 and Th2 helper cells, is not taken into account.

Asking the question of whether an idiotypic network can contribute to self-tolerance represents a reversal in perspective in both traditional immunology and the early work on the network concept itself in the years following Jerne's seminal proposal [Jerne, 1974]. Thus initial work on the network concept sought to examine whether an idiotypic network could account for the immune response itself, for the regulation of that response, and for "immune memory" (i.e., the fact that a secondary response is both faster and of greater magnitude than the primary response). In contrast, in the work to be presented here, the initial focus is on the organization of an autonomous network (i.e., a set of lymphocyte clones that reciprocally activate each other without necessity for stimulation by an external antigen). The coupling of such a network with self-antigens is then conceptualized as the incorporation of antigens into the mode of self-regulating activity characteristic of an interconnected system, i.e., the horizon is clearly defined as that of self-tolerance. Immune responses to foreign antigens are not a major focus; indeed, in our perspective, such responses may well be due to classic clonal selection of mutually independent clones that do not belong to the interconnected network—what we have termed the *peripheral immune system* in contrast to the connected network that forms the *central immune system* [Varela and Coutinho, 1991].

MODEL

The model of the immune network that we have used in this work seeks an optimal compromise between biological realism on the one hand and simplicity on the other. Biological realism has led us, notably, to make a distinction between free soluble immunoglobulin in the serum (the concentration of idiotype i being denoted by f_i) and cell-bound immunoglobulin functioning as a receptor in the membrane of B lymphocytes (denoted by b_i). Within this constraint, maximal simplicity comes from the fact that the production and removal of free and cell-bound immunoglobulins are each represented by single terms in a set of ordinary differential equations. A key element in establishing these equations is that idiotypic interactions between the different clones in the network are mediated by the field or "sensitivity", σ_i, which is defined as the linear sum of the interactions between an idiotype with all the other idiotypes:

$$\sigma_i = \Sigma \, m_{ij} \cdot f_j, \tag{1}$$

where m_{ij} is the affinity coefficient between idiotypes i and j. On this basis, the probability that cells in clone i will maturate to plasma-secreting blasts is given by a bell-shaped function $Mat\ (\sigma_i)$; the probability of proliferation by a similar function $Prol\ (\sigma_i)$. In other words, in this model lymphocyte activation is maximal at intermediate values of the field σ_i; at either high or low levels of σ_i a clone is not activated. A final term, $Meta$ (i), denotes the process of metadynamics by which clones freshly emerged from the bone marrow can be recruited into the network (see Metadynamics and Shapespace, below).

With this notation, the equations that define the basic model are

$$df_i/dt \ = k_1 \cdot f_i \cdot \sigma_i + k_2 \cdot b_i \cdot Mat\ (\sigma_i) \tag{2}$$

$$db_i/dt \ = k_3 \cdot b_i + k_4 \cdot b_i \cdot Prol\ (\sigma_i) + Meta\ (i) \tag{3}$$

[for the initial presentation of this model, see Varela et al., 1988; for a recent study that systematically investigates this general class of models, see De Boer et al., 1992].

DYNAMICS

Equations 2 and 3, taken together, are nonlinear, and in general the dynamics of the system are complex and highly dependent on the structure of the connectivity matrix m_{ij}. To render the perception of this complexity manageable, it is useful to refer to two elementary forms.

The first "reference configuration" is that of a single clone with autoaffinity. If the initial concentrations of f and b are above threshold values, this minimal system has a fixed-point attractor such that the clone displays ongoing self-activation; the equilibrium concentrations of f and b are inversely proportional to the self-affinity m_{11} [Stewart and Varela, 1990]. This minimal system can be extended to a set of completely interconnected clones of arbitrary number (i.e., $m_{ij} = 1$ for all i and all j). Such a set behaves, collectively, like a single clone with autoaffinity, i.e., there is a fixed-point attractor [Bersini, 1992].

The second "reference configuration" is that of two clones that have little or no autoaffinity, but strong mutual affinity with each other; i.e., the affinity matrix has the form

$$\begin{matrix} \delta & 1 \\ 1 & \delta \end{matrix}$$

where $\delta \ll 1$.

It appears that such a system has no nonzero fixed-point attractor. However, for certain parameter settings, this system does possess a cyclic attractor, in which the two clones oscillate out of phase [Stewart and Varela, 1990]. This elementary form can be extended to a "chain" of inter-connected clones (1 has affinity with 2, 2 with 3, 3 with 4, and so forth; i.e., $m_{ij} = 1$ if $(i - j)$ is $+1$ or -1; $m_{ij} = 0$ otherwise). In such a system, the odd-numbered clones tend to behave as a unit, oscillating in phase with each other, but out of phase with the other unit consisting of the even-numbered clones [Stewart and Varela, 1990; Bersini, 1992].

The spirit of the network approach requires that the clones in a network should not be completely independent, but should depend on each other for their mutual activation. The two basic forms described above, taken together, lead to the important suggestion that collectively sustained ongoing activity in a differentiated network is likely to be "oscillatory," not necessarily in the strict sense of a cyclic attractor but in the more general sense of fluctuating rather than being dynamically stable. This suggestion is supported by recent simulations investigating the behavior of the basic model with a variety of connectivity matrices [Bersini, 1992].

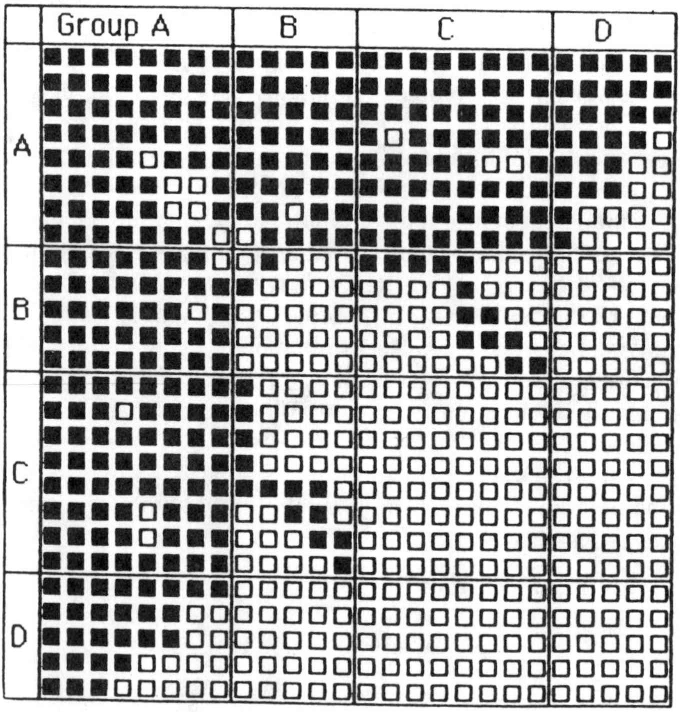

FIGURE 1. The matrix of affinities between 26 immunoglobulins from neonatal mice, as derived from the data of Kearney et al. [1987]. [Redrawn from Stewart and Varela 1989.]

STRUCTURE OF CONNECTIVITY

The behavior of any network clearly depends on the pattern of connections between the nodes. In the case of the idiotypic network, this corresponds to the structure of the affinity matrix m_{ij}. Empirical data on this question are frustratingly sparse, but an important indication is given in the work of Kearney et al. [1987]. Rearrangement of this matrix, taking into account the a priori expectation that the matrix should be symmetrical (if idiotype i interacts with idiotype j, then idiotype j should interact with idiotype i), reveals that this matrix possesses a definite structure (Fig. 1) [Stewart and Varela, 1989]. The clones fall into four groups: A) Clones that are "multi-reactive," having complete affinity with each other (cf. the extended prototype configuration 1) and also having affinity with a high proportion of all other clones; B,C) two "mirror" groups of clones, each group being characterized by the fact that clones have affinity with several clones in the other group but no affinity with any of the clones in the same group (cf. the "chain" configuration referred in the preceding section; and D) poorly connected clones, characterized by the fact that they have affinity neither with each other nor with any of the clones in groups B and C (this being precisely the condition that they should belong to none of these groups), but only with clones in group A.

The dynamic activity of this network, as revealed by computer simulation, shows a satisfying degree of correspondence with the structure of the

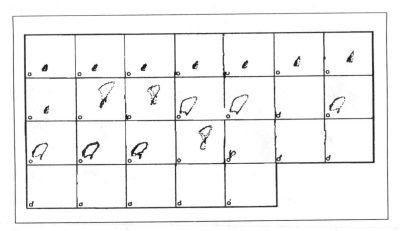

FIGURE 2. The simulated dynamics of a set of lymphocyte clones with the connectivity structure shown in Figure 1. The abscissa of each square represents b_i, the concentration of membrane-bound immunoglobulin; the ordinate represents f_i, the concentration of free immunoglobulin (log scales in each case). The points in each square represent successive dynamic states; a closed loop thus represents a cyclic attractor. [Redrawn from Stewart and Varela, 1989.]

affinity matrix (Fig. 2) [Stewart and Varela, 1989]. Clones in group A have low levels of ongoing activation; they oscillate slightly, but the amplitude of these fluctuations is so small that their behavior is close to that of a fixed-point attractor. Clones in groups B and C show high-amplitude oscillations, in phase within groups and out of phase between groups. Clones in group D are generally not activated.

This model enables a preliminary investigation of the possible relationship between network organization and autoimmunity [Stewart et al., 1989]. Self-antigens are represented by antigens whose presence is constant and unconditional on the field they experience. Antigenic stimulation of the poorly connected clones in group D leads to unlimited proliferation of these clones so that the field produced on the antigen increases indefinitely. This would correspond to autoimmunity. Stimulation of the highly connected clones in group A has little effect. Stimulation of clones in groups B and C is most interesting: The activity of the clone that is directly affected is actually decreased, but concomitantly the activity of many other clones in the network increases (Fig. 3). This provides an image of self-tolerance as an active, positive phenomenon involving an extended network.

METADYNAMICS AND SHAPESPACE

The simulations reported thus far have not taken into account the metadynamics of the system: the fact that the affinity matrix m_{ij} is not given once and for all, but is generated by the processes of recruitment and elimination of clones from the current population. To represent these processes, we

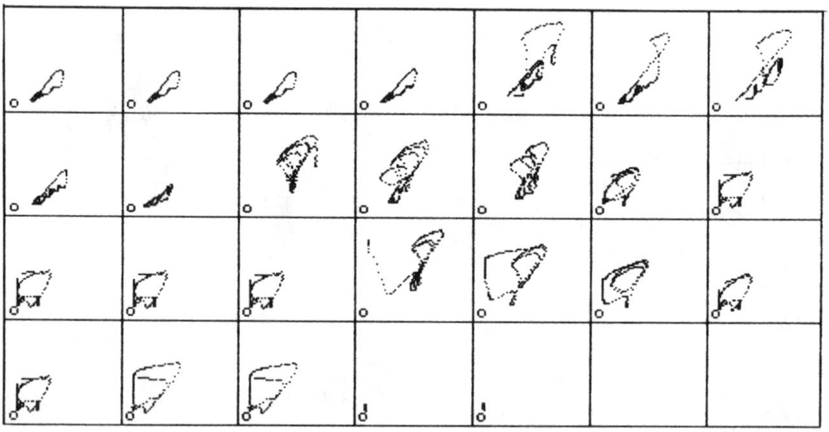

FIGURE 3. The modification of the dynamics shown in Figure 2 in the presence of a "self-antigen" with affinity to clone number 9 (the second square in the second row). The activity of this clone is actually decreased, whereas many other clones show increased activity. [Redrawn from Stewart et al., 1989.]

have adopted a modified version of the "shapespace" concept initially proposed by Perelson and Oster [1979], according to which each point in a two-dimensional shapespace corresponds to a pair of complementary shapes, represented by opposite colors, conventionally "black" and "white" [Stewart and Varela, 1991]. In the preliminary investigations carried out thus far, we have used a rudimentary form of dynamics in which the survival/recruitment of clones requires that the field σ due to idiotypic interactions with other clones should be within a "window" above a lower threshold and below an upper threshold; clones with fields outside this window are eliminated or not recruited.

Briefly, the results of our simulations are as follows. In the absence of antigens, the network constitutes itself and settles into quasistable configurations in shapespace with chains of "black" and "white" clones facing each other (Fig. 4): Such chains will correspond to the "mirror" groups of sections III and IV. If the ontogenesis of the system occurs in the presence of self-antigens, the latter are harmoniously incorporated into the black and

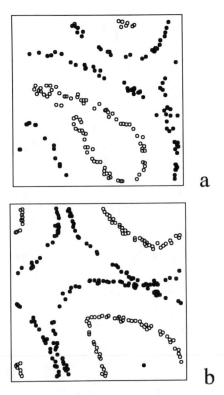

FIGURE 4. Two simulations (**a,b**) showing the quasistable configurations resulting from the self-organizing occupation of shapespace in a simple model of the metadynamics of the immune network. Clones represented by black circles have affinity with neighbouring "white" clones (and vice versa). [Redrawn from Stewart and Varela, 1991.]

white chains (Fig. 5). This corresponds to a potential mechanism for achieving self-tolerance: As can be seen from the fact that the self-antigens are incorporated into viable chains of lymphocytes, the field experienced by these antigens remains within the limits of the "window" and does not reach the high values that are plausibly necessary for triggering destructive reactions by effector mechanisms (complement, macrophages, and so

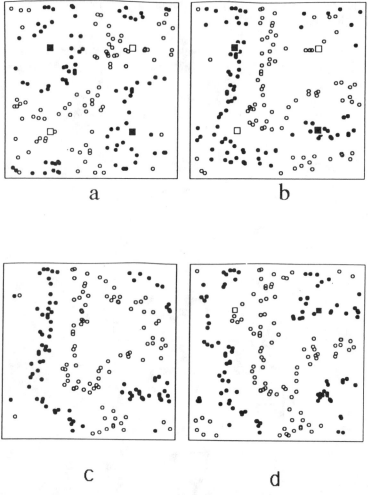

a   b

c   d

FIGURE 5. a,b) Two simulations of the occupation of shapespace when the recruitment of new clones occurs in the presence of four self-antigens represented by two black and two white squares. **c)** The continuation from b when the self-antigens are removed; the pattern is virtually unchanged, illustrating the quasistability of the system. **d)** The readjustment of the pattern when two new self-antigens are introduced in discordant positions: The chains of black and white clones shift in such a way that the new antigens are incorporated. [Redrawn from Stewart and Varela, 1991.]

forth). This point can be emphasized by considering the result if the recruited clones do not interact with each other (cf., Burnetian clonal selection), a situation that can be simulated by recruiting clones of a single color complementary to the antigen. In this case, clones are recruited without limit, producing an indefinitely high field at the point of the antigen. This behavior is that of an immune response: If it were to occur with respect to a self-antigen, the result would be pathological autoimmunity.

RELATION TO EXPERIMENTAL DATA

What are the possibilities for confronting the results of these theoretical investigations with experimental data? The major area in which this has been possible to date comes from observations of the levels of natural antibodies circulating in the serum of nonimmunized mice and humans. The first important observation is that mice raised in "antigen-free" conditions have near-control levels of plasma IgM and of activated, effector lymphocytes in the spleen and internal body surfaces [Varela and Coutinho, 1991]. This clearly indicates that natural antibodies are not directly concerned with responses to environmental antigens, but reflect the autonomous activity of the idiotypic network and/or interaction with self-antigens.

The second observation is that the quantitative levels of natural antibodies fluctuate widely [Lundqvist et al., 1989] (Fig. 6). As already explained (see Dynamics, above), this can be interpreted as a consequence of the fact that these antibodies are produced by differentiated clones incorporated in a largely autonomous, self-activating network. This interpretation is strengthened by the observation that these fluctuations can be strongly influenced by the injection of relatively small amounts of cross-reactive immunoglobulins [Lundqvist et al., 1989].

The third important observation relates to a more detailed analysis of the exact nature of these fluctuations, which are normally neither random nor simply oscillatory. This is graphically shown by calculating the spectral power or Fourier transformation of the fluctuations: A pure oscillation would give rise to a single-peak spectral curve, whereas random noise would give rise to a flat curve. The experimental data typically yield an intermediate condition: wide-band spectra with a tendency to peak around one to two cycles per month (Fig. 6). Furthermore, many of these spectra can be fitted by a curve of the form $1/(\text{frequency})^\delta$, where δ is a constant. Such "$1/f$" spectra suggest that the system is operating near a "chaotic attractor," that is, a complex mixture of various oscillatory modes, which would give it access to a wide array of possible configurations.

The relevance of these spectra to autoimmunity is greatly strengthened by a fourth type of observation showing that the pattern of fluctuations is perceptibly altered in both mice and humans affected by autoimmune disease [Varela et al., 1991]. In autoimmune individuals, the power spectrum

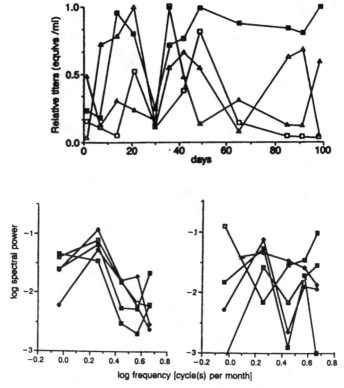

FIGURE 6. **Top)** Representative examples of the fluctuations over time in the serum concentrations of several naturally expressed idiotypes. **Bottom)** Contrast in the spectral patterns of these fluctuations in normal mice (**left**) and strain-, age-, and sex-matched autoimmune mice (**right**). [Redrawn from Varela et al., 1991.]

is disturbed: There is either a single strong peak, or else a flat spectrum corresponding to random fluctuations; this suggests that autoreactive lymphocytes in pathological autoimmunity are characterized by disturbed patterns of network connectivity.

Finally, these observations are prolonged by the effects of intravenous treatment with a balanced set of pooled immunoglobulins from normal individuals (IVIg). It is noteworthy, first, that in a wide range of autoimmune disorders the beneficial effects of such treatment are not simply palliative, but in a substantial proportion of cases actually effect a long-term cure [Imbach, 1991; Dwyer, 1992]. This suggests some sort of systemic effect. What is particularly significant, in the present context, is that such long-term recovery is highly correlated with restoration of a "normal" (1/f) type of power spectrum [Dietrich et al., 1992].

CONCLUSIONS

What are the perspectives for future work? The obvious next step is to consolidate the largely preliminary studies carried out thus far by integrating the aspects described in the previous four sections. In other words, the agenda is to combine metadynamics with a full quantitative dynamics differentiating free and cell-bound immunoglobulins in order to see whether it is possible to reproduce by simulation both the structure of the empirically observed affinity matrices and the precise dynamics of the fluctuations (1/f power spectra) The focal point of this study would be to understand autoimmunity by characterizing the parameter values and initial conditions (notably the distribution of self-antigens in shapespace) such that ontogenesis leads to tolerance to self-antigens, as contrasted with the values and conditions that lead to autoimmune attack on self-antigens. If this consolidation could be achieved as we anticipate, the stage would be set for a major advance in our understanding of autoimmunity, since we would have at our disposal a powerful tool for testing postulates concerning the primary defect (or defects, since etiology may well be multiple) in autoimmune disease. To be successful, any such postulate should make precise predictions on the patterns of network connectivity (the structure of m_{ij}) that correspond to self-tolerance as contrasted with those corresponding to autoimmunity; it should reproduce both types of perturbation in the power spectra of fluctuations in natural antibody levels seen in autoimmune disease (i.e., both single-peak and flat spectra); and it should be able to reproduce the beneficial long-term effects of IVIg treatment. This would open up new perspectives in autoimmunity as regards both prevention and new forms of treatment that could be both more specific and more consistently effective. The importance of such perspectives can hardly be overestimated, since the range of diseases recognized as including an autoimmune component, so recently thought to be restricted to a handful of rarities, is now expanding explosively.

ACKNOWLEDGMENTS

The work described in this paper is based entirely on my collaboration with Antonio Coutinho and Francisco Varela.

REFERENCES

Avrameus S (1991): Natural autoantibodies: From "horror autotoxicus" to "gnothi seauton." Immunol Today 12:154–159.
Bersini H (1992): The interplay between the dynamics and the metadynamics of the

immune network. Artificial Life III Workshop, Sante Fe: IRIDIA Tech Rep TR/ IRIDIA/92-12.

De Boer RJ, Kevrekedis IG, Perlson AS (1992): Immune network behavior. I: From stationary states to limit cycle oscillation. II: From oscillations to chaos and stationary states. Bull Math Biol (in press).

Dietrich G, Varela FJ, Hurez V, Bouanani M, Kazatchkine MD (1992): Manipulating the human immune network with normal immunoglobulin G. Proc Natl Acad Sci USA (in press).

Dwyer JM (1992): Drug therapy: Manipulating the immune system with immune globulin. N Engl J Med 326:107–116.

Imbach P, ed (1991): "Immunotherapy With Intravenous Immunoglobulins." London: Academic Press.

Jerne NK (1974): Towards a network theory of the immune system. Ann Immunol 125C:373–389.

Kearney JK, Vakil M, Nicholson N (1987): Nonrandom V_H gene expression and idiotype–antiidiotype expression on early B cells. In Kelsoe G, Schulze D (eds): "Evolution and Vertebrate Immunity." Austin: Texas University Press, pp 175–190.

Lundqvist I, Coutinho A, Varela F, Holmberg D (1989): Evidence for the functional dynamics in an antibody network. Proc Natl Acad Sci USA 86:5074–5078.

Perelson AS, Oster G (1979). Theoretical studies of clonal selection. J Theor Biol 81:645–670.

Stewart J, Varela FJ (1989): Exploring the meaning of connectivity in the immune network. Immunol Rev 110:37–61.

Stewart J, Varela FJ (1990): Dynamics of a class of immune networks. II. Oscillatory activity of cellular and humoral components. J Theor Biol 144:103–115.

Stewart J, Varela FJ (1991): Morphogenesis in shapespace. J Theor Biol 153:477–498.

Stewart J, Varela FJ, Coutinho A (1989): J Autoimmun 2(Suppl):15–23.

Varela F, Anderssen A, Dietrich G, Sunbland A, Holmberg D, Kazatchkine M, Coutinho A (1991): Population dynamics of natural antibodies in normal and autoimmune individuals. Proc Natl Acad Sci USA 88:5917–5921.

Varela FJ, Coutinho A (1991): Second generation immune networks. Immunol Today 12:159–166.

Varela F, Coutinho A, Dupire B, Vaz NM (1988): Cognitive networks: Immune, neural and otherwise. In Perelson AS (ed): "Theoretical Immunology." New York: Addison-Wesley, Vol. II, pp 359–374.

II

AUTOIMMUNE DISEASE

16

BOUNDARIES BETWEEN PHYSIOLOGICAL AUTOREACTIVITY AND PATHOLOGICAL AUTOIMMUNITY

Michel D. Kazatchkine and Antonio Coutinho

Unité d'Immunopathologie, Hôpital Broussais (M.D.K.); Unité d'Immunobiologie, Institut Pasteur (A.C.), Paris, France

The domain of autoreactivity is that of the relationships between V-region repertoires and components of the individual that produce and express those V regions. Autoreactive V regions include configurations (shapes) that are either complementary to or mimic self-antigenic structures. Molecular mimicries only exist as a function of a third structure that reacts with both. As V regions themselves are self-components, this three-party relationship gives rise to a network of connected molecular species that includes autoantigens together with the expressed antibody and lymphocyte repertoires. Because V-region interactions are degenerate and each V region or self-antigen is large enough to express multiple binding sites, the network is characterized by a high degree of connectivity, each component being capable of interacting with a variety of others in the set. Autoreactive

Autoimmunity: Physiology and Disease, Pages 243–246
© *1994 Wiley-Liss, Inc.*

V regions are thus "more connected" than those related to antigenic structures that are absent from the organism (nonself). The concept of a greater degree of connectivity associated with autoreactivity has been documented by the analysis of V-region complementarities in newborn individuals, germ-free animals, and natural autoreactive antibodies in the adult. Selective connectivity of the autoreactive repertoire is the result of positive cellular selection in ontogeny, indicating the role of V-region connectivity in the establishment of tolerance to the set of antigens that are present during development (self).

The functional significance of the network of autoreactive V regions arises from the fact that its structure has been selected by, and simultaneously supports activities of, the participant lymphocytes, thus resulting in the functional autonomy of this compartment of the immune system. The structure and organization of the network result in a particular dynamic behavior of autoreactive lymphocytes in each individual. A direct manifestation of the functional autonomy of the autoreactive network is the production of natural antibodies in healthy individuals, independent of external antigenic stimuli. The restricted spontaneous temporal patterns of fluctuations of serum autoantibody levels observed in human and mouse reflect such network organization of autoreactive B cells. Evidence for autoreactive T cells and complementarity between their respective V regions and those of natural antibodies and their respective B cells also has been produced. In short, current evidence indicates that autoreactive lymphocytes are present in healthy individuals and that connectivity in this set of V regions simultaneously limits specific clonal expansion and maintains the great diversity that characterizes the expressed repertoire of the normal immune system.

Autoimmune diseases are chronic conditions characterized by organ-specific or systemic symptoms that are associated with selective stimulation of some autoreactive clonal specificities and thus with a defect in the diversity of the expressed repertoire. With time, we have learned that autoimmune diseases are characterized not merely by the expansion of a limited number of autoantibody clones or T cells, but rather by defects in connectivity and/or diversity of the autoreactive repertoire. This concept is extensively supported by many of the authors in the following section of this volume, by Weigert's findings of limited diversity of antibodies in autoimmune conditions, by the analysis of the spontaneous fluctuations of autoantibody concentrations in diseased humans and animals, and by the findings that organ-specific diseases are characterized also by altered patterns of autoantibodies unrelated to the target organ. The network organization of autoreactive repertoires implies that these are recursively selected through connectivity, that is, the expressed repertoires participate in selecting forthcoming diversity. Defective connectivity will result therefore in altered expressed diversity and in the autonomous maintenance (and chronicity) of the altered structure and dynamics of the autoreactive repertoires. Defective connectivity and diversity, currently referred to as "failure in regulation and control mechanisms," therefore provide the basis for understanding the chronic, self-perpetuating, but nevertheless fluctuating (sometimes spontaneously remitting) course of autoimmune diseases. The delicate balance among autoimmune physiology, transient but self-limited episodes of autoimmune symptomatology, and chronic sustained disease relates, according to these views, to the robustness of the autoreactive network and to its susceptibility to perturbations, that is, its ability to regain "dynamic attractors" compatible with normality. The high frequency of individuals with autoimmune symptomatology and disease also suggests the close relationship between physiological autoreactivity and disease.

These concepts, while delineating very subtle boundaries between physiological autoreactivity and autoimmune disease, also provide a single underlying principle for the establishment of self-tolerance, for the emergence of pathological autoimmunity, and for defining therapeutic strategies aimed at restoring physiological tolerance by reinforcing appropriate V-region connectivity. It is immediately apparent that structural and/or genetic analysis of autoreactive antibody or T-cell receptor V regions will fail to provide a demarcation between physiological and pathological states of autoreactivity, except by revealing the limited diversity of the latter. In contrast, these views hold that the difference between health and disease is to be found at levels of supraclonal organization, through quantitative assessment of V-region connectivity, and analyses of dynamic behaviors of autoreactive lymphocytes.

The striking therapeutic effects of infusing intravenously IgG obtained from healthy individuals (IVIg) in a variety of organ-specific and systemic autoimmune diseases appears to provide major support for these novel concepts. Since IVIg preparations are obtained from large pools of healthy individuals, they represent the physiological autoreactive antibody network. Analysis of reactivities present in the therapeutic pools indeed has revealed the presence of complementarities to autoantibodies and of autoantibodies themselves, both kinds of reactivities being present at higher concentrations in the subset of IgG molecules that are most strongly connected to others in the pool. Infusion of IgG into patients demonstrates the functional relevance of the in vitro findings through neutralization of circulating autoantibodies and stimulation or downregulation of specific B-cell subsets expressing antigen receptors connected to V regions present in IVIg. Furthermore, the long-lasting effects of IVIg in some patients, extending far beyond the half-life of the infused IgG, demonstrate that administration of a physiologically selected (in the donors) set of V regions imposes on the diseased immune system (of the recipient) a normal process of endogenous repertoire selection, thus indicating recursivity of autoimmune network operation. These conclusions have been strengthened recently by the restoration of normal dynamic patterns of natural autoantibodies by IVIg in an autoimmune patient. The therapeutic effects of IVIg thus seem to justify strategies that aim at restoring connectivity and diversity in auto-immune patients. Beyond its clinical relevance, IVIg has carried the heuristic value of validating concepts of the emergence of autoimmune disease through failure of regulatory V-region networks. The same is true for other novel therapeutic strategies, such as T-cell vaccination, that have proven effective in several experimental models of autoimmune disease. Indeed, the increased resistance to induction of autoimmune symptoms in animals that have recovered from a first course of experimental disease is a manifestation of the potential importance of vaccinal strategies for autoimmune disease.

Such therapeutic approaches and their results contrast with those that aim at suppressing specific clonal reactivities to putative autoantigenic targets of autoimmune disease. The latter immunosuppressive strategies, including clonotypic suppression, peptide competition, anti-class II major histocompatibility complex, and anti-T-cell receptor V β-family suppression, are based on the alternative view that autoimmune disease is the linear consequence of 1) an abnormal clonal response to a normal self-antigen, 2) a "normal" clonal response to an abnormal autoantigen, or 3) a "normal" clonal response to a "normal" self-antigen that is abnormally presented.

As evidence of the activity of autoreactive T cells in healthy individuals and of the differential implication of functional subsets (CD4/CD8; Th-1/Th-2) in natural tolerance and autoimmunity accumulates, all therapeutic interventions, whether suppressive or stimulatory, should also take into account the regulation of effector class in T-cell responses. Furthermore, these concepts suggest possibilities for novel cytokine or anticytokine therapies in autoimmune disease and support the view that natural tolerance, rather than representing absence of autoreactivity, represents a delicate balance that is actively regulated by the autoreactivities themselves.

In summary, we view natural tolerance as representing the ongoing activity of autoreactive lymphocytes in a mode of equilibrium and non-aggressive effector functions, developmentally selected by V-region-dependent complementarities. In this context, autoimmune disease would represent a primary or secondary deficiency in the structural or functional repertoires of the autoimmune network that normally maintain self-tolerance. Because healthy and diseased immune systems do not differ in their autoreactive components but rather in the organization and dynamics of these components, and because basic and clinical research have essentially analyzed humoral or cellular components, it is not surprising that the boundaries between autoreactivity in health and disease appear to be very subtle. We submit, however, that study of network diversity, dynamics, and organization will sharpen those boundaries and thus help to establish appropriate diagnostic and therapeutic strategies.

17

NEW INSIGHTS ON THE PHYSIOLOGICAL AND PATHOLOGICAL RHEUMATOID FACTORS IN HUMANS

Pojen P. Chen and Dennis A. Carson

Department of Medicine (P.P.C., D.A.C.) and Department of Pathology (P.P.C.), University of California, San Diego, La Jolla, California

INTRODUCTION

Rheumatoid arthritis (RA) is an extravascular immune complex disease of unknown etiology [Harris, 1990]. About 80% of patients with this autoimmune disorder have a characteristic marker in their sera, termed *rheumatoid factor* (RF), and are classified as "seropositive" [Chen et al., 1987b]. Importantly, seropositive RA also differs from seronegative RA in its linkage to HLA DR4-Dw4 and -Dw14, as well as to a more severe clinical outcome [Spector, 1990]. Thus seropositive and seronegative RA may involve distinct pathogenetic mechanisms. Hereafter, *RA* refers to *seropositive RA* only.

RF is an autoantibody that binds to the Fc region of IgG [Chen et al., 1987b; Mannik et al., 1988]. The synovial fluids from the inflamed joints of RA patients contain abundant aggregates of immunoglobulin and depressed

Autoimmunity: Physiology and Disease, Pages 247–266
© *1994 Wiley-Liss, Inc.*

levels of complement components; the aggregates consist of mainly IgG and RFs, which are synthesized and deposited in situ [Winchester et al., 1970; Munthe and Natvig, 1971]. These findings suggest that RFs contribute to immune complex formation, complement consumption, and chronic tissue damage in the rheumatoid synovium [Zvaifler, 1973].

Although RF is a major diagnostic marker for RA and may contribute to the disease process, it is not restricted to RA. The autoantibody has been found in patients with other autoimmune diseases, including Sjögren's syndrome, mixed connective tissue disease, systemic lupus erythematosus, and scleroderma, as well as in apparently healthy individuals, albeit in lower concentrations than in RA [Chen et al., 1987b]. Notably, RF-secreting B-cell lines have been derived from normal human subjects (as reviewed in Chapter 6). Moreover, human RF precursor B cells increase in frequency shortly after a repeat immunization or a recurrent infection. Similar findings are observed in mice. Together, these data show that RF in a healthy individual is a "natural" component of a normal immune system and serves some physiological functions; as such, RFs in normal subjects are termed *physiological RFs;* in contrast, RFs in RA patients are termed *pathogenic RFs* [Chen et al., 1990; Carson et al., 1991].

How can the pathogenic RFs on the one hand contribute toward immunopathogenesis of RA, while the physiological RFs on the other hand serve some immune functions in a normal individual? What are the differences between these two types of RFs? Serologically, physiological RFs in healthy subjects are of low titers and consist of mainly IgM molecules; most of them bind to the IgG–Fc fragment (and a few unrelated antigens) with low affinity. In contrast, RFs in RA patients are usually of higher titer and contain both IgM and IgG components, are enriched in the inflamed joints, and bind monospecifically to Fc with high affinity [Mannik et al., 1988; Carson, 1989; Burastero et al., 1988]. However, what are the structural relationships between the physiological and the pathogenic RFs? Do the high affinity pathogenic RFs in RA patients simply derive from the low affinity physiological RFs in normal individuals? Here, we review the rapid progress in the structural and genetic studies of both physiological and pathogenic RFs in humans.

SEROLOGICAL, STRUCTURAL, AND GENETIC ANALYSES OF IgM RHEUMATOID FACTORS FROM PATIENTS WITH CRYOGLOBULINEMIA

Initially, before the development of hybridoma technology, investigators had no choice but to study monoclonal RFs that occur in patients with mixed cryoglobulinemia. It should be noted that such RFs are indeed involved in the pathogenesis of the disease and thus should be considered as pathogenic RFs [Winfield, 1983]. Using carefully absorbed rabbit polyclonal anti-idiotypes, Kunkel and colleagues [1973] described two major cross-reactive idiotypes (CRIs), termed *Wa* and *Po*. The Wa CRI was expressed by about 60% of monoclonal IgM RFs; all Wa-positive RFs belong to the restricted V_κIIIB sub-subgroup, which constitutes only about 13% of total serum immunoglobulin kappa light (L) chains [Kunkel et al., 1974]. Subsequently, Andrews and Capra [1981] determined the amino acid sequences of two Wa-positive RFs (i.e., Sie and Wol) and found that their L chains were similar.

It is known that complementarity-determining regions (CDRs) are the structural basis of many idiotypic determinants [Davie et al., 1986]. Since 2/2 Wa-positive RF L chains had an identical second CDR, a synthetic peptide corresponding to this CDR (designated PSL2) was prepared and used to immunize rabbits. The resultant anti-PSL2 antisera, without any absorption, bound specifically to RF Sie and its L chain [Chen et al., 1984]. When 30 IgM RFs from different patients were analyzed, 20 (67%) were positive [Chen et al., 1984, 1985b, 1988a]. Significantly, all Wa-positive RFs reacted with the anti-PSL2 antibodies. Combined, these data suggested strongly that the second L chain CDR is the structural basis of the Wa CRI and that, more importantly, all Wa-positive IgM RFs in mixed cryoglobulinemia probably employ a single V_κ germline gene.

Subsequently, we prepared an additional synthetic peptide corresponding to the third CDR of the Wa-positive Sie L chain (designated PSL3) and used this peptide to induce anti-PSL3 antisera [Chen et al., 1985b]. Again, the antibody reacted specifically with Sie and its L chain. When a total of 30 IgM RFs were analyzed, 17 (57%) were positive [Chen et al., 1985b, 1988]. These results corroborated the notion that all Wa-positive RFs in mixed cryoglobulinemia may employ a single V_κ germline gene.

To prove this hypothesis, we collaborated with Drs. Fernando R. Goni and Blas Frangione in New York and with Drs. Marianna M. Newkirk and J. Donald Capra in Dallas to determine the amino acid sequences of several PSL2- and/or PSL3-positive RFs. The results showed that all CRI-positive L chains were extremely homologous in their kappa-variable region (V_κ) gene-encoded area [Goni et al., 1985; Newkirk et al., 1986, 1987]. Based on these data, we derived a consensus sequence and identified a germline V_κ gene that encodes an amino acid sequence identical to the consensus sequence [Chen et al., 1985a, 1986, 1987a; Radoux et al., 1986; Chen, 1990]. The isolated V_κ gene was designated *Humkv325*.

The kv325 amino acid sequence, when compared with 12 PSL2-positive IgM RFs from mixed cryoglobulinemia, is identical to four, but differs from the remaining eight by 1–7 amino acid residues [Chen et al., 1986, 1988a, 1990; Goni et al., 1989; Chen, 1990b]. *This finding demonstrated, for the first time, that some autoantibodies may be encoded directly by inherited immunoglobulin V genes without any somatic modification.* On the other hand, none of the deviated residues in the eight RFs were found in the amino acid sequences of other functional human V_κIII genes, indicating that they are the consequence of somatic mutations. Thus, it should be emphasized here that these early data demonstrate that the majority of monoclonal IgM RFs do contain some somatic mutations [Chen, 1990b]. Moreover, of a total of 25 mutations in the eight RF V_κ regions, 17 are in the antigen-contacting regions, namely, CDRs (encompassing 26 amino acid residues), while eight are in the framework regions (FRs; encompassing 70 amino acid residues) [Chen, 1990b]. The data show that the mutations are significantly more frequent in the CDRs than in the FRs ($P = 0.001$) and suggest that many pathogenic RFs in mixed cryoglobulinemia are antigen driven, presumably by the IgG–Fc fragment.

In addition to recognizing RF L chains, anti-PSL2 and anti-PSL3 also reacts with the L chains of several other autoantibodies, suggesting that the same gene, kv325, may code for different autoantibodies. Indeed, kv325 is identical to the L chain of an autoantibody (Pie) against intermediate filaments and differs by only one amino acid residue each from the L chain of an autoantibody (Son) against low-density lipoprotein and two polyreactive antibodies (i.e., Th-3 and 8E10) that react with IgG and DNA [Pons-Estel et al., 1984; Dersimonian et al., 1989]. Combined, these data showed that kv325 encodes the L chains of several different autoantibodies. This finding provides a structural and genetic basis for the shared CRI among autoantibodies of different antigen specificities and suggests an idiotypic connectivity between autoantibodies.

Several investigators have generated murine monoclonal anti-idiotypic antibodies against human RFs. We used the Wa-positive Sie RF to generate an anti-idiotype termed *17.109* [Carson and Fong, 1983]. The antibody reacted with many PSL2$^+$ RFs and their separated L chains. When 17.109 was used to analyze monoclonal IgM RFs, 30%–50% were positive; importantly, all 17.109$^+$ RF L chains were positive with the anti-PSL2 antibody, indicating that 17.109 was also specific for the gene product of kv325 [Fong et al., 1986]. The conclusion was subsequently verified by DNA sequence analysis of several 17.109-positive cell lines [Kipps et al., 1988]. Since anti-PSL2 and anti-PSL3 were polyclonal rabbit antisera with limited supply, while 17.109 was a monoclonal antibody with unlimited supply, all the subsequent serological analyses of kv325 expression has been done with 17.109.

About 20 years ago, Preud'homme and Seligmann [1972] discovered that about 15% of B-cell chronic lymphocytic leukemia (CLL) had surface immunoglobulin with RF activity. Aware of these data, Kipps et al. [1988] used 17.109 to analyze B-cell CLL and found that nearly 20% of the κ L chain-bearing CLL were positive. As noted earlier, kv325 encodes the L chains of several different autoantibodies. Moreover, several investigators reported that, in both humans and mice, autoreactive B-cell precursors were often in a proliferative state [Fong et al., 1985; Portnoi et al., 1986]. Together, these findings led us to propose that B cells expressing kv325 may be stimulated by autoantigens to proliferate constantly and that the continual cell cycling may render these cells more susceptible to random transformation and subsequent abnormal clonal expansion [Chen et al., 1987a]. This postulate has been corroborated by the extensive overlaps between autoantibody-related V genes and the V genes expressed by the malignant B cells, as reviewed recently [Chen et al., 1990].

In 1986, Mageed et al. generated a murine monoclonal anti-CRI antibody (designated *G6*) from a mouse immunized with the monoclonal IgM RF Kok. They analyzed 12 IgM RFs and found five (42%) to be positive; significantly, G6 reacted with the separated heavy (H) chains of the CRI-positive RFs. Subsequently, Newkirk et al. [1987] determined the H chain amino acid sequences of two G6-positive IgM RFs (i.e., Bor and Kas); they found both V_H1 sequences were very similar to each other and to a rearranged V_H1 gene expressed by the Lr B-cell CLL.

At about the same time, in a separate study of human autoantibodies, we discovered that the reported 18/2 V_H cDNA sequence of an anti-DNA antibody was identical to the germline VH26 gene and to the 30P1 V_H cDNA sequence [Dersimonian et al., 1987; Chen et al., 1988b], which is part of the restricted V_H gene repertoire expressed during early ontogeny in fetal liver [Schroeder et al., 1987]. The data indicated that certain V_H genes that can encode autoantibodies are preferentially expressed during the early development of the antibody repertoire and may play an important role in the formation of the repertoire [Perlmutter, 1987; Yancopoulos et al., 1988; Hillson and Perlmutter, 1990; Siminovitch and Chen, 1990].

In this context, we noted that, among all human V_H1 gene amino acid sequences, 51P1 (another fetal V_H1 cDNA sequence) was most homologous to Bor and Kas, differing from the latter two by only eight residues each; in contrast, all other V_H1 germline genes each differed from both RF H chains by 22–40 residues [Chen et al., 1989]. As noted earlier, about 15% of B-cell CLL express surface IgM with RF activity. Viewed as a whole, these data suggest that G6-positive H chains are encoded by a germline V_H gene that is identical or highly homologous to 51P1 and the rearranged V_H gene in the Lr CLL (designated Humha1Lr). Accordingly, we screened a human genomic library to isolate the hypothetical V_H1 gene.

During these experiments, we found unexpectedly that ha1Lr was actually identical to the 51P1 sequence, except for one base difference near the V–D junction [Chen et al., 1989]. Since ha1Lr and 51P1 derived from two unrelated individuals, the finding indicated that 51P1 was likely to represent the unmutated sequence of the germline V_H1 gene for 51P1 and ha1Lr and that the "51P1/ha1Lr V_H gene" was the V_H gene for the H chains of Bor and Kas, as well as many other G6 CR1-positive RF H chains [Chen et al., 1989]. The conclusion is supported by the subsequent finding that the V_H sequence of two G6-positive B-cell CLL (i.e., And and Nei) were indeed 99% homologous to the 51P1 sequence [Kipps et al., 1989] and by our recent isolation of Humhv1051, which is identical to the V_H-gene-encoded region of 51P1 [Yang et al., 1993].

In addition to the two aforementioned V_κ and V_H genes, similar studies led to identification of Humkv328h5 for the 6B6.6-CRI-positive RFs Les and Pom, and Vg for the L chains of RFs Riv and Sfl [Chen et al., 1987c, 1990; Liu et al., 1989; Schrohenloher et al., 1990; Pech and Zachau, 1984; Newkirk and Capra, 1989]. In summary, analyses of monoclonal RFs from patients with mixed cryoglobulinemia have led to two important findings: 1) autoantibodies (such as RF) may be encoded directly by germline V genes without any somatic mutation; and 2) each autoreactive V gene may encode different autoantibodies, providing a potential molecular genetic basis for the phenomenon of idiotypic connectivity [Chen and Carson, 1991].

MOLECULAR ANALYSES OF PHYSIOLOGICAL RF FROM NORMAL INDIVIDUALS

Insofar as the generation and characterization of RF-secreting B cells from normal individuals is reviewed by Casali et al. (Chapter 6), we here focus on the molecular analysis of physiological RFs. Among many RF B-cell lines derived from several subjects, two (i.e., Kim13.1 and TMC1) have had their H and L chains characterized; in the remaining RFs, only the H chains have been analyzed. Table I summarizes all the published sequence data from RFs; they derive mainly from polyspecific IgM RF B cells, except for one IgG_3 polyspecific RF and one IgA polyspecific RF, as well as one IgM monospecific IgM RF [Sanz et al., 1989a; Cairns et al., 1989; Siminovitch et al., 1990; Schutte et al., 1991; Victor et al., 1991].

The Kim 13.1 RF was derived from the tonsillar lymphocytes of a nonautoimmune donor by direct fusion with a human lymphoblastoid cell line. It reacts with IgG and cardiolipin, but not with DNA or RNA [Siminovitch et al., 1990]. Its H and L chains are 99.7% homologous to hv1051 and Vg, respectively. The TMC1 monospecific RF was generated from blood lymphocytes of a normal donor by Epstein-Barr virus (EBV) transformation. Its H and L chains are 99.6% and 94% homologous to Vh4.21 and Vg, respectively [Victor et al., 1991]. The six Ab* RFs were derived from peripheral blood lymphocytes of different healthy subjects by initial EBV transformation and subsequent fusion with a human–mouse heterohybridoma [Sanz et al., 1989a]. Ab47 reacts with IgG and single-stranded (ss)DNA; all of the others react with IgG, ssDNA, human thyroglobulin and insulin, tetanus toxoid, and various bacterial polysaccharides [Sanz et al., 1989a]. The latter antibodies employ 4 V_H genes: VH26 V_H3 (for 2), $V_H4.21$ (for 2), 71-4 V_H4, and $V_{I-4.1b}$ V_H1 [Sanz et al., 1989a,b; Chen, 1990a; Lee et al., 1987; Shin et al., 1991]. The A455 and ML3 EBV-transformed cell lines were derived from an adult blood and a 19-week-old fetal spleen, respectively; both react with IgG, ssDNA, DNP, TNP, Ars, and tetanus toxoid [Schutte et al., 1991]. A455 expresses a V_H4 gene that is

TABLE I. Immunoglobulin V-gene usage of RFs from normal individuals[a]

Name	H Chain Isotype	Putative Germline V_H Gene	Percent Similarity[b]	Putative Germline V_L Gene	Percent Similarity[b]
Polyspecific					
Ab17	γ^3,κ	$V_H4.21$	87	nd	—
Ab18	μ,κ	VH26 V_H3	99	nd	—
Ab21	μ,κ	VH26 V_H3	93	nd	—
Ab26	μ,λ	71-4 V_H4	91	nd	—
Ab44	α,λ	$V_H4.21$	98	nd	—
Ab47	μ,λ	$V_{I-4.1b}$ V_H1	—	nd	—
Kim13.1	μ,κ	hv1051	99.7	Vg Vk3	99.7
A455	μ,λ	V_H4	—	nd	—
ML3	μ,κ	hv1L1	99.7	nd	—
Monospecific					
TMC	μ,κ	$V_H4.21$	99.6	Vg	94

[a] Humhv1051 is a germline V_H1 gene cloned recently in our laboratory and is identical to 51P1 in the V_H-gene-encoded region [Yang et al., 1993]. All other data are from the literature: Ab17 to Ab47, Sanz et al. [1989a]; Kim13.1, Siminovitch et al. [1990]; A455 and ML3, Schutte et al. [1991]; TMC, Pascual et al. [1990b]; $V_H4.18$, Sanz et al. [1989b]; VH26, Matthyssens and Rabbitts [1980]; and Chen [1990a]; 71-4, Kodaira et al. [1986] and Lee et al. [1987]; $V_{I-4.1b}$, Shin et al. [1991]; and hv1L1, Olee et al. [1992].

[b] The percent similarity after each germline gene denotes its DNA sequence similarity to the V-gene-encoded region in the preceding antibody.

not similar to any known V_H4 germline gene, while ML3 employs the hv1L1 gene [Schutte et al., 1991; Olee et al., 1992].

Overall, the current data show that the physiological RFs employ at least 1 V_κ gene and 7 V_H genes from three different V_H gene families. Significantly, two of two analyzed RF L chains are encoded by Vg, which has been suggested to be preferentially expressed in fetal liver [Hillson and Perlmutter, 1990]. Similarly, VH26 and hv1051 are, respectively, identical to 30P1 and 51P1, while hv1L1 differs from 20P3 by only one double-base at the V–D junction, suggesting that the difference might be due to an imprecise joining of the hv1L1 gene to a rearranged DJ gene; 30P1, 51P1, and 20P3 belong to the restricted fetal antibody repertoire [Schroeder et al., 1987]. In addition, $V_H4.21$ expression has been detected in a 15-week-old fetal spleen by the murine 9G4 monoclonal anti-CRI, which reacts specifically with the $V_H4.21$ gene product [Stevenson et al., 1989; Pascual et al., 1991]. Moreover, hv1L1 (identical to V_{I-2}) and $V_{I-4.1b}$ are, respectively, the second and the fifth V_H genes next to the DJ locus, suggesting that, similar to hv1L1, $V_{I-4.1b}$ may also be frequently expressed during early ontogeny [Shin et al., 1991]. Together, these data suggest that physiological RFs may preferentially use a restricted set of immunoglobulin V_H genes that may also be frequently expressed during early ontogeny.

SEROLOGICAL AND MOLECULAR ANALYSES OF THE PATHOGENIC RF IN RA PATIENTS

To understand the role of RFs in the pathogenesis of RA, several investigators have generated and analyzed monoclonal RFs from patients. Table II summarizes the 22 analyzed RFs derived from 7 RA patients. The RFs consist of 15 monospecific and 7 polyspecific RFs; the monospecific ones include 11 IgM, 1 IgA, and 3 IgG [Soto-Gil et al., 1992; Pascual et al., 1990b; Harindranath et al., 1991; Ezaki et al., 1991; Weisbart et al., 1991; Olee et al., 1992]. HAF10 was generated from rheumatoid synovium by direct fusion with F3B6 human–mouse heterohybridoma [Robbins et al., 1990]; the SJ and TS hybridomas were derived from rheumatoid synovia by initial stimulation with EBV and phytohemagglutinin and subsequent fusion with the murine X63–Ag8.653 cell [Randen et al., 1989]; the mAb hybridomas were produced from the $CD5^+$ B cells in the blood of an RA patient by initial EBV transformation and subsequent fusion with F3B6 [Harindranath et al., 1991]; YES8c was generated from the bone marrow B cells of an RA patient by direct fusion with P3X63–Ag8-U1 [Ezaki et al., 1991]; RF was derived from synovial B cells by EBV transformation [Weisbart et al., 1991]; and D1 and L1 were from synovial fluid B cells by direct fusion with the K6H6/B5 human–mouse heterohybridoma [Olee et al., 1992].

As can be seen in Table II, these RFs employ 15 V_H genes from 3 different V_H gene families, 8 V_λ genes from 4 V_λ families, and 7 V_κ genes from 3 V_κ families. Considering that there are about 100 functional V_H genes, 40 functional V_κ genes, and 50 functional V_λ genes [Berman et al., 1988; Meindl et al., 1990; Combriato and Klobeck, 1991], utilization of 15 (15%) V_H, 7 (18%) V_κ, and 8 (16%) V_λ genes by RFs indicates that the V-gene usage of the pathogenic RFs in RA patients is similar to a normal antibody response to a regular antigen and thus is not restricted. However, among the identified V genes, 4/15 V_H genes are used recurrently, including 1.9III (4 times), 71-2, V_H4.21, and hv1051 (the latter three each accounts for two RFs); 3/8 V_λ genes appear repeatedly, including 1v117, 1v1L1, and 1v418 (each three times), and 1/7 V_κ genes (i.e., Humkv325) is employed recurrently (three times).

Extensive studies in mice have shown that certain V_H genes are expressed preferentially during early ontogenic development and that some of these V_H genes frequently encode autoantibodies [Perlmutter, 1987; Yancopoulos et al., 1988; Holmberg 1987; Bona, 1988]. Similar findings have been noted in humans [Schroeder and Wang, 1990; Cuisinier et al., 1989; Chen et al., 1990; Pascual and Capra, 1991]. For example, the V_H6 gene is expressed frequently during early ontogenic development and is utilized by polyspecific IgM autoantibodies [Berman et al., 1988; Schroeder and Wang, 1990; Cuisinier et al., 1989; Logtenberg et al., 1989; Schutte et al., 1991]. On the other hand, similar to physiological RFs, structural analyses of many natural IgM autoantibodies from normal subjects have revealed that they employ a restricted set of immunoglobulin V genes [Sanz et al.,

TABLE II. Immunoglobulin V-gene usage of RFs from RA patients[a]

Name	H Chain Isotype	Putative Germline V_H Gene	Percent Similarity[b]	Putative Germline V_L gene	Percent Similarity[b]
Monospecific					
HAF10	$\mu\lambda$	hv1f10	99	$V_\lambda 8$	—
SJ1	μ,λ	1.9III $V_H 3$	95	lv117	93
SJ2	μ,λ	hv3005f3	99.4	lv117	96
SJ3	μ,κ	1.9III	99.4	kv325	99
SJ4	μ,κ	71-2 $V_H 4$	96	kv305	100
TS1	μ,κ	hv1051	96	kv325	99.3
TS2	μ,κ	1.9III	98	kv328h5	97
TS3	μ,κ	$V_{1-4.1b}$ $V_H 1$	99.2	A23 $V_\kappa 2$	100
TS5	μ,κ	22-2B $V_H 3$	99.2	$H\kappa 102$ $V_\kappa 1$	98
mAB60	$\alpha 1,\lambda$	VH11 $V_H 3$	92	$V_\lambda 3$	—
mAB61	μ,λ	$V_H 4.18$	98	lv1L1	96
YES8c	μ,κ	hv1051	95	kv325	99
hRF1	$\gamma 4,\kappa$	nd	—	A3 $V_\kappa 2$	99.7
D1	$\gamma 3,\kappa$	$V_H 3$	—	Vg $V_\kappa 3$	99.7
L1	$\gamma 1,\lambda$	hv1L1	97	lv1L1	99
Polyspecific					
mAB63	μ,λ	$V_H 4.21$	100	lv418	99
mAB65	μ,λ	71-2 $V_H 4$	87	lv418	100
mAB67	μ,λ	V79 $V_H 4$	99.3	lv1L1	97
PR-SJ1	μ,λ	$V_H 4.35$	100	$V_\lambda 5$	—
PR-SJ2	μ,λ	1.9III	95	$V_\lambda 4$	—
PR-TS1	μ,λ	hv3005	99.6	lv117	98
PR-TS2	μ,λ	$V_H 4.21$	100	lv418	100

[a] Humhv1051 is a germline $V_H 1$ gene cloned recently in our laboratory and is identical to 51P1 in the V_H-gene-encoded region [Yang et al., 1993]. All other data are from the literature: HAF10RF and hv1f10, Soto-Gil et al. [1992]; both monospecific and polyspecific RFs from SJ and TS, Pascual et al. [1990b], Victor et al. [1991] and Pascual et al. [1992]; mAB60-67, Harindranath et al. [1991]; YES8c, Ezaki et al. [1991]; hRF1, Weisbart et al. [1991]; D1, L1, hv1L1, and lv1L1, Olee et al. [1992]; 1.9III and 22-2B, Berman et al. [1988]; hv3005 and hv3005f3, Chen [1990a] and Olee et al. [1991]; 71-2 and V79, Kodaira et al. [1986] and Lee et al. [1987]; $V_{1-4.1b}$, Shin et al. [1991]; VH11, Rechavi et al. [1982]; $V_H 4.18$ and 4.21, Sanz et al. [1989b]; $V_H 4.35$, Pascual et al. [1992]; Humlv117, Siminovitch et al. [1989]; Humkv305/A11 and kv325/A27, Chen et al. [1987a] and Straubinger et al. [1988]; Humkv328h5, Liu et al. [1989]; A3 and A23, Straubinger et al. [1988]; $H\kappa 102$, Bentley and Rabbitts [1980]; Vg, Pech and Zachau [1984]; and Humlv418/iglv3s1, Daley et al. [1992b]; Frippiat et al. [1990].
[b] The percent similarity after each germline gene denotes its DNA sequence similarity to the V-gene-encoded region in the preceding antibody.

1989a; Chen et al., 1990; Pascual and Capra, 1991]; and several of these V genes, such as hv1051 and VH26, have been found to be expressed preferentially during early ontogenic development [Schroeder et al., 1987; Hillson and Perlmutter, 1990; Schroeder and Wang, 1990; Siminovitch and Chen, 1990; Schutte et al., 1991].

In this context, it is important to note that most reported pathogenic RF V genes are similar to those used by the natural autoantibodies and the fetal antibody repertoire [Chen et al., 1990; Hillson and Perlmutter, 1990; Pascual et al., 1990a; Dersimonian et al., 1990; Chen and Carson, 1991]. For example, four RA-derived RFs (i.e., SJ1, SJ3, and TS2, and PR-SJ2) utilize 1.9III, which also encodes the Kim4.6 natural autoantibody and the FL2-2 fetal-liver-derived cell line [Cairns et al., 1989; Nickerson et al., 1989]; SJ2 uses the most frequently expressed V_H gene in fetal liver (i.e., Humhv3005f3/GL–SJ2/M72 or its homologous 56P1) [Schroeder and Wang, 1990; Olee et al., 1991; Pascual et al., 1990b]; SJ4 employs 71-2, which also encodes the C6B2 natural autoantibody [Hoch and Schwaber, 1987]; TS1 and YES8c employ hv1051, which encodes the H chain of the Kim13.1 natural autoantibody and is part of the restricted fetal antibody repertoire [Pascual et al., 1990b; Ezaki et al., 1991; Chen et al., 1989, 1990; Carson et al., 1991]; TS3 employs $V_{I-4.1b}$, which also encodes the Ab47 natural RF [Sanz et al., 1989a]; mAB61 uses $V_H4.18$, which also encodes the DM1 antiplatelet antibody [Hiraiwa et al., 1990]; L1 utilizes hv1L1, which is also used by the ML3 natural autoantibody from a 19-week-old fetal spleen [Schutte et al., 1991]; mAB63 and PR-TS2 use $V_H4.21$, which also encodes the Ab17 and Ab44 natural RFs and is expressed in a 15-week-old fetal spleen [Sanz et al., 1989a; Stevenson et al., 1989; Pascual et al., 1991]; RFs SJ1 and SJ2 utilize Hum1v117, which also encodes the Kim4.6 L chain [Siminovitch et al., 1989]; TS1, SJ3, and YES8c use Humkv325/A27, which also encodes the L chains of TH3 and 8E10 polyspecific autoantibodies [Chen et al., 1987a; Dersimonian et al., 1989]; TS2 uses Humkv328h5, which is also employed by the C6B2 natural autoantibody and is part of the restricted fetal antibody repertoire [Cairns et al., 1989; Hillson and Perlmutter, 1990]; the 1v1L1 shared by mAB61, L1, and mAB67 also encodes the L chain of the Kim11.4 natural autoantibody [Daley et al., 1992a]; hRF1 uses A3, which is also utilized by FS1 antierythrocyte antibody [Pascual et al., 1991]; and D1 employs Vg, which encodes the Kim13.1 L chain [Siminovitch et al., 1990].

Combined, these data suggest very strongly that the V-gene usage by pathogenic RF, while appearing to be unrestricted, instead is confined to the limited "autoantibody repertoire" that encompasses about 15% of potentially functional human immunoglobulin V genes. In this context, a pathogenic RF may derive from a "physiologic natural autoantibody" (with or without RF activity) that escaped from the normal mechanisms of regulation, possibly during a serious infection and/or transient dysfunction of the immune system of the host, and thus became a monospecific, high affinity RF due to selection by IgG alone or IgG antibody–antigen complexes, as suggested recently [Olee et al., 1992]. However, it should be noted that RF production in RA patients may be induced by different mechanisms, and thus the aforementioned hypothesis may not account for RF secretion in all RA patients.

The recurrent usage of Humkv325 suggests that it may have some intrinsic RF activity or unusual property in conferring Fc binding activity when in conjunction with appropriate V_H genes. In this regard, it was recently reported that the Humkv325 gene product per se indeed has some RF activity [Hay et al., 1991]. Moreover, of nine κ-bearing RFs, six (67%) use $V_\kappa 3$ genes. It is known that only seven to eight of 40 (20%) functional V_κ genes belong to $V_\kappa 3$ subgroup. Together, the data indicate an overutilization of the $V_\kappa 3$ genes by RFs and imply that the common FRs shared by these $V_\kappa 3$ genes may confer some RF activity, as proposed previously [Chen et al., 1987c].

It has been suggested that some IgG RFs in the synovial fluid may self-associate to form large complexes; the resultant complexes can fix complement and bind to IgM RF much more efficiently than does monomeric IgG and, after phagocytosis by neutrophils, activate the inflammation cascade [Mannik et al., 1988]. Thus the self-associating IgG RFs represent the potentially most pathogenic RFs. Considering the possibility that B cells secreting self-associating IgG RFs may be self-stimulated by their own secreted IgG RFs, synovial fluid lymphocytes were cultured alone for 3 days and then fused with the K6H6/B5 human–mouse heterohybridoma. Initially, among 94 resultant hybridomas, 22 (23%) had RF activity [Lu et al., 1992]. Among the RF-secreting hybridomas from patient ML, two clones (designated L1 and L2) were characterized in detail. The results showed that both were monospecific and bound to Fc with high affinity, $K_d = 4.1 \times 10^{-7}$ M [Lu et al., 1992]. More importantly, both precipitated spontaneously, suggesting that the RF may be self-associating. To examine this possibility, both RF and a control human monoclonal IgG antiferritin antibody (each at 0.5 mg/ml in phosphate-buffered saline) were incubated for 30 hours at 37°C, and the resulting antibody solutions were analyzed by fast protein liquid chromatography on a Superose 6 HR 10/30 column, which was calibrated with human IgM and IgG and with ribonuclease A. The results showed that, after incubation, the elution profile of each IgG RF displayed a new population of IgG RF homodimers; in contrast, the elution profile of the control human IgG antiferritin antibody did not change at all [Lu et al., 1992]. The data thus demonstrated that both RFs could self-associate into large complexes. Subsequently, the expressed H and L chain V genes of L1 RF (designated Humha1L1 and Humla1L1), as well as their germline origins (designated Humhv1L1 and Humlv1L1, respectively), were cloned and characterized [Olee et al., 1992].

Generally, during an antigen-driven response, B cells expressing mutated antibodies with higher affinity for the antigen are progressively selected. Frequently, such affinity maturation is associated with the switch from IgM to IgG [Berek and Milstein, 1987]. Previously, to define precisely the induction and sustaining mechanisms for pathogenic RF production, Shlomchik et al. [1987a,b] compared the disease-specific RFs in autoimmune MRL/lpr mice and the mitogen-induced RFs in normal mice. They found that most IgG RFs from MRL/1pr mice had an average of 4.4 somatic mutations per V region, with the most mutated V region having seven mutations; in contrast, most IgM RFs (generated by polyclonal B-cell activation) had an average of only 0.5 mutations per V region, with the most mutated V region having only two mutations [Shlomchik et al., 1987a,b]. Furthermore, the former mutations occurred nonrandomly; they were located much more frequently in the antigen-contacting regions, namely, the CDRs, than in FRs and often led to amino acid substitutions, resulting in an ratio of replacement (R) to silent (S) mutations higher than 2.9, which is the expected figure for random mutation without the pressure of antigen selection [Shlomchik et al., 1987b]. More importantly, in two of the three mice analyzed, the V-region nucleotide sequences of all IgG RFs from each mouse were very similar to each other, demonstrating that all IgG RF-secreting B cells in each autoimmune mouse were clonally related and apparently were the offspring of a single RF B-cell precursor [Shlomchik et al., 1987b]. In the third mouse, the IgG RFs were likely to derive from two ancestor RF B cells, while an IgM RF came from a yet another RF B cell. These data were highly reminiscent of induced antibody molecules in antigen-driven systems. Viewed as a whole, the data demonstrate that disease-specific IgG RFs are induced and driven by the antigen, the Fc fragment of murine IgG.

A comparison of the H and L chain V regions of the L1 RF with their germline counterparts shows that they have 16 and 7 mutations, respectively [Olee et al., 1992]. Strikingly, all eight changes in the CDRs of both V genes caused amino acid substitutions, resulting an R/S ratio of infinity (i.e., 8/0). In contrast, only 6/11 changes in the FRs of both V genes led to amino acid replacements, resulting in an R/S ratio of 1.2. Taken together with the high binding affinity of L1 toward the Fc fragment, these data suggest strongly that L1 RF was selected by the Fc fragment and thus provide the first direct evidence for an Fc-driven immune response in RA synovium.

When the expressed H and L chain V-gene sequences of the L2 RF were analyzed, it was found that they are identical to that of the L1 RF (Lu and Chen, unpublished data). In the second patient, JC, five high affinity, monospecific IgG RFs were obtained and analyzed. Preliminary sequence data indicate that, of the five, three are identical, while the remaining two are different from the first three, but are identical to each other. Together, the data provide further evidence that IgG RFs in rheumatoid synovia are induced and driven by the Fc fragment of human IgG molecules. The conclusion is consistent with the observations that several different antigenic determinants on IgG molecules are recognized by polyclonal RFs in RA patients. It should be pointed out that if RFs in different RA patients are induced by an unknown cross-reacting antigen, then it is extremely unlikely that such RFs would recognize distinct antigenic determinants of IgG molecules in different RA patients. Viewed as a whole, the skewed mutation patterns and mono- or oligoclonality of IgG RFs in an individual RA patient clearly demonstrate that the pathogenic IgG RFs in rheumatoid synovium are driven continuously by the Fc fragment of IgG over a sustained period of time.

CONCLUSION

As reviewed here, intensive studies of human RFs during the last decade have rapidly advanced our understanding of RFs. The combined data indicate that 1) physiological RFs employ a restricted set of autoreactive V genes that account for about 15% of potentially functional V genes and encode autoantibodies of various specificities; 2) pathogenic RFs apparently derive from physiological RFs or autoantibodies, but escape from the normal regulation, possibly during a serious infection and/or a transient dysfunction of the immune system of the host; and 3) in the rheumatoid synovium, the escaped RF B cells may be continuously driven by IgG and become high affinity IgG RF B cells, as well as self-associating IgG RF-secreting B cells. The latter can be self-stimulated, thus resulting in a sustained production of IgG RFs, immune complexes, inflammation, and eventually chronic tissue damage. Further experiments are warranted to verify this hypothesis, which, if proved, may lead to new approaches to interfere with the pathological cascade that leads to self-associating RF production and joint destruction.

ACKNOWLEDGMENTS

The authors gratefully acknowledge the secretarial assistance of Ms. Jane Uhle in the preparation of this manuscript. Funding for this research is supported in part by grants AI32243, AR25443, AR07567, AR40770, and RR00833 from the National Institutes of Health.

REFERENCES

Andrews DW, Capra JD (1981): Complete amino acid sequence of variable domains from two monoclonal human anti-gamma globulins of the Wa cross-idiotypic group: Suggestion that the J segments are involved in the structural correlate of the idiotype. Proc Natl Acad Sci USA 78:3799–3803.

Bentley DL, Rabbitts TH (1980): Human immunoglobulin variable region genes-DNA sequences of two V(κ) genes and a pseudogene. Nature 288:730–733.

Berek C, Milstein C (1987): Mutation drift and repertoire shift in the maturation of the immune response. Immunol Rev 96:23–40.

Berman JE, Mellis SJ, Pollock R, Smith CL, Suh H, Heinke B, Kowal C, Surti U, Chess L, Cantor CR, Alt FW (1988): Content and organization of the human Ig V_H locus: Definition of three new V_H families and linkage to the Ig C_H locus. EMBO J 7:727–738.

Bona CA (1988): V genes encoding autoantibodies: Molecular and phenotypic characteristics. Annu Rev Immunol 6:327–358.

Burastero SE, Casali P, Wilder RL, Notkins AL (1988): Monoreactive high affinity and polyreactive low affinity rheumatoid factors are produced by CD5+ B cells from patients with rheumatoid arthritis. J Exp Med 168:1979–1992.

Cairns E, Kwong PC, Misener V, Ip P, Bell DA, Siminovitch KA (1989): Analysis of variable region genes encoding a human anti-DNA antibody of normal origin: Implications for the molecular basis of human autoimmune responses. J Immunol 143:685–691.

Carson DA (1989): Rheumatoid factor. In Kelley WJ, Harris ED Jr, Ruddy S, Sledge CB (eds): "Textbook of Rheumatology." Philadelphia: WB Saunders, pp 198–207.

Carson DA, Chen PP, Kipps TJ (1991): New roles for rheumatoid factor. J Clin Invest 87:379–383.

Carson DA, Fong S (1983): A common idiotype on human rheumatoid factors identified by a hybridoma antibody. Mol Immunol 20:1081–1087.

Chen PP (1990a): Structural analyses of human developmentally regulated V_h3 genes. Scand J Immunol 32:257–267.

Chen PP (1990b): Molecular genetics of human autoantibodies. In Farid NR, Bona CA (eds): "The Molecular Aspects of Autoimmunity." Orlando, FL: Academic Press, pp 41–58.

Chen PP, Albrandt K, Kipps TJ, Radoux V, Liu F-T, Carson DA (1987a): Isolation and characterization of human $V_\kappa III$ germline genes: Implications for the molecular basis of human $V_\kappa III$ light chain diversity. J Immunol 139:1727–1733.

Chen PP, Albrandt K, Orida NK, Radoux V, Chen EY, Schrantz R, Liu F-T, Carson DA (1986): Genetic basis for the cross-reactive idiotypes on the light chains of human IgM anti-IgG autoantibodies. Proc Natl Acad Sci USA 83:8318–8322.

Chen PP, Carson DA (1991): Molecular and genetic studies of human autoantibodies. In Talal N (ed): "Molecular Autoimmunity: Molecular, Oncologic, Genetic Immunology and Clinical Aspects." London: Academic Press, pp 65–79.

Chen PP, Fong S, Carson DA (1987b): Rheumatoid factor. Rheum Dis North Am 13:545–568.

Chen PP, Fong S, Goni F, Silverman GJ, Fox RI, Liu M-F, Frangione B, Carson DA (1988a): Cross-reacting idiotypes on cryoprecipitating rheumatoid factor. Springer Semin Immunopathol 10:35–55.

Chen PP, Fong S, Normansell D, Houghten RA, Karras JG, Vaughan JH, Carson DA (1984): Delineation of a cross-reactive idiotype on human autoantibodies with antibody against a synthetic peptide. J Exp Med 159:1502–1511.

Chen PP, Goni F, Fong S, Jirik F, Vaughan JH, Frangione B, Carson DA (1985a): The majority of human monoclonal IgM rheumatoid factors express a "primary structure-dependent" cross-reactive idiotype. J Immunol 134:3281–3285.

Chen PP, Goni F, Houghten RA, Fong S, Goldfien R, Vaughan JH, Frangione B, Carson DA (1985b): Characterization of human rheumatoid factors with seven antiidiotypes induced by synthetic hypervariable region peptides. J Exp Med 162:487–500.

Chen PP, Liu M-F, Glass CA, Sinha S, Kipps TJ, Carson DA (1989): Characterization of two Ig V_h genes which are homologous to human rheumatoid factors. Arthritis Rheum 32:72–76.

Chen PP, Liu M, Sinha S, Carson DA (1988b): A 16/6 idiotype positive anti-DNA antibody is encoded by a conserved V_h gene with no somatic mutation. Arthritis Rheum 31:1429–1431.

Chen PP, Olsen NJ, Yang P-M, Soto-Gil RW, Olee T, Siminovitch KA, Carson DA (1990): From human autoantibodies to fetal antibody repertoire to B cell malignancy: It's a small world after all. Int Rev Immunol 5:239–251.

Chen PP, Robbins DL, Jirik FR, Kipps TJ, Carson DA (1987c): Isolation and characterization of a light chain variable region gene for human rheumatoid factors. J Exp Med 166:1900–1905.

Combriato G, Klobeck H-G (1991): Vλ and Jλ–Cλ gene segments of the human immunoglobulin λ light chain locus are separated by 14 kb and rearrange by a deletion mechanism. Eur J Immunol 21:1513–1522.

Cuisinier A-M, Guigou V, Boubli L, Fougereau M, Tonnelle C (1989): Preferential expression of V_H5 and V_H6 immunoglobulin genes in early human B-cell ontogeny. Scand J Immunol 30:493–497.

Daley MD, Olee T, Peng H, Soto-Gil RW, Chen PP, Siminovitch K (1992a): Molecular characterization of the human immunoglobulin $V_\lambda I$ germline gene repertoire. Mol Immunol 29:1031–1042.

Daley DD, Peng H, Misener V, Liu X-Y, Chen PP, Siminovitch K (1992b): Molecular analysis of human immunoglobulin V_λ germline genes: Subgroups $V_\lambda III$ and $V_\lambda IV$. Mol Immunol 29:1515–1518.

Davie JM, Seiden MV, Greenspan NS, Lutz CT, Bartholow TL, Clevinger BL (1986): Structural correlates of idiotopes. Annu Rev Immunol 4:147–165.

Dersimonian H, Long A, Rubinstein D, Stollar BD, Schwartz RS (1990): V_h genes of human autoantibodies. Int Rev Immunol 5:253–264.

Dersimonian H, McAdam KPWJ, Mackworth-Young C, Stollar BD (1989): The recurrent expression of variable region segments in human IgM anti-DNA autoantibodies. J Immunol 142:4027–4033.

Dersimonian H, Schwartz RS, Barrett KJ, Stollar BD (1987): Relationship of human variable region heavy chain germ-line genes to genes encoding anti-DNA autoantibodies. J Immunol 139:2496–2501.

Ezaki I, Kanda H, Sakai K, Fukui N, Shingu M, Nobunaga M, Watanabe T (1991): Restricted diversity of the variable region nucleotide sequences of the heavy and light chains of a human rheumatoid factor. Arthritis Rheum 34:343–350.

Fong S, Gilbertson TA, Hueniken RJ, Singhal SK, Vaughan JH, Carson DA (1985): IgM rheumatoid factor autoantibody and immunoglobulin producing precursor cells in the bone marrow of humans. Cell Immunol 95:157–172.

Fong S, Chen PP, Gilbertson TA, Weber JR, Fox RI, Carson DA (1986): Expression of three cross reactive idiotypes on rheumatoid factor autoantibodies from patients with autoimmune diseases and seropositive adults. J Immunol 137:122–128.

Frippiat J-P, Chuchana P, Bernard F, Buluwela L, Lefranc G, Lefranc M-P (1990): First genomic sequence of a human Ig variable lambda gene belonging to subgroup III. Nucleic Acids Res 18:7134.

Goni FR, Chen PP, McGinnis D, Arjonilla ML, Fernandez J, Carson D, Solomon A, Mendez E, Frangione B (1989): Structural and idiotypic characterization of the L chains of human IgM autoantibodies with different specificities. J Immunol 142:3158–3163.

Goni F, Chen PP, Pons-Estel B, Carson DA, Frangione B (1985): Sequence similarities and cross-idiotypic specificity of L chains among human monoclonal IgM–K with anti-gammaglobulin activity. J Immunol 135:4073–4079.

Harindranath N, Goldfarb IS, Ikematsu H, Burastero SE, Wilder RL, Notkins AL, Casali P (1991): Complete sequence of the genes encoding the V_h and V_l regions of low- and high-affinity monoclonal IgM and IgA1 rheumatoid factors produced by $CD5^+$ B cells from a rheumatoid arthritis patient. Int Immunol 3:865–875.

Harris ED Jr (1990): Rheumatoid arthritis: Pathophysiology and implications for therapy. Mech Dis 322:1277–1290.

Hay FC, Soltys AJ, Tribbick G, Geysen HM (1991): Framework peptides from xIIIb rheumatoid factor light chains with binding activity for aggregated IgG. Eur J Immunol 21:1837–1841.

Hillson JL, Perlmutter RM (1990): Autoantibodies and the fetal antibody repertoire. Int Rev Immunol 5:215–230.

Hiraiwa A, Nugent DJ, Milner ECB (1990): Sequence analysis of monoclonal antibodies derived from a patient with idiopathic thrombocytopenic purpura. Autoimmunity 8:107–113.

Hoch S, Schwaber J (1987): Identification and sequence of the V–H gene elements encoding a human anti-DNA antibody. J Immunol 139:1689–1693.

Holmberg D (1987): High connectivity, natural antibodies preferentially use 7183 and QUPC 52 V_h families. Eur J Immunol 17:399–403.

Kipps TJ, Tomhave E, Chen PP, Carson DA (1988): Autoantibody-associated kappa light chain variable region gene expressed in chronic lymphocytic leukemia with little or no somatic mutation. Implications for etiology and immunotherapy. J Exp Med 167:840–852.

Kipps TJ, Tomhave E, Pratt LF, Duffy S, Chen PP, Carson DA (1989): Developmentally restricted immunoglobulin heavy chain variable region gene expressed at high frequency in chronic lymphocytic leukemia. Proc Natl Acad Sci USA 86:5913–5917.

Kodaira M, Kinashi T, Umemura I, Matsuda F, Noma T, Ono Y, Honjo T (1986): Organization and evolution of variable region genes of the human immunoglobulin heavy chain. J Mol Biol 190:529–541.

Kunkel HG, Agnello V, Joslin FG, Winchester RJ, Capra JD (1973): Cross-idiotypic specificity among monoclonal IgM proteins with anti-gammaglobulin activity. J Exp Med 137:331–342.

Kunkel HG, Winchester RJ, Joslin FG, Capra JD (1974): Similarities in the light chains of anti-gamma-globulins showing cross-idiotypic specificities. J Exp Med 139:128–136.

Lee KH, Matsuda F, Kinashi T, Kodaira M, Honjo T (1987): A novel family of variable region genes of the human immunoglobulin heavy chain. J Mol Biol 195:761–768.

Liu M-F, Robbins DL, Crowley JJ, Sinha S, Kozin F, Kipps TJ, Carson DA, Chen PP (1989): Characterization of four homologous light chain variable region genes which are related to 6B6.6 idiotype positive human rheumatoid factor light chains. J Immunol 142:688–694.

Logtenberg T, Young FM, Van Es JH, Gmelig-Meyling FHJ, Alt FW (1989): Auto-antibodies encoded by the most J_h-proximal human immunoglobulin heavy chain variable region gene. J Exp Med 170:1347–1355.

Lu EW, Deftos M, Tighe H, Carson DA, Chen PP (1992): Generation and characterization of two monoclonal self-associating IgG rheumatoid factors from a rheumatoid synovium. Arthritis Rheum 35:101–105.

Mageed RA, Dearlove M, Goodall DM, Jefferis R (1986): Immunogenic and antigenic epitopes of immunoglobulins. XVII. Monoclonal anti-idiotypes to the heavy chain of human rheumatoid factors. Rheumatoid Int 6:179–183.

Mannik M, Nardella FA, Sasso EH (1988): Rheumatoid factors in immune complexes of patients with rheumatoid arthritis. Springer Semin Immunopathol 10:215–230.

Matthyssens G, Rabbitts TH (1980): Structure and multiplicity of genes for the human immunoglobulin heavy chain variable region. Proc Natl Acad Sci USA 77:6561–6565.

Meindl A, Klobeck H-G, Ohnheiser R, Zachau HG (1990): The V_κ gene repertoire in the human-germline. Eur J Immunol 20:1855–1863.

Munthe E, Natvig JB (1971): Characterization of IgG complexes in eluates from rheumatoid tissue. Clin Exp Immunol 8:249–262.

Newkirk MM, Capra JD (1989): Restricted usage of immunoglobulin variable region genes in human autoantibodies. In Hanjo T, Alt FW, Rabbits T (eds): "Immuno-globulin Genes." Orlando: Academic Press, pp 215–220.

Newkirk M, Chen PP, Carson DA, Posnett B, Capra JD (1986): Amino acid sequence of a light chain variable region of a human rheumatoid factor of the Wa idiotypic group, in part predicted by its reactivity with antipeptide antibodies. Mol Immunol 23:239–244.

Newkirk MM, Mageed RA, Jefferis R, Chen PP, Capra JD (1987): Complete amino acid sequences of variable regions of two human IgM rheumatoid factors, BOR and KAS of the Wa idiotypic family, reveal restricted use of heavy and light chain variable and joining region gene segments. J Exp Med 166:550–564.

Nickerson KG, Berman J, Glickman E, Chess L, Alt FW (1989): Early human IgH gene assembly in Epstein-Barr virus-transformed fetal B cell lines. Preferential utilization of the most J_H-proximal D segment (DQ52) and two unusual V_H-related rearrangements. J Exp Med 169:1391–1403.

Olee T, Lu EW, Huang D-F, Soto-Gil RW, Deftos M, Kozin F, Carson DA, Chen PP (1992): Genetic analysis of self-associating IgG rheumatoid factors from two rheumatoid synovia implicates an antigen driven response. J Exp Med 175:831–842.

Olee T, Yang P-M, Siminovitch KA, Olsen NJ, Hillson J, Wu J, Kozin F, Carson DA, Chen PP (1991): Molecular basis of an autoantibody-associated restriction fragment length polymorphism that confers susceptibility to autoimmune diseases. J Clin Invest 88:193–203.

Pascual V, Andris J, Capra JD (1990a): Heavy chain variable region gene utilization in human antibodies. Int Rev Immunol 5:231–238.

Pascual V, Capra JD (1991): Human immunoglobulin heavy-chain variable region genes: Organization, polymorphism, and expression. Adv Immunol 49:1–74.

Pascual V, Randen I, Thompson K, Sioud M, Forre O, Natvig J, Capra JD (1990b): The complete nucleotide sequences of the heavy chain variable regions of six monospecific rheumatoid factors derived from Epstein-Barr virus-transformed B cells isolated from the synovial tissue of patients with rheumatoid arthritis. J Clin Invest 86:1320–1328.

Pascual V, Victor K, Lelsz D, Spellerberg MB, Hamblin TJ, Thompson KM, Randen I, Natvig J, Capra JD, Stevenson FK (1991): Nucleotide sequence analysis of the V regions of two IgM cold agglutinins. J Immunol 146:4385–4391.

Pascual V, Victor K, Randen I, Thompson K, Natvig JB, Capra JD (1992): IgM rheumatoid factors in patients with rheumatoid arthritis derive from a diverse array of germline immunoglobulin genes and display little evidence of somatic variation. J Rheumatol 19:50–53.

Pech M, Zachau HG (1984): Immunoglobulin genes of different subgroups are interdigitated within the V_κ locus. Nucleic Acids Res 12:9229–9236.

Perlmutter RM (1987): Programmed development of the antibody repertoire. Curr Top Microbiol Immunol 135:96–109.

Pons-Estel B, Goni F, Solomon A, Frangione B (1984): Sequence similarities among kIIIb chains of monoclonal human IgMk autoantibodies. J Exp Med 160:893–904.

Portnoi D, Freitas A, Holmberg D, Bandeira A, Coutinho A (1986): Immunocompetent autoreactive B lymphocytes are activated cycling cells in normal mice. J Exp Med 164:25–35.

Preud'homme JL, Seligmann M (1972): Anti-human immunoglobulin G activity of membrane-bound monoclonal immunoglobulin M in lymphoproliferative disorders. Proc Natl Acad Sci USA 69:2132–2135.

Radoux V, Chen PP, Sorge JA, Carson DA (1986): A conserved human germline V_κ gene directly encodes rheumatoid factor light chains. J Exp Med 164:2119–2124.

Randen I, Thompson KM, Natvig JB, Forre O, Waalen K (1989): Human monoclonal rheumatoid factors derived from the polyclonal repertoire of rheumatoid synovial tissue: Production and characterization. Clin Exp Immunol 78:13–18.

Rechavi G, Bienz B, Ram D, Ben-Neriah Y, Cohen JB, Zakut R, Givol D (1982): Organization and evolution of immunoglobulin V_H gene subgroups. Proc Natl Acad Sci USA 79:4405–4409.

Robbins DL, Kenny TP, Coloma MJ, Gavilondo-Cowley JV, Soto-Gil RW, Chen PP, Larrick JW (1990): Serological and molecular characterization of a human monoclonal rheumatoid factor derived from rheumatoid synovial cells. Arthritis Rheum 33:1188–1195.

Sanz I, Casali P, Thomas JW, Notkins AL, Capra JD (1989a): Nucleotide sequences of eight human natural autoantibody V-H regions reveals apparent restricted use of V-H families. J Immunol 142:4054–4061.

Sanz I, Kelly P, Williams C, Scholl S, Tucker P, Capra JD (1989b): The smaller human V_H gene families display remarkably little polymorphism. EMBO J 8:3741–3748.

Schroeder HW Jr, Hillson JL, Perlmutter RM (1987): Early restriction of the human antibody repertoire. Science 238:791–793.

Schroeder HW Jr, Wang JY (1990): Preferential utilization of conserved immunoglobulin heavy chain variable gene segments during human fetal life. Proc Natl Acad Sci USA 87:6146–6150.

Schrohenloher RE, Accavitti MA, Bhown AS, Koopman WJ (1990): Monoclonal antibody 6B6.6 defines a cross-reactive kappa light chain idiotype of human monoclonal and polyclonal rheumatoid factors. Arthritis Rheum 33:187–198.

Schutte MEM, Ebeling SB, Akkermans KE, Gmelig-Meyling FHJ, Logtenberg T (1991): Antibody specificity and immunoglobulin V_H gene utilization of human monoclonal CD5$^+$ B cell lines. Eur J Immunol 21:1115–1121.

Shin EK, Matsuda F, Nagaoka H, Fukita Y, Imai T, Yokoyama K, Soeda E, Honjo T (1991): Physical map of the 3' region of the human immunoglobulin heavy chain locus: Clustering of autoantibody-related variable segments in one haplotype. EMBO J 10:3641–3645.

Shlomchik MJ, Marshak-Rothstein A, Wolfowicz CB, Rothstein TL, Weigert MG (1987a): The role of clonal selection and somatic mutation in autoimmunity. Nature 328:805–811.

Shlomchik M, Nemazee D, Van Snick J, Weigert M (1987b): Variable region sequences of murine IgM anti-IgG monoclonal autoantibodies (rheumatoid factors). II. Comparison of hybridomas derived by lipopolysaccharide stimulation and secondary protein immunization. J Exp Med 165:970–987.

Siminovitch KA, Chen PP (1990): The biologic significance of human natural autoimmune responses: Relationship to the germline, early immune and malignant B cell variable gene repertoire. Int Rev Immunol 5:265–277.

Siminovitch KA, Misener V, Kwong PC, Song Q-L, Chen PP (1989): A natural autoantibody is encoded by germline heavy and lambda light chain variable region genes without somatic mutation. J Clin Invest 84:1675–1678.

Siminovitch KA, Misener V, Kwong PC, Yang P-M, Laskin CA, Cairns E, Bell D, Rubin LA, Chen PP (1990): A human anti-cardiolipin autoantibody is encoded by developmentally restricted heavy and light chain variable region genes. Autoimmunity 8:97–105.

Soto-Gil RW, Olee T, Klink BK, Kenny TP, Robbins DL, Carson DA, Chen PP (1992): A systematic approach to define the germline gene counterparts of a mutated autoantibody from a rheumatoid arthritis patient. Arthritis Rheum 35:356–363.

Spector TD (1990): Rheumatoid arthritis. Rheum Dis Clin North Am 16:513–537.

Stevenson FK, Smith GJ, North J, Hamblin TJ, Glennie MJ (1989): Identification of normal B-cell counterparts of neoplastic cells which secrete cold agglutinins of anti-I and anti-i specificity. Br J Haematol 72:9–15.

Straubinger B, Huber E, Lorenz W, Osterholzer E, Pargent W, Pech M, Pholenz H-D, Zimmer F-J, Zachau HG (1988): The human VK locus: Characterization of a duplicated region encoding 28 different immunoglobulin genes. J Mol Biol 199:23–34.

Victor KD, Randen I, Thompson K, Forre O, Natvig JB, Fu SM, Capra JC (1991): Rheumatoid factors isolated from patients with autoimmune disorders are derived from germline genes distinct from those encoding the Wa, Po, and Bla cross-reactive idiotypes. J Clin Invest 87:1603–1613.

Weisbart RH, Wong AL, Noritake D, Kacena A, Chan G, Ruland C, Chin E, Chen

ISY, Rosenblatt JD (1991): The rheumatoid factor reactivity of a human IgG monoclonal autoantibody is encoded by a variant $V_\kappa II$ L chain gene. J Immunol 147:2795–2801.

Winchester RJ, Agnello V, Kunkel HG (1970): Gamma globulin complexes in synovial fluids of patients with rheumatoid arthritis: Partial characterization and relationship to lowered complement levels. Clin Exp Immunol 6:689–705.

Winfield JB (1983): Cryoglobulinemia. Hum Pathol 14:350–354.

Yancopoulos GD, Malynn BA, Alt FW (1988): Developmentally regulated and strain-specific expression of murine V_H gene families. J Exp Med 168:417–435.

Yang P, Olee T, Carson DA, Chen PP (1993): Characterization of two highly homologous autoantibody-related $V_H I$ genes in humans. Scand J Immunol 37:504–508.

Zvaifler NJ (1973): The immunopathology of joint inflammation in rheumatoid arthritis. Adv Immunol 13:265.

18

HUMAN AND EXPERIMENTAL MYASTHENIA GRAVIS

Ann Kari Lefvert

Department of Medicine and Immunological Research Laboratory,
Karolinska Hospital, Stockholm, Sweden

INTRODUCTION

The disease myasthenia gravis (MG) is commonly described as the prototype of an autoantibody-mediated, organ-specific autoimmune disease. The disease and the autoimmune response against the acetylcholine receptor on the postsynaptic muscle endplate are regarded as having a simplistic cause and effect relationship. However, the results of recent research must lead to the conclusion that the autoantibodies cannot be the sole or even the main explanation for the neuromuscular symptoms. It is now evident that the autoimmune response and the disease are the results of multifactorial, interconnected chains of events. The recent research on human and experimental myasthenia gravis is reviewed here, and the evidence for the pathogenic mechanisms is examined.

The clinical picture of MG was described in the literature as early as 1685 [1]. Since 1956, the typical muscular symptoms of MG have been attributed to a reduced effect of the neurotransmitter acetylcholine on the motor endplate of striated muscle [2]. The theoretical possibility of an antibody against the acetylcholine receptor was first discussed by Simpson in 1960 [3]. The evi-

Autoimmunity: Physiology and Disease, Pages 267–305
© *1994 Wiley-Liss, Inc.*

dence that the symptoms of MG are mediated via a humoral factor came in 1973 [4], when lymph drainage of patients with MG was shown to induce a marked clinical and electrophysiological improvement. Retransfusions of cell-free lymph and immunoglobulin fractions from lymph precipitated symptoms, while retransfusions of lymph mononuclear cells had no effect [5]. This crucial experiment clearly demonstrated the presence of autoreactive immunoglobulin molecules.

In 1973, Patrick and Lindstrom [6] described a myasthenia-like illness in rabbits immunized with purified acetylcholine receptor from the electric organ of the eel, *Electrophorus electricus*. The electric organs from electric eels and electric rays consist of tissue analogous to skeletal muscle postsynaptic endplates and containing densely packed acetylcholine receptors. Immunization with such purified receptor resulted in production of antibodies that cross-reacted with the rabbit's own endplates. As antibodies appeared, the rabbits developed muscle weakness and fatigability closely resembling the symptoms of MG. This observation began a search for antibodies against cholinergic receptor proteins also in human MG. Such antibodies were indeed found in the majority of patients with MG [7,8], and it was presumed that MG resulted from autoantibody interference with the synaptic transmission by binding to the acetylcholine receptor.

HUMAN MYASTHENIA GRAVIS

The disease is characterized by increased fatigability and weakness of skeletal muscles. The estimated incidence of the disease is 5–10 per 100,000 people. Women are affected twice as often as males. The onset of disease for women is mainly during the reproductive period and for men is typically later in life [9].

In the early stages of the disease, the most frequent manifestations involve muscle groups innervated by cranial nerves such as the ocular muscles resulting in ptosis and diplopia. Generalized muscle fatigue affecting limbs and trunk and bulbar muscles may develop. Which muscle groups that are affected may vary from day to day, and the symptoms are sometimes assymmetrical in distribution. Spontaneous remissions and exacerbations are common. The natural course of the disease is commonly a gradual worsening of symptoms during the first 2–3 years after onset of disease, followed by a more stable phase and often by spontaneous amelioration.

The commonly used clinical classification of MG was designed by Osserman with the modifications of Oosterhuis [10]. MG is thus classified into stages A (complete remission), I (symptoms restricted to one muscle group), IIA (mild generalized), IIB (severe generalized), III (acute fulminating), and IV (chronic severe).

Patients with MG display a high incidence of thymic abnormalities. Hyperplastic changes are found in 60%–70% of the patients and thymomas in

10%–15% [11]. The presence of thymoma is usually associated with a more severe disease and higher concentrations of antibodies against the acetylcholine receptor [7]. MG is the only autoimmune disease in which thymectomy has a proven beneficial effect [12]. Thymectomy is efficient in inducing a remission only in patients with hyperplasia, while removal of a thymoma usually does not affect the symptoms.

MG among white patients is associated with the haplotypes A1B8 and/or DR w3 in young females and A3,B7 and/or DR w2 in old males, although the association between these haplotypes and the disease is rather weak [13]. A study of HLA-DRB and -DQB polymorphism revealed further associations between different haplotypes and thymic histology and also age at onset of disease [14]. Different haplotypes are correlated with MG in other racial groups [15].

The main treatment of MG is with inhibitors of cholinesterase, and this is in most cases enough to achieve an acceptable improvement. Most young patients with thymus hyperplasia benefit from thymectomy, and this operation is—in most medical centers—routinely performed in all cases with generalized symptoms. In resistant cases, immunosuppressive treatment such as corticosteroids, azathioprine, cyclophosphamide, and cyclosporine A is used with good effect. Drainage of thoracic duct lymph and plasmapheresis usually has a rapid effect, and plasmapheresis may be employed in acute situations. Intravenous administration of large quantities of human gammaglobulin (IgG) preparations has been postulated to have some effect, although these studies are generally poorly documented. Our recent results show that IgG treatment has profound effects on the autoimmune repertoire and thus is discussed below. Of the more experimental treatments, infusions of a chimeric (mouse–human) anti-CD4$^+$ antibody has been tried by us with good effect. The immunological effect of this experimental treatment has great bearing on the question of the regulation of the autoimmune process in MG and is discussed below.

EXPERIMENTAL AUTOIMMUNE MYASTHENIA GRAVIS

The first animal model of human MG was the rabbit [6]. Rabbits immunized with purified receptor from the electric organ of electric eels or rays develop a progressive paralysis, usually starting within 1 week after the second immunization. The symptoms initially respond to cholinesterase inhibitors, but most animals die from progressive disease. Since the immunized rabbit is difficult to maintain and the knowledge of rabbit immunology is relatively limited, most research on experimental autoimmune myasthenia gravis (EAMG) has been done using different mouse and rat strains.

Mice immunized with purified receptor from electric organs or from vertebrate muscle together with complete Freund's adjuvant [16–19] generally develop antibodies against the receptor. The concentration of antibodies and development of muscle weakness and other signs of EAMG seem to be highly dependent on the mouse strain [16]. Usually, the muscle weakness is not very marked in mice due to the supposedly large reserve in neuromuscular transmission in mice. Most studies report an association with products by the I-A locus, and EAMG. H-2^b strains are generally highly susceptible and C57BL/6 mice are the most prone to EAMG upon immunization with receptor protein from electric organs. In contrast, mice strains with the haplotype H-2^k and also those with H-2^{d,s,q,f,p,r} are less susceptible [16]. There is generally a positive correlation between EAMG, serum antireceptor antibody levels, loss of receptors at the endplate, amount of immunoglobulin bound to the endplate, and electrophysiological signs of deranged neuromuscular function. It is of interest that one mouse strain, AKR/J, with the haplotype H-2^k, in contrast to other strains with that particular haplotype, developed very high concentrations of receptor antibodies but only in about 10% EAMG. This discrepancy between EAMG and serum antibody level was proposed to be due to the complement C5 deficiency of this strain. Using B10.D2/Sn "old" mice (devoid of hemolytic complement activity) and B10.D2/Sn "new" mice (with detectable hemolytic complement activity) it was shown that complement C5 deficiency protected against EAMG [16]. It is possible to induce EAMG in susceptible mouse strains also without adjuvant [20], although this procedure generally results in a lesser incidence of a milder disease.

In rats, the disease is characteristically biphasic [21]. An acute phase of EAMG occurs about 7 days after immunization with receptor and is self-limiting. It is characterized by macrophage infiltration of the motor endplates [22]. The animals recover from the acute phase after 5 days and appear clinically normal until about 4 weeks after immunization, when most animals experience a second and chronic phase of the disease. The histopathological features of chronic EAMG in rats closely resembles those of human MG [22,23]. Also in rats there is a general correlation between endplate morphology, antireceptor antibodies, and clinical and electrophysiological signs of disease.

The development of EAMG in rats is likewise controlled by genetic factors. Lewis rats are susceptible and Wistar Furth rats resistant to EAMG, although both species produce antibodies against the immunizing receptor. It is, however, possible to produce the disease also in Wistar Furth rats by hyperimmunization, showing that the resistance to EAMG is not absolute [24].

In both rats and mice, passive transfer of receptor antibodies in serum from patients [25,26] and of antireceptor monoclonal antibodies induces EAMG. Monoclonal antibodies against the ligand binding site of the receptor induce a hyperacute development of weakness [27], whereas antibodies against other regions induce a slowly developing disease associated with inflammatory lesions on the endplate [28]. Cells from immunized animals are also able to transfer the symptoms of EAMG, although the efficacy of cell transfers has been low, especially relative to antibody transfers. All experiments in which successful transfers occurred included both T and B cells, and large amounts of purified T cells were completely ineffective in inducing disease in rats [29].

Still another way of inducing EAMG is using immunization with internal images of the acetylcholine receptor (AChR). Using bisQ, a structurally constrained ligand of the AChR, antibodies and EAMG were induced by immunization with anti-bisQ antibodies [30]. A murine monoclonal antiidiotypic antibody raised against a receptor antibody binding to the ligand binding site of the receptor was able to bind cholinergic ligands and also to induce EAMG [31].

ACETYLCHOLINE RECEPTOR

The autoantigen in MG is the AChR. There are two forms of receptors: Extrajunctional receptors that are spread over the surface of the whole muscle and junctional receptors that are located under the nerve terminal. These two forms are different with regard to subunit composition, half-life, channel open time, and pharmacological and immunological properties. Extrajunctional receptors are found during ontogeny and in adult humans and animals after denervation. In adult humans, the AChR is a pentamer composed of four subunits ($\alpha_2\beta(\gamma$ or $\varepsilon)\delta$) [32]. The molecular mass of the receptor is around 250 kD, with the individual subunits around 50 kD each. In mammalian muscle the extrajunctional receptors contain the γ-subunit that after formation of the synaptic junction is replaced with the ε-subunit. There is a large degree of sequence homology between the different subunits within a species, as well as between species [33,34].

The subunit arrangement creates a channel with pentameric symmetry (α-β-α–γ-δ) [35]. Approximately 50% of the receptor is extracellular, 40% spans the membrane, and 10% is intracellular [36].

The acetylcholine binding site of the AChR has been localized to the α-subunit [37]. The binding site for α-bungarotoxin, a high affinity ligand commonly used to identify the receptor, partly overlaps with and extends beyond the acetylcholine binding site [38]. The activation of the receptor and induction of channel opening requires that the agonist bind to both α-subunits. Even though the two α-subunits are identical, they have different affinities for certain antagonists, e.g., d-tubocurarine. As shown by binding studies using monoclonal antibodies and sera from patients with MG, the immunological properties are different and the antibodies block only one of the α-bungarotoxin binding sites [39,40].

Desensitization, a short state of unresponsiveness, of the receptor occurs for a short while (milliseconds) after ligand binding and channel opening [41]. Desensitization is accompanied by conformational changes in the AChR, predominantly in the δ- and γ-subunits. The net results of these events is a less symmetrical configuration of the receptor. Increased rate of receptor desensitization also occurs by the action of different protein kinases [42].

In MG, both the normal and the hyperplastic thymus contain muscle-like "myoid" cells that have been shown to express AChR-like structures both in culture and in situ [43]. According to one theory, as yet unproven, induction of the disease takes place within the thymus, while damage to the receptor on muscle endplate is secondary [29].

CELLULAR IMMUNE RESPONSE IN MYASTHENIA GRAVIS

The synthesis of anti-AChR antibodies is regulated by AChR-specific T-helper cells [44]. These T cells are by most investigators considered to react predominantly with the α-subunit [45] and especially with the NH_2-terminal part, which has a high degree of amphipathicity, an important feature of T-cell epitopes [46].

T-cell reactivity against more than one epitope of the α-subunit is common in MG patients. In one study, the majority of patients responded to more than one peptide in the proliferative assay [47]. Studies of AChR-specific polyclonal and oligoclonal T-helper cell lines have also shown a polyclonal T-cell response to different synthetic peptides [48–50]. In one of these studies, a T-helper cell line from one patient with MG recognized 5 out of 32 tested peptides that each covered 14–20 residues of the human α-subunit [49].

The T-cell determinants generally consist of short peptide sequences of a protein antigen that has been appropriately cleaved and/or unfolded. T cells recognize epitopes of a denatured protein antigen equally well as in their native form. Intracellular processing of an antigen is not always required for T-cell recognition if the antigen is present as smaller peptides [51]. Mapping of the T-cell epitope can thus be approached using small peptide segments of proteins. In a recent work, we employed solid-phase bound overlapping hexapeptides to characterize the T-cell epitopes on the α-chain of the receptor [52]. The T-cell stimulation by 70 hexapeptides, overlapping with one amino acid and representing a 75 amino acid long sequence of the NH_2-terminal part of the α-chain, was detected by the secretion of IFN-γ from single T cells. A polyclonal T-cell response was present in most of the patients. The peptide that induced IFN-γ secretion in the highest number of patients was amino acids 29–34. The peptides covering residues amino acids 28–35 and amino acids 69–76 induced a positive response in 6–9/24 patients (25%–37.5%) as compared to 0–1/24 controls (0%–4.2%).

The results indicate a polyclonal T-cell response to the α-chain of AChR in patients with MG. No dominant T-cell epitope was found. The pattern of the T-cell response indicates that different epitopes and/or multiple T-cell clones are involved in the T-cell recognition of the AChR.

Other studies from our group regarding the cellular immune response in

MG employed the same method for the enumeration of stimulated T cells by the secretion of IL-2 and IFN-γ from single T cells [53]. T cells were stimulated with human monoclonal idiotypic and anti-idiotypic antibodies bearing separate recurrent idiotypes and with affinity-purified human acetylcholine receptor. Incubation with the idiotypic antibody resulted in T-cell stimulation, measured as numbers of IFN-γ-secreting cells, in 78% of patients and in 7% of the healthy controls. The anti-idiotypic antibody activated T cells in 50% of patients and in 4% of the controls. The mean value of the idiotype and anti-idiotype reactive T cells in the patients was $18/10^5$ and $10/10^5$ peripheral blood mononuclear cells (PBMC), respectively. T-cell activation measured as numbers of IL-2-secreting cells showed a difference between patients and controls that was as significant as for IFN-γ secretion. These results demonstrate the presence of idiotypic and anti-idiotypic T cells in MG (Fig. 1).

The prevalence of T cells reactive with the affinity-purified AChR of human skeletal muscle was studied using the same technique [54,55]. AChR-reactive T cells were significantly increased in the peripheral blood of patients compared with healthy individuals. The AChR stimulated T cells in 87.7% of the patients as compared with 7.4% of the controls. The mean value of AChR-reactive T cells in the patients was $19.6/10^5$ PBMC, corresponding to 1/5,102 PBMC (Fig. 1). Comparable results were obtained also for IL-2-secreting cells.

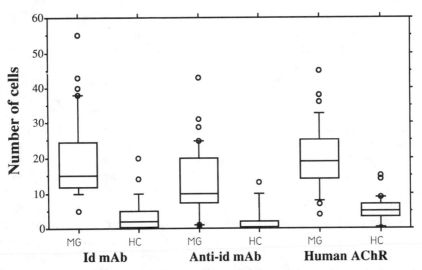

FIGURE 1. Box plot showing median and 90% confidence interval of numbers of T cells stimulated to IFN-γ secretion/10^5 PBMC by incubation with a human monoclonal idiotypic antibody, a human monoclonal anti-idiotypic antibody, and affinity-purified human skeletal muscle AChR in patients with MG and in healthy controls (HC).

T-CELL RECEPTOR

Polymorphism in α- and β-chain T-cell receptor genes have recently been described and—in certain cases—found to correlate with susceptibilities to autoimmune diseases such as insulin-dependent diabetes mellitus and systemic lupus erythematosus (SLE). The distribution of a new polymorphism in the genes encoding for T-cell receptor α-chain was recently described and showed significant differences in the frequency of the polymorphic Vα and Cα markers between patients with multiple sclerosis, MG, Graves' disease, and healthy individuals [56]. In another study, analysis of immunoglobulin and T-cell receptor gene rearrangements in the thymus of MG patients by Southern blot showed no signs of a rearranged T- or B-cell receptor clone [57]. Studies on human T-cell receptor Vα or Vβ genes using monoclonal antibodies that cover around 25% of the total CD3$^+$ T-cell population showed that 4/16 patients with MG had dramatically expanded "clones" of α/β T cells in the circulation. In occasional patients, close to half of all T cells in a CD4 or CD8 subset may have one V gene of α- or β-type, that is, they are oligoclonal or monoclonal [58].

AUTOANTIBODIES IN MYASTHENIA GRAVIS

Disease-Specific Autoantibodies in Myasthenia Gravis

Antibodies binding to the AChR of human muscle are present in 90% of patients with generalized MG and in 70% of patients with localized MG [7]. The assay of these antibodies is routinely performed using detergent-extracted human receptor. A better way of assaying these antibodies would be to measure the binding to an intact receptor in situ on a muscle cell. One such cell line, of rhabdomyosarcoma or neuroblastoma origin, designated TE671, can be used for assay of antibodies against an intact receptor [59].

The antibodies can disturb neuromuscular function in at least three principally different ways. The first is complement-mediated destruction of the endplate, leading to a flattening of the normal postsynaptic folding, increased synaptic junction distance, and a lower concentration of functioning receptors. The terminal complement components, the membrane attached components, can together with immunoglobulins be found bound to the neuromuscular junction both in EAMG during the acute phase and—to a lesser extent—in human MG [60,61]. Depletion of complement by treatment with cobra venom factor [62] as well as blockade of the complement cascade by monoclonal antibodies against complement factor 6 [63], reduced the neuromuscular symptoms and also the loss of receptors in the acute phase of EAMG. Complement-mediated destruction is clearly important in the acute phase of EAMG [60], but probably less so in the human disease. The complement levels in MG are usually not lowered and not correlated with the severity of symptoms [64]. However, the morphological aspect of the end-plate is often simplified and the postsynaptic area reduced in long-standing human MG, suggesting that the complement-mediated destruction might contribute to the receptor loss [60].

According to another proposed mechanism, reduction of AChR density could be caused by antigenic modulation of AChR metabolism resulting in increased internalization rate and ultimately in a relative decrease in receptors. Sera from patients with MG accelerate the rate of receptor internalization on cultured myotubules from embryonal rat muscle two to three times [65,66]. The effect is dependent on an intact $F(ab')_2$ fragment and the cross-linking of receptors [66]. There is a good correlation between the concentration of serum antibodies and increased turnover rate, but no correlation between rate of internalization and clinical symptoms [67]. Moreover, antibodies in unaffected mice immunized with *Torpedo* receptor increased the internalization rate as much as antibodies from severely affected mice immunized with the same antigen [68] Thus the hypothesis rests on observations made on human or animal myotubule cultures grown in presence of myasthenia serum, but there has been no direct demonstration of this pathogenic mechanism in myasthenic muscles.

Clinical and experimental observations also suggest a third mechanism, an immunopharmacological blockade of the receptor by antibodies that sterically inhibit agonist binding [69,70]. The symptoms, especially in early disease resemble those of a transient neuromuscular block and are usually promptly reverted by an adequate anticholinesterase medication. Other indications for such a mechanism are the rapid effect of plasma exchange and drainage of the thoracic duct lymph.

Immunization of mice with a *Torpedo* receptor peptide involved in toxin binding resulted in EAMG with marked muscle dysfunction. The mechanism was supposed to be direct agonist blockade, since antigenic modulation was not observed [71]. In chicken, a mouse monoclonal antibody directed against the ligand binding site of chicken receptor had a very rapid pharmacological blocking effect on the neuromuscular transmission, leading to instant paralysis and death [27].

The prevalence of antibodies directed against the toxin binding site in MG as determined by inhibition of α-bungarotoxin binding to cultured myotubules from chicken or to detergent-extracted human muscle receptor is as high as 80%–98% [69,72]. Such antibodies are able to inhibit 50% of toxin binding [72,73], often belong to IgG subclasses 1 and 3, and are more prevalent in patients with severe disease [69, 72–74]. When interpreting these data it is, however, important to keep in mind that the acetylcholine and the toxin binding sites are not completely identical.

A hypothetical mechanism by which antibody might alter the pharmacological properties of the receptor is receptor desensitization. Conformational changes induced by antibody binding do alter the biological activities of several enzymes [75], and antibody binding to receptor might thus induce the desensitized state, including a conformational change in the receptor. Such a mechanism can be considered a form of immunopharmacological blockade.

The specific autoantibody repertoire in MG also comprises antibodies bearing receptor–antibody-associated idiotypes and anti-idiotypic antibodies against the receptor antibodies [76–80]. The receptor–antibody-associated idiotypic and anti-idiotypic antibodies have been determined by direct binding to murine monoclonal anti-idiotypic and antireceptor antibodies, respectively. The murine monoclonal anti-idiotypic antibody A-I21 was raised against a human antireceptor antibody with specificity for the ligand binding region of the receptor. This monoclonal antibody bound cholinergic ligands and was able to trigger the production of antireceptor antibodies in experimental animals [31]. Thus it can be considered as the internal image of the receptor and as bearing at least part of its epitopes. This monoclonal antibody bears a recurrent idiotype that is recognized by 60% of patients with MG. The other murine monoclonal anti-idiotypic antibodies were raised against affinity-purified antireceptor antibodies from MG patients and designated A-I3, 8, 24, 41, and 45. These monoclonal antibodies bind to immunoglobulins in 14%–38% of MG patients.

The monoclonal antireceptor antibodies TR63, 94, and 105 used for the detection of anti-idiotypic antibodies were raised against the purified receptor of *Torpedo marmorata* and selected for their strong cross-reactivity with human receptor. The monoclonal TR63 recognizes a recurrent idiotype present in 52% of patients and is directed against the ligand binding site of the receptor.

A special kind of anti-idiotypic antibody, an anticholine antibody, was isolated from the serum of patients by a choline affinity column [81]. It was found that the anticholine antibodies bound cholinergic agonists and antagonists with the same rank order potency as the AChR. Thus these anticholine antibodies may be regarded as an internal image of the ligand binding site of the AChR.

Other Autoantibodies

MG is often associated with the presence of other autoantibodies. Most prevalent are antibodies against muscle antigens, found in 30% of the patients. These antigens are present in both heart and skeletal muscle tissue. One of these antigens, a solubilized, citric-acid-extracted fraction of striated muscle, was closely associated with the presence of thymoma, and this antigen has now been identified as titin [82]. Another antigen was extracted from heart muscle with hypertonic sucrose and antibodies against this were found in a majority of MG patients [83]. The importance for such antibodies for cardiac disease, which is proposed to be overrepresentated in MG patients, is unclear [84].

Antinuclear antibodies and antithyroid antibodies are found in 20% and

30%, respectively [85]. Of interest is that MG patients also have antibodies against neuronal antigens, such as antibodies reacting with human neuroblastoma cells [86] and antibodies against presynaptic structures [87].

Antibodies against the β_2-adrenergic receptor (β_2-AR) are found in about 18% of patients with MG [88]. The β_2-AR is present on muscle cells and controls various metabolic functions necessary for muscle activity. Activation of the β_2-AR leads to phosphorylation of the AChR and to an increased rate of receptor desensitization. The β_2-AR is also present on immune cells, and stimulation of the receptor is known to enhance antibody production, as well as activate T cells. Such antibodies might modulate the outcome of MG in a complex network of neurophysiological and neuroimmunological mechanisms.

Properties of the Autoantibodies in MG

Fine Specificity of Antireceptor Antibody Binding to the Receptor. The extracellular part of the α-subunit has been reported to contain a region that is conformation dependent and binds the majority of receptor antibodies from both rats with EAMG and MG patients [89,90]. This region has been termed the *main immunogenic region* (MIR), and most of the mapping studies to define the region have been done using monoclonal antibodies. A further MIR on the human receptor detected by using antibody binding to overlapping peptides was claimed to be restricted to residues 67–76 of the α-subunit [91].

An immunodominant region recognized by rats immunized with whole *Torpedo* receptor accounts for 60% of the antigenicity and is located within residues 330–400 [92]. Based on the clonal prevalence of reactive monoclonal antibodies, another immunodominant region corresponding to residues 351–368 of the intracellular part of the *Torpedo* receptor has been reported [93]. Sera from mice and rabbits immunized with whole *Torpedo* receptor defined eight epitopes on the *Torpedo* receptor extracellular residues 1–210. Two of those (25–36 and 102–114) were immunodominant based on the amount of antibody bound to each peptide [94]. In yet another study, antisera from rats, rabbits, and mice immunized with recombinant human muscle AChR α-subunit extracellular domain 1–210, multiple binding sites were present [95].

In a recent study, we employed binding of antibodies to synthetic peptides of various theoretical flexibility and to overlapping hexapeptides, bound to a solid surface, as a way of mapping the receptor α-subunit residues 10–84 [96,97]. MG sera reacted to two synthetic peptides corresponding to either two regions of high backbone flexibility (residues 28–43 and 44–59) or one region of low theoretical flexibility (residues 66–79). Epitope mapping of the region between residues 10 and 84 allowed the detection of two antigenic sites within residues 20–26 and 64–69. Combining these two studies, a dominant antigenic site located in residues 66–69 can be postulated. This epitope is within the reported location of the human MIR. An interesting observation was that sera from patients regarded as seronegative by the routine assay reacted with these peptides. Thus, with different approaches, many parts of the α-chain were determined to be immunogenic. Since the α-chain accounts for 40% of the total extracellular domain, this is not surprising [98].

These results of all these cited investigations should, however, be interpreted with caution. Studies employing monoclonal antibodies can never exclude the possibility that steric hinderance, with or without cross-linking, accounts for inhibition of binding. A large (290 kD) receptor would be expected to carry a mosaic of epitopes potentially stimulatory for B cells in an outbred, human population. Thus the use of monoclonal antibodies obtained in inbred species introduces a bias in the system. Lastly, most of the epitopes on the receptor are likely to be conformational dependent and not disclosed by studies using small peptide fragments [99].

The importance of fine specificities is also demonstrated by antibodies that distinguish between extrajunctional and junctional AChR [100,101]. The majority of patient sera react much better with AChR obtained from partially denervated human muscle than with AChR from innervated muscle. These findings have important implications for the selection of sources of antigens for the tests used in routine assays of AChR antibodies.

Kinetic Properties. We have earlier shown that the receptor antibodies of patients with severe MG have a short half-life [102]. There is also a good correlation between duration of remission after termination of lymph drainage and $t_{1/2}$ of the receptor antibodies in that patients with long-standing remissions after the drainage was stopped also have a long half-life of their receptor antibodies [103]. This suggests that the antibody populations that are important for neuromuscular symptoms have a faster turnover than other species of antibodies. We have now extended these studies to patients with severe MG and antibodies against the AChR together with other autoantibodies and autoimmune diseases in the active stage or in remission. Four patients had active, severe MG. Two of them had antibodies against gliadin and nuclear antigens, respectively, but no clinical signs of activity of another autoimmune disease than MG. One patient had severe MG as well as active Hashimoto's thyroiditis.

The kinetic parameters $t_{1/2}$, fractional catabolic rate, and rate of synthesis for autoantibodies and for antibodies against microbial antigens were determined during lymph drainage using a mathematical model [102]. The results of the determination of the kinetic parameters of total IgG, IgG$_3$, receptor antibody, and other autoantibodies for all patients are shown in Table I, and the determination of these parameters for receptor antibody activity, different idiotypes, and anti-idiotypic antibodies present in the same patients are in Table II.

All patients had a very short half-life of receptor antibody activity and a rapid rate of synthesis and catabolism, whereas the calculated half-lives for total IgG, IgG$_3$, and antibodies against tetanus toxoid were within the normal

TABLE I. Kinetic parameters for total IgG, IgG_3, receptor antibodies, and other autoantibodies in four patients (patients 1, 2, 3, 5) with severe myasthenia gravis and no other active autoimmune disease and in one patient with severe myasthenia and Hashimoto's thyroiditis (patient 4)

	Patient No.				
	1	2	3	4	5
$t_{1/2}$ (days) total IgG	22	21	18	30	37
$t_{1/2}$ (days) IgG_3	5	6.2	8.3	4.8	4
Fractional catabolic rate (%)	22	18	23	27	16
$t_{1/2}$ (days) receptor antibody	2	2.5	1.2	1.3	8
Fractional catabolic rate (%)	57	74	65	76	48
$t_{1/2}$ (days) (ds)DNA	24				
Fractional catabolic rate (%)	9				
$t_{1/2}$ (days) (ss)DNA	26				
Fractional catabolic rate (%)	4				
$t_{1/2}$ (days) cardiolipin	35				
Fractional catabolic rate (%)	2				
$t_{1/2}$ (days) RF	28				
Fractional catabolic rate (%)	5				
$t_{1/2}$ (days) gliadin		19			
Fractional catabolic rate (%)		4			
$t_{1/2}$ (days) thyroglobulin				4	
Fractional catabolic rate (%)				58	
$t_{1/2}$ (days) tetanus	25	23	18	34	36
Fractional catabolic rate (%)	3	5	6	2	1.4

range. The kinetic parameters for autoantibodies not associated with MG were within the normal range except in the patient with active thyroiditis, who had a rapid turnover also of thyroglobulin antibodies. The turnover rates of MG–associated idiotypes and of anti-idiotypic antibodies varied but were in most cases higher than that of normal IgG and of other autoantibodies.

These findings suggest that antibody species that are relevant for the activity of the disease are eliminated much more rapidly from serum than are antibodies with irrelevant specificities. The elimination can occur by binding to the antigen, cholinergic receptor, and thyroglobulin, respectively, or by binding to complementary anti-idiotypic antibodies followed by elimination of the complexes.

Thus one cause of the bad correlation between serum concentrations of autoantibodies and symptoms is different kinetic characteristics of different antibody populations. In MG, not all species of idiotypes and anti-idiotypic antibodies showed a rapid turnover rate. This further suggests that different antibody populations have different pathogenetic properties. The kinetic properties of different antibody populations may thus be an indication of the relative importance of antibody species for disease symptoms.

TABLE II. Kinetic parameters for receptor antibodies, related idiotypes, and anti-idiotypic antibodies in four patients with severe myasthenia gravis and no other active autoimmune disease (patients 1, 2, 3, 5) and in one patient with severe myasthenia and Hashimoto's thyroiditis (patient 4)

	Patient No.				
	1	2	3	4	5
$t_{1/2}$ (days) receptor antibody	2	2.5	1.2	1.3	8
Fractional catabolic rate (%)	57	74	65	76	48
$t_{1/2}$ (days) idiotype 21	3		1.2		4.5
Fractional catabolic rate (%)	84		87		45
$t_{1/2}$ (days) anti-idiotype 63	13		2.5		
Fractional catabolic rate (%)	22		78		
$t_{1/2}$ (days) idiotype 3	22	6			
Fractional catabolic rate (%)	8	21			
$t_{1/2}$ (days) idiotype 24	3.2			2	
Fractional catabolic rate (%)	68			69	
$t_{1/2}$ (days) anti-idiotype 94		14			3
Fractional catabolic rate (%)		28			87

VARIABLE GENE SEGMENT USAGE BY HUMAN ANTIRECEPTOR AND ANTI-IDIOTYPIC ANTIBODIES

The nucleotide sequence of the heavy and light chains of four human monoclonal antibodies isolated from Epstein-Barr virus-transformed peripheral blood lymphocytes were analyzed [104]. Three of the antibodies, two IgM and one IgG, bound to the AChR; and one was an IgG anti-idiotypic antibody. The IgM antireceptor antibodies were direct copies of germline gene segments, while the structures of the IgG antireceptor antibody and the anti-idiotypic antibody appear to be mutated, suggesting perhaps that they have undergone antigenic selection. Two of the antireceptor antibodies bear the same idiotype, reactive with A-I21. In addition, one of them reacts with A-I3. Structural analysis illustrates that these differ by a single nucleotide in the heavy chain, which leads to a single amino acid substitution in CDR3, and that they are identical at the light chain. This suggest that the subtle differences seen in idiotypic specificities may be determined by the single amino acid substitution within CDR3 of the heavy chain. Thus the structures of the IgM antibodies demonstrate that the expression of unmutated germline gene segments can generate autoreactive antibodies, while analysis of the IgG antibodies suggests that somatic mutation and antigenic selection may contribute to the production of autoantibodies in patients with MG.

DISCOVERY OF ANTIBODY REPERTOIRE IN CELL CULTURE SYSTEMS

Relevant antibody species are not always disclosed by assay of serum samples. The spectrum of myasthenia-specific autoantibodies is more completely disclosed in cell culture supernatants from peripheral lymphocytes after 6 days of culture than in serum [76]. In some patients, antibody species were found only in the cell culture supernatant and not in serum. The correlation with severity of disease and spontaneous production of different antibody species is also much better than the correlation with serum antibody species [105]. Of special interest is the finding that peripheral lymphocytes from almost all patients without antibodies in serum, so-called seronegative patients, produce antibodies in cell culture systems.

Another way of looking at specific B cells is to enumerate the numbers of B cells secreting antibodies binding to AChR and idiotopes on human monoclonal idiotypic and anti-idiotypic antibodies [54,106]. B-cell reactivity was estimated by enumerating cells secreting antibodies binding to affinity-purified AChR and to one idiotypic and one anti-idiotypic antibody. Antibody-secreting cells were detected in the blood of 91% of the patients and in 8% of the controls. The mean value of the antibody-secreting cells in the peripheral blood was 11.7 cells/10^6 PBMC in the patients compared with a mean value in controls of 0.16 cells/10^6 PBMC (Fig. 2).

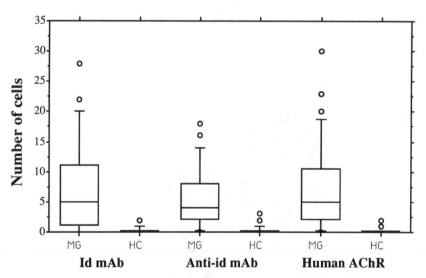

FIGURE 2. Box plot showing median and 90% confidence interval of numbers of B cells/10^6 PBMC secreting IgM antibodies binding to a human monoclonal idiotypic antibody and to a human monoclonal anti-idiotypic antibody and IgG antibodies binding to affinity-purified human skeletal muscle AChR in patients with MG and in healthy controls (HC).

B cells secreting antibodies to the idiotypic antibody were found in 75% of patients and in 12% of controls, while cells secreting antibodies against anti-idiotypic antibody were found in 89% of patients and 16% of controls. The mean values of B cells in patients reacting with idiotypic or anti-idiotypic antibody were 7 cells/10^6 and 6 cells/10^6 PBMC, respectively (Fig. 2).

Epstein-Barr-Virus Transformation of Peripheral Lymphocytes

One way of mapping the disease-specific repertoire of autoantibodies is Epstein-Barr-virus (EBV) transformation of peripheral lymphocytes followed by cloning of antibody-producing cells [107]. Using this approach, we have obtained clones producing monoclonal IgG and IgM antibodies with different specificities, both anti-AChR antibodies and idiotypic and anti-idiotypic antibodies. The repertoire as disclosed by EBV transformation does not represent that found in serum or as produced in cell culture by peripheral lymphocytes with regard to idiotypic specificity and heavy and light chains used.

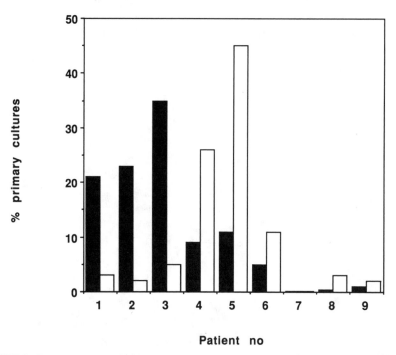

FIGURE 3. Prevalence of idiotypic (closed bars) and anti-idiotypic (open bars) antibodies in primary cultures of 10^5 EBV-transformed peripheral lymphocytes. Patients 1, 2, and 3 have severe MG; patients 4, 5, and 6 have MG in complete remission; and 7, 8, and 9 are healthy individuals.

An important observation made possible using the purified monoclonal antibodies was the existence of complementary idiotypes and anti-idiotypes in the same patient. These two antibodies bound to each other when incubated together and subjected to sucrose density gradient centrifugation [107].

The repertoire in primary cultures of EBV-transformed B cells in patients with severe MG or MG in complete remission and in healthy individuals is shown in Figure 3. There is a quantitative but not absolute difference between MG patients in different stages of disease and between MG patients and healthy controls. In this experiment, the prevalence of lines producing anti-idiotypic antibodies was higher in patients in complete remission.

The autoantibody repertoire as disclosed by EBV transformation varies considerably between patients. Figure 4 shows the prevalence of different antibody species in four patients with moderately severe MG.

IDIOTYPIC NETWORK IN MYASTHENIA GRAVIS

The first indication of the importance of an idiotypic network in MG came from studies of rabbits immunized with the cholinergic ligand bisQ [30]. The anti-bisQ antibodies showed pharmacological and immunological properties similar to those of the AChR and should thus belong to the class of "internal image" anti-idiotypic antibodies that bear some structural similarity to the AChR ligand binding site. A mouse monoclonal anti-idiotype bearing the internal image of the AChR binding site was produced by immunization with purified receptor antibodies against the ligand binding site of the AChR [108]. Immunization with this antibody induced antireceptor antibodies and signs of EAMG [31]. These observations have obvious implications to the etiology of MG, as autoantibody production may result not only from exposure to antigen but also from exposure to an internal image anti-idiotypic antibody.

An anti-idiotype may work in the opposite way by suppressing the disease. Active EAMG induced by administration of an idiotype specific for the AChR was suppressed by administration of the anti-idiotypic antibody [109].

Cross-reactive idiotypes on the AChR antibodies are present in mice with EAMG [110,111], but attempts to regulate the immune response using anti-idiotypes directed against cross-reactive idiotypes has generally failed [110], although cases of successful treatment have been reported [112]. Cross-reactive idiotypes are present in human MG [77], with one particular cross-reactive idiotype binding to the murine monoclonal antibody A-I21 and present in approximately 60% of the patients [78].

Anti-idiotypic antibodies are present in about 50-60% of MG patients [78]. Subpopulations of such antibodies might as discussed above trigger an immune response against the receptor. They might also have a protective role and downregulate the autoimmune response.

There is indirect evidence for a protective role of the anti-idiotypic antibodies in MG. The prevalence of naturally occurring anti-idiotypic antibodies

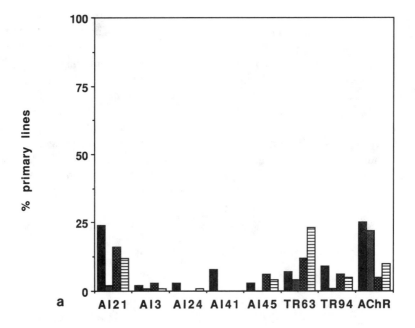

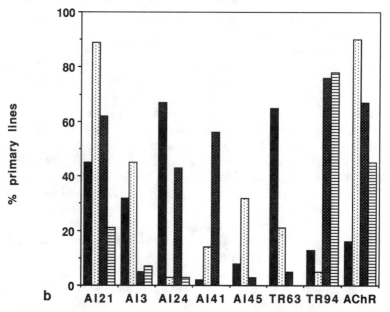

FIGURE 4. Prevalence of IgG (**a**) and IgM (**b**) antibodies in primary cultures of 10^5 EBV-transformed peripheral lymphocytes from four patients with moderately severe MG.

is higher in patients with mild generalized MG (stage IIa) of recent onset (less than 1 month since diagnosis) than in patients with severe generalized MG (stages IIb to IV) with prolonged disease (greater than 5 years) [78]. Studies of the development of anti-idiotypic and antireceptor antibodies showed that anti-idiotypic antibodies precede the receptor antibodies during the evolution of disease [113]. Patients examined before clinical signs of MG were evident had high concentrations of anti-idiotypic antibodies that disappeared when antireceptor antibodies appeared. An example of such a patient is shown in Figure 5. Examination of healthy relatives of MG patients showed a correlation between the presence of antireceptor antibodies and an abnormal single fiber electromyography. In contrast, a normal single fiber electromyography was detected in relatives with circulating anti-idiotypic antibodies, suggesting that the anti-idiotypes were able to inhibit the effect of the antireceptor antibodies [114]. Not one relative had the combination of antireceptor antibodies, anti-idiotypic antibodies, and abnormal single-single fiber electromyography.

The receptor antibodies of healthy children born to myasthenic mothers have a half-life that is significantly shorter than expected for normal IgG, whereas receptor antibodies of children with neonatal MG have an ab-

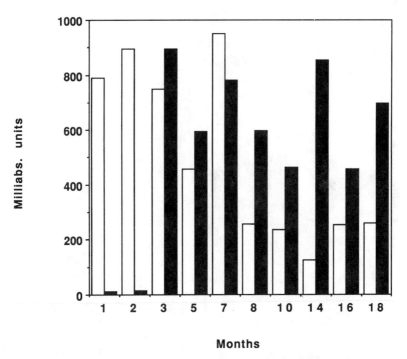

FIGURE 5. Time course of an idiotypic antibody (closed bars) and of an anti-idiotypic antibody (open bars) in a patient during development of spontaneous MG. Clinical symptoms of MG appeared at month 5.

normally long half-life [80,115]. There is also a strong correlation between neonatal myasthenia and the absence of anti-idiotypic antibodies [80], suggesting that anti-idiotypic antibodies in sufficient concentrations can protect the newborn from the effects of the maternal antibodies.

Patients treated with penicillamine sometimes develop a disease that is identical with spontaneous MG. Such patients commonly show a shift from idiotype to anti-idiotype dominance after discontinuation of the drug and clinical recovery as the disease heals [80]. The pattern of idiotypes and anti-idiotypic antibodies is shown in Figure 6 for one patient.

WHAT IS THE CAUSE OF THE BAD CORRELATION BETWEEN AUTOANTIBODIES AGAINST THE ACETYLCHOLINE RECEPTOR AND DISEASE?

In autoimmune disorders, the correlation between clinical symptoms and amount of disease-specific autoantibodies is generally poor. In MG, the antiacetylcholine receptor antibodies do have importance for the neuromuscular symptoms as shown by the effect of plasma exchange and drainage of lymph and the retransfusion experiments. There is a certain statistical correl-

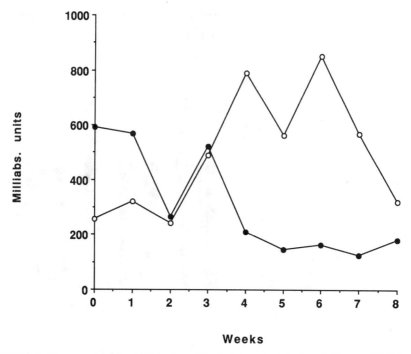

FIGURE 6. Time course of an idiotypic antibody (closed circles) and of an anti-idiotypic antibody (open circles) in a patient recovering from penicillamine-induced MG. Penicillamine treatment was stopped at week 0.

ation between severity of disease and amount of antireceptor antibodies, but there are numerous exceptions. Patients in complete remission may have very high concentrations and patients with severe disease no measurable antibodies at all.

One explanation for this discrepancy is certainly the kinetic properties of the antibodies as discussed earlier. The relevant antibody species are rapidly eliminated by binding to antigen and anti-idiotypic antibodies and thus are not present in serum. The comparison between antibody species produced in cultures of peripheral blood lymphocytes with those in serum also clearly indicates that the autoantibody repertoire in serum does not represent the whole antibody repertoire. The fact that peripheral cells from more than 90% of so-called seronegative patients do produce antibodies in cell culture further supports the assumption that relevant antibody species might not be present in serum.

An especially challenging observation is that autoantibodies regarded as specific for MG are found in numerous other disorders. Examples are first-degree relatives of patients with MG [114], patients with primary biliary cirrhosis [116], monoclonal immunoglobulins [117], thymomas [118], after bone marrow grafting [119], in certain hematological disorders [120], in healthy children of myasthenic mothers [115], and in identical twins discordant for MG [121]. Studies of the properties of the antibodies and of the antibody repertoire in such cases are particularly interesting since they may elucidate the difference between "nonpathogenic" and "pathogenic" auto-antibodies. Studies of the healthy twin in identical twins discordant for MG are particularly interesting since they may elucidate the relative roles of genetic, immune, and environmental factors that regulate the autoimmune process.

We studied a pair of identical twins, 47 years of age, who have been discordant for MG since age 15 years with regard to neuromuscular function and presence and properties of myasthenia-specific autoantibodies [121]. The autoantibody repertoire was tested in serum, as produced by peripheral lymphocytes in culture and as revealed by B-cell lines. The neurological examination of the myasthenic twin showed severely increased fatigability of muscles, accentuated by repetitive movements. Electrophysiological examination showed a pathological SFEMG. The healthy twin had no signs of impaired neuromuscular function on clinical and electrophysiological tests. The serum of the myasthenic twin contained 18.9 and the healthy 20.2 nmol toxin–receptor complex precipitated per liter of serum, and the spectra of antibodies in serum and produced by cultured peripheral blood mononuclear cells were very similar, as was the spectrum of antibodies as revealed in primary cultures of EBV-transformed cells. A Scatchard plot of the affinities of the serum antibodies against the AChR showed in both twins one high affinity antibody population with a K_o of 1.3×10^{-10} and 1.5×10^{-10} for the healthy and myasthenic twin, respectively. Mice injected with immunoglobulins from the twins showed a decrease in concentration of free receptor in their muscles. The amount of free receptor as compared with that of mice transfused with normal immunoglobulin preparations was similar for mice treated with immunoglobulins from the healthy and the myasthenic twin.

The marked similarity of the spectrum of autoantibodies suggests that the twins have a similar B-cell repertoire. The presence of disease-specific auto-antibodies and a high prevalence of B cells committed to make such antibodies in the healthy identical twin is a puzzling phenomenon when taking into account the pathogenetic mechanism of the autoantibodies. Since the spectra of antibodies were very similar in both individuals, differences in autoantibody affinity or idiotypic specificities as a cause of the discrepancy of symptoms should be unlikely, even though such a difference cannot be excluded. Differences in T-cell regulatory mechanisms should not explain the difference in clinical status between the twins, since differences in T-cell regulation should be reflected in autoantibody concentration or B-cell repertoire.

Extensive studies of the properties of the antibodies in primary biliary cirrhosis as compared with those in MG also failed to reveal absolute differences [116, 122–125]. Patients with primary biliary cirrhosis have a higher prevalence of IgM antireceptor antibodies, but usually also IgG antibodies. The affinities of the antibodies are high and similar to those in MG. The primary biliary cirrhosis patients had higher prevalence of antibodies binding to the ligand binding site of the receptor, a puzzling phenomenon since such antibodies are correlated with severe disease in MG. The idiotypic repertoire in serum, and as revealed by EBV-transformed cell lines, showed quantitative differences, but all species of antibodies found in MG were also found in primary biliary cirrhosis.

A study of AChR antibodies in patients with monoclonal gammopathies showed that 14/146 patients had antibody activity against the AChR localized to the monoclonal immunoglobulin [117]. The antireceptor antibodies were of IgG, IgM, and IgA isotypes, and the monoclonal immunoglobulins that were further characterized had similar high affinities for the AChR as antireceptor antibodies from MG patients and also bore the same idiotypes as found in patients with MG. None of the patients with monoclonal immunoglobulins binding to the AChR had any electrophysiological or clinical signs of disturbed neuromuscular function. If antireceptor antibodies were indeed pathological, one would expect the myeloma patients to have noticeable muscle weakness. Others [126,127] have also detected autoreactive monoclonal immunoglobulins in myeloma patients who do not manifest any pathological symptoms.

In healthy first-degree relatives of MG patients, low concentrations of receptor antibodies could be demonstrated in 54% of the 58 relatives, anti-idiotypic antibodies in 37%, and pathological and borderline single fiber EMG in 45%. None of the relatives showed any clinical or electrophysiological signs of muscle weakness [114]. Newborn children of MG mothers always have the same or slightly higher antibody concentration as the mother at birth, but only about 12% show symptoms of transient neonatal MG [115].

There may be several explanations for the discrepancy between symptoms and antibody concentration in serum in a disease that is supposedly antibody mediated. One might be that the antigen usually used for the determination of antireceptor antibodies is detergent extracted from muscle and thus not identical to the antigen in vivo. This prompted us to explore the effects of antibodies from patients with MG on a receptor in situ using the celline TE671 and to compare them with the effects of antibodies found in patients without neuromuscular symptoms. Both the blocking effects on α-bungarotoxin binding and the increase in turnover time of receptors were measured using this cell line. There was, however, no difference between the antibodies in ability either to cause blocking or to increase in internalization between the patients with MG or primary biliary cirrhosis or patients with monoclonal gammopathies.

Differences on the receptor level may encompass individual variations in the multiple adaptive and protective factors operating to maintain neuromuscular transmission by regulating the rate of receptor degradation and synthesis following antibody binding in vivo. Regulatory mechanism such as antiidiotypic antibodies seem to have an affect on receptor antibody expression and on the receptor, as discussed previously. Differences in the antibody species present have never been shown to be a major factor for their pathogenicity, although there is a certain statistical difference between mild and severe disease with regard to idiotype pattern and presence of antibodies against the ligand binding site of the receptor.

Clearly, factors other than the concentration, specificities, idiotypes, avidity, and capacity to transfer neuromuscular blockade to experimental animals must be of importance. Such mechanisms may be individual variations in the adaptive factors that maintain neuromuscular function by regulation of receptor degradation and synthesis following damage by antibody binding or by regulating acetylcholine release.

Another interesting possibility is that the immune response and the binding of antibodies are modulated in other, until now unknown ways. Antibodies against the β_2AR [88] might theoretically have such modulatory effects. Approximately 18% of the MG patients have antibodies against residues 172–197 of the human β_2-AR, and the number of patients having antibodies against the entire receptor are most probably higher. The β_2-AR is present on human skeletal muscle [128] and on the cells of the immune system [129]. The β_2-AR has been postulated as being the mediator by which the sympathetic nervous system interacts with the immune system. Agonists to the β_2-AR increase muscle contractility [130], which is in accordance with the clinical observation that MG patients may benefit from epinephrine derivatives and deteriorate when given β_2-AR-blocking agents. Thus antibodies with antagonist function might lead to increased muscle fatigue.

Addition of the β_2-AR agonist isoproterenol to a muscle cell culture results in an increased rate of AChR desensitization [42]. Antibodies against the β_2-AR with agonist functions might then further decrease the number of functional AChR on the endplate.

The β_2-AR are present in high density on human lymphocytes. These cells are thus subjected to regulation by epinephrine. This implies that antibodies that act as ligands for the β_2-AR may also influence the function of the immune system. Antibodies with agonist action might increase the production of intracellular cAMP, leading to increased antibody synthesis. Stimulation of the β_2-AR is probably important for the activation of suppressor T cells [131]. Thus antagonist-like antibodies to the β_2-AR could suppress suppressor T-cell function, possibly leading to an enhanced immune response. Support for this theory comes from experiments showing that ablation of the sympathetic system results in a more severe form of both EAMG [132] and experimental allergic encephalomyelitis [133]. The possible effects on neuroimmunological and neurophysiological interactions by anti-β_2-AR antibodies in MG leads to the conclusion that these antibodies must be considered as possible participants in the pathological response in MG.

EFFECTS OF TREATMENT OF MG WITH INTRAVENOUS HUMAN IgG OR ANTIBODIES AGAINST CD4⁺ CELLS GIVES NEW INSIGHT INTO THE REGULATION OF THE AUTOIMMUNE PROCESS

Intravenous Human IgG

Treatment with high dose intravenous IgG has been beneficial in many proven or supposedly autoimmune disorders [134]. IgG has also been claimed to be effective in the treatment of MG, although the studies performed thus far are poorly documented with regard to effect on antibody and T-cell response and lack objective evaluation of symptoms [135,136].

Several mechanisms of the action of IgG have been proposed. These include reversible blockade of Fc receptors of the cells of the reticuloendothelial cells, Fc-dependent feedback of autoantibody synthesis by B cells; modulation of T-cell function; interference with complement-mediated tissue destruction; modulation of cytokine secretion; and V-region-dependent modulation of the autoimmune repertoire [134]. The last mechanism has been suggested to be of importance due to several experimental findings, including decreased concentration of autoantibodies during treatment, binding of autoantibodies to a column of IgG, and the fact that IgG contains anti-idiotypic antibodies against several autoantibodies [134]. IgG obtained from healthy individuals has a clear affect on the autoimmune repertoire. Idiotypic suppression of antibodies against the AChR was obtained by treatment of newborn mice with a natural syngeneic anti-idiotypic monoclonal antibody [137]. Infusion of normal mice with pooled normal mouse IgG induced a selective stimulation of peripheral autoreactive CD4⁺ T and B cells [138]. These observations suggest that antibodies from healthy individuals have the ability to modulate the expression of the autoimmune repertoire.

We have treated two patients with MG with IgG 0.4 g/kg body weight for 5 days. One patient reported a moderate subjective improvement that could not be verified using electrophysiological tests. The other patient's condition did not change.

The serum concentration of antibodies against the AChR did not change. There was, however, marked changes in the concentration of different species of idiotypic and anti-idiotypic antibodies (Fig. 7). These changes might partly be explained by complex formation between IgG and autoantibodies, since increased immune complex formation, as detected by sucrose density gradient centrifugation, was present in both patients during and up to 1 week after the treatment period. There was also a marked increase in the T-cell stimulation to DNA synthesis by two murine monoclonal antibodies that recognize recurrent idiotopes on the autoantibodies (Fig. 8). Thus, although we could not objectively verify any clinical improvement, the treatment had marked effects on the autoimmune T- and B-cell repertoire with general stimulation of idiotype- and anti-idiotype-specific T cells and changes in the

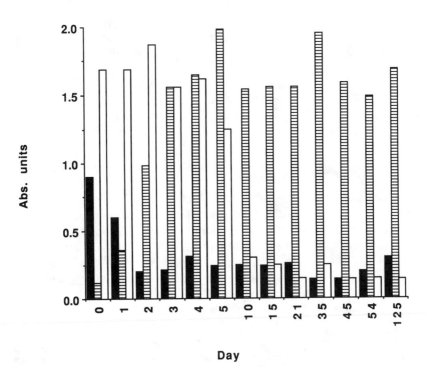

Day

FIGURE 7. Serum levels of two idiotypic antibodies, defined by binding to the murine monoclonal antibodies A-I21 (closed bars) and A-I3 (Hatched bars) and of one anti-idiotypic antibody binding to TR63 (open bars) during and after treatment with human IgG.

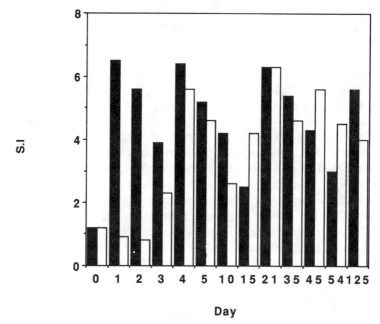

FIGURE 8. Stimulation index obtained by incubating PBMC from one patient with two murine monoclonal antibodies, one idiotypic antibody, A-I21 (closed bars) and one anti-idiotypic antibody TR63 (open bars) during and after treatment with human IgG.

concentration of certain species of idiotypic and anti-idiotypic antibodies in the serum of the patients.

Antibodies Against CD4+ Cells

Monoclonal antibodies against the CD4 antigen on T cells have been proposed to be effective in the treatment of both experimental autoimmune diseases, including experimental autoimmune MG [139] and human autoimmune disorders such as rheumatoid arthritis [140]. Anti-CD4 antibody treatment has thus far been used in human diseases in which there are no good objective verifications either of disease-specific immunity or of clinical improvement. We have recently treated a 57-year-old woman with severe myasthenic symptoms for 7 days with 25 mg/day of a chimeric (human constant regions and murine variable regions) anti-CD4 monoclonal antibody [141]. The therapeutic effect was assessed by muscle function tests and by single fiber EMG and the effects on the immune system by assessing lymphocyte phenotypes and specific and nonspecific T- and B-cell responses.

Clinical and electrophysiological improvement was evident on the fourth day of treatment, was most pronounced during the second to eighth weeks, and was still present at the 5 months follow-up. A progressive deterioration started 3 months after initiation of the treatment. The clinical and electrophysiological effects of the treatments are shown in Figure 9. There was a complete normalization of the EMG. The treatment resulted in rapid decrease in the percentage of $CD4^+$ and $CD8^+$ cells. The $CD4^+$ cells recovered to 50% of pretreatment value at 5 months follow-up. The CD4/CD8 ratio was persistently decreased during 5 months of follow-up. Both spontaneous and stimulated IL-2 production and T-cell proliferation was abolished during the anti-CD4 treatment. During several months after completion of therapy T cells were spontaneously more activated than before therapy (Fig. 10). The idiotypic and anti-idiotypic antibody and the affinity-purified receptor induced a more pronounced T-cell activation during the 5 months of follow-up (Fig. 11).

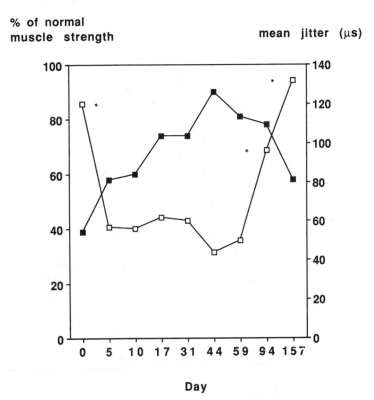

FIGURE 9. Changes in the mean jitter of single fiber EMG (open squares) and changes in the arm muscle strength (closed squares) during and after treatment with an anti-CD4+ antibody. Recordings with a mean jitter above 90 showed significant blocking (*).

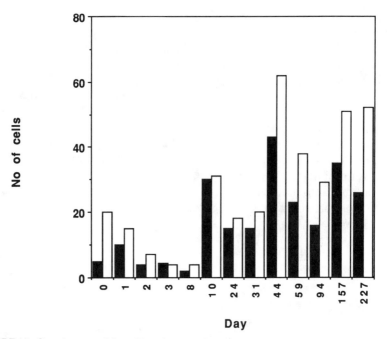

FIGURE 10. Spontaneous (closed bars) and IL-2 (open bars) induced stimulation of PBMC during and after treatment with an anti-CD4$^+$ antibody measured as the numbers of IFN-γ-secreting cells/10^5 PBMC.

The amount of antibodies against the AChR showed a tendency to increase during and after treatment (Fig. 12) and so did the number of B cells producing antibodies against both AChR and idiotypic and anti-idiotypic human monoclonal antibodies. Thus the effect of the treatment seemed to be a stimulation of both disease-specific and -nonspecific B- and T-cell responses rather than a suppression, although the net effect might well be a certain suppression of T-cell-mediated responses. A suppression of T cells would lead to a decrease in cytokine secretion and thus a decreased inflammatory response around the endplate. A recent study has shown that inflammatory cells are indeed present at the endplate in most patients with MG [142]. Such an inflammation might further compromise the deranged neuromuscular function. Part of the beneficial effect of this antibody treatment could thus be to decrease the inflammatory response around the endplate.

CONCLUSIONS

MG is commonly discussed as the prototype of an antibody-mediated autoimmune disease. Studies of disease-specific AChR-specific T and B cells have, however, contributed little to the understanding of the specific disease mechanisms. The fine specificity of the AChR antibodies does not allow distinction

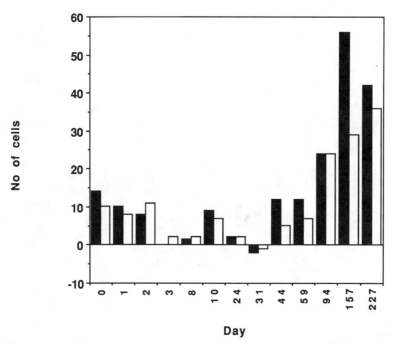

FIGURE 11. T-cell stimulation induced by a human monoclonal idiotypic (closed bars) and a human monoclonal anti-idiotypic antibody (open bars) measured as the numbers of IFN-γ-secreting cells/10^5 PBMC during and after treatment with an anti-CD4$^+$ antibody.

between antibodies that are truly pathogenic. The same kind of antigen and idiotypic specificities are found on antibodies in MG, as well as on antibodies in monoclonal gammopathies, primary biliary cirrhosis, and other conditions not accompanied by neuromuscular symptoms. Thus the concept of pathogenic versus natural autoantibodies has no experimental support.

Interactions between idiotypic and anti-idiotypic antibodies and T cells are probably important for the modulation of the disease. Factors that might modulate both the immune response and the AChR effects include the possible effects of antibodies against the β_2-AR.

The successful treatment of MG using antibodies against CD4$^+$ lymphocytes resulted in long-lasting subjective and objective improvement of a patient and—paradoxically—in an increase in T-cell activation by specific antigens and antibodies and in an increase in production of receptor-associated antibodies. These observations suggest that the current simplistic concept of the autoantibodies against the receptor as the cause of the symptoms does not reveal the whole truth. Undoubtedly, other modulatory systems exist that can interact and alter the immune response or AChR function. The development of successful treatment will depend not only on the characterization of the pathological antibody populations but also on the elucidation of these modulating systems.

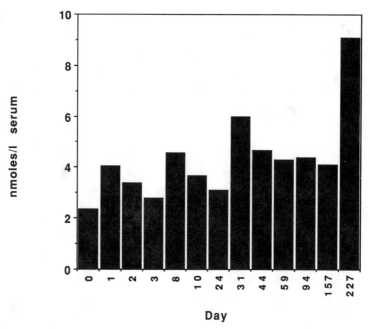

Day

FIGURE 12. Antibodies against the AChR in the serum of a patient during and after treatment with an anti-CD4$^+$ antibody.

REFERENCES

1. Willis T (1685): "The London Practice of Physick." London: Basset & Crooke.
2. Fambrough DM, Drachman DB, Satyamurti S (1973). Neuromuscular junction in myasthenia gravis: Decreased acetycholine receptors. Science 182:293–295.
3. Simpson JA (1960): Myasthenia gravis: A new hypothesis. Scott Med J 5:419–430.
4. Bergström K, Franksson C, Matell G, von Reis G (1973): The effect of thoracic duct lymph drainage in myasthenia gravis. Eur Neurol 9:157–167.
5. Bergström K, Franksson C, Matell G, Nilsson BY, Persson A, von Reis G, Stensman R (1975): Drainage off the thoracic duct lymph in twelve patients with myasthenia gravis. Eur Neurol 13:19–30.
6. Patrick J, Lindstrom J (1973): Autoimmune response to acetylcholine receptors. Science 180:871–873.
7. Lefvert AK, Bergström K, Matell G, Osterman PO, Pirskanen R (1978): Determination of acetylcholine receptor antibodies in myasthenia gravis: Clinical usefulness and pathogenetic implications. J Neurol Neurosurg Psychiatry 41:394–403.
8. Lindstrom J (1977): An assay for antibodies to human acetylcholine receptor in serum from myasthenia gravis patients. Clin Immunol Immunopathol 7:36–43.
9. Cohen MS (1987): Epidemiology of myasthenia gravis. Monogr Allergy 21:246–251.

10. Oosterhuis HJGH (1964): Studies in myasthenia gravis. Part I. A clnical study of 180 patients. J Neurol Sci 1:512–546.

11. Namba T, Brunner NG, Grob D (1978): Myasthenia gravis in patients with thymoma, with particular reference to onset after thymectomy. Medicine 57:411–433.

12. Blalock A, Mason MF, Morgan HJ, Riven S (1939): Myasthenia gravis and tumors of the thymic region. Report of a case in which tumor was removed. Surgery 110:544–561.

13. Compston D, Vincent A, Newsom-Davis J, Batchelor J (1980): Clinical, pathological, HLA antigen and immunological evidence for disease heterogeneity in myasthenia gravis. Brain 103:579–601.

14. Carlsson B, Wallin J, Pirskanen R, Matell G, Smith CIE (1990): Different HLA DR-DQ associations in subgroups of idiopathic myasthenia gravis. Immunogenetics 31:285–290.

15. Christiansen FT, Pollack MS, Garlepp MJ, Dawkins RL (1984): Myasthenia gravis and HLA antigens in American blacks and other races. J Neuroimmunol 7:121–129.

16. Christadoss P (1989): Imunogenetics of experimental autoimmune myasthenia gravis. Crit Rev Immunol 9:247–278.

17. Granato DA, Fulipus BW, Moody JF (1976): Experimental myasthenia gravis in Balb/C mice immunized with rat acetylcholine receptor from rat denervated muscle. Proc Natl Acad Sci USA 73:2872–2880.

18. Berman PW, Patrick J (1980): Experimental myasthenia gravis: a murine system. J Exp Med 151:204—207.

19. Pachner AR, Kantor FS (1983): The relation of clinical disease to antibody titre, proliferative response and neurophysiology in murine experimental autoimmune myasthenia gravis. Clin Exp Immunol 51:543–549.

20. Jermy AC, Fisher CA, Vincent AC, Willcox NA, Newsom-Davis J (1989): Experimental autoimmune myasthenia gravis induced in mice without adjuvant: Genetic susceptibility and adoptive transfer of weakness. J Autoimmun 2:675–688.

21. Lennon VA, Lindstrom JM, Seybold ME (1975): Experimental autoimmune myasthenia gravis: A model in rats and guinea pigs. J Exp Med 141:1365–1375.

22. Engel AG, Tsujihata JM, Lennon VA (1976): The motor endplate in myasthenia gravis and in experimental autoimmune myasthenia gravis, a quantitative ultrastructural study. Ann NY Acad Sci 274:60–79.

23. Engel AG, Santa T (1971): Histometric analysis of the ultrastructure of the neuromuscular junction in myasthenia gravis and in the myasthenic syndrome. Ann NY Acad Sci 183:46–54.

24. Zoda T, Yeh T-M, Krolick KA (1990): Clonotypic analysis of antiacetylcholine receptor antibodies from experimental autoimmune myasthenia gravis–sensitive Lewis rats and experimental autoimmune myasthenia gravis–insensitive Wistar Furth rats. J Immunol 146:663–670.

25. Toyka KV, Drachman DB, Pestronk A, Kao J (1975): Myasthenia gravis: Passive transfer from man to mouse. Science 190:397–399.

26. Lingstrom JM, Engel AG, Seybold ME (1976): Pathological mechanisms in

experimental autoimmune myasthenia gravis: Passive transfer of experimental autoimmune myasthenia gravis in rats with antiacetylcholine receptor antibodies. J Exp Med 144:739–753.

27. Gomez CM, Richman DP (1983): Anti-acetylcholine receptor antibodies directed against the α-bungarotoxin binding site induce a unique form of experimental myasthenia. Proc Natl Acad Sci USA 80:4089–4093.

28. Lennon VA, Lamberg EH (1980): Myasthenia gravis induced by monoclonal antibodies to acetylcholine receptors. Nature 285:238–240.

29. Wekerle H, Hohlfeldt R, Ketelsen UP, Kalden JR, Kalies I (1981): Thymic myogenesis, T-lymphocytes and the pathogenesis of myasthenia gravis. Ann NY Acad Sci 377:455–476.

30. Wasserman NH, Penn AS, Freimuth PI, Treptow N, Wentzel S, Cleveland WL, Erlanger BF (1982): A new route to anti-acetylcholine receptor antibodies and experimental myasthenia gravis. Proc Natl Acad Sci USA 79:4810–4814.

31. Lefvert AK, Fulpius BW (1984): Receptor-like properties of a monoclonal anti-idiotypic antibody against an anti-acetylcholine receptor antibody. Scand J Immunol 19:485–489.

32. Raftery MA, Vandlen RL, Reed KL, Lee T (1976): Characterization of *Torpedo californica* acetylcholine receptor-subunit composition and ligand binding properties. Cold Spring Harbor Symp Quant Biol 40:193–202.

33. Noda M, Furutani Y, Takahashi H, Yoyosato M, Tanabe T, Shimizi S, Kikyotani S, Kayano T, Hirose T, Inayama S, Numa S (1983): Cloning and sequence analysis of calf cDNA and human genomic DNA encoding α-subunit precursor of muscle acetylcholine receptor. Nature 305:818–823.

34. Noda M, Takahashi H, Tanabe T, Toyosato M, Kikyotani S, Furutani Y, Hirose T, Takashima H, Inayama S, Miyata T, Numa S (1983): Structural homology of *Torpedo californica* acetylcholine receptor subunits. Nature 302:528–532.

35. Hamilton SL, Pratt DR, Eaton DC (1985): Arrangement of the subunits of the nicotinic acetylcholine receptor of *Torpedo californica* as determined by α-neurotoxin cross-linking. Biochemistry 1985:2210–2219.

36. Klymkowsky MW, Stroud RM (1979): Immunospecific identification and three-dimensional structure of membrane-bound acetylcholine receptor from *Torpedo californica*. J Mol Biol 128:319–334.

37. Dennis M, Giraudat J, Kotzyba-Hibert F, Goeldner M, Hirth C, Chang JY, Lazure C, Cretien M, Changeux JP (1988): Amino acids of the *Torpedo marmorata* acetycholine receptor α-subunit labeled by a photoaffinity ligand for the acetylcholine binding site. Biochemistry 27:2346–2357.

38. Mishina M, Tobimatsu T, Imoto K, Tanaka K, Fujita Y, Fukuda K, Kurasaki M, Takahashi H, Morimoto Y, Hirose T, Inayama S, Takahashi T, Kuno M, Numa S (1985): Location of functional regions of acetylcholine receptor α-subunit by site-directed mutagenesis. Nature 313:364–369.

39. Dowding AJ, Hall ZW (1987): Monoclonal antibodies specific for each of the two toxin-binding sites of *Torpedo* acetylcholine receptor. Biochemistry 26:6372–6381.

40. Gu Y, Silberstein L, Hall ZW (1985): The effects of a myasthenic serum on the acetylcholine receptors of C2 myotubes. 1. Immunological distinction between the two toxin-binding sites of the receptor. J Neurosci 5:1909–1916.

41. Magleby KL, Pallotta BA (1981): A study of desensitization of acetylcholine receptors using a nerve-released transmitter in the frog. J Physiol 316:225–250.

42. Huganir RL, Delcour AH, Greengard P, Hess GP (1986): Phosphorylation of the nicotinic acetylcholine receptor regulates its rate of desensitization. Nature 321:774–776.

43. Kao I, Drachman DB (1977): Thymic muscle cells bear acetylcholine receptor: Possible relation to myasthenia gravis. Science 195:74–75.

44. Hohlfeld R, Kalies I, Kohleisen B, Heininger K, Conti-Tronconi BM, Toyka KV (1986): Myasthenia gravis: Stimulation of antireceptor autoantibodies by auto-reactive T cell lines. Neurology 36:618–621.

45. Hohlfeld R, Toyka KV, Tzartos SJ, Carson W, Conti-Tronconi BM (1987): Human T-helper lymphocytes in myasthenia gravis recognize the nicotinic receptor α-subunit. Proc Natl Acad Sci USA 84:5379–5383.

46. Hohlfeld R, Toyka KV, Miner LL, Walgrave SL, Conti-Tronconi BM (1988): Amphipathic segment of the nicotinic receptor alpha subunit contains epitopes recognized by T lymphocytes in myasthenia gravis. J Clin Invest 81:657–660.

47. Brocke S, Brautbar C, Steinman L, Abramsky O, Rothbard J, Neuman D, Fuchs S, Mozes E (1988): In vitro proliferative responses and antibody titers specific to human acetycholine receptor synthetic peptides in patients with myasthenia gravis and relation to HLA class II genes. J Clin Invest 82:1894–1900.

48. Harcourt GC, Sommer N, Rithbard J, Willcox HNA, Newsom-Davies J (1988): A juxta-membrane epitope on the human acetylcholine receptor recognized by T cells in myasthenia gravis. J Clin Invest 82:1295–1300.

49. Protti MP, Manfredi AA, Straub C, Wu X, Howard JF, Contini-Tronconi BM (1990): Use of synthetic peptides to establish antihuman acetylcholine receptor CD4$^+$ cell lines from myasthenia gravis patients. J Immunol 144:1711–1720.

50. Newsom-Davis J, Harcourt G, Sommer DB, Willcox N, Rothbard B (1989): T-cell reactivity in myasthenia gravis. J Autoimmun 2(Suppl):101–108.

51. Allen PM, Matsueda GR, Haber E, Unanue ER (1985): Specificity of the T cell receptor: Two different determinants are generated by the same peptide and the I-a^k molecule. J Immunol 135:368–373.

52. Åhlberg R, Yi Q, Eng H, Pirskanen R, Lefvert AK (1992): T cell epitopes on the human acetylcholine receptor alpha-subunit residues 10–84 in myasthenia gravis. Scand J Immunol 36:435–442.

53. Yi Q, Åhlberg R, Lefvert AK (1992): T cells with specificity for idiotypic determinants on human monoclonal autoantibodies in myasthenia gravis. Res Immunol 143:149–156.

54. Qing Yi, Lefvert AK (1993): Acetylcholine receptor specific T and B cells in myasthenia gravis. Ann NY Acad Sci (in press).

55. Yi Q, Lefvert AK (1993): Human muscle acetylcholine receptor reactive T and B lymphocytes in myasthenia gravis. J Neuroimmunol 42:215–222.

56. Oksenberg JR, Sherrit M, Begovich AB, Erlich HA, Bernard CC, Cavaiil-Sforza LL, Steinman L (1989): T cell receptor Vα and Cα alleles associated with multiple sclerosis and myashenia gravis. Proc Natl Acad Sci USA 86:988–992.

57. Tesch H, Hohlfeld R, Toyka KV (1989): Southern blot show no signs of a rearranged T or B cell clone in the thymus of myasthenia gravis patients. J Neuroimmunol 21:169–176.

58. Grunewald J, Åhlberg R, Lefvert AK, Dersimonian H, Wigzell H, Jansson CH (1991): Abnormal T cell expansion and V gene usage in myasthenia gravis patients. Scand J Immunol 34:161–168.

59. Luther MA, Schoepfer R, Whiting P, Casey B, Blatt Y, Montal MS, Montal M, Lindstrom J (1989): A muscle acetylcholine receptor is expressed in the human cerebellar medulloblstoma cell line TE671. J Neurosci 9:1082–1096.

60. Engel AG, Santa T (1971): Histometric analysis of the ultrastructure of the neuromuscular junction in myasthenia gravis and in the myasthenic syndrome. Ann NY Acad Sci 183:46–54.

61. Sahashi K, Engel AG, Lambert EH, Howard FM (1980): Ultrastructural localization of the terminal and lytic ninth complement component (C_9) at the motor end-plate in myasthenia gravis. J Neurol 39:162–172.

62. Lennon VA, Seybold ME, Lindstrom JM, Cochrane C, Ulevitch R (1978): Role of complement in the pathogenesis of experimental autoimmune myasthenia gravis. J Exp Med 147:973–983.

63. Biesecker G, Gomez CM (1989): Inhibition of acute passive transfer experimental autoimmune myasthenia gravis with Fab antibody to complement C6. J Immunol 142:2654–2659.

64. Behan WMH, Behan PO (1979): Immune complexes in myasthenia gravis. J Neurol Neurosurg Psychiatry 42:595–599.

65. Drachman DB, Adams RN, Josifek LF, Self SG (1982): Functional activities of autoantibodies to acetylcholine receptors and the clinical severity of myasthenia gravis. N Engl J Med 307:769–775.

66. Sterz R, Hohlfeld R, Rajki K, Kaul M, Heininger K, Peper K, Toyka KV (1986): Effector mechanisms in myasthenia gravis: End-plate function after passive transfer of IgG, Fab, and F(ab')$_2$ hybrid molecules. Muscle Nerve 9:306–312.

67. Tzartos SJ, Sophianos D, Zimmerman K, Starzinski-Powitz A (1986): Anti-genic modulation of human myotube acetylcholine receptor by myasthenic sera. Serum titer determines receptor internalization rate. J Immunol 136:3231–3238.

68. Berman PW, Heinemann SF (1984): Antigenic modulation of junctional acetylcholine receptor is not sufficient to account for the development of myasthenia gravis in receptor immunized mice. J Immunol 132:711–717.

69. Lefvert AK, Cuenoud S, Fulpius BW (1981): Binding properties and subclass distribution of anti-acetylcholine receptor antibodies in myasthenia gravis. J Neuroimmunol 1:125–135.

70. Lefvert AK, Cuenoud S, Fulpius BW (1981): A new evidence for true immuno-pharmacologic blockade in myasthenia gravis. In Pepeu G (ed): "Cholinergic Mechanisms." New York: Plenum Press, pp 333–343.

71. Takamori M, Okumura S, Nagata M, Yoshikawa H (1988): Myasthenogenic significance of synthetic α subunit peptide 183–200 of *Torpedo californica* and human acetylcholine receptor. J Neurol Sci 85:121–129.

72. Vernet-der Garabedian B, Morel E, Bach JF (1986): Heterogeneity of antibodies directed against the α-bungarotoxin binding site on human acetylcholine receptor and severity of myasthenia gravis. J Neuroimmunol 12:65–74.

73. Lefvert AK, Bergström K (1977): Immunoglobulins in myasthenia gravis: Effect of human lymph IgG$_3$ and F(ab')$_2$ fragments on a cholinergic receptor preparation from *Torpedo marmorata*. Eur J Clin Invest 7:115–119.

74. Rodgaard A, Nielsen FC, Djurup R, Somnier F, Gammeltoft S (1987): Acetyl-choline receptor antibody in myasthenia gravis: Predominance of IgG subclasses 1 and 3. Clin Exp Immunol 67:82–88.

75. Arnon R (1975): Enzyme inhibition by antibodies. Acta Endocrinol 78(Suppl 194):133–153.

76. Lefvert AK, Sundén H, Holm G (1986): Acetylcholine receptor antibodies and anti-idiotypic antibodies produced in blood lymphocyte cultures from patients with myasthenia gravis. Scand J Immunol 23:655–662.

77. Lefvert AK (1988): Anti-acetylcholine receptor related idiotypes in myasthenia gravis. J Autoimmun 1:63–72.

78. Lefvert AK (1988): Anti-idiotype antibodies in myasthenia gravis. In Bona C (ed): "Biological Applications of Anti-Idiotypes." Vol. II. Boca Raton, FL: CRC Press, pp 69–91.

79. Lefvert AK (1987): Idiotypes and anti-idiotypes of human autoantibodies to the acetylcholine receptor. Monogr Allergy 22:57–70.

80. Lefvert AK (1986): Auto-anti-idiotypic immunity and acetylcholine receptors. In Cruse JM (ed): "Concepts in Immunopathology–Immunoregulation." Vol. 3. Basel: Karger, pp 285–310.

81. Eng H, Lefvert AK (1988): Isolation of an anti-idiotypic antibody with acetyl-choline receptor-like binding properties from a myasthenia gravis patients. Ann Inst Pasteur 139:569–580.

82. Aarli JA, Stefansson K, Marton LSG, Wollman RL (1990): Patients with myas-thenia gravis and thymoma have in their sera IgG aiútoantibodies against titin Clin Exp Immunol 82:284–288.

83. Connor RI, Lefvert AK, Benes SC, Lang RW (1990): Incidence and reactivity pattern of skeletal and heart reactive autoantibodies in the sera of patients with myasthenia gravis. J Neuroimmunol 26:147–157.

84. Hofstad H, Ohm OJ, Mork SJ, Aarli JA (1984): Heart disease in myasthenia gravis. Acta Neurol Scand 70:176–184.

85. Levinson AI, Lisak RP, Zweiman B, Kornstein M (1985): Phenotypic and functional analysis of lymphocytes in myasthenia gravis. Springer Semin Immu-nopathol 8:209–233.

86. Müller K, Andersson LC (1984): Antibodies against human neuroblastoma cells in the sera of patients with myasthenia gravis. J Neuroimmunol 7:97–105.

87. Lu C-Z, Link H, Mo Z-A, Xiao B-G, Zhang Y-L, Qin Z (1991): Antipresynaptic membrane receptor antibodies in myasthenia gravis. J Neurol Sci 102:39–45.

88. Eng H, Magnusson Y, Matell G, Lefvert AK, Saponja R, Hoebeke J (1992): β_2-Adrenergic receptor antibodies in myasthenia gravis. J Autoimmun 5:213–227.

89. Tzartos SJ, Lindstrom JM (1980): Monoclonal antibodies used to probe acetyl-choline receptor structure: Localization of the main immunogenic region and detection of similarities between subunits. Proc Natl Acad Sci USA 77:755–759.

90. Tzartos SJ, Seybold ME, Lindstrom JM (1982): Specificities of antibodies to acetylcholine receptors in sera from myasthenia gravis patients measured by monoclonal antibodies. Proc Natl Acad Sci USA 79:188–192.

91. Tzartos SJ, Kolka A, Walgrave SL, Conti-Tronconi BM (1988): Localization of

the main immunogenic region of human muscle acetylcholine receptor to residues 67–76 of the α-subunit. Proc Natl Acad Sci USA 85:2899–2903.

92. Ralston S, Sarin V, Thanh HL, Rivier J, Fox JL, Lindstrom J (1987): Synthetic peptides used to locate the α bungarotoxin binding site and immunogenic regions on α-subunits of the nicotinic acetylcholine receptor. Biochemistry 26:3261–3266.

93. Souroujon MC, Neumann D, Pizzighella S, Safran A, Fuchs S (1986): Localization of a highly immunogenic region on the acetylcholine receptor α-subunit. Biochem Biophys Res Commun 135:82–89.

94. Mulac-Jericevic B, Kurisake J, Atassi MZ (1987): Profile of the continuous antigenic regions on the extracellular part of the α-chain of an acetylcholine receptor. Proc Natl Acad Sci USA 84:3633–3637.

95. Sano M, McCormick DJ, Talib S, Griesmann GJ, Lennon VA (1991): Identification of three extended antibody-binding segments in recombinant human muscle acetylcholine receptor a subunit extracellular domain 1–210. Int Immunol 3:983–989.

96. Eng H, Bergman T, Carlquist M, Jörnvall H, Åhlberg R, Lefvert AK (1992): Antigenic peptides of the nicotinic acetylcholine receptor α-subunit reactive with myasthenia gravis patient sera. In "Autoantibodies in Myasthenia Gravis." Stockholm, Sweden: Karolinska Institute.

97. Eng H, Bergman T, Åhlberg R, Lefvert AK (1992): Fine specificity analysis of myasthenia gravis sera for the human acetylcholine receptor α-subunit residues 10–84. In "Autoantibodies in Myasthenia Gravis." Stockholm, Sweden: Karolinska Institute.

98. Popot JL, Changeux J-P (1984): Nicotinic receptor of acetylcholine: Structure of an oligomeric integral membrane protein. Physiol Rev 64:1162–1239.

99. Lennon VA, Griesmann GE (1989): Evidence against acetylcholine receptor having a main immunogenic region as target for autoantibodies in myasthenia gravis. Neurology 39:1069–1076.

100. Lefvert AK (1982): Differences in the interaction of acetylcholine receptor antibodies with receptor from normal, denervated and myasthenic human muscle. J Neurol Neurosurg Psychiatry 45:70–73.

101. Weinberg CB, Hall ZW (1979): Antibodies from patients with myasthenia gravis recognize determinants unique to extrajunctional acetylcholine receptors. Proc Natl Acad Sci USA 76:504–508.

102. Lefvert AK (1978): Immunoglobulins in myasthenia gravis: Kinetic properties of the receptor antibody studied during lymph drainage. J Clin Exp Immunol 34:111–117.

103. Lefvert AK, Matell G (1978). Thoracic duct lymph drainage in myasthenia gravis: Clinical effect and kinetic studies of the acetylcholine receptor antibody. In Dau PC (ed): "Plasmapheresis and the Immunobiology of Myasthenia Gravis." New York: Houghton-Mifflin, pp 151–160.

104. Victor KD, Pascual V, Lefvert AK, Capra JD (1992): Human anti-acetylcholine receptor antibodies use variable gene segments analogous to those used in autoantibodies of various specificities. Mol Immunol 29:1501–1506.

105. Lefvert AK, Holm G, Sundén H, Pirskanen R (1987): Cellular production of

antibodies related to the acetylcholine receptor in myasthenia gravis: Correlation with clinical stage. Scand J Immunol 25:265–273.

106. Yi Q, Lefvert AK (1993): Idiotypic and anti-idiotypic T and B lymphocytes in myasthenia gravis. J Immunol 149:3423–3426.

107. Lefvert AK, Holm G (1987): Idiotypic network in myasthenia gravis demonstrated by human monoclonal B-cell lines. Scand J Immunol 26:573–579.

108. Lefvert AK, James RW, Alloid C, Fulpius BW (1982): A monoclonal antiidiotypic antibody against myasthenic antibodies. Eur J Immunol 12:790–793.

109. Souroujon MC, Pachner AR, Fuchs S (1986): The treatment of passively transferred experimental myasthenia with anti-idiotypic antibodies. Neurology 36:622–625.

110. Lennon VA, Lambert EH (1981): Monoclonal autoantibodies to acetylcholine receptors: Evidence for a dominant idiotype and requirement of complement for pathogenicity. Ann NY Acad Sci 377:77–96.

111. Schwartz M, Novik D, Givol D, Fuchs S (1978): Induction of anti-idiotypic antibodies by imunization with syngeneic spleen cell education with acetylcholine receptor. Nature 273:543–545.

112. Agius MA, Richman DA (1986): Suppression of development of experimental autoimmune myasthenia gravis with isogeneic monoclonal antiidiotopic antibody. J Immunol 137:2195–2198.

113. Lefvert AK (1988): The start of an autoimmune process: Idiotypic networks during the development of myasthenia gravis. Ann Inst Pasteur 139:633–643.

114. Lefvert AK, Pirskanen R, Svanborg E (1985): Anti-idiotypic antibodies, acetylcholine receptor antibodies and disturbed neuromuscular function in healthy relatives to patients wtih myasthenia gravis. J Neuroimmunol 9:41–53.

115. Lefvert AK, Osterman PO (1983): Neonates to myasthenic mothers: A clinical study and an investigation of kinetic and biochemical properties of the acetylcholine receptor antibodies. Neurology 33:133–138.

116. Sundewall AC, Lefvert AK, Olsson R (1985): Anti-acetylcholine receptor antibodies in primary biliary cirrhosis. Acta Med Scand 217:519–525.

117. Eng H, Lefvert AK, Mellsted H, Österborg A (1987): Human monoclonal immunoglobulins that bind the human acetylcholine receptor. Eur J Immunol 17: 1867–1869.

118. Aarli JA, Lefvert AK, Tönder O (1981): Thymoma-specific antibodies in sera from patients with myasthenia gravis demonstrated with indirect hemagglutination. J Neuroimmunol 1:421–427.

119. Lefvert AK, Bolme P, Lönnqvist B, Ringdén O, Slördahl S, Smith E (1987): Bone marrow transplantation selectively increases the production of acetylcholine receptor antibodies, related idiotypes and antiidiotypic antibodies. Ann NY Acad Sci 505:825–827.

120. Lefvert AK, Björkholm M (1987): Antibodies against the acetylcholine receptor in hematological disorders—implications for the development of myasthenia gravis after bone marrow grafting. N Engl J Med 317:170.

121. Lefvert AK, Pirskanen R, Eng H, Sundewall AC, Svanborg E (1989): B cell and autoantibody repertoire in a pair of monozygotic twins discordant for myasthenia gravis. Clin Immunol Immunopathol 53:161–170.

122. Sundewall AC, Lefvert AK, Norberg R (1987): Characterization of acetylcholine receptor antibody activity in patients with mitochondrial and other autoantibodies. Clin Immunol Immunopathol 45:184–195.

123. Sundewall AC, Lefvert AK (1990): Acetylcholine receptor antibodies in primary biliary cirrhosis: Characterization of antigen and idiotypic specificity. Scand J Immunol 31:477–484.

124. Sundewall AC, Lefvert AK (1990): Autoantibody repertoire in primary biliary cirrhosis studied by monoclonal cellines. In "Anti-acetylcholine Receptor Antiobodies in Primary Biliary Cirrhosis and Myasthenia Gravis." Stockholm: Karolinska Institute.

125. Sundewall AC, Lefvert AK (1990): Repertoire of autoantibodies related to the acetylcholine receptor studied by B cell lines in patients with myasthenia gravis, primary biliary cirrhosis and normal individuals. In "Anti-acetylcholine Receptor Antibodies in Primary Biliary Cirrhosis and Myasthenia Gravis." Stockholm: Karolinska Institute.

126. Avrameas S, Guilbert B, Dighiero G (1981): Natural antibodies against tubulin, actin, myoglobin, thyroglobulin, fetuin, albumin and transferrin are present in normal human sera and monoclonal immunoglobulins from multiple myeloma and Waldenströms macroglobulinemia may express similar antibody specificities. Ann Immunol 132C:231–236.

127. Dighiero G, Guilbert B, Fermand JP, Lymberi P, Danon F, Avrameas S (1983): Thirty-six human monoclonal immunoglobulins with antibody activity against cytoskeleton proteins, thyroglobulin, and native DNA: Immunologic studies and clinical correlations. Blood 62:264–270.

128. Liggett SB, Shah SD, Cryer PE (1988): Characterization of β-adrenergic receptors of human skeletal muscle obtained by needle biopsy. Am J Physiol 254:E795–E798.

129. Williams L, Snyderman R, Lefkowitz RJ (1976): Identification of beta adrenergic receptors in human lymphocytes by $(-)^3$H-alprenolol binding. J Clin Invest 57:149–155.

130. Bowman WC, Nott MW (1969): Actions of sympathomimetic amines and their antagonists on skeletal muscle. Pharmacol Rev 21:27–72.

131. Depelchin A, Letesson JJ (1981): Adrenaline influence on the immune response II: Its effect through action on the suppressor T cells. Immunol Lett 3:207–213.

132. Agius MA, Checinski ME, Richman DP (1987): Sympathectomy enhances the severity of experimental autoimmune myasthenia gravis (EAMG). J Neuroimmunol 16:11–12.

133. Chelmicka-Schorr E, Checinski ME, Arnason BGW (1988): Chemical sympathectomy augments the severity of experimental allergic encephalomyelitis. J Neuroimmunol 17:347–350.

134. Kaveri S-V, Diedrich G, Kazatchine MD (1991): Intravenous immunoglobulin in the treatment of autoimmune disease. Clin Exp Immunol 86:192–198.

135. Arsura E (1989): Experience with intravenous immunoglobulin in myasthenia gravis. Clin Exp Immunol 52:S170.

136. Cosi V, Lombardi M, Piccolo G, Erbetta A (1991): Treatment of myasthenia gravis with high-dose intravenous immunoglobulin. Acta Neurol Scand 84:81–84.

137. Sundblad A, Hauser S, Holmberg D, Cazenave P-A, Coutinho A (1989): Suppression of antibody responses to the acetylcholine receptor by natural autoantibodies. Eur J Immunol 19:1425–1435.
138. Sundblad A, Huetz F, Portnoi D, Coutinho A (1991): Stimulation of B and T cells by in vivo high dose immunoglobulin administration in normal mice. J Autoimmun 4:325–339.
139. Christadoss P, Dauphinee MJ (1986): Immunotherapy for myasthenia gravis: A murine model. J Immunol 136:2437–2440.
140. Herzog C, Walker C, Müller W, Rieber P, Reiter C, Rietmüller G, Wassmer P, Stockinger H, Madic O, Pichler WJ (1989): Anti-CD4 antibody treatment of patients with rheumatoid arthritis. J Autoimmun 2:627–642.
141. Åhlberg R, Yi Q, Pirskanen R, Matell G, Swerup C, Rieber P, Riethmüller G, Holm G, Lefvert AK (1993): Clinical improvement of myasthenia gravis by treatment with a chimaeric anti-CD4 monoclonal antibody. Ann NY Acad Sci (in press).
142. Maselli RA, Richman DP, Wollmann RL (1991): Inflammation at the neuromuscular junction in myasthenia gravis. Neurology 41:1497–1504.

19

IMMUNOREGULATION OF AUTOIMMUNE RESPONSES IN SYSTEMIC VASCULITIS

C. M. Lockwood

*Department of Medicine, Addenbrooke's Hospital,
Cambridge, United Kingdom*

BACKGROUND

Since the discovery of antineutrophil cytoplasm antibodies (ANCA) in 1982 [1], evidence has been growing that they play a pathogenetic role in systemic vasculitis [2]. The basis for this rests on the fact that ANCA are integral to the development of most primary vasculitides [2], that their levels correlate with disease activity, and that there is an association between ANCA isotype and disease expression [3–7]. In vitro studies have demonstrated the effects of ANCA-rich immunoglobulin on neutrophil function and the promotion of endothelial cell cytotoxicity by ANCA [2]. However, those who advocate the pathogenetic effect of ANCA have to account for the fact that circulating B cells capable of ANCA secretion have been isolated from normal individuals and that ANCA are part of the normal immune repertoire and as such are present in pools of normal immunoglobulins [8].

ANCA ANTI-IDIOTYPE ANTIBODIES

The presence of antibodies that recognize idiotypic determinants located on the variable region of autoantibodies has been demonstrated in many auto-

Autoimmunity: Physiology and Disease, Pages 307–314
© *1994 Wiley-Liss, Inc.*

immune diseases such as myasthenia gravis, anti-Factor VIII disease, and systemic lupus erythematosus [9, 10]. It has been suggested that they are important in regulating the autoimmune response. The best evidence for this comes from anti-Factor VIII disease, in which IgG Fab'$_2$ fragments from the sera of patients in remission have been shown to block the action of pathogenic autoantibodies on Factor VIII [11].

Anti-idiotypic activity toward ANCA has been demonstrated in ANCA-negative remission sera, which can be shown to inhibit the binding of auto-antibody to autoantigen in a dose-dependent manner. ANCA in acute sera can also be retained and concentrated by Fab'$_2$ made from remission sera, immobilized on Sepharose beads [12]. As the ANCA anti-idiotypic antibodies from one patient can interact with the ANCA from the acute sera of other patients, some of the ANCA idiotypes must be "public" to so allow such cross reactivity [12]. Subsequent studies by other workers using the purified autoantigens proteinase 3 and myeloperoxidase have produced similar findings [13, 14]. ANCA anti-idiotypic antibodies are also detectable in intravenous immunoglobulin (IVIg). Furthermore the variability in inhibition observed when the different ANCA-positive sera were incubated with the preparations of IVIg suggested a degree idiotypic heterogeneity that in turn, probably explains the differences in clinical response to IVIg [12, 14].

The degree of inhibition of ANCA Fab'$_2$ from one patient by IVIg Fab'$_2$ can be increased by affinity purification of IVIg Fab'$_2$ on Sepharose-bound ANCA-positive Fab'$_2$ from a second patient. The peak inhibition was shown to occur at a 10-fold lower concentration of IVIg Fab'$_2$. This confirmed the presence of cross-reactive idiotypic determinants on ANCA and suggested the possibility of enriching the neutralizing ability of IVIg, which in turn may be of therapeutic importance (D. Jayme, personal communication). In a preliminary report, IVIg Fab'$_2$ were able to inhibit the ability of ANCA to influence neutrophil function in vitro [15].

Surprisingly, the removal of IgM from ANCA-negative remission sera permitted the detection of IgG ANCA; purification of the IgM fraction enabled demonstration of IgM ANCA anti-idiotypic antibodies and the importance of IgM in the regulation of the IgG ANCA response [12]. This may be analogous to the idiotypic control of IgG autoantibodies by IgM reported in a murine model and is also of practical relevance when physical methods to remove immunoglobulin such as plasma exchange or immunoabsorption are employed in therapy [12, 16, 17].

IVIg AND THE PATHOGENESIS OF SYSTEMIC VASCULITIS

The rationale for the use of IVIg in systemic vasculitis is twofold. The first is its proven benefit in preventing coronary aneurysms in Kawasaki disease, which is an ANCA-positive childhood vasculitis. The second is the possible role of ANCA anti-idiotypic antibodies in regulating disease-associated autoantibodies [18, 19]. After IVIg administration in Kawasaki disease, there is a rapid fall in monocyte interleukin (IL)-1 production and endothelial cell activation manifested by a reduction in ELAM-1 expression [20]. In vitro studies have shown that IVIg can reduce monocyte IL-6 release through an Fc-dependent mechanism [21]. IVIg also impairs immunoglobulin production in vitro through Fc-mediated interactions with B cells and monocytes [22].

The ability of IVIg to prevent the development of diabetes in the non-obese diabetic mouse—a pure T-cell disease—confirms an influence of T-cell function suggested by the normalization of T-cell subsets that occurs after IVIg therapy in Kawasaki disease [23, 24]. This effect may result from the manipulation of network regulation because it can be reproduced by a single monoclonal antibody exhibiting polyreactivity to autoantigens and other antibody idiotypic determinants, but not by antibodies with restricted activity to extrinsic antigens [25]. T-cell involvement in vasculitis is implied from the infiltration of affected vessels by activated T cells, the correlation of serum IL-2 receptor levels with disease activity, and the effectiveness of anti T-cell monoclonal antibodies in therapy, but a direct action of IVIg on T-cell activity in vasculitis has not been investigated [26, 27]. The potential effects of IVIg are the reversal of monocyte and neutrophil activation, a reduction in autoantibody production, or an effect on autoreactive T-cell function. The fall in ANCA seen between 10 and 40 days after IVIg in vivo is compatible with inhibition of ANCA production possibly caused by direct effects of ANCA anti-idiotype in IVIg, or idiotype–anti-idiotype dimers formed between IVIg and ANCA B cells, or suppression of ANCA-specific T-cell help [28]. The involvement of T cells has been suggested by workers who have reported the presence of circulating PR3-specific T cells during active disease [29, 30]. In addition, the mechanism of isotype switching and affinity maturation of ANCA reflects T-cell control [31].

Vasculitis with anti-myeloperoxidase (MPO) antibodies is a feature of the autoimmune disease induced in the Brown Norway rat injected with mercuric chloride, when polyclonal B-cell activation is accompanied by the emergence of autoreactive T cells to class 2 molecules [32]. Depending on the time of infusion, IVIg therapy suppresses proteinuria and the increase in IgE [33]. As idiotypic interactions between IVIg and the induced autoantibodies can be demonstrated, stimulation of network function may explain these results.

TREATMENT OF SYSTEMIC VASCULITIS WITH IVIg

Before the use of corticosteroids, systemic vasculitis was usually fatal, but now over 90% of patients are controlled by a combination of corticosteroid and cytotoxic drugs [34]. However, only 50%–70% achieve sustained remission. Treatment is limited by adverse effects and must be sustained long term, since relapse is common following its withdrawal [34–39]. A search for alternative agents has included co-trimoxazole, plasma exchange, cyclosporin A, monoclonal antibodies, and IVIg [27, 28, 40–42].

In an open study of IVIg in patients with either Wegener's granulomatosis or microscopic polyarteritis, a reduction in disease activity was seen in 13 of 14, which led to clinical remission in 8 [43]. Nine had disease refractory to therapy with steroids and cytotoxic drugs, while five were untreated. Patients received Sandoglobulin 2 g/kg over 5 days. Clinical improvement was matched by falls in C-reactive protein (CRP) and erythrocyte sedimentation rate (ESR); the mean CRP and ESR fell from 44 mg/L and 52 mm to 16 mm/L and 43 mm, respectively, at 8 weeks. Pulmonary infiltrates present on chest x-rays of seven resolved in four and quantitative reductions in the degree of inflammation were assessed by paired indium-111 white cell scan. After a follow-up of 10 months, relapses had occurred in two; otherwise, benefit was maintained and immunosuppression reduced from a mean cytotoxic and prednisolone dosage of 64 and 12 mg/day to 60 and 6 mg/day, respectively. Further falls in CRP and ESR to means of 11 mg and 31 mm were seen.

IVIg can cause reversible impairment of renal function in patients with glomerulonephritis and exacerbate renal injury in lupus nephritis [44, 45]. In contrast, beneficial effects of IVIg have been reported in membranous nephropathy [46]; no adverse effect on the serum creatinine was seen in this study, but patients with deteriorating renal function were excluded.

Sequential ANCA levels revealed an unexpected rise in ANCA binding, which peaked at 10 days after infusions commenced. Four patients had transient exacerbations of systemic symptoms at this time, but no adverse effects on renal function or urinary sediment were seen. ANCA subsequently fell to 50% of the pretreatment values, three patients becoming ANCA negative and remaining stable during follow-up. ANCA binding of pretreatment serum was partly inhibitable by preincubation with IVIg Ab_2 fragments in the 10 patients who were ANCA positive at the time of treatment. Correlations were found between the degree to which a patient's ANCA was inhibited by IVIg in vitro and the fall in circulating ANCA and between pretreatment and follow-up samples, seen in vivo, which provides indirect evidence for the functional effect of idiotypic interactions on ANCA and IVIg in vivo [28].

In a further report, IVIg led to clinical remissions in two patients with Wegener's granulomatosis involving the lungs and kidneys, resistant to conventional treatment [47]. Clinical recovery was accompanied by falls in ANCA; one patient, however, relapsed after 3 months.

IMMUNOSTIMULATION WITH IVIg AND SUSTAINED DISEASE REMISSION

Infusions of therapeutic doses of human IVIg into normal Balb/c mice induces stimulation of B- and T-cell activity [48]. Of particular interest was the finding that this stimulation applies to autoantibodies rather than antibodies to extrinsic antigens [48]. In a serial study of sera from 10 patients treated with IVIg, a sustained elevation of IgM was seen after IVIg, accompanied by increases in nondisease associated autoantibody levels, such as anti-DNA and antiactin, over a period when ANCA levels were falling [49]. The explanation of these results is not clear, but it has been proposed that they reflect immunostimulation of the host's idiotypic networks by IVIg that might enable restoration of physiological immunoregulation, indicated in vasculitis patients by the fall in ANCA [48].

CONCLUSIONS

The importance of idiotypic network regulation in autoimmunity is controversial, but there is accumulating evidence for idiotypic interactions at the B-cell level in many autoimmune diseases, including systemic vasculitis, and on T cells in experimental models such as the nonobese diabetic mouse. IVIg has effects at multiple levels on the inflammatory and immune responses, but the restoration of self-tolerance through stimulation of idiotypic regulation is the most plausible hypothesis for its ability to induce long-term remission from autoimmune disease.

The pathogenesis of vasculitis is not clearly understood but involves autoreactive T- and B-cell responses and a complex interaction of leukocytes, inflammatory mediators, and the endothelium. The potential therapeutic targets for IVIg are several, but as yet only the idiotypic interactions with ANCA have been studied. These show ANCA anti-idiotype to be present in IVIg postrecovery sera, that IVIg can induce prolonged suppression of ANCA synthesis, and that this is associated with the stimulation of immunoglobulin production and nondisease-associated autoantibodies. The implication that this stimulation reflects increased idiotypic network activity that may have regulatory importance is supported by other reports of an increase anti-idiotype between acute and remission stages of disease. The role of IVIg as an alternative to conventional immunosuppression at least in vasculitis awaits controlled clinical study.

REFERENCES

1. Davies DJ, Moran JE, Niall JF, Ryan GB (1982): Segmental necrotizing glomerulonephritis with anti-neutrophil antibody: Possible arbovirus aetiology? Br Med J 285:606–609.
2. Lockwood CM (1993): Specificity and pathogenicity of antineutrophil cytoplasm antibodies. Exp Nephrol 1:13–18.
3. Nolle B, Specks U, Ludemann J, Rohrbach MS, Deremee RA, Gross WL (1989): Anticytoplasmic autoantibodies: Their immunodiagnostic value in Wegener's granulomatosis. Ann Intern Med 111:28–40.

4. Cohen Tervaert JW, van der Woude FJ, Fauci AS, Ambrus JL, Velosa J, Keane WF, Meijer S, van der Giessen M, The T, van der Hem GK, Kallenberg CGM (1989): Association between active Wegener's granulomatosis and anticytoplasmic antibodies. Arch Intern Med 149:2461–2465.

5. Jayne DRW, Jones SJ, Severn A, Shaunak S, Murphy J, Lockwood CM (1989): Severe pulmonary haemorrhage and systemic vasculitis in association with circulating anti-neutrophil cytoplasm antibodies of IgM class only. Clin Nephrol 32:101–106.

6. Jayne DRW, Heaton A, Evans DB, Lockwood CM (1990): Sequential ANCA and CRP estimations in the management of patients with systemic vasculitis. APMIS 98(Suppl 19):44.

7. Jayne DRW, Weetman AP, Lockwood CM (1991): IgG subclass distribution of autoantibodies to neutrophil cytoplasmic antigens in systemic vasculitis. Clin Exp Immunol 84:476–481.

8. Mathieson PW, Lockwood CM, Oliveira DBG (1992): T and B cell responses to neutrophil cytoplasmic antigens in systemic vasculitis. Clin Immunol Immunopathol 63:135–141.

9. Kearney JF (1989): Idiotypic networks. In Paul WE (ed): "Fundamental Immunology." 2nd Ed. New York: Raven Press, pp 663–676.

10. Dwyer JM (1992): Manipulating the immune system with immune globulin. N Engl J Med 236:107–116.

11. Sultan Y, Rossi F, Kazatchkine MD (1987): Recovery from anti-VIII:c (anti-haemophilic factor) autoimmune disease is dependent on generation of anti-idiotypes against anti-VIII:c autoantibodies. Proc Natl Acad Sci USA 84:828–831.

12. Rossi F, Jayne DRW, Lockwood CM, Kazatchkine (1991): Anti-idiotypes against anti-neutrophil cytoplasmic antigen autoantibodies in normal human polyspecific IgG for therapeutic use and in the remission sera of patients with systemic vasculitis. Clin Exp Immunol 83:298–303.

13. Richter C, Schnabel A, Scernok E, Reinhold-Keller E, Gross WL (1993): Intravenous immunoglobulin therapy in Wegener's granulomatosis. In Gross WL (ed): "ANCA Associated Vasculitides: Immunodiagnostic and Pathogenetic Value of Antineutrophil Cytoplasmic Antibodies." London: Plenum Press (in press).

14. Pall A, Varagunam M, Smith N, Adu D, Taylor CM, Michael J (1993): Pooled human IgG inhibits the binding of anti-myeloperoxidase antibodies to myeloperoxidase (abstract). Clin Exp Immunol (in press).

15. Fujimoto T, Lockwood CM (1991): Anti-neutrophil cytoplasm antibodies (ANCA) activate protein kinase C in human neutrophils and HL-60 cells (abstract). J Am Soc Nephrol 1:522.

16. Adib J, Ragimbeau J, Avrameas S, Ternynck T (1990): IgG autoantibody activity in normal mouse serum is controlled by IgM. J Immunol 145:3807–3813.

17. Esnault VLM, Soleimani B, Keogan MT, Brownlee AA, Jayne DRW, Lockwood CM (1991): Association of IgM with IgG ANCA in patients presenting with pulmonary haemorrhage. Kidney Int 41(5):1304–1310.

18. Newburger JW, Takashi M, Burns JC, Beiser AS, Chung KJ, Duffy CE, Glode

MP, Mason WH, Reddy V, Sanders SP, Shulman ST, Wiggins JW, Hicks RV, Fulton DR, Lewis AB, Leung DYM, Waldman JD, Colton T, Rosen FS, Melish ME (1986): Treatment of Kawasaki disease with intravenous immunoglobulin. N Engl J Med 315:341–346.

19. Savage COS, Tizard J, Jayne DRW, Lockwood CM, Dillon MJ (1989): Antineutrophil cytoplasm antibodies in Kawasaki disease. Arch Dis Child 64:360–363.

20. Leung DYM, Cotran RS, Kurt-Jones E, Burns JC, Newburger JW, Pober JS (1989): Endothelial cell activation and high interleukin-1 secretion in the pathogenesis of acute Kawasaki disease. Lancet 1:1298–1302.

21. Andersson JP, Andersson UG (1990): Human intravenous immunoglobulin modulates monokine production in vitro. Immunology 71:372–376.

22. Kondo N, Ozawa T, Mushiake K, Motoyoshi F, Kameyama T, Kasahara K, Kaneko H, Yamashina M, Kato Y, Orii T (1991): Suppression of immunoglobulin production of lymphocytes by intravenous immunoglobulin. J Clin Immunol 11:152–158.

23. Forsgren S, Andersson A, Hillorn V, Soderstrom A, Holmberg D (1991): Immunoglobulin-mediated prevention of autoimmune diabetes in the non-obese diabetic (NOD) mouse. Scand J Immunol 34:445–451.

24. Leung DYM, Burns JC, Newburger JW, Geha RS (1987): Reversal of lymphocyte activation in vivo in the Kawasaki syndrome by intravenous gammaglobulin. J Clin Invest 79:468–472.

25. Andersson A, Forsgren S, Soderstrom A, Holmberg D (1991): Monoclonal natural antibodies prevent development of diabetes in the non-obese diabetic mouse. J Autoimmun 4:733–742.

26. das Neves FC, Kaskas B, Hartley B, Cameron JS (1991): Interstitial cellular infiltrate and soluble interleukin 2 receptor in patients with renal vasculitis (abstract). J Am Soc Nephrol 2:592.

27. Mathieson PW, Cobbold SP, Hale G, Clark MJ, Oliveira DBG, Lockwood CM, Waldmann H (1990): Monoclonal antibody therapy in systemic vasculitis. N Engl J Med 323:250–254.

28. Jayne DRW, Black CM, Davies M, Fox C, Lockwood CM (1991): Treatment of systemic vasculitis with pooled intravenous immunoglobulin. Lancet 1:1137–1139.

29. van der Woude FJ, Van Es LA, Daha MR (1990): The role of the c-ANCA antigen in the pathogenesis of Wegener's granulomatosis. A hypothesis based on both humoral and cellular mechanisms. Neth J Med 36:169–171.

30. Petersen J, Rasmussen N, Szpirt W, Hermann E, Hayet W (1991): T lymphocyte proliferation to neutrophil cytoplasmic antigen(s) in Wegener's granulomatosis (WG) (abstract). Am J Kidney Dis 18:73.

31. Esnault VLM, Jayne DRW, Weetman AP, Lockwood CM (1991): IgG subclass distribution and relative functional affinity of anti-myeloperoxidase antibodies in systemic vasculitis at presentation and during follow-up. Immunology 74:714–718.

32. Mathieson PW, Thiru S, Oliveira DBG (1992): Mercuric chloride-treated Brown Norway rats develop widespread tissue injury including necrotizing vasculitis. Lab Invest 67:121–129.

33. Rossi F, Bellon B, Vial MC, Druet P, Kazatchkine MD (1991): Beneficial effect of human therapeutic intravenous immunoglobulins (IVIg) in mercuric-chloride-induced autoimmune disease of Brown-Norway rats. Clin Exp Immunol 84:129–133.

34. Fauci AS, Katz P, Haynes BF, Wolff SM (1979): Cyclophosphamide therapy of severe systemic necrotizing vasculitis. N Engl J Med 301:235–238.

35. Leib ES, Restivo C, Paulus HE (1979): Immunosuppressive and corticosteroid therapy of polyarteritis nodosa. Am J Med 67:941–945.

36. Cohen J, Pinching AJ, Rees AJ, Peters DK (1982): Infection and immunosuppression: A study of the infective complications of 75 patients with immunologically mediated disease. Q J Med 51:1–15.

37. Bradley JD, Brandt KD, Katz BP (1989): Infectious complications of cyclophosphamide treatment for vasculitis. Arthritis Rheum 32:45–53.

38. Cohen-Tervaert JW, Huitema MG, Hene RJ, Sluiter WJ, The T, van der Hem GK, Kallenberg CGM (1990): Prevention of relapses in Wegener's granulomatosis by treatment based on antineutrophil cytoplasmic antibody titre. Lancet 2:709–711.

39. Neild GH (1991): Infectious complications in the management of systemic vasculitis and rapidly progressive glomerulonephritis. APMIS 98(Suppl 19):56–60.

40. Deremee RA (1989): The treatment of Wegener's granulomatosis with trimethoprim/sulfamethoxazole: Illusion or vision? Arthritis Rheum 31:1068–1073.

41. Lockwood CM, Pinching AJ, Sweny P, Peters DK (1977): Plasma exchange and immunosuppression in the treatment of fulminating immune-complex nephritis. Lancet 1:63–67.

42. Gremmel F, Druml W, Schmidt P, Graninger W (1988): Cyclosporin in Wegener granulomatosis. Ann Intern Med 108:491.

43. Jayne DRW, Esnault VLM, Lockwood CM (1993): ANCA anti-idiotype antibodies and treatment of systemic vasculitis with intravenous immunoglobulin. J Autoimmun 6:207–219.

44. Schifferli J, Leski M, Favre H, Imbach P, Nydegger U, Davies K (1991): High-dose intravenous IgG treatment and renal function. Lancet 1:457–458.

45. Jordan SC (1989): Intravenous gammaglobulin therapy in systemic lupus erythematosus and immune complex disease. Clin Immunol Immunopathol 53:S164–S169.

46. Palla R, Cirami C, Panichi V, Bianchi AM, Parrini M, Grazi G (1991): Intravenous immunoglobulin therapy of membranous nephropathy: Efficacy and safety. Clin Nephrol 35:98–104.

47. Moudgil A, Tuso P, Kamil E, Koyyana R, Jordan SC (1991): Treatment of Wegener's granulomatosis with pooled intravenous immunoglobulin (abstract). J Am Soc Nephrol 2:600.

48. Sundblad A, Huetz F, Portnoi D, Coutinho A (1991): Stimulation of B and T cells by in vivo high does immunoglobulin administration in normal mice. J Autoimmun 4:325–339.

49. Jayne DRW, Lockwood CM (1991): Stimulation of autoantibodies by intravenous immunoglobulin in patients with systemic vasculitis (abstract). J Am Soc Nephrol 3:596.

20

IMMUNOLOGICAL DISTURBANCES RESPONSIBLE FOR GRAVES' DISEASE

John M. Dwyer

Division of Medicine and Department of Immunology, Prince Henry and Prince of Wales Hospitals, University of New South Wales, Sydney, Australia

INTRODUCTION

The human thyroid gland (*thyroid* from the Greek meaning *oblong shield*) consists of two lobes connected by an isthmus wrapped around the trachea in the anterior compartment of the neck. With an adult weight of 15–20 g, it is the largest of the endocrine organs. The gland is designed to produce two hormones vital to numerous metabolic processes and is active from the 11th week of fetal life. It is composed of innumerable discreet follicles (cysts) clustered to resemble a bunch of microscopically tiny grapes. The cells lining the follicles produce thyroid hormones that are stored in the lumen of the follicle for subsequent controlled release. When the gland is resting, the cells lining the follicles are flat and the lumen large. During periods of intense activity, the height of the cells increases (columnar epithelium) and the lumen becomes smaller [Hoffenberg, 1987].

Thyroid follicles slowly produce the protein thyroglobulin, a glycoprotein with a molecular weight of 660,000. A small number of specific

Autoimmunity: Physiology and Disease, Pages 315–338
© *1994 Wiley-Liss, Inc.*

tyrosine residues within this protein may become iodinated to produce two modified amino acids with hormone activity: thyroxine (T_4) and triiodothyronine (T_3) (terminology that is a potential source of confusion in an immunological review!). Coupling of iodotyrosines produces either T_3 or T_4, the final steps in the production line occurring as the hormones are about to be secreted. The production of these hormones is dependent on the daily ingestion of at least 150 μg of iodine by the owner of the gland. An active transport process allows the cells lining thyroid follicles to ingest avidly the iodide produced by the reduction of dietary iodine. Once inside the cells, iodine is bound to tyrosyl residues of thyroglobulin by a peroxidase/hydrogen peroxidase system [Chopra et al., 1983].

The follicle's activity is controlled by an anterior pituitary hormone, thyroid-stimulating hormone (TSH), released in typical "feedback" manner when the serum levels of T_3 and T_4 fall. TSH, after binding to its receptor on follicular cells, activates AMP-dependent mechanisms that lead to the recovery of some of the iodoprotein stored in the follicles. Microvilli project from the apices of the cells into the lumen, where they envelope a small amount of colloid to produce an intracellular "colloid droplet." Proteolytic enzymes in the cells complete the degradation of thyroglobulin, releasing T_3 and T_4 into the cells from where they diffuse into the bloodstream. Normally, the thyroid gland secretes 80 μg of T_4 and 5 μg of T_3 daily. (The latter is the more biologically active hormone.)

TSH is a glycoprotein with a molecular weight of 14,000 and consists of two subunits, α and β, linked by disulfide bridges. TSH release is at least partially controlled by a hormone from the median eminence of the hypothalamus: thyrotropin-releasing hormone (TRH) [Larsen, 1988].

GRAVES' DISEASE

There are two major forms of autoimmune thyroid disease, chronic autoimmune thyroiditis (Hashimoto's disease) and Graves' disease [Charreire, 1989; Utiger, 1991]. While the basic immunopathogenic mechanisms involved in the production of both diseases appear to be similar, though certainly not identical, their affect on the thyroid gland is very different. In Hashimoto's disease, hypothyroidism develops as the secretions of T_3 and T_4 fall. The opposite is true in Graves' disease. Occasionally, there is a transition from one disease to another, and both can occur within members of the same family [Tamai et al., 1987]. As we do not have therapeutic strategies that reliably and safely correct the underlying defects present in autoimmune thyroid disease, therapy is directed at reducing or replacing thyroid hormones to correct any metabolic imbalance that may result.

An undisciplined, excessive production of T_3/T_4 by the thyroid gland produces severe metabolic disturbances that collectively provoke a clinical state known as *thyrotoxicosis*. There are very rare causes of this state, such as TSH-producing tumors of the pituitary gland or the occasional production of T_3 and T_4 by thyroid or nonthyroid malignant cells, but 99% of all cases of thyrotoxicosis result from one of two conditions. By far the less common of the two is Plummer's disease, in which just one or a few follicles at most hypertrophy to produce "nodules" secreting excessive amounts of hormone [Volpé, 1985]. The more common situation involves the hyperplasia and hypertrophy of all the gland's follicles to produce the diffuse, "smooth" enlargement of the thyroid gland characteristic of the disease first described by the Irish physician Robert Graves in the 19th century.

Clinical Picture

Virtually every system in the body is influenced by T_3/T_4. In a typical case, excessive amounts of circulating thyroid hormone will produce an agitated, restless, shaking, and tremulous patient, with bounding pulses, a rapid heart rate, and a visible enlargement of the thyroid gland itself (a goiter). Weight loss despite a good appetite, fatigue, nervousness, increased sweating and heat intolerance, palpitations, breathlessness, diarrhea, and proximal muscle weakness will be complained of frequently.

Ocular involvement is an essential feature of the clinical syndrome that is Graves' disease [Wall et al., 1991]. However, the typical ocular manifestations can occur in Hashimoto's thyroiditis and even in euthyroid states [Salvi et al., 1990]. Patients complain that their eyes have become more prominent, painful, or "gritty." Double vision is not uncommon, as is the increased production of tears. The ocular manifestations are associated with the retro-orbital deposition of mucopolysaccharides with edema and lymphocytic infiltration into retro-orbital tissues [Dwyer et al., 1991]. The extraorbital muscles may not function normally. They may thicken, with muscle elements being replaced by fibrous tissue. Any explanation of the immunopathology of Graves' disease must address the eye disturbances seen, for they cannot be explained by the direct effect of increased levels of T_3 or T_4 found in the circulation, and indeed not infrequently become more florid and disturbing as excess levels of thyroid hormones are reduced by treatment.

Epidemiology

Graves' disease occurs in all populations, is seven times more common in women, and usually presents during the third or fourth decade of life [Andreoli et al., 1990]. No obvious precipitating cause has been discovered. The disorder belongs to the thyrogastric cluster of autoimmune diseases [Brostoff et al., 1991]. An individual who has Graves' disease and family members are more likely than would be expected by chance to experience other disturbances of endocrine function thought to result from autoaggressive immune pathology. Diabetes and primary failure of adrenal, parathyroid, ovarian, and testicular function are not uncommon. Pernicious anemia, produced by the destruction of the parietal cells in the stomach necessary to produce "intrinsic factor," which will promote the absorption of vitamin B_{12} in the lower bowel, also cluster with the above diseases [Taylor, 1976]. All these disorders, for reasons that are unclear, are more common in individuals in whom patches of skin depigmentation produce the condition known as vitiligo, and/or premature greying of the hair occurs. Interestingly, vitiligo may be prominent over the neck and anterior chest wall in patients with thyrotoxicosis. Myasthenia gravis clusters with both this group of autoimmune disorders, and the "lupus" cluster of diseases typified by systemic lupus erythematosus itself. In whites with Graves' disease, the HLA haplotype most frequently displayed features B8 and DR3 histocompatibility antigens [Farid and Bear, 1981].

Autoimmunity

Any modern student of autoimmunity presented with the above facts for the first time, but given the clue that the pathology in the thyroid gland of patients with Graves' disease features an intense infiltration of both T and B lymphocytes, with many of the latter maturing in situ to plasma cells, would be likely to theorize as follows. As tolerance to one's own tissues is a complex, multifactorial, and capricious affair, involving many gene products in numerous interactive "failsafe" mechanisms, genetic variability would be expected to provide some individuals with better (more reliable) mechanisms for preserving self-tolerance, particularly during times of immunological stress (infection?). As evolutionary pressures have yet to provide us with the immunological security that would be associated with the clonal aborption of all T and B cells capable of "recognizing" self-antigens, we must live with a system of tight controls on autoreactive cells that are normally present and normally reactive [Sinha et al., 1990].

Therefore one would expect to find in the circulation of healthy individuals T and B cells with receptors whose variable regions would have a "best-fit" for numerous thyroid-associated autoantigens. One would expect in these same healthy individuals to find small amounts of circulating auto-antibody (mainly IgM) to thyroid autoantigens and antibody to those antibodies (anti-idiotypic antibodies) [Rossi et al., 1989]. The latter would be expected to influence antigen-specific regulatory T cells (either the $CD4^+$ suppressor inducer lymphocytes or CD8 regulatory cells), thus minimizing the activity of cytotoxic T cells capable of reacting to thyroid autoantigens, as well as neutralizing potentially dangerous antibodies by complexing with them in the form of an easily removed idiotype–anti-idiotype dimer.

As selective pressures would favor the conservation of some simplicity in such a complex arrangement of control mechanisms, it would not be surprising to find that such anti-idiotypic antibodies recognize determinants shared by a large number of autoantibodies [Rossi and Kazatchkine, 1989]. Any autoimmune response to elements of the thyroid gland, in a manner that would lead to the pathology associated with Graves' disease, would require the above control mechanisms to fail.

Our student would be correct in presuming that if thyroid antigens were displayed as processed peptides bound to MHC class I and class II proteins on the surface of thyrocytes, then a dangerous situation indeed could develop. In a pathological state, the class I and class II antigens would be vividly and uncharacteristically displayed on thyroid cells, suggesting that cytokines such as interferon-α (IFN-α), which can upregulate the expression of MHC molecules, would be found in abundance within the gland [Bottazzo et al., 1983]. Those adhesion molecules, which may be expressed on both lymphocytes and endothelial cells to help direct immunological traffic into an area under attack, would be expected to be displayed prominently both on the lymphoid cells migrating into the thyroid and on the walls of the blood and lymph vessels supplying the gland.

On purely theoretical grounds, it is unlikely that Graves' disease could be caused by an attack of either T or B cells on nonfunctional antigenic components of the follicles, for destruction per se would only release into the circulation precursors of T_3 and T_4. Whatever the immune response responsible, it would be reasonable to predict that it must be capable of driving forward those physiological mechanisms responsible for the release of T_3/T_4 into the circulation. Clearly, the development of an immune response featuring the production of a thyroid hormone-releasing agonist, but not TSH itself, would seem most likely. Such a conclusion is strengthened by the knowledge that the level of TSH in the circulation of patients with Graves' disease is low indeed. An antibody with TRH properties could produce the symptoms, but TSH levels would then be high rather than low. An immune response that activated TSH receptors on follicular cells would appear to best explain all but the ophthalmological phenomena described above.

Thus the receptor for TSH or peptides very closely linked to that receptor would appear likely to provide the antigen(s) driving the autoimmune process in Graves' disease. The production of a T-cell dependent IgG anti-TSH receptor antibody (TRab) would provide the necessary agonist.

Why should the normally harmless, low intensity recognition and response to determinants of the receptor for TSH turn nasty? A viral infection of the follicular cells could attract cells of the immune system into the gland. Cytokines released during the response could so upregulate the expression of MHC class I and class II proteins on the surface of the thyroid epithelial cells that they may become adequate antigen-presenting cells and indeed present themselves by providing a display of TSH receptor peptides linked to MHC peptides in a format that may prove irresistible to potential autoaggressive T and B cells. The suppression of regulatory mechanisms during the response to an invading microorganism may alter the balancing act normally preventing autoaggression against follicular cells for sufficient time to allow autoaggressive cells to respond to extreme provocation.

Alternatively, infection could so alter "self" that both active and passive mechanisms normally producing tolerance to "self" fail. No provocation at all would be essential if a genetically determined failure occurred in those antigen-specific regulatory cells provided to prevent the development of Graves' disease. Which of the above concepts are supported by observations?

FROM THEORY TO FACT

That the receptor for TSH provides the major antigenic determinants provoking an autoimmune response in thyrotoxicosis is certain [McGregor, 1990]. In 1956, a "long-acting thyroid stimulator" was found in the sera of patients with Graves' disease [Adams, 1988] and by 1964 it had been established that this nonphysiological molecule was in fact an immunoglobulin [Kriss et al., 1964]. Indeed in the same year it became clear that the transient hyperthyroidism that may occur in neonates born to mothers with Graves' disease was caused by the transplacental passage of these IgG thyroid-stimulating molecules [McKenzie, 1964].

Many years were to pass before, in 1989, the TSH receptor itself was finally cloned [Libert et al., 1989]. It was then possible to demonstrate that the disease-causing immunoglobulins did bind to and activate receptors for TSH. The receptor contains 744 amino acids, and the region containing amino acids 350–400 is the most hydrophilic and potentially therefore the most immunogenic. TSH receptors have either multiple subunits or consist of several different TSH receptors each associated with a different level of activity [Wilkin, 1990]. A reliable, commercially available radioassay in which the capacity of the TRab to block the binding of ^{125}I-labeled TSH to a thyroid cell membrane preparation has replaced older bioassays and stimulated much research [Smith and Hall, 1974].

Such competitive inhibition assays soon revealed that two types of antibodies to TRab can be found in human disease states [Konishi et al., 1983]. In thyrotoxicosis, antibodies act as agonists with TSH-like properties. In autoimmune thyroiditis producing severe hypothyroidism, antibodies to the receptor for TSH bind but fail to stimulate. They do of course prevent TSH binding and thyroid function fails. These autoantibodies are analogous to those denying acetylcholine its binding site at the neuromuscular junction in patients with myasthenia gravis, and they may cause transient hypothyroidism in neonates. Some patients with Graves' disease proceed to develop hypothyroidism, not because the gland itself is eventually destroyed by autoreactive cells, but because the nature of the TRab produced switches from agonist to antagonist [Drexhage and van der Gaag, 1986]. With the receptor cloned, it should not be long before we understand the molecular interactions that determine activation or blocking of TSH receptor function.

Patients with both Hashimoto's thyroiditis and Graves' disease often have significant titers of antithyroid peroxidase (thyroid microsomal) antibodies [Burman and Baker, 1985]. Theoretically, these antibodies could inhibit the enzyme's activity and facilitate the killing of antibody-coated thyrocytes by an antibody-dependent cell-mediated cytotoxic reaction. While both mechanisms have been demonstrated in Hashimoto's disease, neither seems to develop in patients with Graves' disease [Utiger, 1991].

TRab are present in the serum of 90% of patients with Graves' disease and are the likely cause of their hyperthyroidism [Wilkin, 1990]. However, a small percentage of patients with Graves' disease do not have detectable levels of such antibody, and it is possible that they may have a different immunological mechanism activating their thyroid gland [Wilkin, 1990]. Equally, this discrepancy could be explained by insufficient sensitivity in the current assay for TRab.

Not all patients with hyperthyroidism develop a goiter. Preparations of immunoglobulins from the sera of patients with Graves' disease who had developed a goiter stimulated the synthesis of DNA in thyroid tissue from guinea pigs, while preparations from patients with Graves' disease who did not have a goiter did not [Drexhage et al., 1980]. The titer of these "thyroid growth-stimulating" antibodies correlates well with goiter size in such an assay. However, a strong correlation between thyroid growth-stimulating antibodies and TRab is frequently absent. Thus it would appear that the antibodies involved are binding to quite different epitopes [van der Gaag et al., 1985].

The detection of TRab is at the end rather than the beginning of the immunological story of Graves' disease. Obviously, these antibodies fail to provoke an adequate (disarming) anti-idiotypic response. What do we know of the mechanisms that have gone astray to allow the production of such disease-producing immunoglobulins?

CELLS INVOLVED IN THE PRODUCTION OF GRAVES' DISEASE

A number of techniques have analyzed the phenotypic profile of the lymphoid cells that enter the thyroid gland during the development of Graves' disease and the autoimmune thyroiditis that destroys the gland to produce hypothyroidism. It might have been expected that CD8 cytotoxic cells would predominate in the thyroid gland of patients with Hashimoto's thyroiditis, for cytotoxic destruction of thyrocytes is a feature of the pathology. In Graves' disease, theoretical considerations might have suggested that CD4 helper lymphocytes would predominate, for it would appear essential that their presence would be required to stimulate the production of autoantibody by B cells. However, a mixed picture is found in both conditions [Weetman and McGregor, 1984]. In Graves' disease, some T cells display the cluster differentiation antigen CD8, suggesting that they are either immunoregulatory or cytotoxic T cells, or that a combination of both is present. There are indeed CD4 lymphocytes present, which could be cells capable of helping locally abundant B cells to produce antibodies, but equally those CD4 lymphocytes could in fact be attempting to induce suppressor cell activity. That at least some of the cells are engaged in such activity is strengthened by the recent finding that some CD4 cells also display the $CD4CD5RA^+$ markers characteristic of cells inducing suppressor cell activity [Davies et al., 1991b]. It seems likely that these phenotypes would have been displayed on the cells as they entered the gland, but it is impossible to be certain that they did not mature after the cells had taken up residency. Animal models have certainly demonstrated the importance of T cells in the development of autoimmune thyroiditis, and there is no doubt that the disease can be adoptively transferred into normal animals by T cells alone [Romball and Weigle, 1987].

What has attracted to the thyroid the T cells found in the glands of a patient with Graves' disease? During secondary immune responses, all manner of bystander lymphoid cells may be recruited to come to the antigen-attacking party; the response thus features polyclonal cells in the sense that many of the cells present will not have T-cell receptors capable of binding to the antigen that initiated the immune response (in our case, thyroid autoantigens). If, on the other hand, the majority of T cells present in the gland of a patient with thyroid disease do indeed have receptors capable of recognizing the receptor for TSH, for example, it would be hard to argue that such cells were not present because a primary immune response, albeit an unfortunate one, was underway with TSH receptor proteins as targets [Margolick et al., 1984].

It has been difficult to harvest the T cells from the glands of patients with thyroid disease, clonally expand them, and then have them survive in culture long enough to study whether their receptors have binding properties specific for thyroid autoantigens [Mackenzie et al., 1987]. However, new technology has supplied strong, albeit indirect, evidence that suggests that the T cells present in the gland of patients with Graves' disease are likely to be thyroid-reactive cells involved in a primary immune response.

The T-cell receptor consists of an α- and a β-chain with constant and variable regions akin to those found on an immunoglobulin [Ben-Nun et al., 1991]. The three-dimensional configuration of the variable region determines what antigenic determinant (epitope) will have a best fit with that particular T cell. T-cell receptor genes undergo rearrangement only in T cells, just as the genes responsible for the production of immunoglobulins undergo rearrangement only in B cells [Oksenberg et al., 1990]. Not surprisingly therefore different clones of T cells whose receptors are interested in the same epitope tend to use the same T-cell receptor variable genes expressing a restricted number of products from the 18 genes available for the variable region of the α-chain of the T-cell receptor [Davies et al., 1991b].

With polymerase chain reaction (PCR) technology, it has been possible to show that the T cells in the thyroid gland of patients with thyroid disease have a restricted heterogeneity [Davies et al., 1991b]. They are not innocent wanderers that happen to be passing through the gland or cells lured in by the cytokines released during a primary immune response in the gland. These T cells in the gland of patients with thyroid disease are focused, aggressive, antigen-specific cells for some reason turned on to antigens expressed on thyroid epithelial cells. Although for obvious reasons the theory cannot be tested in humans, it thus seems likely that T cells must play an initiating role in the production of Graves' disease, just as they do in producing disease when adoptively transferred into normal animals.

A restriction fragment length polymorphism of the T-cell receptor constant β-chain gene has been shown to be associated with Graves' disease in a patient population from Newfoundland [Demaine et al., 1987]. However, a more recent study failed to find any significant association of such genes with Graves' disease in patients in the United Kingdom [Weetman et al., 1987].

While T cells in the thyroid gland of individual patients with Graves' disease show a restriction in the expression of Vα gene products, all patients do not display the same Vα profile. Indeed, the heterogeneity of α-gene expression from patient to patient may indicate that individuals need certain gene rearrangements for the homing of particular cells to their target organ and the ability to passage such cells through endothelial cells into the thyroid gland [Davies et al., 1991b]. Specific HLA haplotypes may require distinct Vα-gene rearrangements if T-cell receptor, antigen, and essential histocompatibility profiles are to interact. Similar studies of the T-cell receptor gene rearrangements on the lymphocytes found in the eyes of patients with Graves' disease will be important.

An increase in the number of circulating B cells with a CD5 phenotype (leu1 in humans and Ly1 in mice) has been noted in the circulation of patients with Graves' disease. CD5$^+$ B cells appear to represent a major subset of the normal human B-cell repertoire capable of either producing autoantibodies or acting as helper cells for those B lymphocytes that may mature to autoantibody-secreting plasma cells [Casali et al., 1987]. CD5$^+$ cells are markedly increased (greater than 9% above the normal range) in hyperthyroid patients with Graves' disease prior to treatment [Iwatani et al., 1989]. No such increase is noted in patients with Hashimoto's disease. The number of circulating CD5 lymphocytes returns to normal after treatment of the hyperthyroidism, and the fall correlates well with a fall in TRab. It seems likely that high levels of thyroid hormone itself directly affect the number of circulating CD5$^+$ cells [Iwatani et al., 1989].

In summary, the above evidence obtained with the cells from the thyroid glands of patients with Graves' disease strongly suggests that invading T cells are reacting to defined sequences of the TSH receptor but do not establish that concept as fact. To date, cloning studies on intrathyroidal cells have detected T cells capable of reacting to the thyroid cell antigens, thyroglobulin, and thyroid peroxidase, but not to the receptor for TSH itself [Fisfalen et al., 1988; Londei et al., 1985].

As CD4, CD8, and B cells are present in diseased glands, all the elements necessary for initiating humoral and cellular immune attacks on thyroid epitopes are in place. CD4 cells could "help" B cells make antibodies, such as TRab, while CD8 cells could attack thyroid elements in a cytotoxic fashion after receiving permission from CD4 inducer cells in the form of interleukin-2 (IL-2). Clearly, the same data make it equally possible that moderating influences on both T and B lymphocytes in the form of CD4$^+$ suppressor inducer cells, and CD8 regulatory T cells, may also be present. Disease or nondisease could well be a matter of the balance of such activated forces. Further studies are needed to clarify the matter.

DO THYROID EPITHELIAL CELLS MAKE THEMSELVES TARGETS FOR AUTOIMMUNE PHENOMENA BY EXPRESSING CLASS I AND CLASS II MHC ANTIGENS?

On normal human thyroid epithelial cells, only trace amounts of class I (HLA-A, -B, -C) antigens have been found [Lucas-Martin et al., 1988]. Class II antigens (HLA-DR, -DP, -DQ) have not been detected [Hanafusa et al., 1983]. Conversely, the epithelial cells from the thyroid gland of patients with Graves' disease and autoimmune (destructive) thyroiditis display an increased density of class I antigens and do express class II antigens [Londei et al., 1985]. Studies from several laboratories have suggested that the appearance of class II antigens allows increased CD4 lymphocyte recognition of autoantigens, with subsequent help being provided to B cells to make autoantibodies [Davies, 1985; Eguchi et al., 1987].

Helper/inducer CD4 lymphocytes only respond to antigen if the binding to the T-cell receptor incorporates binding of HLA-DR peptides. With the discovery that the thyroid cells of patients with Graves' disease express class II antigens, the previously presented data become less surprising. Any number of thyroid autoantigens may be recognized by the cells accumulating in the thyroid, while the recognition of determinants of the receptor for TSH could lead to the production thyroid-stimulating immunoglobulins. The important question relates to the reason the thyroid cells would do something so potentially dangerous and abnormal as to display the molecules that allow these normally hormone-producing cells to become antigen-presenting cells, in this case presenting themselves. Indeed, it has been reported that thyroid epithelial cells expressing class II antigen can present foreign antigen to T cells [Davies and Piccinini, 1987].

A number of reports have demonstrated the ability of interferon-γ (IFN-γ) to induce the expression on thyroid epithelial cells of class II antigens [Todd et al., 1985; Weetman et al., 1985]. The process is facilitated by TSH itself and by tumor necrosis factor-α (TNF-α) [Buscema et al., 1989].

Certainly, the thyroid epithelial cells in patients with autoimmune thyroiditis can produce IFN-γ and TNF-α, as well as IL-1 and IL-6 [Turner et al., 1987].

In vitro exposure of normal thyroid epithelial cells to specific concentrations of IFN-γ for 3 days will lead to the expression of both class I and class II antigens. While IFN-α is maintained in the cell cultures, class II antigen will continue to be expressed. Such antigens rapidly disappear if IFN-γ is removed [Todd et al., 1985; Weetman et al., 1985]. TNF-α alone can enhance the expression of class I but not class II antigens. It can, however, act synergistically with IFN-γ to enhance the expression of all HLA antigens [Migita et al., 1990]. A similar synergistic effect has been reported in studies looking at the expression of class II antigens on pancreatic β cells where TNF-α actually stimulates activated T cells to produce IFN-γ [Pujol-Borrell et al., 1987].

Another cytokine that has no effect on the expression of HLA antigens on thyroid epithelial cells without a partner is IL-1. A synergistic effect has however been noted if IL-1 and IFN-γ are combined [Turner et al., 1987]. Of importance, studies have demonstrated that the cytokines thus far mentioned, either alone or in combination, are not directly cytotoxic for thyroid epithelial cells [Migita et al., 1990]. IL-6 does not enhance thyroid cell expression of HLA antigens but can drive B cells to antibody production and thus could enhance the local production of TRab [Grubeck-Loebenstein et al., 1989].

Thus to date we have observed that the thyroid gland in patients with Graves' disease contains numerous activated T cells. The similarity of the T-cell receptors on such cells suggests that a primary immune response is underway. These cells together with the abundant dendritic (? antigen presenting) cells present in the gland seem to produce numerous cytokines. The net effect is to upregulate the expression of HLA I or II antigens, thus creating a situation in which self-tolerance could fail and an autoaggressive primary immune response develop.

WHY ARE THYROID EPITHELIAL CELLS TURNED INTO ANTIGEN-PRESENTING CELLS?

The simple answer here is "we do not know," but two theories are popular. The first is that all the autoimmune phenomena are secondary to infection occurring within the thyroid gland [Ingbar et al., 1987]. This scenario presents as follows. An infection of thyroid epithelial cells by, for example, a virus would lead to the expression on the surface of the infected cells of viral proteins. Some of these proteins would be secreted into the extracellular fluid where they could be picked up and presented to antigen-specific CD4 lymphocytes by antigen-presenting cells, such as macrophages or B cells. The production of specific antiviral antibodies may follow, but the earlier interactions would involve the release of numerous cytokines. These cytokines would upregulate the expression of class I and class II antigens, as well as adhesion molecules (see below), on the surface of the thyroid epithelial cell infected with virus. The infected cells now become targets for antigen-specific lymphocytes. They are destroyed, and the initiating virus is eliminated.

However, in genetically susceptible individuals, the presence in the thyroid gland of these lymphokines would lead to such significant upregulation of the expression of class I antigens and the aberrant expression of class II antigens on thyrocytes that antigenic determinants presented on the surface of *nonvirus*-infected epithelial cells would provoke a response. Viral antigens themselves, or the cytokine cocktail released because of the infection, leads to decreased surveillance by immunoregulatory T cells in genetically susceptible individuals, and the disease process persists. A chronic autoimmune disease results.

An alternative variation on this theme would suggest that viral proteins could either damage self-antigens on the surface of thyroid epithelial cells or bind to them in such a way that they are recognized as "altered self" [Weigle, 1977]. An appropriate but self-damaging immune response would follow. Finally, it is possible that some viral proteins may have a three-dimensional configuration that mimics that of an autoantigen. Because determinants of the virus are present that do not mimic self, an immune response will follow, with the cytokine release described above leading to the generation of a response against both the viral antigens that mimic self and the self-antigens themselves [Weigle, 1977].

While this theory is attractive, there is virtually no evidence to support it, for there has been no convincing demonstration of an infection within the thyroid epithelial cells of patients with Graves' disease or, for that matter, in any part of the gland. However, it is interesting that for many years it has been noted that a number of patients with Graves' disease do frequently complain that they have had an unusually large number of infections prior to developing their thyroid disease [Andreoli et al., 1990].

Recently, attention has been focused once again on the gram-negative bacillus *Yersinia enterocolitica,* first linked to thyroid disease in 1974 [Bech et al., 1974]. Humans are infected with *Yersinia* by direct spread from animals, and a chronic enterocolitis may develop. Autoimmune phenomena such as skin eruptions and arthralgia are not uncommon in humans infected with *Yersinia.* Of great interest but uncertain biological significance is the fact that *Y. enterocolitica* contains a saturable binding site for human TSH. Such hormone binding sites seems to be well conserved among such organisms, for gonadotropin and bovine TSH can be bound to other members of the family. It has thus been suggested that *Y. enterocolitica* must contain antigenic determinants that cross-react with human thyroid autoantigens. Studies have suggested that as many as 80% of patients with Graves' disease have in their serum IgG antibodies to *Yersinia* plasmid proteins [Weiss et al., 1987]. It may be, however, that it is not *Yersinia* infection that stimulates the production of TRab; rather, it is the abnormal process responsible for Graves' disease that ensures that antibodies will be produced that can bind to the cross-reacting sequences within the bacillus. This interpretation is supported by a recent prospective study of patients with Graves' disease, all of whom were negative for plasmid protein antibodies at the time of diagnosis, although they had developed TRab at that stage. Six months after the diagnosis, however, all patients had developed antibodies that could react with *Yersinia* plasmid protein [Wenzel and Heesemann, 1987].

One other environmental factor deserves mention. There are reports of an association between stressful life events and Graves' disease [Winsa et al., 1991]. As stress has been frequently related to disturbed immune performance, it is conceivable that in a genetically susceptible individual inadequate coping skills or unavoidable stress produces, through connections existing between the central nervous system and lymphocytes, a disturbance in immunoregulation that initiates Graves' disease. It is of interest that an increased incidence of Graves' disease has been observed during each major war this century. In the 1939–45 war, hospital admissions for Graves' disease increased fivefold in Scandinavia but quickly returned to normal after the war [Kracht and Kracht, 1952; Rosch, 1992].

ADHESION MOLECULES AND THE INDUCTION OF GRAVES' DISEASE

The migration of lymphocytes into an area where antigen awaits recognition and attack is not a random affair [Shimizu and Shaw, 1991]. Receptors on the surface of lymphocytes interact with adhesion molecules on the endothelial cells lining a blood vessel and move through the vessel wall into an extracellular matrix where they are again guided to a target [Springer, 1990]. Once a T cell reaches a potential target, it must recognize antigen bound to cell surface MHC antigens. However, while this specific recognition is needed for activation, other mechanisms produce a necessarily tight adhesion of the T-cell surface membrane to its target that is at least 10 times stronger than that achieved by T-cell receptor-antigen binding [Dustin et al., 1988]. In addition to increasing the efficiency of binding, there is good evidence that interaction of adhesion molecules on the surface of a T cell and an antigen-processing cell may involve the generation of signaling cascades, important to the generation of an efficient response [Springer et al., 1987].

The major molecules producing these immunological "bear hugs," without which neither helper nor cytotoxic function will ensue, are members of the integrin and immunoglobulin supergene families, respectively. Lymphocyte function-related antigen (LFA-1) is present on the surface of T cells, while an intercellular cell adhesion molecule (ICAM-1) is present on many antigen-presenting cells and cells pressed into that function by cytokines such as IFN-γ and TNF-α, which are capable of upregulating the expression of ICAM-1 on a cell membrane, as well as HLA-DR [Springer, 1990]. A thyroid epithelial cell displaying its receptor for TSH, in association with HLA class II antigen and the adhesion molecule ICAM-1, would be a provocative target indeed for even the most disciplined T cell attempting to remain tolerant.

The presence or absence of ICAM-1 molecules on the surface of thyroid epithelial cells from patients with Graves' disease is controversial because of conflicting data. Two studies have reported that ICAM-1 was either present on the surface of thyroid epithelial cells stained for the molecule using indirect immunofluorescent techniques and monoclonal antibodies or after the exposure of the cells to IFN-γ and TNF-α in vitro [Weetman et al., 1989; Zheng et al., 1990]. Of interest, a second adhesion molecule, LFA-3, appeared on the surface of thyroid epithelial cells from patients with Graves' disease exposed to these cytokines. This molecule is known to interact with the CD2 antigen present on the surface of both helper and cytotoxic T cells and is an integrin thought to be important in the signaling processes mentioned earlier [Zheng et al., 1990]. Cells from the thyroid glands of patients with nontoxic goiters could not be persuaded to display LFA-3 in the presence of IFN-γ and TNF-α. The rapid disappearance of adhesion molecules from the surface of the thyroid epithelial cells after cytokines were withdrawn may explain why cells harvested from patients with Graves' disease did not display ICAM-1 or LFA-3 until cytokines were introduced into the tissue culture fluids. The staining techniques referred to above were able to demonstrate both ICAM-1 and LFA-3 at the basal surface of thyroid epithelial cells from patients with Graves' disease.

In contrast to these studies, a further examination of the question using frozen sections of tissue, monoclonal antibodies, and immunofluorescence failed to find ICAM-1 on the thyroid epithelial cells from 30 patients with Graves' disease but did find a vivid display of the molecule on the epithelial cells of 75% of patients with autoimmune thyroiditis [Bagnasco et al., 1991]. The methodology and the sensitivity used in these varying studies were dissimilar but it seems certain that ICAM-1 expression is much stronger on the cells of patients with Hashimoto's thyroiditis. Thyroid epithelial cells may be able to present antigens (both exogenous and self-antigens) in Graves' disease, thus stimulating the production of TRab while escaping destruction by cytotoxic T cells because of a relative lack of ICAM-1 and perhaps LFA-3.

DOWNREGULATION OF THE EXPRESSION OF CLASS II ANTIGENS ON THYROID EPITHELIAL LYMPHOCYTES FROM PATIENTS WITH GRAVES' DISEASE

In immunology, one can be confident that if molecules can be found to upregulate the expression of a cell's surface protein, somewhere in the cytokine cocktail will be molecules that will downregulate the same structure.

Thus it is not surprising that molecules capable of both upregulating and downregulating the expression of class II antigens on thyroid epithelial cells have been discovered. Epidermal growth factor and the closely related transforming growth factor-α can suppress the induction of HLA class II antigens on thyroid epithelial cells exposed to IFN-γ and TNF-α [Todd et al., 1990]. The downregulation occurs both at the time of attempted induction and after class II antigens have been expressed. It is relatively easy to overcome the downregulatory effects of these molecules by adding additional IFN-γ. It may well be that a disturbance in the critical balance of these regulatory forces develops in patients with autoimmune diseases in general and Graves' disease in particular.

DISTURBED IMMUNOREGULATION AND GRAVES' DISEASE

For many years it has been suggested that a failure of antigen-specific immunoregulatory T cells would be pivotal in the development of Graves' disease [Volpé, 1987]. Among autoreactive T lymphocytes one would expect to find in healthy individuals CD4 helper and CD8 cytotoxic lymphocytes with receptors for determinants within the receptor for TSH. But in such individuals one would also expect to find antigen-specific T cells recognizing the same determinants but with the responsibility for ensuring that any potentially autoaggressive lymphocytes remain quiescent. CD4 suppressor inducer and CD8 suppressor cells programmed to recognize but downregulate any response to TSH receptor antigens would be a feature of any normal regulatory network primed to prevent autoimmunity. A failure of this regulatory mechanism induced by genetic and/or environmental factors could explain the onset of Graves' disease. While plausible, even likely, the concept remains unproven.

To date, no T cells with receptors for any of the determinants associated with the receptor for TSH have been identified. T cells capable of recognizing many other thyroid antigens, especially thyroglobulin, have, however, been observed [Fisfalen et al., 1988; Londei et al., 1985]. However, it is of interest to note that when patients with thyrotoxicosis are treated with methiazole, which blocks the release of T_3 and T_4, there is a decrease in the number of intrathyroidal CD4 cells and an increase in CD8 cells. The latter may well be immunosuppressive in nature. Hypothyroidism itself affects CD8 suppressor cell performance, and thus the thyrotoxic state could help to perpetuate the disease process [Volpé, 1986].

In both Graves' disease and Hashimoto's thyroiditis, reductions in the number and function of circulating suppressor T cells have been reported, with the most convincing studies examining the function of antigen-specific immunoregulatory T cells [Tomer and Shoenfeld, 1989]. It has been demonstrated, for example, that in Graves' disease and insulin-dependent diabetes mellitus a defect exists in the ability of suppressor T cells from patients to suppress lymphocyte migration in response to thyroid and islet cell antigens, respectively [Topliss et al., 1983]. However, the defect in suppressor cell response to islet cell antigens in diabetes can be corrected by adding suppressor cells from patients with Graves' disease, while the defect in the suppressor cell response to thyroid antigens in Graves' disease can be corrected by adding suppressor cells from patients with diabetes. Such findings strongly suggest that the suppressor T-cell defects in Graves' disease and diabetes are antigen specific and different. Recent complementary reports suggest that the activity of suppressor inducer cells in the thyroid gland of patients with Graves' disease is decreased [Ueki et al., 1987].

Another disturbance in immunoregulation may be important for inducing the pathogenetic mechanisms that lead to Graves' disease and indeed many other autoimmune conditions. A failure of anti-idiotypic mechanisms to prevent the production or function of pathology-inducing autoantibodies may be a central feature of autoaggressive disease.

Two separate anti-idiotypic networks have been characterized, one found only in healthy people and the other occurring in those who have avoided autoimmune-induced pathology by making a supranormal immunoregulatory response or recovering from such an insult by the production of immunoregulatory anti-idiotypic antibodies [Varela et al., 1991].

Normal individuals produce autoantibodies against a host of self-antigens. These are normally IgM in class, and antibodies to these antibodies, usually of the IgG class, are detectable in the serum of healthy individuals [Rossi et al., 1989]. This normal idiotype–anti-idiotype interaction helps to keep our immunological house in order. For autoimmune disease to occur, it appears that T and B cells must respond to *different antigenic determinants* on self-tissues than those that provoke the production of natural autoantibodies. In the disease situation, self-determinants complexed to an individual's MHC antigens tempt immunocytes capable of responding to the complex. Anti-idiotypic antibodies should be produced in response to any autoantibodies that follow, particularly if they are likely to produce tissue damage.

In general, research to date suggests that anti-idiotypic antibodies capable of binding to disease-producing immunoglobulin idiotypes are not found in patients with active autoimmune disease [Varela and Coutinho, 1991]. Such protective antibodies are found in the serum of many relatives of patients with autoimmune diseases, suggesting that some may have avoided disease by their production. Anti-idiotypic antibodies, however, capable of down-regulating the production of disease-associated autoantibodies are most easily found in the serum of patients enjoying a remission from disease [Dietrich et al., 1991]. Of interest, such anti-idiotypic antibodies have a broad specificity that enables them to neutralize a number of disease-producing autoantibodies [Rossi and Kazatchkine, 1989].

In patients with thyroid disease, T and B cells responsive to thyroid autoantigens are plentiful. Antibodies to thyroglobulin provoke anti-idiotypic antibodies in patients with quiescent disease [Rossi et al., 1991], and there is some evidence that antibody to TRab helps to control Graves' disease in humans [Paschke et al., 1990].

A number of authors have argued that TRab may themselves be anti-idiotypic antibodies to autoantibodies against TSH itself [Hill and Erlanger, 1988]. This seems to be unlikely for a number of reasons. Internal image anti-idiotypic antibodies would be required, and these are known to represent only a minor portion of an immune response to idiotype [Roitt et al., 1985]. TSH binding antibodies are found in only a very small percentage of patients with Graves' disease [Raines et al., 1985]. Moreover, if TRab bound antibodies to TSH, TSH itself should be detectable in the sera of patients with Graves' disease but in fact it is usually markedly suppressed.

If we accept that TRab are primary autoantibodies produced in response to the receptor for TSH itself, then some anti-idiotypic antibodies to TRab might be expected to be capable of binding to TSH. Several groups have reported the presence of antibodies in the serum of patients with Graves' disease that will bind to bovine TSH; however, these are not anti-idiotypic antibodies and are not thought to be of any clinical significance [Biro, 1981].

One study does suggest that remission sera from patients with Graves' disease contain antibody to TRab that can prevent this antibody from binding to the receptor for TSH. The methodology used involves the transplantation of thyroid tissues from patients with Graves' disease into athymic nude mice with subsequent studies of the effects of remission sera on the blocking of the biological activity of exacerbation sera [Davies et al., 1991a].

Regulatory mechanisms involving anti-idiotypic antibodies are not necessarily distinct from those involving sensitized suppressor T cells. Anti-idiotype can directly neutralize antibody and, via a direct effect on B cells, either upregulate or downregulate their production of antibody [Kaveri et al., 1991], but they can also interact with suppressor T cells [Dwyer 1992], thus allowing both mechanisms to be interactive in a protective network. Studies on the suppression or prevention of autoimmune disease, for example, experimental allergic encephalomyelitis, after vaccination with T lymphocytes suggest a regulatory role for an idiotypic T-cell network on the expression of autoreactivity, integrated with complex physiological regulatory interactions that occur among lymphocytes and between lymphocytes and antibodies [Varela et al., 1991].

THYROID-ASSOCIATED EYE DISEASE

Progressive inflammation of the extraocular muscles and the surrounding orbital connective tissues occurs in most patients with Graves' disease and in a small proportion of those with Hashimoto's thyroiditis. There are several possible explanations for the unique association of ophthalmopathy and thyroid disease, none of which are entirely satisfactory. One explanation invokes the proximity of the orbit to the thyroid gland, and there is evidence for the existence of lymphatic channels between the two tissues [Rusznyak et al., 1967]. The transfer of antibodies, cytokines, or mononuclear cells from the thyroid gland to the orbit may thus be facilitated, and it is of interest that the eye disease is sometimes worse on the side on which a patient habitually sleeps [Wall et al., 1991]. However, most of the evidence suggests that the possibility of immunological cross-reactivity, that is, antigenic determinants that are shared on thyroid epithelial cells and the cells of the extraocular eye muscles, is best supported by the experimental data [Salvi et al., 1988]. Indeed, convincing support for the hypothesis has recently been obtained from cloning and sequencing eye muscle and thyroid proteins that are targets for autoantibodies in the serum of patients with thyroid-associated eye disease [Wall et al., 1991]. Various epitopes shared by soluble and membrane-associated thyroid and eye muscle antigens have been recognized by monoclonal antibodies. The correlation between eye muscle disease and anti-eye muscle antibodies is best for an antibody against a 64 kD antigen [Wall et al., 1991]. Sera from 50% of unselected patients with thyroid eye disease and 75% of those with severe eye disease of recent onset have antibodies that react with an immunodominant 64 kD antigen in eye muscle membranes that is also expressed on thyroid membranes.

Antibodies reactive with the 64 kD antigen might cause eye disease because they are cytotoxic to both thyroid and eye muscle cells, evoking antibody-dependent cell-mediated cytotoxicity. Alternatively, such antibodies may only be markers of the thyroid eye muscle autoimmune reaction, with tissue damage being mediated by cytotoxic antibodies reactive with related antigens. The possible involvement of cytotoxic T cells that bind to the 64 kD protein in association with an appropriate MHC class I molecule is another possible mechanism.

A currently unexplainable discrepancy in all these theories has been mentioned earlier, namely, the worsening of the thyroid eye disease as thyrotoxicosis and antibodies against thyroid antigen decline. The ability of intravenously administered IgG to suppress the retro-orbital inflammatory response associated with thyroid eye disease, even in situations in which standard immunosuppressive regimens have failed, makes it reasonable to suggest that anti-idiotypic antibodies may be present in pooled human gammaglobulin that are capable of suppressing the inflammatory response whatever its cause [Dwyer et al., 1991].

FINAL THOUGHTS

Many of the changes anticipated if Graves' disease is indeed produced by autoimmune pathology have been readily demonstrated. We are, however, left with tantalizing questions that are important but difficult to answer. Clearly, our ultimate frustration at this stage is ignorance at the molecular level of the initiating event that leads to an attack on the receptor for TSH. Do some genetically prone individuals have T cells that can react with expressed autoantigens not associated with class II antigens, thus starting a cascade that secondarily involves the upregulation of class I and class II antigens and the subsequent perpetuation of the immunopathology? Is there an unrecognized infectious agent involved in the triggering of Graves' disease? Can, in some individuals, antigen-presenting cells not involved in a specific immune response be triggered to release cytokines in the thyroid gland in a manner analogous to the activation of complement cascades by an alternative pathway? Such de novo cytokine release could initiate pathology. One imagines that there must be an efficient mechanism operating at the tissue level that protects cells from being attacked themselves when locally cytokines must be released to facilitate a response to foreignness. In autoimmune diseases in general and in Graves' disease in particular, are such mechanisms failing?

While such questions cannot currently be answered, the techniques available to modern immunologists should help Graves' disease surrender its mysteries in the near future. In so doing, it is certain that a much better understanding of autoimmune diseases in general will follow, thus increasing the likelihood that safe, efficient, and curative therapeutic strategies can be developed.

REFERENCES

Adams DD (1988): Long-acting thyroid stimulator: How receptor autoimmunity was discovered. Autoimmunity 1:3–9.

Andreoli TE, Carpenter CCJ, Plum F, Smith LH Jr (1990): The thyroid. In Andreoli TE, Carpenter CCJ, Plum F, Smith LH Jr (eds): "Cecil Essentials of Medicine." 2nd Ed. Philadelphia: WB Saunders, pp 456–466.

Bagnasco M, Caretto A, Olive D, Pedini B, Canonica GW, Betterle C (1991): Expression of intercellular adhesion molecule-1 (ICAM-1) on thyroid epithelial cells in Hashimoto's thyroiditis but not in Graves' disease or papillary thyroid cancer. Clin Exp Immunol 83:309–313.

Bech K, Larsen JH, Hansen JM, Nerup J (1974): *Yersinia enterocolitica* infection and thyroid disorders. Lancet 2:951–952.

Ben-Nun A, Liblau RS, Cohen L, Lehmann D, Tornier-Lasserve E, Rosenzweig A, Zhang JW, Raus JC, Bach MA (1991): Restricted T cell receptor V beta usage by myelin basic protein-specific T cell clones in multiple sclerosis: predominant genes vary in individuals. Proc Natl Acad Sci USA 88:2466–2470.

Biro J (1981): Specific binding of thyroid-stimulation hormone by human serum globulins. J Endocrinol 88:339–349.

Bottazzo GF, Pujol-Borell R, Hanafusa T, Feldmann M (1983): Role of aberrant HLA-DR expression and antigen presentation in induction of endocrine autoimmunity. Lancet (ii):1115–1159.

Brostoff J, Scadding GK, Male DK, Roitt IM (1991): Endocrine disorders. In Brostoff J, Scadding GK, Male DK, Roitt IM (eds): "Clinical Immunology." London: Gower Medical Publishing, diagrams 7.1–7.13.

Burman KD, Baker JR (1985): Immune mechanisms in Graves' disease. Endocrine Rev 6:183–232.

Buscema M, Todd I, Deuss V, Hammond L, Mirukian R, Pujol-Borrell R, Bottazzo GF (1989): Influence of tumor necrosis factor-x on the modulation by IFN-γ of

HLA class II molecules in human thyroid cells and its effect of interferon-γ binding. J Clin Endocrinol Metab 69:433–439.

Casali P, Burastero SE, Nakamura M, Inghirami G, Notkins AL (1987): Human lymphocytes making rheumatoid factor and antibody to ssDNA belong to Leu-1[+] B cell subset. Science 236:77–81.

Charreire J (1989): Immune mechanisms in autoimmune thyroiditis. Adv Immunol 46:263–334.

Chopra IJ, Hershman JM, Pardridge WM, Nicoloff JT (1983): Thyroid function in nonthyroidal illness. Ann Intern Med 98:946–957.

Davies TF, Kimura H, Fong P, Kendler D, Shultz LD, Thung S, Martin A (1991a): The SCID-hu mouse and thyroid autoimmunity: Characterization of human thyroid autoantibody secretion. Clin Immunol Immunopathol 60:319–330.

Davies TF (1985): Cocultures of human thyroid monolayer cells and autologous T cells: Impact of HLA class II antigen expression. J Clin Endocrinol Metab 61:418–422.

Davies TF, Martin A, Concepcion ES, Graves P, Cohen L, Ben-Nun A (1991b): Evidence of limited variability of antigen receptors on intrathyroidal T cells in autoimmune thyroid disease. N Engl J Med 325(4):238–244.

Davies TF, Piccinini LA (1987): Intrathyroidal MHC class II antigen expression and thyroid autoimmunity. Endocrinol Metab Clin North Am 16:247–268.

Demaine AG, Welsh KI, Hawe BS, Farid NR (1987): Polymorphism of the T cell receptor beta chain in Graves' disease. J Clin Endocrinol Metab 65:643–646.

Dietrich G, Piechaczyk M, Pau B, Kazatchkine MD (1991): Evidence for restricted epitopic and idiotypic specificity of anti-thyroglobulin autoantibodies. Eur J Immunol 21:811–814.

Drexhage HA, Bottazzo GF, Doniach D, Bitensky L, Chayen J (1980): Evidence for thyroid-growth-stimulating immunoglobulins in some goitrous thyroid diseases. Lancet 2:287–292.

Drexhage HA, van der Gaag RD (1986): Immunoglobulins affecting thyroid growth. In McGregor AM (ed): "Immunology of Endocrine Disease." Lancaster: MTP Press Ltd., pp 51–70.

Dustin ML, Staunton DL, Springer TA (1988): Supergene families meet in the immune system. Immunol Today 9:213–215.

Dwyer JM (1992): Manipulating the immune system with immune globulin. N Engl J Med 326(2):107–116.

Dwyer JM, Benson EM, Currie JN, O'Day J (1991): Intravenously administered IgG for the treatment of thyroid eye disease. In Imbach P (ed): "Immunotherapy With Intravenous Immunoglobulins." London: Academic Press, pp 387–394.

Eguchi K, Otsubo T, Kawabe Y, Ueki Y, Fukuda T, Matsunaga M, Shimomura C, Ishikawa N, Tezuka H, Nakao H, Ito K, Morimoto C, Nagataki S (1987): The remarkable proliferation of helper T cell subsets in response to autologous thyrocytes and intrathyroidal T cells from patients with Graves' disease. Clin Exp Immunol 70:403–410.

Farid NR, Bear JC (1981): The human major histocompatibility complex and endocrine disease. Endocrine Rev 2:50–86.

Fisfalen ME, DeGroot LJ, Quintans J, Franklin WA, Soltani K (1988): Microsomal antigen-reactive lymphocyte lines and clones derived from thyroid tissues of patients with Graves' disease. J Clin Endocrinol Metab 66:776–784.

Grubeck-Loebenstein B, Buchan B, Chantry D, Kassal H, Londei M, Pirich K, Barrett K, Turner M, Waldhausl W, Feldmann M (1989): Analysis of intrathyroidal cytokine production in thyroid autoimmune disease: Thyroid follicular cells produce interleukin-1α and interleukin-6. Clin Exp Immunol 77:324–330.

Hanafusa T, Pujol-Borrell R, Chiovato L, Russell RCG, Doniach D, Bottazzo GF (1983): Aberrant expression of HLA-DR antigen on thyrocytes in Graves' disease. Lancet 2:1111–1115.

Hill BL, Erlanger BF (1988): Monoclonal antibodies to the thyrotropin receptor raised by an autoantiidiotypic protocol and their relationship to monoclonal antibodies from Graves' patients. Endocrinology 6:2840–2850.

Hoffenberg R (1987): Thyroid disorders. In Weatherall DJ, Ledingham JGG, Warrell DA (eds): "Oxford Textbook of Medicine." 2nd Ed. Oxford: Oxford University Press, pp 10.30–10.50.

Ingbar SH, Weiss M, Cushing GW, Kasper DL (1987): A possible role for bacterial antigens in the pathogenesis of autoimmune thyroid disease. In Pinchera A, Ingbar SH, McKenzie JM, Fenzi GF (eds): "Thyroid Immunity." New York: Plenum Press, pp 35–44.

Iwatani Y, Amino N, Kaneda T, Ichihara K, Tamaki H, Tachi J, Matsuzuka F, Fukata S, Kuma K, Miyai K (1989): Marked increase of CD5$^+$ B cells in hyperthyroid Graves' disease. Clin Exp Immunol 78:196–200.

Kaveri S-V, Dietrich G, Hurez V, Kazatchkine MD (1991): Intravenous immunoglobulins (IVIg) in the treatment of autoimmune diseases. Clin Exp Immunol 86:192–198.

Konishi J, Iida Y, Endo K, Misaki T, Nohara Y, Matsoura N, Mori T, Torizuka K (1983): Inhibition of thyrotropin-induced adenosine 3′,5′-monophosphate increase by immunoglobulins from patients with primary myxoedema. J Clin Endocrinol Metab 57:544–549.

Kracht J, Kracht U (1952): Zur histopathologie und therapie de schreckthyrotoxicosis der wildkaminchens. Virchows Arche 321:238–274.

Kriss JP, Pleshakov V, Chien JR (1964): Isolation and identification of the long-acting thyroid stimulator and its relation to hyperthyroidism and circumscribed pretibial myxoedema. J Clin Endocrinol Metab 24:1005–1028.

Larsen PR (1988): The thyroid. In Wyngaarden JB, Smith LH Jr (eds): "Cecil Textbook of Medicine." 18th ed. Philadelphia: WB Saunders, pp 1315–1340.

Libert F, Lefort A, Gerard C, Parmentier M, Perret J, Ludgate M, Dumont JE, Vassart G (1989): Cloning, sequencing and expression of the human thyrotropin (TSH) receptor: Evidence for binding of autoantibodies. Biochem Biophys Res Commun 165:1250–1255.

Londei M, Bottazzo GF, Feldmann M (1985): Human T cell clones from autoimmune thyroid glands: Specific recognition of autologous thyroid cells. Science 228:85–89.

Lucas-Martin A, Foz-Sala M, Todd I, Bottazzo GF, Pujol-Borrell R (1988): Occurrence of thyrocyte HLA class II expression in a wide variety of thyroid disease: Relationship with lymphocytic infiltration and thyroid autoantibodies. J Clin Endocrinol Metab 66:367–375.

Mackenzie WA, Schwartz AE, Friedman EW, Davis TF (1987): Intrathyroidal T cell clones from patients with autoimmune thyroid disease. J Clin Endocrinol Metab 64:818–824.

Margolick JB, Hsu S-M, Volkmann DJ, Burman KD, Fauci AS (1984): Immunohisto-chemical characterisation of intrathyroid lymphocytes in Graves' disease. Am J Med 76:815–821.

McGregor AM (1990): Autoantibodies to the TSH receptor in patients with autoim-mune thyroid disease. Clin Endocrinol 33:683–685.

McKenzie JM (1964): Neonatal Graves' diseases. J Clin Endocrinol Metab 24:660–668.

Migita K, Eguchi K, Otsubo T, Kawakami A, Nakao H, Ueki Y, Shimomura C, Kurata A, Fukuda T, Matsunaga M, Ishikawa N, Ito K, Nagataki S (1990): Cy-tokine regulation of HLA on thyroid epithelial cells. Clin Exp Immunol 82:548–552.

Oksenberg JR, Stuart S, Begovich AB, et al. (1990): Limited heterogeneity of rear-ranged T cell receptor Vα transcripts in brains of multiple sclerosis patients. Nature 345:344–346.

Paschke R, Teuber J, Enger I, Schmeidl R, Schwedes U, Usadel KH (1990): Evidence for a role of anti-idiotypic antibodies in the induction of remission in Graves' disease. J Autoimmun 3:441–448.

Pujol-Borrell T, Todd T, Doshi I, Bottazzo GF, Sutton R, Gray D, Adolf GR, Feldmann M (1987): HLA class II induction in human islet cells by interferon-γ plus tumor necrosis factor or lymphotoxin. Nature 326:304–306.

Raines KB, Baker JR, Lukes YG, Wartofsky L, Burman KD (1985): Antithyrotropin antibodies in the sera of Graves' disease patients. J Clin Endocrinol Metab 61:217–222.

Roitt IM, Thanavala YM, Male DK, Hay FC (1985): Antiidiotypes as surrogate antigens: Structural considerations. Immunol Today 6:265–267.

Romball CG, Weigle WO (1987): Transfer of experimental autoimmune thyroiditis with T cell clones. J Immunol 138:1092–1098.

Rosch PJ (1992): Stress and Graves' disease. Lancet (i):428.

Rossi F, Dietrich G, Kazatchkine MD (1989): Anti-idiotypes against autoantibodies in normal immunoglobulins: Evidence for network regulation of human autoimmune responses. Immunol Rev 110:135–149.

Rossi F, Jayne DR, Lockwood CM, Kazatchkine MD (1991): Anti-idiotypes against anti-neutrophil cytoplasmic antigen autoantibodies in normal human polyspecific IgG for therapeutic use and in the remission serum of patients with systemic vasculitis. Clin Exp Immunol 83:298–303.

Rossi F, Kazatchkine MD (1989): Anti-idiotypes against autoantibodies in pooled normal human polyspecific Ig. J Immunol 143:4104–4109.

Rusznyak I, Foldi M, Szabo G (1967): Relationship between the eye and the lym-phatic system. In Youlten L (ed): "Lymphatics and Lymph Circulation: Physiol-ogy and Pathology." 2nd Ed. New York: Pergamon Press, p 187.

Salvi M, Fukazawa H, Bernard N, Hiromatsu Y, How J, Wall JR (1988): Role of autoantibodies in the pathogenesis and association of endocrine autoimmune dis-orders. Endocrinol Rev 9:450–466.

Salvi M, Zhang Z-G, Haegert D, Woo M, Liberman A, Cadarso L, Wall JR (1990): Patients with endocrine ophthalmopathy not associated with overt thyroid disease have multiple thyroid immunological abnormalities. J Clin Endocrinol Metab 70:89–94.

Shimizu Y, Shaw S (1991): Lymphocyte interactions with extracellular matrix. FASEB J 5:2292–2299.

Sinha AA, Lopez MT, McDevitt HO (1990): Autoimmune diseases: The failure of self tolerance. Science 248:1380–1388.

Smith BR, Hall R (1974): Thyroid-stimulating immunoglobulins in Graves' disease. Lancet 2:427–431.

Springer TA (1990): Adhesion receptors of the immune system. Nature 346:425–434.

Springer TA, Dustin ML, Kishimoto TK, Marlin SD (1987): The lymphocyte function-associated LFA-1, CD2, and LFA-3 molecules: Cell adhesion receptors of the immune system. Annu Rev Immunol 5:223–252.

Tamai H, Hirota Y, Kasagi K, Matsubayashi S, Kuma K, Iida Y, Konishi J, Okimura MC, Walter RM, Kumagai LF, Nagataki S (1987): The mechanism of spontaneous hypothyroidism in patients with Graves' disease after antithyroid drug treatment. J Clin Endocrinol Metab 64:718–722.

Taylor KB (1976): Immune aspects of pernicious anaemia and atrophic gastritis. Clin Haematol 5:497–519.

Todd I, Hammond LJ, James RFL, Feldmann M, Bottazzo GF (1990): Epidermal growth factor and transforming growth factor-alpha suppress HLA class II induction in human thyroid epithelial cells. Immunology 69:91–96.

Todd I, Pujol-Borrell R, Hammond LJ, Bottazzo GF, Feldmann M (1985): Interferon-γ induces HLA-DR expression by thyroid epithelium. Clin Exp Immunol 61:265–273.

Tomer Y, Shoenfeld Y (1989): The significance of T suppressor cells in the development of autoimmunity. J Autoimmun 2:739–758.

Topliss D, How J, Lewis M, Row V, Volpé R (1983): Evidence for cell-mediated immunity and specific suppressor T lymphocyte dysfunction in Graves' disease and diabetes mellitus. J Clin Endocrinol Metab 57:700–705.

Turner M, Londei M, Feldmann M (1987): Human T cells from autoimmune and normal individuals can produce tumor necrosis factor. Eur J Immunol 17:1807–1814.

Ueki Y, Eguchi K, Fukuda T, Otsubo T, Kawabe T, Shimomura C, Matsunaga M, Tezuka H, Ishikawa N, Ito K (1987): Dysfunction of suppressor T cells in thyroid glands from patients with Graves' disease. J Clin Endocrinol Metab 65:922–928.

Utiger R (1991): The pathogenesis of autoimmune thyroid disease. N Engl J Med 325(4):278–279.

van der Gaag RD, Drexhage HA, Wiersinga WM, Brown RS, Docter R, Bottazzo GF, Doniach D (1985): Further studies on thyroid growth-stimulating immunoglobulins in euthyroid nonendemic goitre. J Clin Endocrinol Metab 60:972–979.

Varela F, Andersson A, Dietrich G, Sundblad A, Holmberg D, Kazatchkine M, Coutinho A (1991): The population dynamics of antibodies in normal and autoimmune individuals. Proc Natl Acad Sci USA 88:5917–5921.

Varela F, Coutinho A (1991): Second generation immune networks. Immunol Today 12:159–166.

Volpé R (1985): "Autoimmunity and Endocrine Disease." New York: Marcel Dekker, pp 109–285.

Volpé R (1986): The role of immune dysregulation in the pathogenesis of autoimmune thyroid disease. In Drexhage HA, Wiersinga WM (eds): "The Thyroid and Autoimmunity." Amsterdam: Elsevier, pp 283–293.

Volpé R (1987): Immunoregulation in autoimmune thyroid disease. N Engl J Med 316(1):44–46.

Wall JR, Salvi M, Bernard NF, Boucher A, Haegert D (1991): Thyroid-associated ophthalmology—A model for the association of organ-specific autoimmune disorders. Immunol Today 12(5):150–153.

Weetman AP, Cohen S, Magkoba MW, Barysiewicz LK (1989): Expression of an intracellular adhesion molecule, ICAM-1, by human thyroid cells. J Endocrinol 122:185–191.

Weetman AP, McGregor AM (1984): Autoimmune thyroid disease: Developments in our understanding. Endocrinol Rev 5:309–353.

Weetman AP, So AK, Roe C, Walport MJ, Foroni L (1987): T cell receptor alpha chain V region polymorphism linked to primary autoimmune hypothyroidism but not Graves' disease. Hum Immunol 20:167–173.

Weetman AP, Volkman DJ, Burman KD, Gerrard TL, Fauci AP (1985): The in vitro regulation of human thyrocyte HLA-DR antigen expression. J Clin Endocrinol Metab 61:817–824.

Weiss M, Ingbar S, Winblad S, Kasper DL (1987): Demonstration of a saturable binding site for thyrotropin in *Yersinia enterocolitica*. Science 219:1331–1333.

Wenzel BE, Heesemann J (1987): Enteropathogenic *Yersinia* and thyroid autoimmune disease share antigen homologies, abstracted. Immunobiology 175:262.

Weigle WO (1977): Cellular events in experimental autoimmune thyroiditis, allergic encephalomyelitis, and tolerance to self. In Talal N (ed): "Autoimmunity." New York: Academic Press, pp 141–170.

Wilkin TJ (1990): Receptor autoimmunity in endocrine disorders. N Engl J Med 323(19):1318–1324.

Winsa B, Karlsson A, Adami H-O, Bergström R (1991): Stressful life events and Graves' disease. Lancet (ii):1475–1479.

Zheng RQH, Abney ER, Grubeck-Loebenstein B, Dayan C, Maini RN, Reldmann M (1990): Expression of intercellular adhesion molecule-1 and lymphocyte function-associated antigen-3 on human thyroid epithelial cells in Graves' and Hashimoto's diseases. J Autoimmun 3:727–736.

21

SPECIFIC REGULATION OF EXPERIMENTAL AUTOIMMUNE THYROIDITIS: TOWARD A NEW CONCEPTION OF AUTOIMMUNE REACTIVITY

Karine Mignon-Godefroy, Marie-Pierre Brazillet, and
Jeannine Charreire

INSERM U.283, Hôpital Cochin, Paris, France

INTRODUCTION

Experimental models of autoimmune diseases have been useful in elucidating some of the pathogenic mechanisms involved in the triggering and development of autoimmune reactivity.

Experimental autoimmune thyroiditis (EAT) is an autoimmune thyroid disorder induced in suceptible strains of mice, i.e., CBA/J [Vladutiu and Rose, 1971], and by porcine thyroglobulin (pTg) or murine Tg (mTg) emulsified in adjuvants as originally described by Rose and Witebsky [1956]. The disease, which results in hypothyroidism, is assessed by both circulating anti-Tg autoantibodies (A-Abs) and infiltrations of the thyroid gland by T lymphocytes, mainly of the CD8 phenotype [Creemers et al., 1984; Conaway et al., 1989].

Autoimmunity: Physiology and Disease, Pages 339–352
© *1994 Wiley-Liss, Inc.*

Briefly, we 1) defined one peptide (F40D) from human thyroglobulin (hTg) inducing EAT and 2) produced monoclonal antibodies (mAbs) to mTg, some of which, such as 3B8G9, recognized F40D peptide. Then 3B8G9 was used to develop Ab2β and Ab2α monoclonal anti-idiotypic (anti-id) antibodies. We then 3) selected one cytotoxic T-cell hybridoma specific for F40D in a class I–restricted context and 4) studied the in vivo biological effects of those reagents on EAT. In that respect, recent advances made in our laboratory allow us to propose a new conception of autoimmune reactivity.

We discuss here the advances we made during the last years in the mechanism of induction, immunological diagnosis, and prevention of EAT and Hashimoto's thyroiditis. Lastly, we propose a new hypothesis to explain the occurrence and the perpetuation of EAT and, to a larger extent, of autoimmune reactivity.

F40D, AN EAT-INDUCER PEPTIDE, BEARS EPITOPES RECOGNIZED BY T AND B CELLS

The recent characterization of one peptide from hTg, F40D, inducing EAT in CBA/J mice [Téxier et al., 1992b], led us to investigate whether this peptide expressed epitopes that would be recognized by the B- and T-cell hybridomas related to EAT we simultaneously selected.

Briefly, we demonstrated that monoclonal anti-Tg A-Abs selected using a standard ELISA test with Tg from various species could also be functionally characterized using a T-cell proliferative assay on syngeneic thyroid epithelial cells (TEC) [Yeni and Charreire, 1981; Charreire, 1982], such T-helper cells being able to transfer EAT when injected into normal syngeneic recipients [Charreire and Michel-Béchet, 1982]. Through this approach, a first set of murine monoclonal anti-Tg A-Abs, including 3B8G9, were further defined upon their ability to block this T-cell proliferative response, whereas other monoclonal anti-Tg A-Abs, such as 4B10 E12, could not do so [Salamero et al., 1987]. Lastly, 3B8G9 and 4B10E12 were also tested for their ability to bind to F40D peptide. As shown in Table I, only 3B8G9 monoclonal anti-Tg A-Ab could also bind to F40D.

As we had characterized one cytotoxic T-cell hybridoma, HTC2, specific in a class I–restricted context for pTg or hTg [Rémy et al., 1989] and demonstrated that HTC2 cells could prevent further EAT induction when 10^6 inactivated cells were injected i.v. 3 weeks before Tg immunization [Roubaty et al., 1990], we investigated if HTC2 cells could recognize the F40D peptide. As shown in Table I, HTC2 cells were able to induce lysis of syngeneic macrophages pulsed with F40D peptide, whereas macrophages pulsed with control peptides were never lysed (data not shown). From these two sets of experiments we concluded that the 40 amino-acid peptide from hTg, which induces EAT in CBA/J mice, expresses epitopes recognized by Tg-specific B- and T-cell hybridomas.

TABLE I. F40D, an EAT-inducer peptide, bears epitopes recognized by Tg-specific T and B cells

	Recognition of		
	pTg	hTg	F40D
B-cell hybridomas[a]			
3B8G9	+	+	+
4 B10E12	+	+	−
T-cell hybridoma[b]			
HTC$_2$	+	+	+

[a] Binding in ELISA.
[b] Cytotoxicity toward CBA/J macrophages pulsed with the various antigens.

B AND T CELLS SPECIFIC FOR F40D PEPTIDE BEAR IDIOTOPES THAT BEHAVE AS EAT MARKERS

When CBA/J and C57Bl/6 mice are immunized with pTg emulsified in adequate adjuvants, CBA/J mice develop severe EAT 4 weeks later, whereas C57Bl/6 do not. Briefly, in both strains of animals similar levels of anti-Tg A-Abs are detected, but only thyroid glands from CBA/J animals are infiltrated with T lymphocytes [Vladutiu and Rose, 1971; Tang et al., 1990]. Evaluation of the levels of anti-id A-Abs in the sera of these two strains of mice was performed on day 28 post-Tg-immunization, during the acute phase of the disease in CBA/J (Table II). Anti-id A-Abs specific for polyclonal anti-Tg A-Abs or for 4B10 E12 (a monoclonal anti-Tg A-Ab that does not recognize F40D peptide) were at similar levels in the two strains of animals, with or without EAT. Anti-id A-Abs binding to 3B8G9 (the monoclonal anti-Tg A-Ab that specifically recognizes F40D peptide), behaved quite differently. Briefly, they were only detected in sera from CBA/J mice, the strain that develops EAT, whereas they were never found in C57Bl/6 sera, independent of the time post-Tg immunization they were tested [Tang et al., 1990].

In a second set of experiments, we investigated the percentages of T cells expressing a T-cell receptor (TCR) specific for F40D peptide in spleen and lymph node cells from pTg-immunized CBA/J mice. As shown in Table II, such T cells, evidenced using the mAb anticlonotypic antibody AG7 [Téxier et al., 1992a], increased with time postimmunization and were at maximal levels (1.38% approximately) on day 28 post-Tg immunization. When such cells were enumerated in naive CBA/J mice or in counterpart lymphoid organs from Tg-immunized C57Bl/6 mice, no significant modification was observed after immunization, and background levels (approximately 0.4% of the cells) of the AG7$^+$ T cells were invariably observed.

TABLE II. B and T cells specific for F40D peptide bear idiotopes that behave as EAT markers[a]

| | Strains of Immunized Mice | |
	CBA/J	C57 Bl/6
EAT anti-id antibodies to	+	−
Polyclonal anti-Tg	450[b] ± 50	548 ± 55
Monoclonal anti-Tg-Ab 4B10E12	506 ± 65	552 ± 78
Monoclonal anti-Tg-Ab 3B8G9	711 ± 52**	313 ± 34
Percent AG7$^+$ CD8$^+$ T cells in		
Spleen	1,38[c]	0,05
Lymph node	1,35	0,32

[a] Mean ± SEM of five to seven determinations on day 28 post-Tg immunization.
[b] o.d. at 405 nm.
[c] Net percentage of AG7$^+$CD8$^+$ T cells calculated as follows: percentages in Tg-immunized mice minus counterpart percentages in only adjuvant-injected mice. Evaluation was made by FACS analysis on 10.00 cells.
** $P < 0.02$ compared with counterpart titer in C57Bl/6 mice.

T- AND B-CELL HYBRIDOMAS SPECIFIC FOR F40D PEPTIDE PREVENT EAT INDUCTION

Since the network theory of the immune system was elaborated [Jerne 1974; Jerne et al., 1982], there has been increasing evidence that interactions between id and anti-id are crucial in the regulation of the immune response to self-antigens. Thus autoimmunity may appear when the steady stade of the immune system is disturbed not only by an autoantigen but also by id or anti-id antibodies. In the last years, the ability of anti-id antibodies to prevent several autoimmune diseases has been demonstrated in EAT [Zanetti et al., 1986], collagen-induced arthritis (CIA) [Arita et al., 1987], uveoretinitis [de Kozak et al., 1987], murine lupus [Carteron et al., 1989; Morland et al., 1991], interstitial nephritis [Neilson and Philips, 1982], and myasthenia gravis [Agius and Richman, 1986].

In addition to the protections induced by anti-id antibodies specific for the adequate autoantigens, the prevention of EAT [Maron et al., 1983], experimental autoimmune encephalomyelitis [Sun et al., 1988; Lider et al., 1988; Ellerman et al., 1988], CIA [Kakimoto et al., 1988; Chiocchia et al., 1993], and murine lupus [de Alboran et al., 1992] was observed after admnistration of antigen-specific T-cell lines or clones belonging to the CD4 T-cell subset and specific for the respective autoantigen (except in CIA, where CD8 T cells were used).

Taking these data into account, B- and T-cell hybridomas specific for F40D peptide were tested for their ability to prevent EAT induction in CBA/J mice. One million of inactivated (irradiated or mitomycin-treated) hybridomas were

TABLE III. T or B cells specific for F40D peptide prevent EAT induction

Cells Injected[a]	Specificity for F40D	Tg Challenge	EAT Incidence	Mean Infiltration Indexes[b]
T cells				
0	0	+	8/8	4, 2
BW5147	−	+	8/8	3, 1
HTC2	+	+	3/8	1, 0
142	−	+	8/8	3, 1
B cells				
0	0	0	0/5	0
3B8G9	+	+	0/5	0
4B10E12	−	+	3/5	2, 1
3B8H7	−	+	3/5	1, 9

[a] Inactivated cells (1×10^6) were i.p. inoculated 21 days before Tg challenge.
[b] Evaluated on day 28 after Tg immunization.

injected i.p. into syngeneic naive recipients 21 days before pTg challenge. As shown in Table III, only F40D-specific T or B hybridomas were able to prevent EAT induction in CBA/J mice, whereas the other Tg-specific T- or B-cell hybridomas that do not recognize F40D peptide were unable to do so. It is noteworthy that HTC2 hybridoma cells do not belong to the CD4 subset but to the CD8 class I–restricted cytotoxic T subset.

TABLE IV. Anti-idiotype and anticlonotypic monoclonal antibodies can also prevent EAT induction

Monoclonal Antibodies Injected[a]	Tg Challenge	Incidence	Infiltration Indexes[b]
Experiment A			
0	0	0/5	0
0	+	4/5	4
control mAb	+	4/5	3,8
H2 (Ab2-β)	+	2/5	1,1
A1 (Ab2-α)	+	4/5	3,6
Experiment B			
0	+	4/5	3,0
AG7 (200 μg)	+	0/5	0
AG7 (40 μg)	+	0/5	0
AG7 (1 μg)	+	2/4	2,6
Ig2b (200 μg)	+	4/4	3,2

[a] Monoclonal antibodies (40 μg/mouse) were injected i.p. on days 7 and −1 in experiments A and B, respectively.
[b] Evaluated on day 28 after Tg immunization.

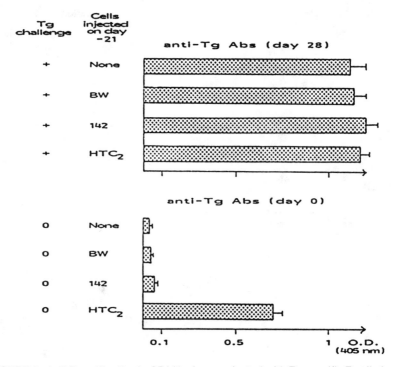

FIGURE 1. Anti-Tg antibodies in CBA/J mice vaccinated with Tg-specific T-cell clones.

IDIOTYPIC REGULATION OF EAT

Anti-id or Anticlonotypic mAb Can Also Prevent EAT Induction

Since 10^6 of inactivated T- and B-cell hybridomas specific for epitope(s) located in F40D peptide were able to prevent further EAT induction, we hypothesized that protection could result from in vivo production of anticlonotypic or anti-id antibodies, respectively. To test this hypothesis, such reagents were developed and injected i.p. prior to pTg immunization. As shown in Table IV, anti-id mAb2β was able to prevent EAT induction, whereas anti-id mAb2α or isotype-matched irrelevant mAbs could not. Similarly, the anticlonotypic mAb AG7 specific for HTC2-TcR was also able to prevent EAT induction specifically when injected 1 day prior to pTg immunization. Therefore, these data strengthen our hypothesis that protections achieved by F40D-specific B- and T-cell hybridomas resulted from in vivo productions of anti-id or anticlonotypic antibodies.

Idiotypic Regulation of EAT Prevention by HTC2 Cells

In a last series of experiments we further demonstrated the existence of idiotypic regulation in EAT through serological studies of EAT prevention

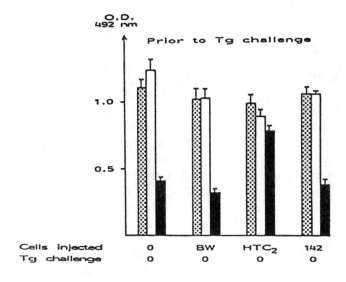

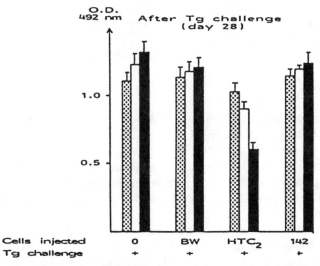

FIGURE 2. Anti-id responses to polyclonal and monoclonal Tg-specific idiotypes in mice vaccinated with the HTC2 T cell clone. Anti-id antibodies were determined against polyclonal anti-Tg antibody (stippled bars), anti-Tg mAb 4B10E12 (open bars), or anti-Tg mAb 3B8G9 (closed bars).

obtained after inoculation of HTC2 cells into CBA/J mice [Roubaty et al., 1990]. In these animals, evaluation of anti-Tg and anti-id A-Abs were performed on day 0 (3 weeks after injection of 10^6 inactivated HTC2 cells and prior to pTg immunization) and on day 28 post-pTg challenge, when EAT was in the acute phase. On day 28, high levels of anti-Tg A-Abs were found in each group of mice immunized with pTg, whatever the specificity of the T-cell hybridomas inoculated. In contrast, on day 0 before pTg challenge, only mice having received HTC2 cells developed an anti-Tg antibody response (Fig. 1).

This unexpected detection of anti-Tg A-Abs in mice inoculated with HTC2 cells only and that had never met Tg in the past led us to hypothesize that these were Ab3. Therefore we investigated the presence of anti-id antibodies in these sera (Fig. 2), their fine specificities being defined by the use of polyclonal anti-Tg and of the monoclonal anti-Tg A-Abs 3B8G9 and 4B10E12, described above. Anti-id antibodies specific for polyclonal anti-Tg antibodies or for the F40D unrelated monoclonal anti-Tg Ab 4B10E12 were at similar levels in the various groups of mice studied before Tg challenge. The only striking difference we found concerned the specific anti-3B8G9 responses in mice inoculated with HTC2 cells: whereas control animals showed background levels of anti-3B8G9 anti-id antibodies in their sera, HTC2-injected mice exhibited an increase of more than 200% in the levels of these A-Abs (Fig. 2a). Study of the same anti-id responses on day 28 post-Tg challenge showed no differences in anti-id responses to polyclonal antibodies or to mAb 4B10E12 (a mAb not related to a pathogenic epitope of F40D). The only variations we detected were great decreases in anti-3B8G9 Ab concentrations in sera from mice inoculated with HTC2 cells leading back to background levels comparable with those detected in control sera from naive CBA/J animals (Fig. 2b).

DISCUSSION

The characterization of the F40D peptide from hTg able to induce EAT in the susceptible strain of mice CBA/J allowed us to investigate the specific immunological mechanisms occurring during EAT. To address this issue, we developed B- and T-cell hybridomas that specifically recognized this peptide, produced their anti-id and anticlonotypic mAbs, respectively, and used these reagents to test the involvement of T and B cells specific for the F40D peptide during EAT.

F40D peptide is located at the end of the second third of the Tg molecule (660 kD) in a domain defined as "type 3a" and repeated twice in human [Malthiéry and Lissitzky, 1987] and bovine [Mercken et al., 1985] Tg molecules. Despite its great hydrophobicity [Kyte and Doolittle, 1982] and its poor antigenicity [Jameson and Wolf, 1988], this peptide bears epitopes recognized by both Tg-specific T and B cells. The presence of epitopes recognized by B and T cells on the same peptide is surprising. However, a sequence of 40 amino acids is large enough to contain several epitopes, as assessed by the multiple overlapping [Hannum and Margoliash, 1985] or distinct [Shastri et al., 1986] T-cell epitopes described in cytochrome *c* and lysozyme, respectively. More precisely, Hannum et al. [1985] demonstrated that the B10A mouse B-cell response to pigeon cytochrome *c*, a well-known and widely studied protein [Brautigan et al., 1978], is directed to the area of the protein that is also recognized by B10A T cells in association with I-E molecules. This property of F40D hTg peptide to bear T- and B-cell epitopes is the pivotal element of our new conception of autoimmune triggering and development, now exposed.

Recently, one thyroxine-containing peptide from the mTg molecule was described as an EAT inducer [Hutchings et al., 1992]. However, contrasting with our approach, EAT was induced by T-cell clones specific for the thyroxine-containing peptide and not by the peptide alone. It must be noted that in the past these T cells were reported by the same authors as unable to induce thyroid lesions in normal recipients [Champion et al., 1985; Champion et al., 1987] and that EAT induction by thyroid-specific T-cell lines [Charreire and Michel-Béchet, 1982; Maron et al., 1983] or clones [Romball and Weigle, 1987] is quite different from EAT induction by antigen, i.e., Tg [for review, see Charreire, 1989].

The pathogenic role of F40D peptide was directly and indirectly demonstrated. Direct proofs were provided by the detection of anti-id antibodies that behave as mirror images of F40D and then of T cells bearing a TCR specific for F40D in sera and lymphoid organs from CBA/J mice with EAT exclusively. In these experiments, anti-id antibodies represent the first serological marker of EAT, since a lack of correlation between anti-Tg A-Abs and the severity of EAT assessed by lymphocytic infiltration was widely reported [for review, Charrreire, 1989]. Along the same line, T cells bearing a TCR similar to HTC2 cells were detected only in the lymphoid cells from CBA/J mice suffering from EAT. Moreover, their percentages, which reached approximately 1.4%, were highest when EAT was in the acute phase (Brazillet et al., in preparation). Indirect demonstrations of the basic role played by F40D in EAT were brought through experiments aimed at preventing EAT induction. These experiments were achieved by injecting either 10^6 inactivated F40D-specific T or B cells or 40 μg of mAb specific for the Ig or the TCR of these F40D-specific T and B cells into naive CBA/J mice.

Our experiments clearly showed that specific regulation of EAT occurs through a physiological idiotypic network bridging T and B lymphocytes specific for one pathogenic epitope of the hTg molecule. Idiotypic regulation of EAT by anti-Tg and their anti-id antibodies was expected, since it was previously demonstrated in mice and humans. Indeed, spontaneously occurring or in vitro induced [Zanetti and Bigazzi, 1981; Zanetti et al., 1983a] anti-id A-Abs to anti-Tg antibodies were obtained in the BUF rats. They were shown to be highly cross-reactive [Zanetti et al., 1983b, 1985], able to block the Tg–anti-Tg interaction in vitro, and to decrease the levels of anti-Tg antibodies [Glotz and Zanetti, 1986] when injected in vivo. In humans, they were detected in 10% of Hashimoto's thyroiditis patients' sera [Sikorska, 1986]. Moreover, a monoclonal anti-id A-Ab was detected in the serum of one patient with multiple myeloma [Zouali et al., 1984]. More recently, such anti-id antibodies were found in pooled normal human polyspecific immunoglobulin [Rossi and Kazatchkine, 1989; Rossi et al., 1990; Dietrich and

Kazatchkine, 1990]. These last series of data, along with the study of dynamics of natural antibodies in normal and autoimmune individuals [Varela et al., 1991], led to successfull therapeutic approaches directed at reestablishing normal antibody dynamics through alterations in connectivity [Gelfand, 1989; Nydegger et al., 1989].

The interference of a T-cell subset, or its anticlonotypic A-Ab, in the B-cell idiotypic network was much less expected. Nonetheless, it was postulated by Male [1986] and Male et al. [1983, 1985] that the D8 idiotype could be borne as well by anti-Tg A-Abs as by Tg-specific T cells, in particular CBA/J. Therefore Tg-specific T and B cells would be able to recognize an identical epitope on the Tg molecule. Even if this hypothesis has been cautioned in the past [Binz et al., 1976; Eichmann et al., 1978; Coutinho and Meo, 1983; Pereira et al., 1989], our preliminary results (data not shown) rather support that F40D peptide bears at least two distinct or slightly overlapping epitopes recognized either by T or B cells.

From our point of view, such a peptide may play a basic role in autoimmune reactivity: The simultaneous breakdown of the silent self–antiself B- and T-cell idiotypic networks would lead to the occurrence, development and perpetuation of autoimmune disorders. In contrast, the dysregulation of only one of these, the B or the T idiotypic network, would lead to transient autoimmune disorder.

ACKNOWLEDGMENTS

This work was supported in part by a grant from "la Fondation pour la Recherche Médicale," Paris, and "l'Association pour la Recherche sur le Cancer," Villejuif, France.

REFERENCES

Agius MA, Richman DP (1986): Suppression of development of experimental autoimmune myasthenia gravis with isogeneic monoclonal antiidiotypic antibody. J Immunol 137:2195–2198.

Arita C, Kaibara N, Jingushi S, Takagishi K, Hotokebuchi T, Arai K (1987): Suppression of collagen arthritis in rats by heterologous anti-idiotypic antisera against anticollagen antibodies. Clin Immunol Immunopathol 43:374–381.

Binz H, Wigzell H, Bazin H (1976): T-cell idiotypes are linked to immunoglobulin heavy chain genes. Nature 264:639–642.

Brautigan DL, Ferguson-Miller S, Margoliash E (1978): Mitochondrial cytochrome c: Preparation and activity of native and chemically modified cytochrome c. Methods Enzymol 53:128–164.

Carteron NL, Schimenti CL, Wofsy D (1989): Treatment of murine lupus with F(ab')$_2$

fragments of monoclonal antibody to L3T4. Suppression of autoimmunity does not depend on T helper cell depletion. J Immunol 142:1470–1475.

Champion BR, Rayner DC, Byfield PGH, Page KR, Chan CTJ, Roitt IM (1987): Critical role of iodination for T cell recognition of thyroglobulin in experimental murine thyroid autoimmunity. J Immunol 139:3665–3670.

Champion BR, Varey AM, Katz D, Cooke A, Roitt IM (1985): Autoreactive T-cell lines specific for mouse thyroglobulin. Immunology 54:513–519.

Charreire J (1982): Syngeneic sensitization of mouse lymphocytes on monolayers of thyroid epithelial cells. II. T and B cell involvement in primary responses. Eur J Immunol 12:416–421.

Charreire J, Michel-Béchet M (1982): Syngeneic sensitization of mouse lymphocytes on monolayers of thyroid epithelial cells. III. Induction of thyroiditis by thyroid-sensitized T lymphoblasts. Eur J Immunol 12:421–425.

Charreire J (1989): Immune mechanisms in autoimmune thyroiditis. Adv Immunol 46:263–334.

Chiocchia G, Boissier MC, Manoury B, Fournier C (1993): T cell regulation of collagen-induced arthritis in mice. II. Immunomodulation of arthritis by cytotoxic T cell hybridomas specific for type II collagen. Eur J Immunol 23:327–332.

Conaway DH, Giraldo AA, David CS, Kong YCM (1989): In situ kinetic analysis of thyroid lymphocyte infiltrate in mice developing experimental autoimmune thyroiditis. Clin Immunol Immunopathol 53:346–353.

Coutinho A, Meo T (1983): Immunoglobulin gene expression by T lymphocytes. Scand J Immunol 18:79–100.

Creemers P, Giraldo AA, Rose NR, Kong YCM (1984): T-cell subsets in the thyroids of mice developing autoimmune thyroiditis. Cell Immunol 87:692–697.

de Alboran IM, Gutierrez JC, Gonzalo JA, Andreu JL, Marcos MAR, Kroemer G, Martinez-A C (1992): lpr T cells vaccinate against lupus in MRL/lpr mice. Eur J Immunol 22:1089–1093.

de Kozak Y, Mirshahi M, Boucheix C, Faure JP (1987): Prevention of experimental autoimmune uveoretinitis by active immunization with autoantigen-specific monoclonal antibodies. Eur J Immunol 17:541–547.

Dietrich G, Kazatchkine MD (1990): Normal immunoglobulin G (IgG) for therapeutic use (intravenous Ig) contain antiidiotypic specificities against an immunodominant, disease-associated, cross-reactive idiotype of human anti-thyroglobulin autoantibodies. J Clin Invest 85:620–625.

Eichmann K, Falk I, Rajewsky K (1978): Recognition of idiotypes in lymphocyte interaction. II. Antigen-independent cooperation between T and B lymphocytes that possess similar and complementary idiotypes. Eur J Immunol 8:853–857.

Ellerman KE, Powers JM, Brostoff SW (1988): A suppressor T-lymphocyte cell line for autoimmune encephalomyelitis. Nature 331:265–267.

Gelfand EW (1989): Intervention in autoimmune disorders: Creation of a niche for intravenous γ-globulin therapy. Clin Immunol Immunopathol 53:S1–S6.

Glotz D, Zanetti M (1986): Detection of regulatory idiotype on a spontaneous neonatal self-reactive hybridoma antibody. J Immunol 137:223–227.

Hannum CH, Margoliash E (1985): Assembled topographic antigenic determinants of pigeon cytochrome c. J Immunol 135:3303–3313.

Hannum CH, Matis LA, Schwartz RH, Margoliash E (1985): The B10.A mouse B cell response to pigeon cytochrome c is directed against the same area of the protein that is recognized by B10.A T cells in association with the $E_\beta^k : E_\alpha^k$ Ia molecule. J Immunol 135:3314–3322.

Hutchings PR, Cooke A, Dawe K, Champion BR, Geysen M, Valerio R, Roitt IM (1992): A thyroxine-containing peptide can induce murine experimental autoimmune thyroiditis. J Exp Med 175:869–872.

Jameson BA, Wolf H (1988): The antigenic index: A novel algorithm for predicting antigenic determinants. Comput Appl Biosci 4:181–186.

Jerne NK (1974): Towards a network theory of the immune system. Ann Immunol (Inst Pasteur) 125C:373–389.

Jerne NK, Roland J, Cazenave PA (1982): Recurrent idiotopes and internal images. EMBO J 1:243–247.

Kakimoto K, Katzuki M, Hirofuji T, Iwata H, Koga T (1988): Isolation of T cell line capable of protecting mice against collagen-induced arthritis. J Immunol 140:78–83.

Kyte J, Doolittle RF (1982): A simple method for displaying the hydropathic character of a protein. J Mol Biol 157:105–132.

Lider O, Reshef T, Beraud E, Ben-Nun A, Cohen IR (1988): Anti-idiotypic network induced by T cell vaccination against experimental autoimmune encephalomyelitis. Science 239:181–183.

Male DK (1986): Idiotypes and autoimmunity. Clin Exp Immunol 65:1–9.

Male D, Pryce G, Quartey-Papafio R, Roitt I (1983): The occurrence of defined idiotypes on autoantibodies to mouse thyroglobulin. Eur J Immunol 13:942–947.

Male D, Pryce G, Roitt I (1985): Molecular analysis of induced idiotypes associated with autoanti-thyroglobulin. Mol Immunol 22:255–263.

Malthiéry Y, Lissitzky S (1987): Primary structure of human thyroglobulin deduced from the sequence of its 8448-base complementary DNA. Eur J Biochem 165:491–498.

Maron R, Zerubavel R, Friedman A, Cohen IR (1983): T lymphocyte line specific for thyroglobulin produces or vaccinates against autoimmune thyroiditis in mice. J Immunol 131:2316–2322.

Mercken L, Simons MJ, Swillens S, Massaer M, Vassart G (1985): Primary structure of bovine thyroglobulin deduced from the sequence of its 8,431-base complementary DNA. Nature 316:647–651.

Morland C, Michael J, Adu D, Kizaki T, Howie AJ, Morgan A, Staines NA (1991): Anti-idiotype and immunosuppressant treatment of murine lupus. Clin Exp Immunol 83:126–132.

Neilson EG, Phillips SM (1982): Suppression of interstitial nephritis by auto-anti-idiotypic immunity. J Exp Med 155:179–189.

Nydegger UE, Sultan Y, Kazatchkine MD (1989): The concept of anti-idiotypic regulation of selected autoimmune diseases by intravenous immunoglobulin. Clin Immunol Immunopathol 53:S72–S82.

Pereira P, Bandeira A, Coutinho A (1989): V-region connectivity T cell repertoires. Annu Rev Immunol 7:209–249.

Rémy JJ, Téxier B, Chiocchia G, Charreire J (1989): Characteristics of cytotoxic thyroglobulin-specific T cell hybridomas. J Immunol 142:1129–1133.

Romball CG, Weigle WO (1987): Transfer of experimental autoimmune thyroiditis with T cell clones. J Immunol 138:1092–1098.

Rose NR, Witebsky E (1956): Studies on organ specificity. V. Changes in the thyroid glands of rabbits following active immunization with rabbit thyroid extracts. J Immunol 76:417–427.

Rossi F, Kazatchkine MD (1989): Anti idiotypes against autoantibodies in pooled normal human polyspecific Ig. J Immunol 143:4104–4109.

Rossi F, Guilbert B, Tonnelle C, Ternynck T, Fumoux F, Avrameas S, Kazatchkine MD (1990): Idiotypic interactions between normal human polyspecific IgG and natural IgM antibodies. Eur J Immunol 20:2089–2094.

Roubaty C, Bédin C, Charreire J (1990): Prevention of experimental autoimmune thyroiditis through the anti-idiotypic network. J Immunol 144:2167–2172.

Salamero J, Rémy JJ, Charreire J (1987): Primary syngeneic sensitization on monolayers of thyroid epithelial cells. X. Inhibition of T-cell proliferative response by thyroglobulin-specific monoclonal antibodies. Clin Immunol Immunopathol 43:34–47.

Shastri N, Gammon G, Horvath S, Miller A, Sercarz E (1986): The choice between two distinct Tcell determinants within a 23-amino-acid region of lysozyme depends on their structural context. J Immunol 137:911–915.

Sikorska HM (1986): Anti-thyroglobulin anti-idiotypic antibodies in sera of patients with hashimoto's thyroiditis and Graves' disease. J Immunol 137:3786–3795.

Sun D, Qin Y, Chluba J Epplen JT, Wekerle H (1988): Suppression of experimentally induced autoimmune encephalomyelitis by cytolytic T-T cell interactions. Nature 332:843–845.

Tang H, Bédin C, Téxier B, Charreire J (1990): Auto antibody specific for a thyroglobulin epitope inducing experimental autoimmune thyroiditis or its anti-idiotype correlates with the disease. Eur J Immunol 20:1535–1539.

Téxier B, Bédin C, Roubaty C, Brézin C, Charreire J (1992a): Protection from experimental autoimmune thyroiditis conferred by a monoclonal antibody to T cell receptor from a cytotoxic hybridoma specific for thyroglobulin. J Immunol 148:439–444.

Téxier B, Bédin C, Tang H, Camoin L, Laurent-Winter C, Charreire J (1992b): Characterization and sequencing of a 40 amino-acid peptide from human thyroglobulin inducing experimental autoimmune thyroiditis. J Immunol 148:3405–3411.

Varela F, Andersson A, Dietrich G, Sundblad A, Holmberg D, Kazatchkine M, Coutinho A (1991): Population dynamics of natural antibodies in normal and autoimmune individuals. Proc Natl Acad Sci USA 88:5917–5921.

Vladutiu AO, Rose NR (1971): Autoimmune murine thyroiditis: Relation to histocompatibility (H-2) type. Science 174:1137–1139.

Yeni P, Charreire J (1981): Syngeneic sensitization of mouse lymphocytes on monolayers of thyroid epithelial cells. I. Study of proliferative response. Cell Immunol 62:313–323.

Zanetti M, Barton RW, Bigazzi PE (1983a): Anti-idiotypic immunity and autoimmunity. II. idiotypic determinants of autoantibodies and lymphocytes in spontaneous and experimentally induced autoimmune thyroiditis. Cell Immunol 75:292–299.

Zanetti M, Bigazzi PE (1981): Anti-idiotypic immunity and autoimmunity. I. In vitro and in vivo effects of anti-idiotypic antibodies to spontaneously occuring autoantibodies to rat thyroglobulin. Eur J Immunol 11:187–195.

Zanetti M, de Baets M, Rogers J (1983b): High degree of idiotypic cross-reactivity among murine monoclonal antibodies to thyroglobulin. J Immunol 131:2452–2457.

Zanetti M, Liu FT, Rogers J, Katz DH (1985): Heavy and light chains of a mouse monoclonal autoantibody express the same idiotype. J Immunol 135:1245–1251.

Zanetti M, Glotz D, Rogers J (1986): Perturbation of the autoimmune network. II. Immunization with isologous idiotype induces auto-anti-idiotypic antibodies and suppresses the autoantibody response elicited by antigen: a serologic and cellular analysis. J Immunol 137:3140–3146.

Zouali M, Fine JM, Eyquem A (1984): A human monoclonal IgG1 with anti-idiotypic activity against anti-human thyroglobulin autoantibody. J Immunol 133:190–194.

22

IS EXPERIMENTAL ALLERGIC ENCEPHALOMYELITIS A MODEL OF MULTIPLE SCLEROSIS?

Ellen Heber-Katz

The Wistar Institute, Philadelphia, Pennsylvania

WHY IS EAE CONSIDERED TO BE A MODEL OF MULTIPLE SCLEROSIS?

The history of experimental allergic encephalomyelitis (EAE) is interestedly tied to the Pasteur antirabies vaccine. This vaccine, when given to patients, caused many cases of encephalitis, and it was originally thought that this was due to the activity of the rabies virus. However, the lesions did not look like those due to rabies. In fact, the lesions found in the white matter of the brain resembled lesions found in other viral diseases such as measles, vaccinia, and influenza, but most importantly they resembled lesions found in multiple sclerosis (MS). It was subsequently realized that the virus was grown in rabbit brain, and it was the brain itself that was the cause of the acute paralysis in patients. This was perhaps the first case of human EAE [Raine and Schaumburg, 1977].

Autoimmunity: Physiology and Disease, Pages 353–364
© *1994 Wiley-Liss, Inc.*

The finding that postrabies vaccine encephalitis (human EAE) was caused by brain tissue led to the isolation of a protein known as *myelin basic protein* (MBP), which when injected in adjuvant was shown to cause paralysis in experimental animals accompanied by a T-cell infiltrate in the lesions found in the brain and spinal cord. T cells generated from such animals were MBP specific, and the T cells alone could be reinjected and had the same effects as MBP in adjuvant.

Because of these findings, the study of MBP reactivity in MS patients has been of major interest. MBP-reactive T cells have been found in peripheral blood of MS patients, a fact that has driven these studies even further. In this review we discuss some of our own studies of MBP-reactive, EAE-specific T cells and how they may or may not strengthen the relationship between EAE and MS.

THE ANTIGENS THAT CAUSE EAE—IS THERE SOMETHING SPECIAL ABOUT MBP?

As stated above, based on the early studies of postrabies infection encephalitis, MBP became the focus of studies on EAE. However, recent studies have indicated that any myelin-associated antigen is able to cause EAE. The second component of myelin to be found to be encephalitogenic was proteolipoprotein (PLP) [Cambi et al., 1982; Satoh et al., 1987; Tuohy et al., 1988]. Recently Weerth et al. [1992] showed that two other myelin proteins, myelin-associated glycoprotein (MAG) and myelin oligodendrocyte glycoprotein (MOG), result in inflammation and encephalomyelitis. Finally, results with transgenes in which chloramphenicol acetyltransferase (CAT) is expressed on the MBP promotor indicate that this nonmyelin-associated antigen does generate a specific T-cell response that causes EAE [Esch et al., 1992]. CAT is expressed like MBP and acts immunologically like MBP. Responsiveness to CAT in the normal mouse and in the transgene seem identical and are unlike the tolerance results obtained in the VSV system of Zinkernagel [1990].

On the other hand, another CNS antigen that is nonmyelin associated, the astrocyte antigen GFAP, does not induce a strong inflammatory response (H. Lassman, personal communication). Thus it may be the location of the antigen and possibly the sensitivity of the target tissue that is important and the reason why EAE is caused only by myelin-associated antigens implying no special status for MBP.

EAE-CAUSING T CELLS USE SIMILAR TCR V REGIONS

Protection studies using an attenuated line of MBP-reactive T cells that could vaccinate against disease suggested that these cells shared an idiotypic determinant with the cells in vivo that caused EAE [Ben-Nun, et al., 1981). Thus beyond T-cell vaccination the hope of therapeutics directed against this shared idiotypy (via T-cell receptor [TCR] components) seemed a possibility. Soon after this finding, support was presented for limited idiotypic determinants present on T cells from studies of restricted TCR usage by T cells in the response to a very different antigen, cytochrome c. These T cells responded to the single dominant antigenic determinant of cytochrome c and used a restricted set of TCR V regions and restricted junctional regions [Hedrick et al., 1984; Fink et al., 1986; Winoto et al., 1986]. Similar data followed from other systems [e.g., Tan et al., 1988; Danska et al., 1990].

In the case of MBP, it was shown that the response to a self-antigen followed the same rules as that of a response to a nonself-antigen. Thus injection of self-antigen (MBP) in complete Freund's adjuvant (CFA) resulted in a potent T-cell proliferative response to a dominant determinant selected by the MHC haplotype of the injected animal [Hashim, 1978; Fritz et al., 1983]. Thus animals of different MHC haplotypes responded to different regions or dominant determinants of the MBP molecule.

Analysis of the TCR gene usage in response to dominant MBP determinants in the rat and the mouse in EAE has also been examined in T-cell-mediated autoimmune disease states, and similar delimited usage patterns have been found [Acha-Orbea et al., 1988; Urban et al., 1988; Zamvil et al., 1988; Burns et al., 1989; Chluba et al., 1989]. In principle, then, this result was indeed compatible with the potential for idiotypic regulation of a restricted antiself-response at both the cellular and humoral level.

In our own studies of the Lewis rat EAE-specific T-cell repertoire, the encephalitogenic T cells were found to be mainly reactive to residues 68–88 of MBP, the dominant encephalitogenic determinant [Happ and Heber-Katz, 1987). The TCRs from all these T cells in the primary response were found to use the same β-chain variable region, Vβ8.2 [Burns et al., 1989]. However, when individually analyzed, none were identical as determined by TCR β-chain rearrangements and then sequencing [Happ et al., 1988; Zhang and Heber-Katz, 1992], indicating that these cells were derived not from a single progenitor, but rather from multiple cells. The same T cells, when analyzed for TCR α-chain usage, were found in the majority of cases to use Vα2 (approximately 70% [Burns et al., 1989]. Similar TCR β-chain gene usage was reported in the Lewis rat EAE system by a second group [Chluba et al., 1989], and Vα4 usage was seen in MBP-reactive T cells from a related rat strain, LeR (Blankenhorn, unpublished data).

Sequencing of a panel of the Lewis rat EAE-inducing T cells revealed β-chains with identical V regions and similar junctional or CDR3 regions [Zhang and Heber-Katz, 1992] and α-chains using six different Vα-family members and junctional regions with a large degree of diversity (Zhang, unpublished data). Thus one might conclude that idiotypic therapy in the Lewis rat should be directed at the β-chain junctional (CDR3) region.

EAE-INDUCING T CELLS FROM DIFFERENT SPECIES SHARE V REGIONS

Similar studies were carried out in the murine EAE-specific T-cell response. In H-2^u–positive strains of mice, the encephalitogenic determinant of MBP is residues 1–11. The encephalitogenic T cells generated to this determinant were found to use Vβ8.2 in approximately 80% of the cases and to use Vα2 or 4 [Acha-Orbea et al., 1988; Urban et al., 1988]. In all of these cells, the joining regions were identical within each VαVβ combination, indicating highly conserved gene and nucleotide (N)-addition usage.

When comparing the mouse and rat T-cell responses in EAE, one is struck by the similarities in TCR V gene usage [Heber-Katz and Acha-Orbea, 1989]. Here, the *same* Vα and Vβ gene families in combination are used in response to the encephalitogenic MBP determinant, though different MHC class II molecules and different MBP peptide fragments are recognized. Since TCR gene usage is thought to be related to the antigen and the MHC being recognized, it is not easy to understand this relationship of encephalitogenicity and V gene usage in the absence of similarities in antigen specificity and MHC restriction. The possibility of functional antigenic cross-reactivity has been examined and excluded and does not appear to explain the similarities in V gene usage.

This relationship of T-cell encephalitogenicity and TCR V gene usage (the Vα2Vβ8 gene combination) has been extended to encephalitogenic T cells from five different strains of rats that recognize different and noncross-reactive antigenic determinants and MHC class II molecules [Heber-Katz and Acha-Orbea, 1989]. This also applies to Lewis T cells specific for a subdominant encephalitogenic determinant of MBP (87–99) recognized in association with I-E rather than with the Lewis I-A MHC isotype associated with the MBP 68–88 response [Offner et al., 1989].

SHARED V REGIONS OF T CELLS INVOLVED IN OTHER AUTOIMMUNE DISEASES

Our findings that pathogenic EAE-inducing T cells utilize the same V region combination (Vα2Vβ8) irrespective of antigen specificity were extended to other autoimmune diseases. Experimental allergic neuritis (EAN) is a T-cell-mediated disease and involves the peripheral nervous system (unlike EAE, which is CNS specific). The T cells recognize the P2 protein, which is a component of the myelin sheath, made by Schwann cells, and is unrelated to MBP [Rostami et al., 1984]. T cells in the Lewis rat that respond to the neuritic determinant of P2 predominantly use the TCR V region combination Vα2Vβ8 [Clark, et al., 1992], though the junctional regions are different from those used by MBP-specific T cells (Zhang et al., in preparation). Experimental allergic uveoretinitis (EAU) is also a T-cell mediated disease. The T cells respond to peptides derived from the retinal S antigen or a second antigen, interphotoreceptor retinoid binding protein both nervous system–derived proteins, and use Vα2Vβ8 in both cases as well [Gregorson et al., 1991; Merryman et al., 1991; Egwuagu et al., 1991].

These findings led us to propose that there is a relationship between V region sharing and tissue (neural-derived) specificity and pathology [Heber-Katz and Acha-Orbea, 1989]. However, the T-cell-mediated disease adjuvant arthritis (AA), which can be induced by purified protein derivative (PPD) in the Lewis rat, is not nervous system related, but here again there are T cells that use the same Vα2Vβ8 combination (van Eden and Cohen, personal communication; Wekerle, personal communication; Clark and Heber-Katz, unpublished data).

WHY ARE Vα and Vβ REGIONS SHARED WHEN ANTIGEN REACTIVITY IS NOT?

We have considered several possibilities to explain the V region sharing that we see in EAE in different strains and species (in EAN, EAU, and AA) in spite of the fact that antigen and the MHC clearly are not shared. One possibility is that there is another ligand that is being recognized other than antigen + MHC. Another possibility is that this Vα2Vβ8 combinatorial structure is the target for antiidiotypic regulation through T cells and/or B cells.

For the first possibility, the idea of a ligand other than antigen + MHC was supported by studies of antigen-presenting cell (APC) + antigen–activated MBP-specific T-cell killing of oligodendrocytes [Kawai and Zweiman, 1988]. These experiments were repeated with MBP-specific, class II–restricted rat T-cell hybridomas in which similar specific killing of oligodendrocytes was seen in the absence of any activation by exogenous antigen and endogenous class II molecules [Kawai, et al., 1991]. We proposed "the V-region disease hypothesis," suggesting that the TCR had two binding sites with two independent binding events leading to specific autoimmune disease [Heber-Katz and Acha-Orbea, 1989; Heber-Katz, 1990]. Thus the CDR3 region was involved in antigen + MHC specificity, leading to cell activation, migration, and retention at specific disease sites. The second region, or the V region, was involved in the recognition of a molecule present on autoimmune disease target tissue that led to pathogenicity. Thus, once the class II–restricted T cells were at their specific locations where antigen + MHC was present, they could then interact with target tissue such as the oligodendrocyte in the *absence* of class II.

A recent finding in our laboratory indicates that soluble TCR β-chain, derived from an MBP-specific Lewis rat T cell, by itself can bind to MBP in the absence of class II (Zhang and Heber-Katz, unpublished observations). It is unclear where MBP is binding; however, the specificity of binding is not identical to the specificity of T-cell activation. Thus if this binding is related to the MHC-restricted binding, then one would have to propose that the α-chain is modifying MHC-independent β-chain binding activity. On the other hand, binding may be occurring outside the MHC-restricted binding site and MBP may be acting as a V-region binding ligand that is selecting Vβ8. Since MBP is made by both oligodendrocytes and Schwann cells, this may explain why T cells involved in neurological autoimmune diseases use Vβ8. Such V-region binding activity may play a role in selection at a stage in development when only the β-chain is expressed [Groettrup et al., 1992]. Though an intriguing finding, other ligands that bind both Vβ8 and Vα2 are being analyzed.

For the second possibility of explaining V-region sharing, support for idiotype regulation comes from the EAE T-cell vaccination experiments [Ben-Nun et al., 1981] suggesting that the T cells involved in EAE are idiotypically related. Further support for this notion came from antibody studies in Lewis rats in which the antibody used appears to be specific for a combinatorial idiotype (we believe that it is not anti-V region and is only present on activated EAE-, EAN-, and EAU-causing T cells). This antibody (10.18) could both depress and enhance disease [Owhashi and Heber-Katz, 1988].

Recent experiments have *not* supported the idea of idiotypic regulation through a combinatorial Vα2Vβ8 determinant, however. Howell et al. [1989] used synthetic peptides from two different regions of the Lewis rat MBP TCR [Burns et al., 1989]: 1) the third complementarity region (CDR3) of the EAE TCR β-chain containing the VDJ region and 2) the J region of the EAE TCR α-chain, projected to be a commonly used J region in Lewis rat EAE. Preimmunization with either peptide could induce resistance to disease. The mediator of this resistance could not be identified. In a second study also done in the Lewis rat and examining resistance to EAE [Vandenbark et al., 1989], a synthetic peptide with the sequence of the second complementarity region (CDR2) of the EAE-inducing TCR β-chain V region was used. Potent protection from EAE was obtained. In this case, however, the authors were able to isolate TCR peptide-specific T cells that could recognize EAE-inducing T cells in vitro. They made T-cell lines from these resistant rats that were specific for the Vβ8-CDR2 peptide and showed that, upon adoptive transfer, these cells confer resistance. The obvious importance of these studies was the potential to regulate disease and, by extension, MS.

So what are we left with? This VαVβ combination is 1) unrelated to antigen + MHC and 2) unrelated to combinatorial idiotypic regulation. The most likely explanation is a selecting ligand. And what the V-region disease hypothesis proposes is that in general V-region selections may generate V-region binding sites outside and independent of antigen–MHC binding sites. We furthermore propose that these binding sites may be biologically significant in both nonimmune phenomena as well as in autoimmune phenomena. Thus every VαVβ combination may potentially generate ligand binding sites. The antigen–MHC binding site in conjunction with relevant tissue ligand binding sites are the most potent in mediating autoimmune responses, and this double requirement naturally serves to limit autoimmune TCR responses.

IS MS A DISEASE OF REGULATION?

In our own studies on the effects of TCR peptides on EAE, we used the same peptides as the other groups and found that the injection of these peptides before MBP resulted not in suppression but in disease enhancement [Desquenne-Clark et al., 1991]. We were unable to find T cells that could respond to the TCR peptides or antibody that could bind to the immunizing peptides. Thus we could not identify the mediator of the enhancement. These results were confirmed by other groups [Kawano et al., 1992; Sun, 1992].

This finding is still consistent with the notion of the existence of TCR peptide-specific regulatory cells. The absence of an in vitro response to peptide could be explained by a population of otherwise downregulatory cells being in the "off" state with a concomitant deregulation of EAE (seen as enhancement rather than suppression). To tolerize the TCR peptide-specific regulatory population intentionally, we injected peptide into neonatal Lewis rats. It had been previously shown that MBP injected into neonatal rats induced tolerance [Quin et al., 1989]. We found that the animals, as adults, when injected with MBP showed severe disease, sometimes resulting in death, and chronic relapsing EAE similar to that seen in MS.

This finding is compatible with tolerance of a regulatory cell. Since this tolerance is long term and since the renewal of regulatory T cells from the thymus is probably constant, it is likely that this is an infectious form of tolerance, namely, suppression or the generation of an anti-idiotypic network.

Thus the possible elimination of a regulatory population results in EAE that presents with early onset of disease, more severe symptoms, chronic disease, and, most interestingly, a cycling of symptoms indicating a network of interacting units. Studies in the mouse have indicated that the elimination of the CD8 population and by extension the suppressor population results in cycling of disease as well [Koh et al., 1992; Jiang et al., 1992].

T-CELL RECEPTORS INVOLVED IN EAE SEEN EARLY DURING DEVELOPMENT AND IN NUDE RATS, SUGGESTING EXTRATHYMIC MATURATION

Upon sequencing the TCR mRNA from the rat MBP clones, examination of the junctional region revealed two things. First, there was a dominant serine at residue 97 in all of the sequences. The dominant junctional amino acid sequence was DSS, though only the first serine was constant. Second, the number of N-region additions was low compared with normal junctional regions [Zhang and Heber-Katz, 1992].

Low usage or absence of N regions has been considered to be a phenotype of cells that have been generated early in ontogeny [Gu et al., 1990; Feeney, 1991; Bogue et al., 1991]. Low N-region addition has been attributed to lack of TDT in neonates so that T- or B-cell receptors are unable to add nontemplate-directed nucleotides; thus we proposed that the EAE T cells were derived early during development. To determine if low N-region addition were a property of developing rat T cells, we examined rat neonatal thymus, liver, and spleen. Surprisingly, in the rat neonatal spleen the EAE β-chain sequence DSS was found in 20% of the sequences obtained, whereas none were seen in the neonatal thymus. Neonatal spleen showed no evidence of TCR cell surface expression by FACS analysis using the R73 antirat TCR antibody, which seems to only bind to TCR heterodimers [Hunig et al., 1989]. Such a finding suggested to us 1) that this EAE sequence was present early in spleen in the absence of a complete surface receptor and perhaps was being selected by its being expressed on the surface of a T cell as a β-homodimer [Groetrupp et al., 1992]; and 2) that the neonatal splenic cells were not derived from thymocytes, this sequence was not in the thymus, and maturation may be taking place outside the thymus.

To determine the Vβ8 + T-cell receptor repertoire that could be generated in the absence of a thymus, we used Lewis nude rats. Sequencing of Vβ8 mRNA from Lewis nude spleen again revealed the DSS sequence in association with Vβ8.2 as well as with Vβ8.1. The origin and activity of these cells remain to be determined but such data may yield information on a selecting ligand.

SEARCH FOR SHARED TCR V REGIONS IN MS PATIENTS

The degree of V-region sharing seen in EAE, both within a set of T cells from a given strain for a given antigenic determinant and among T cells specific for different antigens from different strains and species, suggested that the same may be true for humans. For most of the human studies, the assumption that MBP is an important component of the MS T-cell response appears to be an accepted fact, though there is really no solid evidence that MBP is involved. It should be noted that normal individuals respond to MBP, with no difference in the MBP-specific repertoire.

The results of TCR analyses of patients' MBP-reactive T cells have been extremely diverse. There are studies showing V-region sharing by MBP clones in different patients though the V regions identified by each group were different [Hafler et al., 1988; Wucherpfennig et al., 1990; Kotzin et al., 1991]. In one group, shared V regions used were independent of MHC and antigenic determinant. In another group, V-region sharing was seen in clones derived from a single patient but different between patients [Ben-Nun et al., 1991]. And, finally, one study showed no V-region sharing by MBP clones in individual patients [Giegerich et al., 1992).

Studies analyzing MS brain lesions without the bias of any antigen have yielded as confusing results as those seen with MBP-specific T-cell clones [Oksenberg et al., 1990; Wucherpfennig et al., 1992]. The issue of nonspecifically recruited inflammatory cells is probably a major one. Studies have also shown an association between Vβ restriction fragment length polymorphisms and disease susceptibility again independent of antigen [Beall et al., 1989; Oksenberg et al., 1989; Seboun et al., 1989]. All in all, the picture is getting continually more complex.

One interesting approach has been the adoptive transfer of cerebrospinal fluid cells from patients into severely compromised immunodeficient mice [Saeki et al., 1992]. This type of experiment may finally provide information on the cells involved in demyelination and inflammation in MS.

REFERENCES

Acha-Orbea H, Mitchell DJ, Timmerman L, Wraith DC, Taich GS, Waldor MK, Zamvil S, McDevitt H, Steinman L (1988): Limited heterogeneity of TcRs from lymphocytes mediating autoimmune encephalomyelitis allows specific immune intervention. Cell 54:263.

Beall SS, Concannon P, Charmley P, McFarland HF, Gatti RA, Hood LE, McFarlin DE, Biddison WE (1989): The germline repertoire of T cell receptor β chain genes in patients with chronic progressive multiple sclerosis. J Neuroimmun 21:59.

Ben-Nun A, Wekerle H, Cohen IR (1981): Vaccination against EAE with T-lymphocyte lines and cells reactive against myelin basic proteins. Nature 292:60.

Ben-Nun A, Liblau RS, Cohen L, Lehmann D, Tournier-Lasserve E, Rosensweig A, Jingwu Z, Raus JCM, Bach MA (1991): Restricted T cell receptor Vβ gene usage by myelin basic protein-specific T cell clones in multiple sclerosis: Predominant genes vary in individuals. Proc Natl Acad Sci USA 88:2466.

Bogue M, Canderas S, Benoist C, Mathis D (1991): A special repertoire of α and β T cells in neonatal rats. EMBO J 10:3647.

Burns F, Li X, Shen N, Offner H, Chou YK, Vandenbark AA, Heber-Katz E (1989): Both rat and mouse TcRs specific for the encephalitogenic determinant of MBP use similar Vα and Vβ chain genes even though the MHC and encephalitogenic determinants being recognized are different. J Exp Med 169:27.

Cambi F, Lees MB, Williams RM, Macklin WB (1982): Chronic EAE induced in rabbits with bovine white matter proteolipid protein. J Neuropathol Exp Neurol 41:508.

Clark L, Heber-Katz E, Rostami A (1992): T cells which cause EAN and EAE share T cell receptor V regions. Ann Neurol, 31:587.

Chluba J, Steeg C, Becker A, Wekerle H, Epplen JT (1989): TcR b chain usage in MBP specific rat T lymphocytes. Eur J Immunol 19:279.

Danska JS, Livingstone AM, Paragas V, Ishihara T, Fathman CG (1990): The presumptive CDR3 regions of both T cell receptor a and b chains determine T cell specificity for myoglobin peptides. J Exp Med 172:27.

Desquenne-Clark L, Esch TR, Otvos L Jr, Heber-Katz E (1991): T cell receptor peptide immunization leads to enhanced and chronic experimental allergic encephalomyelitis. Proc Natl Acad Sci USA 88:7219.

Egwuagu CE, Chow C, Beraud E, Caspi R, Mahdi RM, Brezin AP, Nussenblatt RB, Gery I (1991): T cell receptor β chain usage in EAU. J Autoimmun 4:315.

Esch T, Miskimins R, Heber-Katz E (1993): CAT induces encephalomyelitis in MBP-CAT transgenic mice expressing CAT in oligodendrocytes. Transgene 1:11.

Feeney A (1991): Lack of N regions in fetal and neonatal mouse thymus. J Exp Med 172:1377.

Fink PJ, Matis L, McElliott DL, Bookman M, Hedrick S (1986). Correlations between T cell specificity and the structure of the antigen receptor. Nature 312:219.

Fritz RB, Chou C-HJ, McFarlin DE (1983): Induction of EAE in PL/J and (SJL × PL/J)F$_1$ mice by myelin basic protein and its peptides: Localization of a second encephalitogenic determinant. J Immunol 130:191.

Giegerich G, Pette M, Meinl E, Epplen JT, Wekerle H, Hinkanen A (1992): Diversity of TcR α and β chain genes expressed by human T cells specific for similar MBP/MHC complexes. Eur J Immunol 22:1331.

Gregorson DS, Fling SP, Merryman CF, Zhang X, Li X, Heber-Katz E (1991): Conserved TcR V gene usage by uveitogenic T cells. Clin Immunol Immunopathol 58:154.

Groetrupp M, Baron A, Griffiths G, Palacios R, von Boehmer H (1992): T cell receptor β chain homodimers on the surface of immature but not mature α,γ,δ chain deficient T cell lines. EMBO J 11:2735.

Gu H, Forrester I, Rajewsky K (1990): Sequence homologies, N sequences insertion, and JH gene utilization in VHDJH joining: Implications for the joining mechanism and the ontogenic timing of Ly1 B cell and B-CLL progenitor generation. EMBO J 9:2133.

Hafler DA, Duby AD, Lee SJ, Benjamin D, Seidman JG, Weiner HL (1988): Oligoclonal T lymphocytes in the cerebrospinal fluid of patients with multiple sclerosis. J Exp Med 167:1313.

Happ MP, Heber-Katz E (1987): Differences in the repertoire of the Lewis rat T cell response to self and non-self MBPs. J Exp Med 167:502.

Happ MP, Kiraly AS, Offner H, Vandenbark A, Heber-Katz E (1988): The autoreactive T cell population in experimental allergic encephalomyelitis: T cell receptor β chain rearrangements. J Neuroimmunol 19:191.

Hashim G (1978): Myelin basic protein: Structure, function, and antigenic determinants. Immunol Rev 39:60.

Heber-Katz E (1990): The autoimmune T cell receptor: Epitopes, idiotopes, and malatopes. Clin Immunol Immunopathol 55:1.

Heber-Katz E, Acha-Orbea H (1989): The V-region hypothesis: Evidence from autoimmune encephalomyelitis. Immunol Today 10:164.

Hedrick SM, Cohen DI, Nielson EA, Davis MM (1984): Isolation of cDNA clones encoding T-cell specific membrane associated proteins. Nature 308:149.

Howell MD, Winters ST, Olee T, Powell HC, Carlo DJ, Brostoff SE (1989): Vaccination against experimental allergic encephalomyelitis with T cell receptor peptides. Science 246:668.

Hunig TH, Wallny J, Hartley JK, Lawetzky A, Tiefenthaler G (1989): A monoclonal antibody to a constant determinant of the rat T cell antigen receptor that induces T cell activation: Differential reactivity with subsets of immature and mature T lymphocytes. J Exp Med 169:73.

Jiang H, Zhang XM, Pernis B (1992): Role of CD8 T cells in murine EAE. Science 256:1213.

Kawai K, Heber-Katz E, Zweiman B (1991): Cytotoxic effects of myelin basic protein-reactive T cell hybridoma cells on oligodendrocytes. J Neuroimmunol 32:75.

Kawai K, Zweiman B (1988): Cytotoxic effects of myelin basic protein-reactive T cells on cultured oligodendrocytes. J Neuroimmunol 19:159.

Kawano Y-I, Sasamoto Y, Kotake S, Thurau SR, Wiggert B, Gery I (1991): Trials of vaccination against EAU with a T cell receptor peptide. Curr Eye Res 10:789.

Koh D-R, Fung-Leung W-P, Ho A, Gray D, Acha-Orbea H, Mak T-W (1992): Less mortality but more relapses in EAE in CD8-/- mice. Science. 256:1210.

Kotzin BL, Karuturi S, Chou YK, Lafferty J, Forrester JM, Better M, Nedwin GE, Offner H, Vandenbark A (1991): Preferential T cell receptor beta chain variable gene use in myelin basic protein reactive T cell clones from patients with multiple sclerosis. Proc Natl Acad Sci USA 88:9161.

Merryman CF, Donoso LA, Zhang XM, Heber-Katz E, Gregorson D (1991): Characterization of a new potent immunopathogenic epitope in S-antigen which elicits T cells expressing $V\beta8$ and $V\alpha2$ genes. J Immunol 146:75.

Oksenberg JR, Sherritt M, Begovich AB, Erlich HA, Bernard CC, Cavalli-Sforzi LL, Steinman L (1989): T cell receptor Va and Ca alleles associated with multiple sclerosis and myasthenia gravis. Proc Natl Acad Sci USA 86:988.

Oksenberg JR, Stuart S, Begovich AB, Bell RB, Erlich HA, Steinman L, Bernard CCA (1990): Limited heterogeneity of rearranged T cell receptor $V\alpha$ transcripts in brain of multiple sclerosis patients. Nature 345:344.

Offner H, Hashim GA, Celnick B, Galang A, Li X, Burns FR, Shen N, Heber-Katz E, Vandenbark AA (1989): T cell determinants of myelin basic protein include a unique encephalitogenic I-E restricted epitope for Lewis rats. J Exp Med 170:355.

Owhashi M, Heber-Katz E (1988): Protection from EAE conferred by a monoclonal antibody against a shared idiotype on rat TcRs specific for MBP. J Exp Med 168:2153.

Quin Y, Sun D, Goto M, Meyermann R, Wekerle H (1989): Resistance to experimental autoimmune encephalomyelitis induced by neonatal tolerization to myelin basic protein: Clonal elimination vs. regulation of autoaggressive lymphocytes. Eur J Immunol 19:373.

Raine CS, Schaumburg HH (1977): Neuropathology of myelin diseases. In Morell P (ed): "Myelin." New York: Plenum Press, p 271.

Rostami AM, Brown MJ, Lisak R (1984): The role of myelin P2 protein in the production of experimental allergic neuritis. Ann Neurol 16:680.

Saeki Y, Mima T, Sakoda S, Fujimura H, Arita N, Nomura T, Kishimoto T (1992): Transfer of MS into severe combined immunodeficiency mice by mononuclear cells from cerebrospinal fluid of the patients. Proc Natl Acad Sci USA 89: 6157.

Satoh JK, Sakai M, Endoh F, Koike T, Kunishita T, Namikawa T, Yamamura T, Tabira T (1987): EAE mediated by murine encephalitogenic T cell lines specific for myelin proteolipid apoprotein. J Immunol 138:179.

Seboun E, Robinson MA, Doolittle TH, Ciulla TA, Kindt TJ, Hauser SL (1989): A susceptibility locus for multiple sclerosis is linked to the T cell receptor β chain complex. Cell 57:1095.

Sun D (1992): Synthetic peptides of rat $V\beta8$ TcR fail to elicit regulatory T cells reactive with $V\beta8$ TcR on rat encephalitogenic T cells. Cell Immunol 141:200.

Tan K-N, Datlot BM, Gilmore JA, Kronman AC, Lee JH, Maxam MM, Rao A (1988):

The T cell receptor Vα3 gene segment is associated with reactivity to azobenene-arsonate. Cell 54:247.

Tuohy VK, Sobel RA, Lees MB (1988): Myelin proteolipid protein-induced EAE: Variations of disease expression in different strains of mice. J Immunol 140:1868.

Urban J, Kumar V, Kono D, Gomez C, Horvath SJ, Clayton J, Ando, DG, Sercarz EE, Hood L (1988): Restricted use of TcR V genes in murine autoimmune encephalomyelitis raises possibilities for antibody therapy. Cell 54:577.

Vandenbark AA, Hashim G, Offner H (1989): Immunization with a synthetic T cell receptor V region peptide protects against experimental autoimmune encephalomyelitis. Nature 341:541.

Weerth S, Lassman H, Perry L, Linington C (1992): Pathogenic autoimmune T cell responses to multiple myelin antigens: MBP, MAG and MOG, abstracted. In Neuroimmune Interactions and Their Regulation. p 66.

Winoto A, Urban JL, Lan NC, Governman J, Hood L, Hansburg D (1986): Predominant use of a Vα gene segment in mouse T cell receptors for cytochrome c. Nature 324:679.

Wucherphennig K, Newcombe J, Li H, Keddy C, Cuzner ML, Hafler DA (1992): T cell receptor VαVβ repertoire and cytokine gene expression in active MS lesions. J Exp Med 175:993.

Wucherphennig K, Ota N, Endo JG, Seidman H, Rosenzweig L, Weiner HL, Hafler DA (1990): Shared human T cell receptor Vβ usage to immunodominant regions of myelin basic protein. Science 248:1016.

Zamvil SS, Mitchell DJ, Lee NE, Moore AC, Waldorf MK, Saki K, Rothbard JB, McDevitt HO, Steinman L, Acha-Orbea H (1988): Predominant expression of a T cell receptor Vβ gene subfamily in autoimmune encephalomyelitis. J Exp Med 167:1586.

Zhang X-M, Heber-Katz E (1992): Encephalitogenic T cells in adult Lewis rats appear to be products of early ontogeny. J Immunol 148:746.

Zinkernagel RM, Cooper S, Chambers J, Lazzarini RA, Hengartner H, Arnheiter H (1990): Virus-induced autoantibody response to a transgenic viral antigen. Nature 345:68.

23

AUTOIMMUNITY AND AUTOIMMUNE DIABETES MELLITUS

Alan G. Baxter and Anne Cooke

*Department of Pathology, Division of Immunology, Cambridge University,
Cambridge, United Kingdom*

INTRODUCTION

Insulin-dependent diabetes mellitus (IDDM) is an autoimmune disease in which the β-cells of the pancreas are selectively destroyed by cells of the immune system. The exact mechanism by which the β-cell is destroyed remains to be clarified. While class I–restricted destruction by $CD8^+$ T cells is an attractive hypothesis, it is also possible that macrophages, either alone or together with T cells, may destroy β-cells via local cytokine or free radical release.

WHAT INITIATES AUTOIMMUNITY?

It has often been suggested that tolerance to β-cells may break down as a result of viral infection. The dramatic increase in incidence of diabetes in the Western world over the last decade [Bingly and Gale, 1989] confirms a strong environmental influence, and the observation that IDDM appears to have a seasonal pattern of onset and sometimes arises after viral infection

Autoimmunity: Physiology and Disease, Pages 365–375
© *1994 Wiley-Liss, Inc.*

supports the proposition of a viral etiology. Much attention has been focused on the possible role of enteroviruses, particularly group B coxsackieviruses, in precipitating β-cell destruction [Coleman et al., 1973]. Between 7% and 76% of newly diabetic patients have IgM antibodies to Coxsackie B virus in their blood [Banatvala, 1987; Eggers et al., 1983], and the finding of Coxsackie B4 virus in the pancreas of a diabetic child [Yoon et al., 1979] was also for some time used to support the viral trigger hypothesis; however, more recent findings suggest that the β-cell destruction had preceded the infection.

HOW COULD A VIRUS TRIGGER AUTOIMMUNITY?

Tolerance to self-antigens may be achieved during ontogeny by deletion of autoreactive T or B cells with receptors capable of a high affinity interaction with self-antigen [Kappler et al., 1987], and autoreactive lymphocytes that escape into the periphery may only be capable of low affinity interactions. Additional mechanisms of peripheral tolerance such as anergy or suppression may further reduce autoreactivity. However, T cells that recognize viral antigens may provide help for other T cells or for B cells in an autoimmune response, a so-called T-cell bypass [Weigle, 1971; Allison, 1971]. Viral infection of a cell could result in the expression of immunogenic neoantigens that could be either virally encoded or self-antigens modified by viral attachment or virally encoded proteases. Possible examples of virus-related T-cell bypasses are the DNA polymerases of Epstein-Barr and hepatitis viruses, which bear homologous sequences to myelin basic protein, a target antigen in multiple sclerosis [Fujinami and Oldstone, 1985; Jahnke et al., 1985], and the capsid protein VP2 of polioviruses, which contains sequences similar to those of the acetylcholine receptor, the target antigen in myasthenia gravis [Oldstone, 1987]. Friend leukemia virus infection of rats has been shown to result in the development of a Coombs'-positive hemolytic anemia possibly arising through T-helper recognition of viral antigen budding from the surface of erythroblasts. Such virus-specific T-helper cells could provide help for B cells with specificity for antigens on the surface of normal erythrocytes. B-cell affinity maturation developed through somatic mutation could lead to the emergence of high affinity B-cell clones with specificity for self-antigens. T cells would be required for the maintenance of the autoreactive B-cell response, and once the infection had been cleared the autoantibody response should recede. For example, influenza, measles, infectious mononucleosis, and herpes simplex virus infections are sometimes followed by self-limiting autoimmune thrombocytopenia or hemolytic anemia. However, tissue destruction associated with the initial insult may result in activation of other autoreactive T cells and spreading of autoimmunity to other immunogenic self-determinants [Lehmann et al., 1992], maintaining tissue destruction after clearance of the viral trigger.

Although this scenario has been presented in the context of virus infection, it may be envisaged with other cross-reactive stimuli such as bacterial or parasitic infections or pharmacological agents. For example, in genetically predisposed individuals, quinine derivatives, thiazide diuretics and sulfonamides can induce thrombocytopenia; D-penicillamine can cause thrombocytopenia, systemic lupus erythematosus, and myasthenia gravis, and dopamine derivatives and mefanamic acid can trigger hemolytic anemia [Lee and Chase, 1975; Stein et al., 1980; Delamere et al., 1983]. While some of the immune complex disorders initiated by such drugs may be attributable to effects on the complement cascade [Sim, 1989], modification of self-proteins and thus genesis of neoantigens also contributes to the observed pathology. Again, autoimmune disease usually remits on withdrawal of the offending drug.

The recent experiments of Ohashi and colleagues [1991] suggest a possible mechanism by which exogenous antigens may induce autoimmunity. In their experimental model the majority of the T cells in double transgenic mice expressed a T-cell receptor with specificity for a transgenic lymphocyte choriomeningitis virus (LCMV) glycoprotein restricted to pancreatic β-cells. These transgenic mice did not develop IDDM spontaneously despite the presence of large numbers of antigen-specific $CD8^+$ T cells. Following infection with LCMV, the mice developed autoimmune diabetes that was dependent on both $CD4^+$ and $CD8^+$ T cells. The experiment nicely demonstrated that $CD8^+$ T cells with the potential capability of destroying self-antigen failed to do so in the absence of the requisite help. The failure to recognize stimulatory antigens in the absence of costimulators has been described as T-cell ignorance. In this case, help was induced by viral infection and presumably required presentation of viral products on highly effective antigen-presenting cells such as dendritic cells at the site of tissue destruction. Similar results were obtained by Oldstone et al. [1991] in mice transgenic for LCMV glycoproteins or nuclear proteins. Experiments by Jacques Miller and colleagues [Heath et al., 1992] may cast further light on the nature of this requisite help, as $CD8^+$ T cells with specificity for a transgene (RIP-K^b) expressed by β-cells did not attack the β-cells unless provided with high local concentrations of interleukin (IL)-2. This could be interpreted as suggesting that T cells with low enough avidity to escape into the periphery may be activated by coincidental production of IL-2. Such cells could not attack the majority of somatic cell types, which rarely express sufficiently high levels of MHC and accessory molecules required for normal T-cell triggering unless local inflammation resulted in effective presentation, activation of T-helper cells, and IL-2 production.

DOES PERIPHERAL TOLERANCE PREVENT AUTOIMMUNE DISEASE?

There is good evidence to suggest that, in addition to the above-mentioned mechanisms of central tolerance or ignorance, other processes exist to modify responsiveness to self-antigens. Since Witebsky et al. [1957] induced chronic thyroiditis in rabbits by injection of thyroglobulin extracts, several other groups have produced similar models of autoimmune tissue destruction by injection of tissue extracts or tissue-specific proteins, usually in the presence of adjuvant. These experiments demonstrated that $CD4^+$ T cells that recognize native self-antigens were present in normal mice and were capable of causing autoimmune pathology when activated. T cells cloned from such immunized animals could transfer autoimmune pathology. This approach has been used to demonstrate that T cells exist with specificity for thyroglobulin, thyroid peroxidase, myelin basic protein, and collagen type II. These cells do not normally express their pathological potential, but it is elicited following immunization, and they retain their autoaggressive behavior following activation and maintenance in vitro.

It is possible that under normal conditions the autoaggressive T cells that have avoided purging by central tolerance are unable to respond because they

1. Express low levels of T-cell receptor (TCR) or accessory molecules
2. Are anergic
3. Are held in check by a peripheral regulatory mechanism

PERIPHERAL TOLERANCE ACHIEVED BY DOWN MODULATION OF TCR

There are several double transgenic experiments demonstrating that tolerance to self (H-Y) [Uematsu et al., 1988; Bluthmann et al., 1988] or neoself-antigens (e.g., transgenic K^b) [Heath et al., 1992; Husbands et al., 1992] may be achieved by deletion of T cells expressing high levels of antigen-specific TCR. T cells bearing the transgenic TCR can be found in the periphery of mice expressing the ligand, but the levels of TCR or accessory molecules are reduced, suggesting that T cells with only a poor ability to interact with the antigen and MHC escape negative selection. Thus in the experiments of Schonrich and colleagues [1991] T cells expressing a transgenic TCR specific for the alloantigen K^b could be found in the periphery of mice expressing K^b under the control of the glial fibrillary acidic protein promoter. These T cells did not appear to recognize K^b in vivo but could respond to the alloantigen in vitro. The peripheral T cells of these double transgenic mice appeared to have lower levels of expression of both the TCR and the CD8 molecule, but normal expression and functional activity were regained after culture in vitro. Experiments described above by Jacques Miller and his collaborators [Heath et al., 1992] suggested a similar situation since they found tolerance in vivo to K^b expressed in the β-cells of the pancreas that could be reversed in vitro by addition of IL-2. Thus there is evidence to support tolerance to self-antigens being achieved by clonal deletion and escape into the periphery achieved only by those autoreactive T cells unable to respond to self-antigens.

A ROLE FOR ANERGY IN PREVENTING AUTOIMMUNITY?

Anergic lymphocytes display a robust state of unresponsiveness. There are many experimental systems in which anergy seems to be implicated. However, it is not always clear that the effects observed are not attributable to elimination of autoreactive cells, a lack of costimulator function, or an active suppressor mechanism. An example of anergy is the "T-cell dormant" state induced in nonobese diabetic (NOD) mice treated with complete Freund's adjuvant [Sadelain et al., 1990; Ulaeto et al., 1992]. Injected mice did not spontaneously develop diabetes, and islet grafts in diabetic recipients could be protected by complete Freund's adjuvant injection. The anergic state was robust as transfer of diabetes by injection of spleen cells from diabetic donors was markedly inhibited in Freund's-treated mice; however, autoreactive T cells had not been eliminated from treated mice, as their splenocytes were able to induce diabetes when transferred into male NOD mice [Ulaeto et al., 1992].

IS PERIPHERAL TOLERANCE MAINTAINED BY AN ACTIVE PROCESS?

Since the early work of Gershon and Kondo [1970], many experiments have demonstrated the presence of T cells that are able to prevent the induction of immune responses, including those to autoantigens. Thus following immunization of mice with high doses of rat red blood cells (RBC) to induce autoantibodies against mouse RBC, T cells are also generated that can be shown in transfer experiments to prevent the induction of such autoantibodies in naive individuals [Cooke et al., 1978]. Experimental allergic thyroiditis (EAT) and autoantibody formation against thyroglobulin (Tg) was prevented in mice when Tg was administered in high doses intravenously prior to immunization with Tg and adjuvant [Kong et al., 1982]. $CD4^+$ T cells are generated in such tolerized mice that are able on transfer to prevent the induction of EAT in recipient mice [Parish, et al., 1988]. These $CD4^+$ T cells have been shown to be of the CD45R0 phenotype (Hutchings, Lightstone, Cooke, and Marvel, unpublished observations). The presence of such regulatory T cells has been demonstrated in many experimental autoimmune conditions. A thymus is not necessary for peripheral tolerance induction by many of these protocols, suggesting that the antigen acts directly on a peripheral T cell to elicit its regulatory function.

In all the situations thus far described the cells develop as a result of an active immunization protocol. Is there any evidence that such cells may be present under normal conditions to prevent disease? The observation that thymectomy of normal mice at 2–4 days of age results in the development of a variety of organ-specific autoimmune disorders and the elaboration of autoantibodies is highly suggestive that this is the case [Sakaguchi et al., 1985]. Autoimmunity is prevented by transfer of normal adult T cells into such thymectomized mice, and depletion data suggest that the cell type mediating protection is an $Ly1^+$ T cell.

NOD mice spontaneously develop IDDM as a result of an autoimmune attack on their pancreatic β-cells [Makino et al., 1980]. Female mice have a much higher spontaneous incidence of disease than male mice, but the disease can be prematurely induced in female mice and induced in male mice with high doses of cyclophosphamide [Harada and Makino, 1984]. The exact mechanism by which this drug acts remains to be clarified, but an effect on endogenous suppressor cells has been proposed [Yasunami and Bach, 1988]. Charlton and colleagues [1989] have shown that $CD4^+$ splenic T cells from nondiabetic mice were able to prevent disease induction by cyclophosphamide. It was also concluded from the experiments of Yasunami and Bach [1988] and Hutchings and Cooke [1990] that a population of $CD4^+$ T cells may be able to regulate IDDM induced in NOD mice by passive transfer of diabetic spleen cells.

The presence of a $CD4^+$ T-cell population that is capable of regulating the spontaneous occurrence of autoimmune pathology is also indicated by the experiments of Fowell et al. [1991]. Rat $CD4^+$ T cells may be subdivided into two populations on the basis of the levels of expression of the CD45RC isoform. When athymic nude rats were reconstituted with T cells consisting predominantly of $CD4^+$ T cells that expressed high levels of the CD45RC isoform, the rats developed a wasting disease with inflammatory infiltrates present in many organs, including the liver, lung, and thyroid. In contrast, rats reconstituted with both T-cell populations or just $CD4^+$ T cells expressing low levels of CD45RC were healthy and developed no inflammation of the lung and liver and showed a much reduced incidence of thyroid pathology. Penhale et al. [1975] have shown that $PVG.RT1^c$ rats subjected to thymectomy followed by several doses of irradiation developed thyroiditis. Fowell et al. [1991] applied this protocol to PVG rats with a different MHC ($RT1^u$), and the animals spontaneously developed diabetes and not thyroiditis. The development of disease in these rats was prevented when $CD4^+$ T cells were introduced into the irradiated rats after their last dose of irradiation. The $CD4^+$ T cells that mediated this suppression of induced diabetes expressed only low levels of the CD45RC isoform.

It has previously been shown by workers in several laboratories that primed or nonprimed $CD4^+$ T cells can prevent the occurrence of autoimmunity. The recent experiments from Fowell and colleagues [1991] and the unpublished observations of Marvel and colleagues mentioned above show that this function may be restricted to a subpopulation of CD4$^+$ T cells. In the rat these T cells have been shown to reside within a pool that has been shown to secrete IL-4 and IL-10 and may therefore be T-helper 2 cells.

CAN THE IMMUNE SYSTEM BE REEDUCATED TO PREVENT AUTOIMMUNITY?

As it is now clear that not all autoreactive T and B cells are purged from the peripheral repertoire, it is possible that such cells may be induced to express their pathogenetic potential. Such autoreactive responses can be regulated. When high responder mouse strains are immunized with mouse Tg and complete Freund's adjuvant, they develop a thyroiditis that spontaneously resolves [Rose et al., 1971] and when Tg-specific T cells are transferred to naive mice they develop a thyroiditis that, although severe, is self-limiting [Vladutiu and Rose, 1975]. Recent evidence from experiments in mice suggests that one of the major thyroiditogenic epitopes on Tg is iodinated [Champion et al., 1985, 1987, 1991]. It is interesting to note that when iodination of Tg is prevented by treatment with amino triazole, Tg-reactive T cells do not accumulate in the thyroid, suggesting that the target antigen needs to be seen in the gland [Champion et al., 1987]. One possible explanation for the resolution of the thyroid inflammatory response is that presentation of autoantigen by thyroid epithelial cells may render naive T cells anergic, despite being stimulatory to T hybridomas.

A further level of control may be mediated by regulatory cells. For example, administration of antigen together with anti-CD4 antibody has been shown to be capable of inducing antigen-specific tolerance [Cobbold et al., 1990], and with nondepleting anti-CD4 antibodies it has been possible to demonstrate successful prevention of both spontaneous and experimentally induced autoimmune conditions [Hutchings et al., 1992]. The mechanisms by which these therapeutic protocols work are currently being elucidated, but there are some data to suggest that tolerance is not obtained simply through anergy of autoreactive T cells, but, at least in the case of experimentally induced autoimmune disease, by the development of T cells capable of preventing autoreactivity.

The way in which an antigen is presented to the immune system may also determine the subsequent outcome of the immune response. Administration of antigen orally or as an aerosol has been shown to lead to suppression of the response to that antigen. The recent data from Weiner's lab suggests that, at least in the case of orally administered antigen, it may be T-cell production of TGF-β that leads to suppression of the immune response [Khoury et al., 1992]. Another interesting aspect of this latter work is the observation that local TGF-β production may downregulate responses to other antigens by a bystander effect. This implies that if an organ can be targeted by T cells elaborating inhibitory cytokines, then they should be able to inhibit all immune cells in the neighborhood. This possibility can be readily tested in the model of experimentally induced thyroiditis, since $CD4^+$ T cells that regulate thyroiditis induced by Tg should then also be capable of regulating thyroiditis induced by thyroid peroxidase. In the case of IDDM, the induction of regulatory T cells recognizing insulin may suffice to prevent the spontaneous development of disease. Indeed, oral tolerance to insulin has been shown to protect NOD mice from diabetes [Zhang et al., 1991] despite having been demonstrated not to be the primary target antigen of immune destruction [Hurtenbach and Maurer, 1989]. In summary, it may be possible to reestablish tolerance to self-antigens by employing an organ-targeting strategy such that inhibitory cytokine production (TGF-β or IL-10) prevails at the site of inflammation. The advantage of such a strategy is that it will not be necessary to determine the pathologically relevant epitopes on the target organ but just any organ-specific antigen.

REFERENCES

Allison AC (1971): Unresponsiveness to self antigens. Lancet 2:1401–1403.

Banatvala JE (1987): Insulin dependent diabetes mellitus: Coxsackie B viruses revisited. Prog Med Virol 34:33–54.

Bingly PJ, Gale EAM (1989): Rising incidence of IDDM in Europe. Diabetes Care 12:289–295.

Bluthmann H, Kisielow P, Uematsu Y, Malissen M, Krimpenfort P, Berns A, von Boehmer H, Steinmetz M (1988): T cell-specific deletion of T-cell receptor transgenes allows functional rearrangement of endogenous α- and β-genes. Nature 334:156–159.

Champion BR, Page KR, Parish N, Rayner DC, Dawe K, Biswas-Hughes G, Cooke A, Geysen M, Roitt IM (1991): Identification of a thyroxine-containing self-epitope of thyroglobulin which triggers thyroid autoreactive T cells. J Exp Med 174:363–370.

Champion BR, Rayner DC, Byfield PGH, Page KR, Chan CTJ, Roitt IM (1987): Critical role of iodination for T cell recognition of thyroglobulin in experimental murine thyroid autoimmunity. J Immunol 139:3665–3670.

Champion BR, Vary AM, Katz D, Cooke A, Roitt IM (1985): Autoreactive T-cell lines specific for mouse thyroglobulin. Immunology 54:513–519.

Charlton B, Bacelj A, Slattery RM, Mandel TE (1989): Cyclophosphamide-induced diabetes in NOD/Wehi mice: Evidence for suppression in spontaneous autoimmune diabetes mellitus. Diabetes 38:441–447.

Cobbold SP, Qin S, Waldmann H (1990): Reprogramming the immune system for tolerance with monoclonal antibodies. Semin Immunol 2:377–387.

Coleman TJ, Gamble DR, Taylor KW (1973): Diabetes in mice after coxsackie B4 infection. Br Med J 3:25–27.

Cooke A, Hutchings P, Playfair JHL (1978): Suppressor T cells in experimentally autoimmune haemolytic anaemia. Nature 273:154–155.

Delamere JP, Jobson S, Mackintosh LP, Wells L, Walton KW (1983): Penicillamine-induced myasthenia gravis in rheumatoid arthritis: Its clinical and genetic features. Ann Rheum Dis 42:500–504.

Eggers HJ, Mertens TH, Gruneklee D (1983): Coxsackie infection and diabetes. Lancet 2:631–633.

Fowell D, McKnight AJ, Powrie F, Dyke R, Mason D (1991): Subsets of CD4$^+$ T cells and their roles in the induction and prevention of autoimmunity. Immunol Rev 123:37–64.

Fujinami RS, Oldstone MBA (1985): Amino acid homology between encephalitogenic sites of myelin basic protein and virus: Mechanism for autoimmunity. Science 230:1043–1045.

Gershon RK, Kondo K (1970): Cell interactions in the induction of tolerance: The role of thymic lymphocytes. Immunology 18:723–737.

Harada M, Makino S (1984): Promotion of spontaneous diabetes in nonobese diabetes-prone mice by cyclophosphamide. Diabetologia 27:604–606.

Heath WR, Allison J, Hoffmann MW, Schonrich G, Hammerling G, Arnold B, Miller JFAP (1992): Autoimmune diabetes as a consequence of locally produced interleukin-2. Nature 359:547–549.

Hurtenbach U, Maurer C (1989): Type 1 diabetes in NOD mice is not associated with insulin-specific autoreactive T cells. J Autoimmun 2:151–161.

Husbands SD, Schonrich G, Arnold B, Chandler PR, Simpson E, Philpott KL, Tomlinson P, O'Reilly L, Cooke A, Mellor AL (1992): Expression of major histocompatibility complex class I antigens at low levels in the thymus induces T cell tolerance via a non-deletional mechanism. Eur J Immunol 22:2655–2611.

Hutchings PR, Cooke A (1990): The transfer of autoimmune diabetes in NOD mice can be inhibited or accelerated by distinct cell populations present in normal mice. J Autoimmun 3:175–185.

Hutchings P, O'Reilly L, Parish NM, Waldmann H, Cooke A (1992): The use of a non-depleting anti-CD4 monoclonal antibody to re-establish tolerance to β cells in NOD mice. Eur J Immunol 22:1913–1918.

Jahnke U, Fisher EH, Aylord AC (1985): Sequence homology between certain viral proteins and proteins in encephalitomyelitis and neuritis. Science 229:282–284.

Kappler JW, Roehm N, Marrack P (1987): T cell tolerance by clonal elimination in the thymus. Cell 49:273–280.

Khoury SJ, Hancock WW, Weiner HL (1992): Oral tolerance to myelin basic protein and natural recovery from experimental autoimmune encephalitis are associated with down regulation of inflammatory cytokines and differential upregulation of transforming growth factor β, interleukin 4, and prostaglandin E expression in the brain. J Exp Med 176:1355–1364.

Kong YM, Okayasu I, Giraldo AA, Beisel KW, Rose NR (1982): Tolerance to thyroglobulin by activating suppressor mechanisms. Ann NY Acad Sci 392:191.

Lee SL, Chase PH (1975): Drug-induced systemic lupus erythematosus: A critical review. Semin Arthritis Rheum 5:83–103.

Lehmann PV, Forsthuber T, Miller A, Sercarz EE (1992): Spreading T cell autoimmunity to cryptic determinants of an autoantigen. Nature 358:155–157.

Makino S, Kunimoto K, Muraoka Y, Mizushima Y, Katagiri K, Tochino Y (1980): Breeding of a nonobese diabetic strain of mouse. Exp Anim 29:1–13.

Ohashi PS, Oehen S, Buerki K, Pircher H, Ohashi CT, Odermatt B, Malissen B, Zinkernagel RM, Hengartner H (1991): Ablation of "tolerance" and induction of diabetes by virus infection in viral antigen transgenic mice. Cell 65:305–317.

Oldstone MBA (1987): Molecular mimicry and autoimmune disease. Cell 50:819–820 and Erratum 51:878.

Oldstone MBA, Nerenberg M, Southern P, Price J, Lewicki H (1991): Virus infection triggers IDDM in a transgenic model: Role of anti-self (virus) immune response. Cell 65:319–331.

Parish NM, Roitt IM, Cooke A (1988): Phenotypic characteristics of cells involved in induced suppression to murine experimental autoimmune thyroiditis. Eur J Immunol 18:1463–1467.

Penhale WJ, Farmer A, Irvine WJ (1975): Thyroiditis in T cell depleted rats. Influence of strain, radiation dose, adjuvants and antilymphocyte serum. Clin Exp Immunol 21:362–375.

Rose NR, Twarog FJ, Crowle (1971): Murine thyroiditis: The importance of adjuvant and mouse strain for the induction of thyroid lesions. J Immunol 106:698–705.

Sadelain MWJ, Quin HY, Lauzon J, Singh B (1990): Prevention of type 1 diabetes in NOD mice by adjuvant immunotherapy. Diabetes 39:583–589.

Sakaguchi S, Fukuma K, Kuribayashi K, Masuda T (1985): Organ-specific autoimmune diseases induced in mice by elimination of T cell subset. J Exp Med 161:72–87.

Schonrich G, Kalinke U, Momburg F, Malissen M, Scmitt-Verhulst A-M, Malissen B, Hammerling GJ, Arnold B (1991): Down regulation of T cell receptors on self-reactive T cells as a novel mechanism for extrathymic tolerance induction. Cell 65:293–304.

Stein HB, Paterson AC, Offer RC, Atkins CJ, Teufel A, Robinson HS (1980): Adverse effects of D-penicillamine in rheumatoid arthritis. Ann Intern Med 92:24–29.

Sim E (1989): In Kammuller ME, Bloksma N, Seinen W (eds): "Autoimmunity and Toxicology." Amsterdam: Elsevier, pp 267–291.

Uematsu Y, Ryser S, Dembic Z, Borgulya P, Krimpenfort P, Berns A, von Boehmer H, Steinmetz M (1988): In transgenic mice the introduced functional T cell receptor β gene prevents expression of endogenous β-genes. Cell 52:831–841.

Ulaeto D, Lacy PE, Kipnis DM, Kanagawa O, Unanue ER (1992): A T-cell dormant state in the autoimmune process of nonobese diabetic mice treated with complete Freund's adjuvant. Proc Natl Acad Sci USA 89:3927–3931.

Vladutiu AO, Rose NR (1975): Cellular basis of the genetic control of immune responsiveness to murine thyroglobulin in mice. Cell Immunol 17:106–111.

Weigle WO (1971): Recent observations and concepts in immunological unresponsiveness and autoimmunity. Clin Exp Immunol 92:437–447.

Whittingham S, McNeilage LJ, Mackay IR (1987): Epstein-Bar virus as an etiological agent in primary Sjögren's syndrome. Med Hypoth 22:373–386.

Witebsky E, Rose RR, Kerplan K, Paine JR, Egan RW (1957): Chronic thyroiditis and autoimmunisation. JAMA 164:1439–1447.

Yasunami R, Bach J-F (1988): Anti-supressor effect of cyclophosphamide on the development of spontaneous diabetes in NOD mice. Eur J Immunol 18:481–484.

Yoon J-W, Austin M, Onodera T, Notkins AL (1979): Virus induced diabetes mellitus. Isolation of a virus from the pancreas of a child with diabetic ketosis. N Engl J Med 300:1173–1179.

Zhang ZJ, Davidson L, Eisenbarth G, Werner ML (1991): Suppression of diabetes in nonobese diabetic mice by oral administration of porcine insulin. Proc Natl Acad Sci USA 88:10252–10256.

24

NATURAL AND THERAPEUTIC CONTROL OF OCULAR AUTOIMMUNITY: RODENT AND MAN

Rachel R. Caspi and Robert B. Nussenblatt

Laboratory of Immunology, National Eye Institute, NIH, Bethesda, Maryland

EXPERIMENTAL AUTOIMMUNE UVEORETINITIS (EAU): A MODEL FOR OCULAR AUTOIMMUNITY

Experimental autoimmune uveoretinitis (EAU) has served for many years as a model for human ocular inflammations of presumed autoimmune etiology. EAU is traditionally induced in susceptible animals (primates and rodents) by immunization with purified retinal antigens in complete Freund's adjuvant or by adoptive transfer of retinal antigen-specific activated $CD4^+$ lymphocytes. To date, three uveitogenic proteins from the photoreceptor cell layer have been identified and characterized: the retinal soluble antigen (S-Ag), the interphotoreceptor retinoid-binding protein (IRBP), and rhodopsin. The diseases induced by different uveitogenic proteins appear to share essential characteristics, such as similar pathology and cellular mechanisms. Characteristic histopathological features of EAU include serous retinal detachment, inflammatory cell infiltration of the vitreous cavity, retina, and choroid,

Autoimmunity: Physiology and Disease, Pages 377–405
Published 1994 Wiley-Liss, Inc.

vasculitis, granuloma formation, and photoreceptor damage of varying intensity. Although frequently accompanied by anterior segment infiltration, tissue damage occurs mainly in the posterior segment. A typical adjunct to EAU is inflammation of the pineal gland ("third eye"), which shares tissue-specific antigens with the retina [Gery et al., 1986], but no other organs appear to be affected.

Studies of cellular mechanisms, in which uveitogenic T-helper (Th) cell lines have played an important role, indicate that pivotal to EAU expression is a delayed-type hypersensitivity response mediated by retinal antigen-specific Th-1-like lymphocytes. It is believed that pathogenesis is initiated by the migration of these uveitogenic Th cells to the eye, where they elicit an inflammatory amplification cascade involving lymphokine production, mast cell degranulation, induction of class II and adhesion molecules on ocular vasculature, and recruitment of nonantigen-specific leukocytes that serve as the final mediators of tissue damage [for review, see Caspi, 1989] (Fig. 1). The importance of antibodies in the pathogenesis of EAU appears to be secondary, because although high titers of antibodies are elicited in animals immunized for EAU induction, typical EAU pathology is induced by adoptive transfer of uveitogenic T-lymphocyte lines without elicitation of detectable serum antibodies [Caspi et al., 1986]. Thus EAU can be classified as a cell-mediated, organ-specific autoimmune disease, similarly to experimental allergic encephalomyelitis and adjuvant arthritis.

TOLERANCE TO OCULAR ANTIGENS: CENTRAL, PERIPHERAL, OR NONE?

The issues surrounding the induction and maintenance, or the breakdown, of a state of tolerance to ocular antigens are colored by the special status of the eye in relation to the immune system. It has long been known that the eye is an "immunologically privileged" organ in that histoincompatible grafts

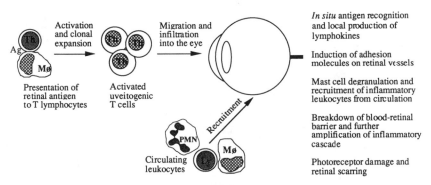

FIGURE 1. Cellular mechanisms in EAU.

placed inside the eye are not rejected in the same fashion as they would be at other sites of the body [Barker and Billingham, 1977]. Historically, the immune privilege phenomenon was explained on the basis of sequestration of antigens: The interior of the eye has no lymphatic drainage and is separated from the immune system by a blood–retinal barrier that restricts free passage of cells and even of proteins into and out of the eye [Bill, 1975; Barker and Billingham, 1977]. Because the eye becomes a closed organ early in fetal development, it was thought that lack of autoaggression against ocular antigens is due to the fact that the immune system never became "aware" of them. Therefore, exposure of the immune system to ocular antigens following a breach of the blood–ocular barrier would result in autoimmunization and termination of the tolerant state. This notion derived its support from a clinical entity that is known as sympathetic ophthalmia, in which a penetrating injury to one eye is followed within weeks or months by a destructive inflammation in the contralateral, uninjured eye.

In light of current knowledge about the role of thymic repertoire selection and postthymic mechanisms in the development of self-tolerance, we would rephrase these concepts to mean a lack of "true" tolerance to ocular antigens. Due to lack of representation of these organ-specific antigens in the thymus, and their early sequestration behind the blood–ocular barrier during ontogeny, T cells reactive to ocular antigens would not be subject to clonal deletion or inactivation. Indeed, lymphocytes reactive to retinal antigens are present in the peripheral blood of healthy individuals, with a clonal frequency of about $1/5 \times 10^6$, and become considerably more numerous in uveitis patients, as detected by in vitro proliferation assays [Hirose et al., 1988a,b; de Smet et al., 1990].

However, it must be pointed out that the pineal gland, which shares antigenic components with the retina [Gery et al., 1986], has no blood–organ barrier and is therefore accessible to the immune system. Moreover, it is now clear that antigens placed in the eye manage to reach the circulation and are recognized by the immune system, although the response evoked is a deviant one (discussed further below) [Streilein, 1987]. Recently, an argument in favor of a role for thymic deletion in the development of tolerance to ocular antigens was provided by Ichikawa et al. [1991], who reported spontaneous induction of uveitis in athymic (nude) mice grafted at 4 weeks of age with embryonic rat thymus. The uveitis could be adoptively tranferred into syngeneic nude mice with CD4$^+$ splenocytes. On the basis of similarities between this model and the one described by Smith et al. [1989], in which T cells that would normally be deleted are shown to persist in neonatally thymectomized mice, the authors propose that the xenogeneic thymus fails to eliminate autoreactive T-cell clones that would be deleted in normal individuals. On the other hand, these data could also be interpreted to suggest a lack of positive selection of T-suppressor cells rather than lack of a negative selection of autoreactive T cells. The finding mentioned above, that lymphocytes reactive to retinal antigens are readily and consistently detectable in healthy individuals, suggests that at least some autoreactive clones escape deletion. That ocular autoimmunity is an exception, rather than the rule, suggests that postthymic mechanisms must exist to prevent their activation. The nature of these mechanisms, i.e., peripheral inactivation, active suppression, lack of antigen recognition (possibly due to lack of coexpression with class II molecules on the same cell), or some combination of the above, continues to be the subject of active investigation.

In the following paragraphs we explore the experimental evidence that might provide clues as to the nature of the mechanisms that play a role in maintaining the homeostasis of ocular tolerance. We next examine immunotherapeutic manipulations in experimental models designed to reinforce such mechanisms and restore immunological balance, with the purpose of overcoming ocular autoimmunity. In the final section, we attempt to draw parallels between the animal models and uveitic diseases in humans and describe the efforts to incorporate into clinical medicine those lessons that have been learned through immunomanipulation of the experimental disease.

NATURAL MECHANISMS THAT MIGHT MAINTAIN OCULAR NONAGGRESSION

Systemic: Immune Privilege, ACAID, and Suppressor T cells

In recent years, the immune privilege phenomenon was shown to consist not of the immune system remaining "blind" to antigens placed within the eye, but rather to be an aberrant form of immunity, characterized by a depressed delayed-type hypersensitivity (DTH) response, together with an intact cytotoxic cell response and a skewing of the humoral response toward production of noncomplement binding immunoglobulins. The depressed cell-mediated immunity was found to be due to induction of antigen-specific suppressor cells, several populations of which were identified in different experimental systems [Streilein, 1987]. Because this deviant immune response was traditionally elicited by introduction of antigen through the anterior chamber of the eye, it was dubbed ACAID (anterior chamber associated immune deviation). However, immune privilege is also afforded to antigens introduced through the posterior portion of the eye [Streilein, 1987] and under some conditions even to histoincompatible retinal transplants [Jiang and Streilein, 1990].

ACAID is consistently inducible to a variety of cell-bound, as well as soluble, antigens placed in the eye, such as histocompatibility and tumor-specific antigens, cell-conjugated haptens, and bovine serum albumin. The mechanism of induction of this phenomenon was found to require an intact oculosplenic axis, with a tolerogenic signal leaving the eye and inducing antigen-specific suppressor cells in the spleen. The nature of the tolerogenic signal is still controversial. Wilbanks and Streilein [1991] were able to demonstrate the presence of a blood–borne signal associated with cells that were subsequently identified as F4/80$^+$ macrophages, a resident population in the anterior uvea. In contrast, Ferguson et al. [1989] demonstrated a soluble signal transferable with serum that could be removed by monoclonal antisuppressor factor antibodies. This apparent contradiction may stem from the fact that the former group has used the soluble antigen BSA, whereas the latter group used hapten-modified self (TNP-coupled splenocytes), and may suggest that the phenomenon of ACAID can be induced through more than one pathway. Notwithstanding the nature of the tolerogenic signal, afferent- as well as efferent-acting antigen-specific suppressor cells are elicited in the spleen and can adoptively transfer suppression of DTH to naive recipients.

It is therefore tempting to hypothesize that an ACAID-like suppression phenomenon could be implicated in systemic tolerance to ocular antigens. Support for this hypothesis was provided by experiments showing that induction of ACAID to S-Ag or to IRBP could prevent EAU in rats and mice, respectively [Mizuno et al., 1989; Hara et al., 1992b]. Spleens of mice in which ACAID to IRBP has been induced contain T lymphocytes that can adoptively transfer protection from EAU [Hara et al., 1992b]. Furthermore, long-term T-suppressor cell lines can be derived from spleens of rats inoculated with S-Ag into the anterior chamber of the eye. Such a line was able to suppress proliferation of uveitogenic T-cell lines in vitro and protected against EAU induction in vivo [Caspi et al., 1988]. These findings argue in favor of a role for suppressor T cells in maintaining a state of tolerance to ocular antigens. Although suppressor T cells specific to ocular antigens have not been identified in unmanipulated animals or in humans, and infusion of normal spleen cells is unable to prevent EAU, such suppressor cells may exist in precursor form, to be activated upon exposure to antigens released from the eye, or in numbers too low to be detected by conventional assays.

Local: Blood–Retinal Barrier and Suppression by Ocular Resident Cells and Intraocular Fluids

Although the eye has a very rich supply of blood through an intricate network of retinal and uveal blood vessels, the inside of the eye is separated from the circulation by a blood–ocular barrier [Bill, 1975]. Early in development, tight junctions form between adjacent cells comprising the layer of retinal pigment epithelium and between the endothelial cells of blood vessels in the retina and the iris/ciliary body, effectively restricting leakage even of substances as small as sucrose and sodium fluorescein. The blood–ocular barrier has always been considered to constitute the first line of defense against intraocular inflammation, and a breakdown of this barrier (measurable as leakage from blood vessels by fluorescein angiography, or by presence of increased amounts of protein in intraocular fluids) is regarded as diagnostic of a disease process [Nussenblatt and Palestine, 1989].

Data obtained in the rat EAU model show that an "artificial" breach of the blood–retinal barrier, by cryopexy, promotes induction of uveitis [de Bara et al., 1989], and the "natural" breakdown of the barrier during uveitis facilitates massive recruitment of specific and nonspecific lymphocytes from the circulation [Lightman et al., 1987]. Mast cell degranulation in the posterior and anterior portions of the eye has been observed early in the process of EAU, before measurable infiltration of the ocular tissues occurs, and is assumed to contribute to the process of breakdown of the blood–ocular barrier [de Kozak et al., 1981; Li et al., 1992]. This assumption is supported by data showing that administration of mast cell inhibitors suppresses EAU [de Kozak et al., 1983]. Also in line with this notion is the observed association between the number of mast cells in ocular tissues of rodents and their susceptibility to EAU: Choroid and anterior uvea of susceptible rat strains are rich in mast cells, whereas resistant strains have a paucity of ocular mast cells [Mochizuki et al., 1984; Li et al., 1992]. Similarly, mast-cell-deficient mutant mice Sl/Sld and W/Wv are less susceptible to EAU than their wild-type counterparts [Bahmanyar et al., 1991].

However, even when the blood–ocular barrier is breached, the eye is not necessarily rendered defenseless against inflammation. In 1987, we showed that retinal glial Müller cells act as potent suppressor cells, capable of inhibiting antigen-driven as well as interleukin (IL)-2-dependent proliferation of uveitogenic Th cells, and we suggested that this function may be involved in preserving the integrity of ocular structure during inflammatory episodes [Caspi et al., 1987]. Subsequently, many other ocular cells were shown to possess a similar capability. In the anterior chamber, ciliary body epithelial cells [Helbig et al., 1990], iris/ciliary body parenchymal cells [Streilein and Bradley, 1991], corneal fibroblasts [Donnelly et al., 1989], and corneal endothelial cells [Kawashima et al., 1992] were reported to have lymphocyte-inhibitory properties. In the posterior part of the eye choroid preparations were similarly suppressive [Hooper et al., 1991]. Different mechanisms are used by these cell types to accomplish immunosuppression: Müller cells and corneal endothelial cells inhibit by contact, iris/ciliary body parenchymal cells and choroidal cells suppress by means of soluble factors, whereas ciliary body epithelial cells suppress by means of both soluble mediators and direct contact. The multiple cell types and diverse means of exerting suppression within the eye are strongly suggestive of the importance of this phenomenon for maintaining ocular integrity.

The precise molecular nature of the membrane-bound suppressive molecule(s) of Müller cells, corneal endothelial cells, or the ciliary body epithelium has not been elucidated, other than that it may be a protein removable by trypsinization [Roberge et al., 1988; Helbig et al., 1990]. However, all have been found to share remarkable functional similarities [Caspi et al., 1987; Helbig et al., 1990; Kawashima et al., 1992]. Suppression of proliferation affects normal lymphocytes irrespective of antigenic specificity, but not malignantly transformed lymphoid cells. The suppression does not involve a cytotoxic effect and does not result in the suppressed cells becoming anergic to subsequent antigenic stimulation. In the case of Müller cells and ciliary body epithelial cells (not reported for corneal endothelial cells), removal of the suppressive molecule by trypsin unmasks an antigen-presenting ability, provided that MHC class II molecules were previously induced by incubation with interferon (IFN)-γ [Roberge et al., 1988; Helbig et al., 1990]. In contrast, the suppressive function is MHC class II independent and can cross allogeneic and even xenogeneic barriers, suggesting an evolutionarily conserved mechanism [Caspi and Roberge, 1989; Helbig et al., 1990].

Cells that inhibit by contact are strategically positioned in areas through which blood–borne lymphocytes must pass in order to inifiltrate the eye [Caspi et al., 1987; Helbig et al., 1990]. In the posterior part of the eye, Müller cells ensheathe the retinal blood vessels. In the anterior part of the eye, ciliary body epithelial cells form a layer covering the richly vascularized ciliary body processes. These cells with their lymphocyte-inhibitory effects could therefore be considered as a second line of defense after the blood–ocular barrier. During immunogenic inflammation, Müller cells and ciliary body epithelial cells express adhesion and MHC class II molecules [Kim et al., 1987; Okumura et al., 1990; Helbig et al., 1991; DeBarge et al., 1992]. Interestingly, class II–positive Müller cells were more efficient than class II–negative Müller cells in suppressing the IL-2–dependent proliferation of uveitogenic Th cells, provided that the specific antigen was present [Caspi and Roberge, 1989]. The enhancement in suppression was accompanied by increased Müller–Th aggregation, and both were largely reversible with anti-class II antibodies. This phenomenon has been suggested to represent a "fly trap" effect: The Th cells bind to antigen (presented in the context of class II) on the surface of Müller cells, whereupon they come in contact with the inhibitory molecule. However, it must be pointed out that there are distinct "holes" in the protection the Müller cells might afford against uveitogenic T cells. Although proliferation, IL-2 production, and high affinity IL-2 receptor expression by T lymphocytes are strongly suppressed, inhibition of IL-3 production is marginal, and there is no inhibition of IFN-γ production [Caspi and Roberge, 1989]. Nevertheless, an in vivo role for the Müller cells in protection against EAU is suggested by the observation that selective "poisoning" of the Müller cells in the naturally resistant Wistar-Furth strain of rats, by intravitreal injection of the gliotoxic agent L-alpha amino adipic acid, doubles the incidence of EAU in the injected eyes [Chan et al., 1991].

The third line of defense against lymphocytes that have successfully penetrated the blood–ocular barrier and the barrier of Müller cells or ciliary body epithelial cells is provided by the immunosuppressive environment of the intraocular fluids. Both the aqueous and the vitreous humors contain soluble factors that suppress lymphocyte activation and proliferation [Koker et al., 1985; Kaiser et al., 1989; Cousins et al., 1991; Yoshitoshi and Shichi, 1991]. The suppressive properties of intraocular fluids can, at least in part, be attributed to the factors produced by the ocular cells lining those cavities [Streilein and Bradley, 1991]. Characterization of the lymphocyte-inhibitory activity of intraocular fluids and of supernatants from cultures of resident ocular cells revealed a number of distinct low to medium molecular weight suppressor factors [Helbig et al., 1990; Hooper et al., 1991; Streilein and Bradley, 1991; Yoshitoshi and Shichi, 1991; Kawashima et al., 1992]. Two of these factors were identified as prostaglandin and transforming growth factor (TGF)-β. However, additional mediators are present, because only partial or no reversal of suppression (depending on the experimental system) could be achieved with indomethacin or with monoclonal antibodies to TGF-β [Helbig et al., 1990; Cousins et al., 1991; Hooper et al., 1991; Streilein and Bradley, 1991; Yoshitoshi and Shichi, 1991].

The primary role of TGF-β in the ocular microenvironment might in fact lie not in direct inhibition of infiltrating lymphocytes, but in promoting ACAID. Studies in the mouse revealed that in the presence of supernatant from cultured iris/ciliary body cells, or aqueous humor (or fluids from other immune privileged sites), the antigen-presenting function of F4/80$^+$ macrophages is altered toward activation of suppressor, rather than helper, T cells [Wilbanks and Streilein, 1992; Wilbanks et al., 1992]. The soluble factor responsible for this functional alteration was identified as TGF-β. Adoptive transfer of as few as 20 such supernatent-treated, BSA-pulsed macrophages was able to induce ACAID to BSA in mice, and supernatant-treated macrophages pulsed with IRBP were able to prevent the induction of EAU [Hara et al., 1992a]. Thus the *local* microenvironment of the eye appears to be involved in triggering what may be a pathway toward induction of *systemic* tolerance to ocular antigens, closing the regulatory circle.

THERAPEUTIC INTERVENTION IN EXPERIMENTAL OCULAR AUTOIMMUNITY: A TREND TOWARD INCREASINGLY SPECIFIC THERAPIES

In the past, pharmacological therapy of immunologically mediated eye diseases consisted primarily of broad spectrum immunosuppressive agents, such as cytotoxic compounds and steroids [Nussenblatt and Palestine, 1989]. As we learn more about the mechanisms involved in ocular autoimmunity in animal models, attempts are being made to target specific stages in the cascade of events that leads to expression of disease (Fig. 2). Without question, a clinically useful immunotherapeutic regimen must be able to target the efferent, or effector, arm of the autopathogenic response, since the patient arrives at the clinic already ill. However, regimens that target the afferent, or induction, stage are not to be dismissed and may be useful as adjuncts, since activation of additional T-cell clonotypes may continuously be occurring during the disease process. These could represent recent thymic emigrants or secondary mobilization of lymphocytes capable of responding to various autoantigens that are released from the damaged tissue. Ideally, immunotherapy should not only selectively target the autopathogenic cells while leaving

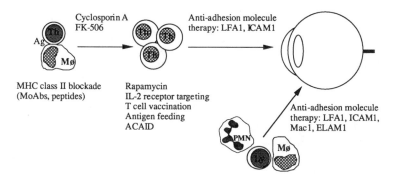

FIGURE 2. Immunological approaches to EAU therapy.

alone other components of the immune system, but should also reinforce the natural regulatory mechanisms with the purpose of ultimately "working itself out of a job." Such is the idea behind the various manipulations designed to enhance the suppressor cell response, to be discussed below.

Direct and Indirect Targeting of Autopathogenic Cells

MHC Class II Blockade. Because activation of uveitogenic lymphocytes begins with recognition of antigen, an early step in the pathogenic process that might be targeted is that of antigen presentation. In addition, local antigen presentation in the eye, by infiltrating macrophages and local cells such as retinal pigment epithelium that aberrantly express class II molecules, might also be involved in the perpetuation of the disease process [Chan et al., 1986b; Percopo et al., 1990]. Wetzig et al. [1988] have shown that treatment of S-Ag immunized Lewis rats with a monoclonal antibody to MHC class II molecules results in downregulation of EAU. Another approach to blocking antigen presentation, by using peptides with high affinity to MHC class II as competitive inhibitors of antigen binding, is currently being explored with promising results [Kozhich et al., 1992].

T Cell-Targeting Macrolides: CsA, FK506, Rapamycin. The fungal macrolide antibiotics cyclosporin A (CsA) and its close relative FK506 are agents that primarily target T lymphocytes [Schreiber and Crabtree, 1992]. They suppress an early stage in T-cell activation, involving the transcription of lymphokine genes and other early genes. Both agents protect against induction of EAU in the Lewis rat model as well as in primates [Nussenblatt et al., 1981b; Mochizuki and Kawashima, 1990; Fujino et al., 1991]. Not unexpectedly, suppression is more dramatic when treatment is started during the afferent stage of the disease [Nussenblatt et al., 1981b]. However, both CsA and FK506 are also able to suppress disease when administered after immuni-

zation, although a higher dose is required. Because of their effect on lymphokine production, CsA and FK506 would be expected to interfere not only
with activation of T cells but also with the process of lymphokine-dependent
recruitment of nonspecific effector leukocytes, which serve as the final mediators of tissue damage in EAU.

The downside of CsA, as well as of FK506, is the systemic toxicity
encountered at therapeutically effective doses [Palestine et al., 1986; Fujino
et al., 1991]. This is particularly problematic in view of the need for chronic
treatment in order to keep uveitis under control, as both these drugs have
only cytostatic effects. Furthermore, evidence obtained in experiments with
a uveitogenic T-cell line indicates that functional triggering of pathogenic
lymphocytes may occur even in the presence of cyclosporin, to be expressed
as soon as the drug is withdrawn [Caspi et al., 1988b]. Although some studies
suggest that antigen-specific suppressor cells may be generated under cover
of CsA or FK506 treatment [Fujino et al., 1988; Kawashima et al., 1990],
more often the disease recurs, and may even rebound, when medication is
reduced or discontinued [Nussenblatt et al., 1982b; Fite et al., 1986; Palestine
et al., 1986; Pasternak et al., 1987; Sai et al., 1988].

A new entrant into the arena of anti-T-cell drugs is another macrolide
antibiotic, rapamycin, which has recently been reported to be highly effective
against EAU [Roberge et al., 1993]. Despite stuctural similarity to FK506 and
CsA, rapamycin targets a later stge of the T-cell activation process, that of
response to IL-2 and to other cytokines [Thomson, 1991]. This difference in
the T-cell activation stage affected by rapamycin in comparison with the
other macrolides, and in comparison with steroids (still today the therapy of
choice for clinical uveitis), can be exploited to design combination therapies
whose purpose is to use lower doses of each drug in order to minimize
systemic toxicity while maintaining optimal levels of therapeutic efficacy
[Roberge et al., 1993; Rubin et al., 1992]. However, none of these drugs
specifically targets the autopathogenic T-cell population.

IL-2R Targeting. The concept of anti-IL-2 receptor (IL-2R) therapy goes
one step further than fungal macrolides toward interrupting the autoimmune
process. Although the targeted population is still the same, i.e., all activated
T lymphocytes, it opens the possibility of permanently eliminating the targeted cells. This can be done through the use of anti-IL-2R antibodies or
through the use of toxins coupled to antibodies or to IL-2. Potential limitations of such therapy (lack of complement binding by antibody, high immunogenicity or toxicity of treatment agent and so forth) can be overcome by
genetic engineering strategies [Waldmann et al., 1992]. Two types of anti-
IL-2R therapy were tested in the Lewis rat EAU model. Roberge et al. [1989]
used the recombinant chimeric toxin IL2-PE40, constructed of the IL-2
moelcule joined to pseudomonas exotoxin that had been stripped of its cell
binding domain. The treatment was able to suppress EAU induced by active
immunization with S-Ag when initiated 7–10 days after immunization, a time

considered to represent the efferent stage of the response. The data indicated that pathogenic lymphocytes were indeed eliminated by the treatment. Higuchi et al. [1991] used the anti-IL-2R monoclonal antibody ART18 to treat efferent stage EAU successfully, as represented by the adoptive transfer of a uveitogenic T-cell line. The therapy was particularly effective when combined with a subtherapeutic dose of CsA. Although the ART18 is not a complement binding antibody, a reduction of the number of uveitogenic lymphocytes in the spleen of treated recipients was apparent. Additional studies are needed to address the question whether long-term remission of disease can result from anti-IL2R treatment.

Adhesion Molecule Blockade. The immunopathology of uveitis is highly dependent on recruitment of inflammatory cells from the circulation, a process that appears to be precipitated by only a few uveitogenic lymphocytes that have gained initial access to the eye [Caspi, 1989; Caspi et al., 1993]. Adhesion molecules are induced early in the process of EAU on the ocular vasculature and on various resident cells in the eye [DeBarge et al., 1992] and are believed to play an important role in the resulting inflammatory amplification cascade. Recent work in our laboratory has explored the utility of adhesion molecule blockade by monoclonal antibodies as a therapeutic approach, using the mouse EAU model. Administration of anti-ICAM-1 or anti-LFA-1 antibodies to IRBP-immunized mice was able to afford measurable protection against development of EAU [Whitcup et al., 1993]. Experiments are currently in progress to assess the efficacy of antiadhesion molecule treatment on suppression of preexisting disease.

Cytokine Network Perturbation. IFN-γ has profound proinflammatory effects when present locally in the eye, an effect that has been attributed to its macrophage-activating properties and induction of MHC class II antigens in the tissue [Hamel et al., 1990]. However, systemic effects of this lymphokine appear to be the opposite from its local effects. We have recently reported that expression of EAU in B10.A mice is exacerbated by systemic depletion of IFN-γ through treatment with a monoclonal anti-IFN-γ antibody [Caspi et al., 1991]. Conversely, augmentation of systemic levels of IFN-γ, through administration of the recombinant cytokine, had an ameliorating effect on disease, despite widespread induction of class II antigens on the ocular tissues (Caspi et al., submitted). It therefore appears that, in contrast to locally produced IFN-γ, systemic IFN-γ acts to downregulate EAU in the mouse. The mechanism of this protection is currently unknown and could include direct and indirect effects on the inflammatory cascade. One cause might be the inhibitory effect of IFN-γ on chemotaxis and migration of macrophages, which normally would serve to retain these cells at the site of inflammation [Wahl et al., 1991]. However, premature exposure of macrophages to IFN-γ while still in the circulation could inhibit their homing toward the eye. In addition, IFN-γ was reported to act as a differentiation factor for suppressor T lymphocytes and for natural suppressor cells [el Masry et al., 1987; Holda et al., 1988].

Therapies Aimed at Restoring Natural Control Mechanisms

Although there is a paucity of data that would implicate surveillance by T-suppressor cells in preventing a first episode of autoimmunization to ocular antigens, experimental evidence suggests that T-suppressor cells do make an appearance after uveitis is induced. In the Lewis rat EAU model, there is an increase with time in the relative number of CD8$^+$ T cells in the eye and a corresponding decrease of CD4$^+$ T cells [Chan et al., 1985b]. This has been interpreted as a reflection of a suppressor cell response. Indeed, treatment of S-Ag–immunized rats with a monoclonal anti-CD8 antibody has the effect of upregulating EAU expression (Higuchi and Caspi, unpublished). Finally, the presence of specific suppressor cells in uveitic rats treated with CsA at doses reported to spare suppressor cells [Hess et al., 1986] can be demonstrated in vitro, as well as in vivo, by adoptive transfer of EAU resistance to untreated animals (Fujino et al., 1988). On the premise that T-suppressor cells do indeed have a role in controlling ocular autoimmunity, various strategies have been explored that attempt to reinforce the suppressor arm of the immune response.

Idiotypic Network Manipulation. Idiotypic networks, in which each idiotype in its turn elicits an anti-idiotypic response, have been proposed to constitute a major mechanism controlling normal immune and pathological autoimmune responses [Jerne, 1984; Rossi et al., 1989]. Evidence for idiotypic regulation of retinal autoimmunity has been presented by de Kozak et al. based on the ability of preimmunization with monoclonal antibodies (id) directed against a particular epitope of S-Ag to suppress induction of S-Ag–induced EAU in guinea pigs and rats [de Kozak and Mirshahi, 1990]. A similar effect could also be elicited by preimmunization with polyclonal anti-id [de Kozak, 1990]. Protection from EAU could be adoptively transferred with lymphocytes of antibody-pretreated donors, but not with the immunoglobulin fraction of their sera [de Kozak et al., 1989]. In addition, lymph node cells from antibody-immunized donor were able to suppress the proliferation of S-Ag–primed lymphocytes in vitro. The suppression therefore appears to be mediated by anti-idiotypic suppressor cells rather than directly by anti-id antibodies. The idiotypic relationship between the putative suppressor cells and uveitogenic Th cells is unclear: The target epitope of the antibody used to elicit anti-id immunity is not a pathogenic one (and is actually located at the opposite end of the S-Ag molecule from the currently known major pathogenic epitopes). Moreover, coinjection of the lymphocytes together with the Ig serum fraction from id-immunized donors actually enhanced EAU in the recipients. Nevertheless, the suppression of disease obtained by successful manipulation of the idiotypic network is quite dramatic and merits further investigation.

T-Cell Vaccination, TCR Peptide Vaccination. Another approach toward elicitation of an antiidiotypic suppressor response has been to immunize directly with the uveitogenic T cells, using a method that has previously been successfully employed in the experimental autoimmune encephalomyelitis (EAE) model [Lider et al., 1988]. Injection of subpathogenic doses of Th-line cells specific to the major pathogenic epitope of IRBP was able to protect rats partially from a subsequent challenge with a uveitogenic dose of the same cells [Beraud et al., 1992]. We were able to show induction of proliferative responses against idiotypic and ergotypic (activation) specificities of the injected Th cells in the vaccinated rats, that presumably represented the suppressor cells responsible for downregulating the disease. Because adoptive transfer of uveitogenic T cells is considered to represent efferent-stage disease, this type of idiotypic network manipulation could have practical clinical implications. However, it is of note that the identical regimen of vaccination had been much more successful in inducing protection from EAE than it was in the case of EAU. This might be due to a more central role for recruited nonantigen-specific cells in the pathogenesis of EAU as compared with EAE [Lightman et al., 1987; Sedgwick et al., 1987; Kim et al., 1988], permitting such cells to escape the anti-idiotypic regulation.

Vaccination against T-cell receptor (TCR) epitopes of the Vb8.2 subfamily, which had been implicated as a pathogenic T-cell clonotype in EAU as well as in EAE [Egwuagu et al., 1991; Gregerson et al., 1991; Merryman et al., 1991], was minimally effective in protecting from S-Ag–induced EAU and was ineffective in protecting from, or was even stimulatory, in IRBP-induced EAU and EAE [Kawano et al., 1991]. This was true for treatment instituted either before or 7–11 days after the immunization. These results are at variance with the data obtained earlier by another group, who were able to suppress both afferent- and efferent-stage EAE by using the identical TCR peptide [Burns et al., 1989; Vandenbark et al., 1989]. This variability in the outcome of the same vaccination protocol in different laboratories and in similar, but distinct, models of autoimmunity underscores the caution that must be used when attempting to manipulate delicately balanced immunological systems.

Induction of ACAID to Retinal Antigens. The important finding that ACAID can be induced by antigen-pulsed macrophages incubated in vitro with TGF-β or TGF-β–containing biological fluids [Wilbanks and Streilein, 1992; Wilbanks et al. 1992], has opened the possibility to exploit this phenomenon for immunotherapy of ocular autoimmunity. We have recently demonstrated in the mouse EAU model that such an approach is indeed feasible. Mice that had received an infusion of splenic macrophages, pulsed with IRBP in the presence of supernatants from cultured iris/ciliary body cells, were significantly protected from subsequent induction of EAU [Hara et al., 1992a]. Because infusion of ACAID-induced suppressor cells can inhibit the efferent stage of EAU induction and can even abort ongoing disease [Hara et al., 1992b], the therapeutic potential of this form of experimental immunotherapy is obvious. Finally, it is of practical implications that ACAID-inducing cells can be generated from peripheral blood monocytes and that the ability of biological fluids to confer ACAID-inducing potential on macrophages is not genetically restricted, i.e., allogeneic and xenogeneic supernatants or TGF-β can be used [Wilbanks and Streilein, 1991, 1992; Wilbanks et al., 1992].

Oral Administration of Antigen. Presentation of antigens through the gut has been shown in a variety of systems to result in the induction of active antigen-specific suppression, mediated by afferent as well as efferent CD8[+] T cells, that effectively inhibits both primary and established immune responses [Silverman et al., 1983; Gautam and Battisto, 1985; Lamont et al., 1988]. The utility of this form of immunomanipulation in the therapy of autoimmunity has initially been shown in the rat EAE model, in which feeding with myelin basic protein (MBP) either before or after immunization suppressed development of disease [Higgins and Weiner, 1988]. Spleens and mesenteric lymph nodes of orally tolerized animals contained antigen-specific CD8[+]T cells, which could transfer protection to unfed recipients, as well as inhibit in vitro proliferative responses to MBP.

Using a similar protocol, we were able to achieve effective suppression of EAU induction in Lewis rats by oral administration of S-Ag [Nussenblatt et al., 1990]. The S-Ag–fed animals, but not the BSA-fed animals, were protected from development of EAU after a subsequent challenge with a uveitogenic regimen of immunization with S-Ag. Furthermore, spleens from S-Ag–fed animals contained antigen-specific suppressive activity, attributable to CD8[+] cells, that could inhibit in vitro proliferation of an S-Ag–specific T-cell line. Significant protection from EAU could also be achieved if feeding was started during the efferent stage of disease induction, 7 days after immunization [Thurau et al., 1991a]. It is interesting to note that suppression to the whole molecule may be achieved by feeding a synthetic peptide containing the dominant pathogenic epitope, but not by feeding subdominant pathogenic eiptopes [Nussenblatt et al., 1990; Thurau et al., 1991b]. In this respect, suppression appears to follow the same hierarchy of immunodominance as uveitogenicity, suggesting involvement of the same epitope in both responses.

The mediator of suppression in orally induced tolerance has recently been shown to be TGF-β, an antigen-nonspecific factor secreted by antigen-specific suppressor T cells [Miller et al., 1992]. The role of TGF-β in oral tolerance, taken together with its demonstrated involvement in induction of the ACAID phenomenon, is suggestive of the importance of this factor in the regulation of tolerance to ocular antigens. In this context, it is perhaps significant that a soluble, antigen-nonspecific factor (TGF-β?) was found to be secreted by a long-term T-suppressor lymphocyte line that inhibits EAU in rats, a line that was selected from the spleen of an animal that had received anterior chamber immunization with retinal S-Ag [Caspi et al., 1988].

As we learn more about the mechanisms involved in the regulation of tolerance and immunity to ocular antigens, the various manipulations described above might converge to provide a basis for a rational regimen of immunotherapy, to restore and to stabilize the natural balance between immunity and suppression. It is perhaps somewhat revealing to observe how many of the strategies described above have been aimed at inducing suppressor cell responses. For a discipline that in recent years has been given to questioning the significance, and even the existence, of suppressor T cells [Möller, 1988; Möller et al., 1990], we certainly appear to be exerting an inordinate amount of effort in designing strategies to reinforce their function.

CLINICAL EXPERIENCE

Human Uveitides of a Putative Autoimmune Nature

Intraocular inflammatory disease (uveitis) is a clinical problem encountered very frequently by the clinician. *Uveitis* is a generic term and does not indicate where in the eye the inflammation is mainly centered, nor does it indicate what is causing the problem. Therefore the disease may be due to a parasite such as toxoplasmosis with a propensity for retinal tissue, or to cytomegalovirus retinitis as a result of the immunosuppression due to the acquired immunodeficiency syndrome (AIDS). Other disorders were initially thought to mediated by infectious processes, particularly syphilis and tuberculosis [Schlaegel, 1969]. With time such diagnoses have not fully explained the clinical syndromes or their course.

Though the concept of autoimmune-driven ocular disease is a old one, harking back to at least Uhlenhuth [1903] and Elschnig [1910], the hypothesis became firmly entrenched in the clinical mind by the late 1960s and early 1970s. The disease entities usually included under the autoimmune rubric are quite varied and encompass the entities classified as "endogenous uveitis," in which a microbial etiology has not been definitely shown. This would include diseases such as symphathetic ophthalmia, pars planitis, and birdshot retinochoroidopathy, which may have only ocular manifestations, to such entities as the Vogt-Koyanagi-Harada syndrome and Behçet's disease, which have multiple systemic complications [Nussenblatt and Palestine, 1989].

Clinical Appearance and Histology of Human Uveitis and How It Compares With Animal Models

Unlike the brain, whose relationship with the immune system in many ways parallels that of the eye, the inside of the globe is accessible to visual inspection. In this regard, ophthalmology is more fortunate than all other internal medical disciplines, as Nature has provided a "window" through which the entire course of disease can be readily followed and documented. In addition, when medically justified, the retina and other ocular tissues may be biopsied, or occasionally a decision may be reached to enucleate the uveitic eye, making the tissue available for laboratory analysis.

The diagnosis of the various disease entities can be visualized by the ophthalmologist by using a variety of tools in the clinic. The presence of a cellular infiltrate in the eye can be recorded, and standardized methods for these observations have been described over the years [Hogan et al., 1959; Kimura et al., 1959; Nussenblatt et al., 1985b; Hirose et al., 1986]. In addition to the presence of the inflammatory cellular infiltrate, one can observe evidence of the breakdown of the blood–ocular barrier with the presence of an increased amount of protein in the eye. The amount of protein in the eye is normally less than in the serum and reflects the fact that the retinal as well as anterior segment vasculature is usually impermeable; this can change dramatically with disease and hence a large increase in the amount of protein in the eye.

Other sequelae from the inflammation can be seen on clinical examination with the help of ancillary tests such as fluorescein angiography and an electroretinogram. Clinical examination can show marked alterations in the retinal vascular architecture. This can be manifested by occlusion of the vessels and subsequent hemorrhage, as well as by sheathing of the vessels. Fluorescein angiography will show not only the retinal vasculature alterations that are sometimes not overtly obvious to simple observation but will also document the presence of cystoid macular edema, a major cause for the loss of vision in uveitic eyes, and neovascularization coming from the optic disc head, the retinal vessels, or from below the retina itself. The electroretinogram can confirm the profound global effect of the uveitis on retinal functioning, even when the clinical changes noted may appear to be very localized.

Many of the clinical and histological aspects seen in human disease have been observed in animal models. The disorder induced by S-Ag immunization in the Lewis rat is an acute disease involving the whole retina very rapidly. Large retinal detachments, massive leukocyte infiltration of the anterior and posterior parts of the eye, and diffuse photoreceptor destruction are hallmarks of this model. The lesions seen after IRBP immunization in mice tend to be more localized and less fulminant, representing a largely granulomatous disease; anterior chamber involvement is minimal. Murine EAU can be recurrent and can have subretinal neovascularization as its sequel, two important features of human uveitis [Chan et al., 1990]. The model that is perhaps the most strikingly reminiscent of human disease is EAU in the monkey [Faure et al., 1981; Nussenblatt et al., 1981a; Hirose et al., 1986]. The disease in nonhuman primates will often have a concomitant anterior segment inflammation, mimicking that seen in the human condition. The inflammation noted posteriorly also has typical features of human disease, including vitreal haze, sheathing of vessels, retinal infiltrates, hemorrhages, as well as retinal vascular leakage noted on fluorescein angiography. EAU in the monkey is chronic, old lesions healing and new lesions appearing as the disease waxes and wanes, with striking similarity to human uveitis. Although none of the animal models of EAU reproduces the full spectrum of human uveitis, each model offers some unique properties, making it suitable for the study of specific aspects of human ocular inflammatory disease.

Systemic Immune Responses

Humoral Immunity. Before the development of the experimental uveitis model, type III hypersensitivity responses were hypothesized to constitute the primary mechanism of intraocular inflammatory disease [O'Connor, 1983]. Despite the fact that no real evidence was available to support this concept other than the circumstantial one that circulating immune complexes have been found in patients with uveitis, this school of thought still has its followers. Studies in the experimental uveitis model demonstrated that immune complexes developed late in the disease and appeared to be a mechanism by which debris is cleared from the eye [Sakai, 1983]. We have seen no decrease, and sometimes even an increase, in levels of circulating immune complexes in patients with Behçet's disease, whose condition is well controlled on immunosuppressive therapy [Nussenblatt et al., 1985a]. Moreover, lupus erythromatosus patients with high circulating immune complex levels do not tend to develop uveitis. A number of investigators who have studied the levels of antiretinal antibodies in uveitis patients compared with healthy controls have found them to be remarkably similar [Doekes et al., 1987; Forrester et al., 1989; Hylkema and Kujlstra, 1989; Hoekzema et al., 1990]. On this basis, the suggestion has been made that these antibodies in fact represent a natural regulatory phenomenon, possibly of protective value against retinal disease [Hylkema and Kijlstra, 1989]. Taken together with data showing that experimental uveitis can be adoptively transferred by retinal antigen-specific T-cell lines without eliciting detectable serum antibody titers [Caspi et al., 1986], these findings do not support a primary role for humoral immunity in the pathogenesis of either the human or the experimental disease.

Cell-Mediated Responses to Retinal Antigens. Circulating lymphocytes in patients with intermediate and posterior uveitis show proliferative responses to purified retinal antigens, with S-Ag responsiveness first having been demonstrated [Nussenblatt et al., 1980; Matsuo et al., 1986]. The percentage of patients responding to S-Ag varies considerably depending on the disease, with essentially all birdshot retinochoroidopathy patients having circulating lymphocytes that respond [Nussenblatt et al., 1982a], while from 40%–60% of patients with other disorders will have a response [Nussenblatt, 1991].

The immunodominant fragments recognized by uveitis patients appear to be different from the ones that are immunodominant in animals. In the rat uveitis model, a major immunodominant and immunopathogenic epitope, encompassing amino acids 352–364, was reported by Gregerson et al.

[1990]. Another immunopathogenic epitope, 339–352, was reported to lie adjacent to this site [Merryman et al., 1991]. Additional immunopathogenic sites include the M and N fragments [Donoso et al., 1987; Singh et al., 1988a]. It is notable that the M fragment was found to be immunopathogenic in other species as well besides the rat, specifically, the guinea pig and the monkey [Singh et al., 1988b; Hirose et al., 1989]; however, this fragment was poorly recognized by human lymphocytes. Recently, de Smet and coworkers [1990, 1991] examined the responses of uveitis patients and of Lewis rats to overlapping peptides representing the complete human S-Ag molecule. It is clear that patients recognize multiple antigenic epitopes and these epitopes are distinct from the ones that rat lymphocytes appear to recognize.

It remains to be resolved whether responses of patients to retinal proteins are reflective of the etiology of their disease or whether they are a secondary phenomenon of autoimmunization to antigens released from damaged tissue, and what is their actual involvement in immunopathogenesis. Nevertheless, based on the fact that different retinal proteins induce what is essentially the same disease in a number of animal species, it seems reasonable to conclude that the findings in animal models can be generalized to the human.

Local Immunological Aspects

The development of uveitogenic, S-Ag–specific T-cell lines constituted an important step in understanding some of the basic mechanisms leading to experimental uveitis [Caspi et al., 1986]. One of the arguments for a direct role of retinal antigen-specific Th cells in the pathogenesis of uveitis has been the observation that they appear to recognize retinal antigens in situ and to be preferentially retained in the uveitic eye. Moreover, IRBP-specific lines derived from the eyes of mice with EAU are strongly uveitogenic, showing that these cells are not only present in the eye but also are functionally competent (Rizzo and Caspi, in preparation). As has been described above, retinal antigen-specific cells are present in the blood of patients with uveitis, but perhaps more significantly these cells are also found in the eye. S-Ag–specific T-cell clones have been grown from the vitreous fluid of uveitis patients, indicating that potentially autoaggressive cells are localized to the area of presumed activation [Nussenblatt et al., 1984].

In the Lewis rat EAU model, a dynamic change in the infiltrating T-cell subsets occurs as the uveitis progresses from a predominantly $CD4^+$ to a predominantly $CD8^+$ population [Chan et al., 1985b]. This could be confirmed to occur in at least one tragic case of human uveitis, in which both eyes were ultimately obtained. In this case of sympathetic ophthalmia, the eye enucleated early in the disease process had mainly $CD4^+$ cells, whereas the eye enucleated almost a year later was infiltrated with mostly $CD8^+$ cells [Chan et al., 1985a].

Not only the T-cell dynamics, but also the responses of ocular tissues in human uveitis and in animal EAU appear to parallel each other. The expression of cell membrane markers was one of the early events to be seen in experimentally induced uveitis. Class II molecules are similarly expressed on the cell surface of many ocular resident cells in human uveitis, including the retinal pigment epithelium, Müller cells, and vascular endothelial cells [Nussenblatt and Palestine, 1989]. Recently, a similar widespread response has been seen with respect to the expression of adhesion molecules [De-Barge et al., 1992; Whitcup et al., 1992]. The immunosuppressive properties of ocular resident cells that have been described in animal models [Caspi et al., 1987; Helbig et al., 1990; Hooper et al., 1991; Kawashima et al., 1992] appear to hold true also for human ocular tissues. Cloned human ciliary body epithelial cells exhibit potent inhibitory effects against uveitogenic rat T-cell lines, and human corneal fibroblasts were reported to suppress mixed lymphocyte reactions [Donnelly et al., 1989; Helbig et al., 1990]. In human eyes stained with Müller cell-specific antibodies, the Müller cells appear to be resistant to the inflammatory cell attack. They survive and even proliferate, forming gliotic scars, while the surrounding retina may be markedly atrophic as a result of the inflammation [Yanoff et al., 1971; Nork et al., 1986; Chan et al., 1986a]. Gliosis is also a typical sequel of EAU in animal models [Rao et al., 1986]. These observations appear to be in line with the in vitro studies in the rat EAU model, showing that Müller cells not only "turn off" activated T lymphocytes but actually thrive on the soluble mediators that they produce [Roberge et al., 1985; Caspi et al., 1987; Caspi and Roberge, 1989].

Therapeutic Strategies in Clinical Uveitis

One of the most important roles that the animal model has played has been that of a template for the development of immunosuppressive strategies for the clinical treatment of uveitis. To date the most common mode of therapy is that of systemic steroids [Nussenblatt and Palestine, 1989]. However, the side effects and the fact that many cases are refractory to steroid therapy are spurring a constant search for newer and better therapeutic modalities. The use of cyclosporine in the clinic stems directly from its successful use in the experimental uveitis model [Nussenblatt et al., 1981b, 1982b]. Cyclosporine has now been used in clinical practice for some time and has been highly successful in treating severe sight-threatening disease, including Behçet's disease [Nussenblatt et al., 1985a; Nussenblatt and Palestine, 1989]. The validation of this approach was thus achieved. Using this logic, FK506, which is also an effective immunosuppressive agent in EAU [Kawashima et al., 1990; Mochizuki and Kawashima, 1990; Fujino et al., 1991], is now being used in clinical trials [Nussenblatt and Palestine, 1989]. Additional medications that have already been successfully tested in the EAU model are currently awaiting controlled clinical trials, including rapamycin and mycophenilate mofetil [Roberge et al., 1993; Rubin et al., 1992; Nussenblatt, unpublished].

Of the immunospecific, nonpharmacological methods of therapy that have been tested in the experimental uveitis model, oral administration of antigen is now being evaluated in clinical trials at the NIH. Enhancement of natural suppressive mechanisms by a treatment that is easily applied and presents no hazard to the patient is an extremely attractive therapeutic approach. However, it must be remembered that although uveitis patients do exhibit immunological responses to S-Ag and to IRBP [Nussenblatt et al., 1980, 1982a; Matsuo et al., 1986; Doekes et al., 1987], the putative eliciting antigens in human uveitis have not yet been identified. Thus the scientific approach of feeding purified retinal proteins, characterized as being uveitogenic in animals, may not be the best approach in a clinical setting. In the long term, the successful application of this therapy will require a better understanding of the retinal antigens and the epitopes being responded to by patients.

Genetic Control of Susceptibility

Strong HLA associations have been observed in many types of human uveitic diseases [Nussenblatt and Palestine, 1989]. Perhaps the most striking association is seen between birdshot retinochoroidopathy and HLA-A29, carrying a relative risk of 50–224 [Nussenblatt et al., 1982a; Baarsma et al., 1990]. As mentioned before, this disease is one that is especially associated with cell-mediated responses to the S-Ag [Nussenblatt et al., 1982a]. In addition, various studies have shown increased frequency of certain types of uveitis in specific ethnic groups or families [Nussenblatt and Palestine, 1989]. Genetic dependence of susceptibility to experimental uveitis is seen in inbred rodents, opening the possibility to study genetic mechanisms affecting predisposition to ocular autoimmunity in genetically well-defined populations, under controlled experimental conditions [for review, see Caspi, 1992]. Studies in the mouse model of EAU have revealed that primary control of susceptibility is defined by MHC genes of the class II (I-A) subregion, implicating recognition of pathogenic epitopes as a major mechanism. In contrast, expression of the class II I-E gene product had an ameliorating influence on disease [Caspi et al., 1992b]. Secondary control of susceptibility appeared to be due to the genetic background, with some backgrounds completely preventing expression of EAU despite the presence of a susceptible MHC haplotype. Non-MHC influences on susceptibility could include such diverse mechanisms as hormonal, mast cell/ vascular, and lymphokine responses, which show genetic variability in susceptible versus nonsusceptible rodent strains [Caspi et al., 1992a]. Further study of the genetic control of EAU in rodent models could help to explain the hereditary factors involved in human uveitis and to identify the individuals at risk for uveitic disease.

CONCLUSIONS

Immunospecific therapy in autoimmune diseases will ultimately be based on understanding how the normal immune system maintains unresponsiveness to self and how this state of self-tolerance is broken. The experimental models that simulate human uveitis have been of enormous importance in helping to understand the basic mechanisms of uveitic disease. The experimental disease is remarkably similar with respect to clinical and immunological parameters to the human intermediate and posterior uveitic entities that require systemic immunotherapy. Successful immunomodulation of the experimental disease has served as a good predictor of clinical success of a given therapeutic modality. Whether the responsiveness of cells from uveitis patients to the currently known uveitogenic proteins is reflective of disease etiology or represents an epiphenomenon is a question that we still cannot answer. This question will probably continue to fuel the debate surrounding the role of autoimmunity in clinical uveitis for some time to come. However, with the experimental autoimmune uveitis model, endogenous uveitis now meets all the criteria for an autoimmune disease as put forward by Milgrom and Witebsky [see Shoenfeld and Isenberg, 1989].

REFERENCES

Baarsma GS, Priem HA, Kijlstra A (1990): Association of birdshot retinochoroidopathy and HLA-A29 antigen. Curr Eye Res 9(Suppl):63–68.

Bahmanyar S, Grubbs BG, Chan CC, Li Q, Wiggert B, Nussenblatt RB, Caspi RR (1991): The role of mast cells in experimental autoimmune uveoretinitis. Invest Ophthalmol Vis Sci 32(Suppl):934.

Barker C, Billingham R (1977): Immunologically privileged sites. Adv Immunol 25:1–54.

Beraud E, Kotake S, Caspi RR, Oddo SM, Chan CC, Gery I, Nussenblatt RB (1992): Control of experimental autoimmune uveoretinitis by low dose T cell vaccination. Cell Immunol 140:112–122.

Bill A (1975): Blood circulation and fluid dynamics in the eye. Physiol Rev 55:383–417.

Burns FR, Li XB, Shen N, Offner H, Chou YK, Vandenbark AA, Heber-Katz E (1989): Both rat and mouse T cell receptors specific for the encephalitogenic determinant of myelin basic protein use similar V alpha and V beta chain genes even though the major histocompatibility complex and encephalitogenic determinants being recognized are different. J Exp Med 169:27–39.

Caspi RR (1989): Basic mechanisms in immune-mediated uveitic disease. In Lightman SL (ed): "Immunology of Eye Disease." Lancaster, England: Kluwer Academic Publishers, pp 61–86.

Caspi RR (1992): Immunogenetic aspects of clinical and experimental uveitis. Reg Immunol 4:321–330.

Caspi RR, Chan C-C, Fujino Y, Oddo S, Najafian F, Bahmanyar S, Heremans H, Wilder RL, Wiggert B (1992a): Genetic factors in susceptibility and resistance to experimental autoimmune uveoretinitis. Curr Eye Res 11(Suppl):81–86.

Caspi RR, Grubbs BG, Chan CC, Chader GJ, Wiggert B (1992b): Genetic control of susceptibility to experimental autoimmune uveoretinitis in the mouse model: Concomitant regulation by MHC and non-MHC genes. J Immunol 148:2384–2389.

Caspi RR, Fujino Y, Najafian F, Grover S, Hansen CB, Wilder RL (1993): Recruitment of antigen-nonspecific cells plays a pivotal role in the pathogenesis of a T cell-mediated organ-specific autoimmune disease, experimental autoimmune uveoretinitis. J Neuroimmunol (in press).

Caspi RR, Kuwabara T, Nussenblatt RB (1988): Characterization of a suppressor cell line which downgrades experimental autoimmune uveoretinitis in the rat. J Immunol 140:2579–2584.

Caspi RR, Parsa C, Chan CC, Grubbs BG, Bahmanyar S, Heremans H, Billiau A, Wiggert B (1991): Neutralization of endogenous interferon-γ exacerbates experimental autoimmune uveoretinitis in the mouse model. Invest Ophthalmol Vis Sci 32(Suppl):790.

Caspi RR, Roberge FG (1989): Glial cells as suppressor cells: characterization of the inhibitory function. J Autoimmun 2:709–722.

Caspi RR, Roberge FG, McAllister CG, el Saied M, Kuwabara T, Gery I, Hanna E, Nussenblatt RB (1986): T cell lines mediating experimental autoimmune uveoretinitis (EAU) in the rat. J Immunol 136:928–933.

Caspi RR, Roberge FG, Nussenblatt RB (1987): Organ-resident, nonlymphoid cells suppress proliferation of autoimmune T-helper lymphocytes. Science 237:1029–1032.

Chan CC, Benezra D, Rodrigues MM, Palestine AG, Hsu SM, Murphree AL, Nussenblatt RB (1985a): Immunohistochemistry and electron microscopy of choroidal infiltrates and Dalen-Fuchs nodules in sympathetic ophthalmia. Ophthalmology 92:580–590.

Chan CC, Caspi RR, Ni M, Leake WC, Wiggert B, Chader GJ, Nussenblatt RB (1990): Pathology of experimental autoimmune uveoretinitis in mice. J Autoimmun 3:247–255.

Chan CC, Fujikawa LS, Rodrigues MM, Stevens GJ, Nussenblatt RB (1986a): Immunohistochemistry and electron microscopy of cyclitic membrane. Report of a case. Arch Ophthalmol 104:1040–1045.

Chan CC, Hooks JJ, Nussenblatt RB, Detrick B (1986b): Expression of Ia antigen on retinal pigment epithelium in experimental autoimmune uveoretinitis. Curr Eye Res 5:325–330.

Chan CC, Mochizuki M, Nussenblatt RB, Palestine AG, McAllister C, Gery I, BenEzra D (1985b): T-lymphocyte subsets in experimental autoimmune uveitis. Clin Immunol Immunopathol 35:103–110.

Chan CC, Roberge FG, Ni M, Zhang W, Nussenblatt RB (1991): Injury of Müller cells increases the incidence of experimental autoimmune uveoretinitis. Clin Immunol Immunopathol 59:201–207.

Cousins SW, McCabe MM, Danielpour D, Streilein JW (1991): Identification of transforming growth factor-beta as an immunosuppressive factor in aqueous humor. Invest Ophthalmol Vis Sci 32:2201–2211.

de Bara R, Kusuda M, Caspers-Velu L, Sanui H, Chan CC, Kuwabara T, Nussenblatt RB, Gery I (1989): Cryopexy enhances experimental autoimmune uveoretinitis (EAU) in rats. Invest Ophthalmol Vis Sci 30:2165–2173.

DeBarge L, Chan C, Caspi RR, Harning R, Nussenblatt R, Whitcup S (1992): Expression of cell adhesion molecules in mice with experimental autoimmune uveitis. Invest Ophthalmol Vis Sci 33(Suppl):796.

de Kozak Y (1990): Regulation of retinal autoimmunity via the idiotypic network. Curr Eye Res 9(Suppl):193–200.

de Kozak Y, Mirshahi M (1990): Experimental autoimmune uveoretinitis: idiotypic regulation and disease suppression. Int Ophthalmol 14:43–56.

de Kozak Y, Mirshahi M, Boucheix C, Faure JP (1989): Modulation of experimental autoimmune uveoretinitis by adoptive transfer of cells from rats immunized with anti-S antigen monoclonal antibody. Reg Immunol 2:311–320.

de Kozak Y, Sainte-Laudy J, Benveniste J, Faure JP (1981): Evidence for immediate hypersensitivity phenomena in experimental autoimmune uveoretinitis. Eur J Immunol 11:612–617.

de Kozak Y, Sakai J, Sainte-Laudy J, Faure JP, Benveniste J (1983): Pharmacological modulation of IgE-dependent mast cell degranulation in experimental autoimmune uveoretinitis. Jpn J Ophthalmol 27:598–608.

de Smet M, Bitar G, Wiggert B, Chader G, Gery I, Nussenblatt R (1991): Immunogenicity and pathogenicity of human S-antigen peptide determinants in the Lewis rat. Invest Ophthalmol Vis Sci 34(Suppl):933.

de Smet MD, Wiggert GJ, Mochizuki CM, Gery I, Nussenblatt RR (1990): Cellular immune responses to fragments of S-antigen in patients with uveitis. In Usui M, Ohno S, Aoki K (eds): "Ocular Immunology Today (Proceedings of the 5th International Symposium on the Immunology and Immunopathology of the Eye)." Amsterdam: Elsevier Science Publishers B.V., pp 285–288.

Doekes G, van der Gaag R, Rothova A, van Kooyk Y, Broersma L, Zaal MJ, Dijkman G, Fortuin ME, Baarsma GS, Kijlstra A (1987): Humoral and cellular immune responsiveness to human S-antigen in uveitis. Curr Eye Res 6:909–919.

Donnelly J, Xi M-S, Rockney J (1989): Inhibition of mixed lymphocyte responses by human corneal fibroblasts. Invest Ophthalmol Vis Sci 30(Suppl):440.

Donoso LA, Merryman CF, Sery TW, Shinohara T, Dietzschold B, Smith A, Kalsow CM (1987): S-antigen: characterization of a pathogenic epitope which mediates experimental autoimmune uveitis and pinealitis in Lewis rats. Curr Eye Res 6:1151–1159.

Egwuagu CE, Chow C, Beraud E, Caspi RR, Mahdi RM, Brezin AP, Nussenblatt RB, Gerry I (1991): T cell receptor beta-chain usage in experimental autoimmune uveoretinitis. J Autoimmun 4:315–324.

el Masry MN, Fox EJ, Rich RR (1987): Sequential effects of prostaglandins and interferon-gamma on differentiation of $CD8^+$ suppressor cells. J Immunol 139:688–694.

Elschnig A (1910): Studien sur sympathischen ophthalmis. Die antigene wirkung des augenpigmentes. Albrecht von Graefe's Arch Ophthalmol 76:509–546.

Faure JP, Phuc LH, Takano S, Sterkers M, Thillaye B, de Kozak Y (1981): [Experimental uveoretinitis induced in monkeys by retinal S antigen. Induction, histopathology.] J Fr Ophtalmol 4:465–472.

Ferguson TA, Hayashi JD, Kaplan HJ (1989): The immune response and the eye. III. Anterior chamber-associated immune deviation can be adoptively transferred by serum. J Immunol 143:821–826.

Fite KV, Pardue S, Bengston L, Hayden D, Smyth JJ (1986): Effects of cyclosporine in spontaneous, posterior uveitis. Curr Eye Res 5:787–796.

Forrester JV, Stott DI, Hercus KM (1989): Naturally occurring antibodies to bovine and human retinal S antigen: A comparison between uveitis patients and healthy volunteers. Br J Ophthalmol 73:155–159.

Fujino Y, Mochizuki M, Chan CC, Raber J, Kotake S, Gery I, Nussenblatt RB (1991): FK506 treatment of S-antigen induced uveitis in primates. Curr Eye Res 10:679–690.

Fujino Y, Okumura A, Nussenblatt RB, Gery I, Mochizuki M (1988): Cyclosporine-induced specific unresponsiveness to retinal soluble antigen in experimental autoimmune uveoretinitis. Clin Immunol Immunopathol 46:234–248.

Gautam SC, Battisto JR (1985): Orally induced tolerance generates an efferently acting suppressor T cell and an acceptor T cell that together down-regulate contact sensitivity. J Immunol 135:2975–2983.

Gery I, Mochizuki M, Nussenblatt RB (1986): Retinal specific antigens and immunopathogenic processes they provoke. Prog Retinal Res 5:75–109.

Gregerson DS, Fling SP, Merryman CF, Zhang XM, Li XB, Heber-Katz E (1991): Conserved T cell receptor V gene usage by uveitogenic T cells. Clin Immunol Immunopathol 58:154–161.

Gregerson DS, Merryman CF, Obritsch WF, Donoso LA (1990): Identification of a potent new pathogenic site in human retinal S-antigen which induces experimental autoimmune uveoretinitis in LEW rats. Cell Immunol 128:209–219.

Hamel CP, Detrick B, Hooks JJ (1990): Evaluation of Ia expression in rat ocular tissues following inoculation with interferon-gamma. Exp Eye Res 50:173–182.

Hara Y, Caspi RR, Wiggert W, Dorf M, Streilein J (1992a): Analysis of an in vitro-generated signal that induces immune deviation similar to that elicited by antigen injected into the anterior chamber of the eye. J Immunol 149:1524–1530.

Hara Y, Caspi RR, Wiggert B, Chan CC, Wilbanks GA, Streilein JW (1992b): Suppression of experimental autoimmune uveitis in mice by induction of anterior chamber-associated immune deviation with interphotoreceptor retinoid-binding protein. J Immunol 148:1685–1692.

Helbig H, Gurley RC, Palestine AG, Nussenblatt RB, Caspi RR (1990): Dual effect of ciliary body cells on T lymphocyte proliferation. Eur J Immunol 20:2457–2463.

Helbig H, Kittredge KL, Coca-Prados M, Nussenblatt RB (1991): [Differential expression of HLA DR, DP and DQ in cultivated, human ciliary body epithelial cells.] Fortschr Ophthalmol 88:295–298.

Hess AD, Colombani PM, Esa AH (1986): Cyclosporine and the immune response: Basic aspects. Crit Rev Immunol 6:123–149.

Higgins PJ, Weiner HL (1988): Suppression of experimental autoimmune encephalomyelitis by oral administration of myelin basic protein and its fragments. J Immunol 140:440–445.

Higuchi M, Diamantstein T, Osawa H, Caspi RR (1991): Combined anti-interleukin-2 receptor and low-dose cyclosporine therapy in experimental autoimmune uveoretinitis. J Autoimmun 4:113–124.

Hirose S, Kuwabara T, Nussenblatt RB, Wiggert B, Redmond TM, Gery I (1986): Uveitis induced in primates by interphotoreceptor retinoid-binding protein. Arch Ophthalmol 104:1698–1702.

Hirose S, McAllister C, Mittal K, Vistica B, Shihohara T, Gery I (1988a): A cell line and clones of lymphocytes from a healthy donor, with specificity to S-antigen. Invest Ophthalmol Vis Sci 29:1636–1641.

Hirose S, Singh VK, Donoso LA, Shinohara T, Kotake S, Tanaka T, Kuwabara T, Yamaki K, Gery I, Nussenblatt RB (1989): An 18-mer peptide derived from the retinal S antigen induces uveitis and pinealitis in primates. Clin Exp Immunol 77:106–111.

Hirose S, Tanaka T, Nussenblatt RB, Palestine AG, Wiggert B, Redmond TM, Chader GJ, Gery I (1988b): Lymphocyte responses to retinal-specific antigens in uveitis patients and healthy subjects. Curr Eye Res 7:393–402.

Hoekzema R, Hwan SB, Rothova A, van Haren M, Donoso LA, Kijlstra A (1990): Serum antibody response to human and bovine IRBP in uveitis. Curr Eye Res 9:1177–1183.

Hogan M, Kimura S, Thygeson P (1959): Signs and symptoms of uveitis: I. Anterior uveitis. Am J Ophthalmol 47:155–170.

Holda JH, Maier T, Claman HN (1988): Evidence that IFN-gamma is responsible for natural suppressor activity in GVHD spleen and normal bone marrow. Transplantation 45:772–777.

Hooper P, Bora NS, Kaplan HJ, Ferguson TA (1991): Inhibition of lymphocyte proliferation by resident ocular cells. Curr Eye Res 10:363–372.

Hylkema HA, Kijlstra A (1989): Circulating immune complexes in uveitis patients. Int Ophthalmol 13:253–257.

Ichikawa T, Taguchi O, Takahashi T, Ikeda H, Takeuchi M, Tanaka T, Usui M, Nishizuka Y (1991): Spontaneous development of autoimmune uveoretinitis in nude mice following reconstitution with embryonic rat thymus. Clin Exp Immunol 86:112–117.

Jerne NK (1984): Idiotypic networks and other preconceived ideas. Immunol Rev 79:5–24.

Jiang LQ, Streilin JW (1990): Immunologic privilege evoked by histoincompatible intracameral retinal transplants. Reg Immunol 3:121–130.

Kaiser CJ, Ksander BR, Streilein JW (1989): Inhibition of lymphocyte proliferation by aqueous humor. Reg Immunol 2:42–49.

Kawano Y, Sasamoto Y, Kotake S, Thurau SR, Wiggert B, Gery I (1991): Trials of vaccination against experimental autoimmune uveoretinitis with a T-cell receptor peptide. Curr Eye Res 10:789–795.

Kawashima H, Fujino Y, Mochizuki M (1990): Antigen-specific suppressor cells induced by FK506 in experimental autoimmune uveoretinitis in the rat. Invest Ophthalmol Vis Sci 31:2500–2507.

Kawashima H, Obritsch F, Evangelista T, Ketcham J, Holland E, Gregerson D (1992): Inhibitory effects of corneal endothelial cells on autoimmune T cells in vitro. Invest Ophthalmol Vis Sci 33(Suppl):986.

Kim MK, Caspi RR, Nussenblatt RB, Kuwabara T, Palestine AG (1988): Intraocular trafficking of lymphocytes in locally induced experimental autoimmune uveoretinitis (EAU). Cell Immunol 112:430–436.

Kim MK, Chan CC, Belfort RJ, Farah M, Burnier MP, Nussenblatt RB, Kuwabara T, Palestine AG (1987): Histopathologic and immunohistopathologic features of subretinal fibrosis and uveitis syndrome. Am J Ophthalmol 104:15–23.

Kimura S, Thygeson P, Hogan M (1959): Signs and symptoms of uveitis: II. Classification of the posterior manifestations of uveitis. Am J Ophthalmol 47:171.

Koker P, Eisenstein R, Schumacher B, Christianson G, Grant D (1985): Ocular tissues contain inhibitors of lymphocyte mitogenesis. Curr Eye Res 4:807–810.

Kozhich A, Vistica P, Gery I, Berzofsky J, Wauben M, Eden Wv (1992): Inhibition of experimental autoimmune uveoretinitis (EAU) by synthetic peptides. Invest Ophthalmol Vis Sci 33(Suppl):1025.

Lamont AG, Bruce MG, Watret KC, Ferguson A (1988): Suppression of an established DTH response to ovalbumin in mice by feeding antigen after immunization. Immunology 64:135–139.

Li Q, Fujino Y, Caspi RR, Najafian F, Nussenblatt R, Chan CC (1992): Association between mast cells and the development of experimental autoimmune uveitis in different rat strains. Clin Immunol Immunopathol 65:294–299.

Lider O, Reshef T, Beraud E, Ben-Nun A, Cohen IR (1988): Anti-idiotypic network induced by T cell vaccination against experimental autoimmune encephalomyelitis. Science 239:181–183.

Lightman SL, Caspi RR, Nussenblatt RB, Palestine AG (1987): Antigen-directed retention of an autoimmune T-cell line. Cell Immunol 110:28–34.

Matsuo T, Nakayama T, Koyama T, Koyama M, Fujimoto S, Matsuo N (1986): Immunological studies of uveitis. 3. Cell-mediated immunity to interphotoreceptor retinoid-binding protein. Jpn J Ophthalmol 30:487–494.

Merryman CF, Donoso LA, Zhang XM, Heber-Katz E, Gregerson DS (1991): Characterization of a new, potent, immunopathogenic epitope in S-antigen that elicits T cell expressing V beta 8 and V alpha 2-like genes. J Immunol 146:75–80.

Miller A, Lider O, Roberts AB, Sporn MB, Weiner HL (1992): Suppressor T cells generated by oral tolerization to myelin basic protein suppress both in vitro and in vivo immune responses by the release of transforming growth factor beta after antigen-specific triggering. Proc Natl Acad Sci USA 89:421–425.

Mizuno K, Clark AF, Streilein JW (1989): Ocular injection of retinal S antigen: Suppression of autoimmune uveitis. Invest Ophthalmol Vis Sci 30:772–774.

Mochizuki M, Kawashima H (1990): Effects of FK506, 15-deoxyspergualin, and cyclosporine on experimental autoimmune uveoretinitis in the rat. Autoimmunity 8:37–41.

Mochizuki M, Kuwabara T, Chan CC, Nussenblatt RB, Metcalfe DD, Gery I (1984): An association between susceptibility to experimental autoimmune uveitis and choroidal mast cell numbers. J Immunol 133:1699–1701.

Möller E, Böhme J, Valugerdi MA, Ridderstad A, Olerup O (1990): Speculations on mechanisms of HLA associations with autoimmune diseases and the specificity of "autoreactive" T lymphocytes. Immunol Rev 118:5–19.

Möller G (1988): Do suppressor T cells exist? Scand J Immunol 27:247–250.

Nork TM, Ghobrial MW, Peyman GA, Tso MO (1986): Massive retinal gliosis. A reactive proliferation of Müller cells. Arch Ophthalmol 104:1383–1389.

Nussenblatt RB (1991): Proctor Lecture. Experimental autoimmune uveitis: Mechanisms of disease and clinical therapeutic indications. Invest Ophthalmol Vis Sci 32:3131–3141.

Nussenblatt RB, Caspi RR, Mahdi R, Chan CC, Roberge F, Lider O, Weiner HL (1990): Inhibition of S-antigen induced experimental autoimmune uveoretinitis by oral induction of tolerance with S-antigen. J Immunol 144:1689–1695.

Nussenblatt RB, Gery I, Ballintine EJ, Wacker WB (1980): Cellular immune responsiveness of uveitis patients to retinal S-antigen. Am J Ophthalmol 89:173–179.

Nussenblatt RB, Kuwabara T, de Monasterio FM, Wacker WB (1981a): S-antigen uveitis in primates. A new model for human disease. Arch Ophthalmol 99:1090–1092.

Nussenblatt RB, Mittal KK, Ryan S, Green WR, Maumenee AE (1982a): Birdshot retinochoroidopathy associated with HLA-A29 antigen and immune responsiveness to retinal S-antigen. Am J Ophthalmol 94:147–158.

Nussenblatt RB, Palestine AG (1989): "Uveitis: Fundamentals and Clinical Practice." Chicago: Year Book Medical Publishers, Inc.

Nussenblatt RB, Palestine AG, Chan CC, Mochizuki M, Yancey K (1985a): Effectiveness of cyclosporin therapy for Behçet's disease. Arthritis Rheum 28:671–679.

Nussenblatt RB, Palestine AG, Chan CC, Roberge F (1985b): Standardization of vitreal inflammatory activity in intermediate and posterior uveitis. Ophthalmology 92:467–471.

Nussenblatt RB, Palestine AG, El Saied M, Meyers S, Lando Z, Mullenberg C, Rozenszajn LA (1984): Long-term antigen specific and non-specific T-cell lines and clones in uveitis. Curr Eye Res 3:299–305.

Nussenblatt RB, Rodrigues MM, Salinas-Carmona M, Gery I, Cevario S, Wacker W (1982b): Modulation of experimental autoimmune uveitis with cyclosporin A. Arch Ophthalmol 100:1146–1149.

Nussenblatt RB, Rodrigues MM, Wacker WB, Cevario SJ, Salinas-Carmona M, Gery I (1981b): Cyclosporin A. Inhibition of experimental autoimmune uveitis in Lewis rats. J Clin Invest 67:1228–1231.

O'Connor GR (1983): Factors related to the initiation and recurrence of uveitis. XL Edward Jackson memorial lecture. Am J Ophthalmol 96:577–599.

Okumura A, Mochizuki M, Nishi M, Herbort CP (1990): Endotoxin-induced uveitis (EIU) in the rat: A study of inflammatory and immunological mechanisms. Int Ophthalmol 14:31–36.

Palestine AG, Austin H3, Balow JE, Antonovych TT, Sabnis SG, Preuss HG, Nussenblatt RB (1986): Renal histopathologic alterations in patients treated with cyclosporine for uveitis. N Engl J Med 314:1293–1298.

Pasternak RD, Wadopian NS, Wright RN, Siminoff P, Gylys JA, Buyniski JP (1987): Disease modifying activity of HWA 486 in rat adjuvant-induced arthritis. Agents Actions 21:241–243.

Percopo CM, Hooks JJ, Shinohara T, Caspi R, Detrick B (1990): Cytokine-mediated activation of a neuronal retinal resident cell provokes antigen presentation. J Immunol 145:4101–4107.

Rao NA, Brown CJ, Marak GE (1986): Ultrastructural analysis of experimental allergic uveitis in rabbit. Ophthalmic Res 18:15–20.

Roberge FG, Caspi RR, Chan CC, Kuwabara T, Nussenblatt RB (1985): Long-term culture of Muller cells from adult rats in the presence of activated lymphocytes/monocytes products. Curr Eye Res 4:975–982.

Roberge FG, Caspi RR, Nussenblatt RB (1988): Glial retinal Müller cells produce IL-1 activity and have a dual effect on autoimmune T helper lymphocytes. Antigen presentation manifested after removal of suppressive activity. J Immunol 140:2193–2196.

Roberge FG, Lorberboum-Galski H, Le Hoang P, de Smet M, Chan CC, Fitzgerald D, Pastan I (1989): Selective immunosuppression of activated T cells with the chimeric toxin IL-2-PE-40. Inhibition of experimental autoimmune uveoretinitis. J Immunol 143:3498–3502.

Roberge FG, Xu D, Chan CC, de Smet MD, Nussenblatt RB, Chen H (1993): Treatment of autoimmune uveoretinitis in the rat with rapamycin, an inhibitor of lymphocyte growth factor signal transduction. Curr Eye Res 12:197–203.

Rossi F, Dietrich G, Kazatchkine MD (1989): Anti-idiotypes against autoantibodies in normal immunoglobulins: Evidence for network regulation of human autoimmune responses. Immunol Rev 110:135–149.

Rubin B, Najafian F, Caspi R, Sehgal S, Nussenblatt R (1992): Synergistic interactions of cyclosporine and rapamycin to inhibit EAU in the Lewis rat. Invest Ophthalmol Vis Sci 33(Suppl):934.

Sai P, Maugendre D, Loreal O, Maurel C, Pogu S (1988): Effects of cyclosporin on autoimmune diabetes induced in mice by streptozotocin: Beta cell-toxicity and rebound of insulitis after cessation of treatment. Diabetes Metab 14:455–462.

Sakai J (1983): [Immune complexes in experimental autoimmune uveo-retinitis.] Nippon Ganka Gakkai Zasshi 87:1288–1299.

Schlaegel TJ (1969): "Essentials of Uveitis." Boston: Little, Brown and Co.

Schreiber SL, Crabtree GR (1992): The mechanism of action of cyclosporin A and FK 506. Immunol Today 13:136–142.

Sedgwick J, Brostoff S, Mason D (1987): Experimental allergic encephalomyelitis in the absence of a classical delayed-type hypersensitivity reaction. Severe paralytic disease correlates with the presence of interleukin 2 receptor-positive cells infiltrating the central nervous system. J Exp Med 165:1058–1075.

Shoenfeld Y, Isenberg D (1989): The mosaic of autoimmunity. In "Research Monographs in Immunology." Elsevier, Amsterdam, p ix.

Silverman GA, Peri BA, Fitch FW, Rothberg RM (1983): Enterically induced regulation of systemic immune responses. II. Suppression of proliferating T cells by an Lyt-1[+], 2-T effector cell. J Immunol 131:2656–2661.

Singh VK, Nussenblatt RB, Donoso LA, Yamaki K, Chan CC, Shinohara T (1988a): Identification of a uveitopathogenic and lymphocyte proliferation site in bovine S-antigen. Cell Immunol 115:413–419.

Singh VK, Yamaki K, Donoso LA, Shinohara T (1988b): S-antigen: Experimental autoimmune uveitis induced in guinea pigs with two synthetic peptides. Curr Eye Res 7:87–92.

Smith H, Chen I-M, Kubo R, Tung K (1989): Neonatal thymectomy results in a repertoire enriched in T cells deleted in adult thymus. Science 245:749.

Streilein JW (1987): Immune regulation and the eye: A dangerous compromise. FASEB J 1:199–208.

Streilein JW, Bradley D (1991): Analysis of immunosuppressive properties of iris and ciliary body cells and their secretory products. Invest Ophthalmol Vis Sci 32:2700–2710.

Thomson AW (1991): The immunosuppressive macrolides FK-506 and rapamycin. Immunol Lett 29:105–111.

Thurau SR, Caspi RR, Chan CC, Weiner HL, Nussenblatt RB (1991a): [Immunologic suppression of experimental autoimmune uveitis.] Fortschr Ophthalmol 88:404–407.

Thurau SR, Chan CC, Suh E, Nussenblatt RB (1991b): Induction of oral tolerance to S-antigen induced experimental autoimmune uveitis by a uveitogenic 20mer peptide. J Autoimmun 4:507–516.

Uhlenhuth P (1903): Zur lehre von der unterscheidung verschiedener eiweissarten mit hilfe spezifischer sera. In "Fetschrift zum 60 geburstag von Robert Koch." Jena, German Democratic Republic: Fischer, pp 49–74.

Vandenbark AA, Hashim G, Offner H (1989): Immunization with a synthetic T-cell receptor V-region peptide protects against experimental autoimmune encephalomyelitis. Nature 341:541–544.

Wahl SM, Allen JB, Ohura K, Chenoweth DE, Hand AR (1991): IFN-gamma inhibits inflammatory cell recruitment and the evolution of bacterial cell wall-induced arthritis. J Immunol 146:95–100.

Waldmann TA, Pastan IH, Gansow OA, Junghans RP (1992): The multichain interleukin-2 receptor: A target for immunotherapy. Ann Intern Med 116:148–160.

Wetzig R, Hooks JJ, Percopo CM, Nussenblatt R, Chan CC, Detrick B (1988): Anti-Ia antibody diminishes ocular inflammation in experimental autoimmune uveitis. Curr Eye Res 7:809–818.

Whitcup SM, Chan CC, Li Q, Nussenblatt RB (1992): Expression of cell adhesion molecules in posterior uveitis. Arch Ophthalmol 110:662–666.

Whitcup SM, DeBarge LR, Caspi RR, Harning R, Nussenblatt RB, Chan CC (1993): Monoclonal antibodies against ICAM-1 (CD54) and LFA-1 (CD11a/CD18) inhibit experimental autoimmune uveitis. Clin Immunol Immunopathol 67:143–150.

Wilbanks GA, Mammolenti M, Streilein JW (1992): Studies on the induction of anterior chamber-associated immune deviation (ACAID). III. Induction of ACAID depends upon intraocular transforming growth factor-beta. Eur J Immunol 22:165–173.

Wilbanks GA, Streilein JW (1991): Studies on the induction of anterior chamber-associated immune deviation (ACAID). 1. Evidence that an antigen-specific, ACAID-inducing, cell-associated signal exists in the peripheral blood. J Immunol 146:2610–2617.

Wilbanks GA, Streilein JW (1992): Fluids from immune privileged sites endow macrophages with the capacity to induce antigen-specific immune deviation via a mechanism involving transforming growth factor-beta. Eur J Immunol 22:1031–1036.

Yanoff M, Zimmerman LE, Davis RL (1971): Massive gliosis of the retina. Int Ophthalmol Clin 11:211–229.

Yoshitoshi T, Shichi H (1991): Immunosuppressive factors in porcine vitreous body. Curr Eye Res 10:1141–1149.

25

CELLULAR AND MOLECULAR ASPECTS OF SYSTEMIC AUTOIMMUNITY

Michel Goldman and Paul-Henri Lambert

Service d'Immunologie, Hôpital Erasme, Université Libre de Bruxelles, Belgium (M.G.); WHO Immunology Research and Training Center, Geneva/Lausanne, Switzerland (P.-H.L.)

INTRODUCTION

In contrast with organ-specific autoimmune diseases, the self-antigens involved in systemic autoimmune disorders are widespread throughout the body [Roitt, 1991]. Consequently, almost every tissue or organ can be injured by the autoimmune process. This is most apparent in systemic lupus erythematosus (SLE), the prototype of systemic autoimmune diseases. During the last years, the investigation of experimental models of systemic autoimmunity by new tools derived from molecular biology allowed significant advances in understanding the pathobiology of SLE and related autoimmune diseases. In this review, we focus on the cellular and molecular interactions leading to abnormal B-cell activation in SLE.

B-CELL ACTIVATION IN SLE: POLYCLONAL OR OLIGOCLONAL?

Autoantibodies found in the serum of lupus patients include antibodies directed to DNA and other nuclear antigens (i.e., histones, RNA, ribonucleo-

Autoimmunity: Physiology and Disease, Pages 407–422
© *1994 Wiley-Liss, Inc.*

proteins), as well as antibodies to IgG (rheumatoid factors), phospholipids (lupus anticoagulant), or blood cells (erythrocytes, platelets, lymphocytes). These patients also display increased numbers of B lymphocytes producing antibodies to self- and nonself-antigens [Jasin and Ziff, 1975; Blaese et al., 1980; Kumagai et al., 1982; Steinberg et al., 1990]. All these features suggest that nonspecific (polyclonal) B-cell activation is responsible for autoantibody production in SLE.

However, the generation of monoclonal antibodies from lupus mice or derived from SLE patients demonstrated that lupus autoantibodies are often reactive with several self-antigens [Schoenfeld et al., 1983b; Zouali et al., 1988] and share common idiotypes [Rauch et al., 1982; Shoenfeld et al., 1983a], suggesting that a limited number of B-cell clones might be responsible for the autoantibodies spectrum. Along the same line, probing the B-cell repertoire of lupus patients with Epstein-Barr virus, Nakamura et al. [1988] found high frequencies of high affinity monoreactive IgG autoantibodies. Similar observations were made by Zouali et al. [1991], when they quantitated the B-cell repertoire using the spot-ELISA technique. Interestingly, both studies demonstrated the presence in the circulation of normal B-cell precursors producing low affinity polyreactive IgM autoantibodies, including anti-DNA autoantibodies. The occurrence of pathogenic anti-DNA autoantibodies could therefore result from antigen-driven stimulation of naturally occurring polyreactive B-cell clones [Zouali et al., 1988]. Occasionally, they might also arise from point mutations in the V-gene sequences of antibacterial antibodies [Diamond et al., 1992]. Although $CD5^+$ B cells in man and their $Ly1^+$ B cell counterparts in mouse represent a major source of natural polyreactive autoantibodies [Hayakawa et al., 1984; Casali et al., 1987], their role in the production of pathogenic anti-DNA autoantibodies has not been clearly established [Steinberg et al., 1990]. The nature of the pathogenic antibodies in SLE is beyond the scope of this review. However, it is relevant to mention here the putative roles of the net electric charge and of the isotype of the autoantibodies. Thus cationic anti-DNA antibodies [Datta et al., 1987], IgG_{2a} antibodies [Theofilopoulos and Dixon, 1985], and more recently IgG3 antibodies in the MRL/lpr strain [Takahashi et al., 1991] proved to be particularly nephritogenic.

Although the respective roles of polyclonal versus antigen-driven B-cell activation in SLE remain a matter of debate, it is likely that both processes are operative at different stages of the disease as indicated by kinetic studies in mice with spontaneous lupus [Steinberg et al., 1990]. In the early phase, B-cell activation is clearly polyclonal since lupus-prone mice produce autoantibodies directed against a variety of self- and nonself-antigens and possess more immunoglobulin-containing cells and more clonable B cells than do normal mice [Izui et al., 1978; Theofilopoulos et al., 1980; Kincade et al., 1979; Klinman and Steinberg, 1987]. Consistent with this, the immunoglobulin V_H genes used by autoimmune strains are not restricted [Kastner et al.,

1989; Kofler et al., 1985; Dersimonian et al., 1987]. This early polyclonal B-cell activation is followed later on by—and possibly favors—the oligoclonal expansion of B cells producing autoantibodies characteristic of SLE; this second wave of B-cell activation is thought to be driven by nuclear self-antigens or cross-reacting exogenous antigens [Steinberg et al., 1990, Zouali et al., 1991].

Several factors might be involved in the B-cell hyperactivity characteristic of SLE. First, there is evidence of intrinsic B-cell changes in certain lupus mice. For example, B cells in the NZB/W, NZB, and BXSB strains display an increased sensitivity to T-cell-derived proliferation and differentiation factors [Prud'homme et al., 1983; Herron et al., 1988; Umland et al., 1989], presumably as a consequence of genetically determined B-cell defects (Prud'homme and Palfrey, 1988]. Second, bacterial substances inducing polyclonal B-cell activation might also participate in the progression of lupus disease. Indeed, bacterial lipopolysaccharide (LPS) has been shown to induce SLE-like features in normal mice and to accelerate the disease in mice spontaneously developing SLE [Izui et al., 1977; Hang et al., 1985]. More recently, bacterial DNA was found to induce B cell proliferation in vitro, suggesting that it might also act as a polyclonal B-cell activator [Messina et al., 1991]. Third, there is compelling evidence that T cells play a central role in the pathobiology of SLE. As discussed below, the precise identification of the T cells responsible for the activation of autoreactive B cells might lead in the near future to the development of new therapeutic strategies of systemic autoimmune diseases.

INVOLVEMENT OF T CELLS IN THE PATHOGENESIS OF EXPERIMENTAL SLE

In this section, we consider genetically determined SLE-like syndromes and experimental allogeneic diseases that might help to understand the role of T cells in SLE.

Genetically Determined Murine SLE

(NZB × NZW) Or (NZB × SWR) F$_1$ Mice. The (NZB × NZW) and (NZB × SWR) F$_1$ mouse strains develop several immunopathological features characteristic of human SLE, including antidouble-stranded DNA autoantibodies and severe lupus glomerulonephritis [Lambert and Dixon, 1968; Datta et al., 1978; Theofilopoulos and Dixon, 1985]. Both strains will be considered together here, although there are some differences between them. Indeed, the NZW parents of the (NZB × NZW) F$_1$ produce autoantibodies and express high levels of retrovirus, whereas the SWR parents of the (NZB × SWR) crosses are perfectly normal in these respects [Datta, 1989].

In addition, a large deletion within the T-cell receptor (TCR) β-chain gene complex of the NZW mouse had been identified, although the contribution of this abnormality to the pathology of (NZB × NZW) F_1 mice remains elusive [Yanagi et al., 1986].

The in vivo effects of a depleting anti-CD4 monoclonal antibody in (NZB × NZW) F_1 mice provided clear evidence that the occurrence of anti-DNA antibodies and the development of glomerulonephritis in this strain was critically dependent on $CD4^+$ cells [Wofsy and Seaman, 1985]. Later it was shown that $CD4^+$ cells from nephritic (NZB ×NZW) F_1 mice elicited anti-DNA antibody production by syngeneic B cells in vitro [Ando et al., 1987]. The phenotype, TCR gene usage, and specificity of the $CD4^+$ cells inducing the production of cationic pathogenic IgG anti-DNA autoantibodies in (NZB × SWR) F_1 mice have been extensively studied by Datta [1989] and coworkers. By analyzing panels of T-cell lines, they found two sets of cells: The first set consists of autoreactive $CD4^+$ helper T cells that preferentially interact with antigen-presenting cells (APC) bearing unique F_1-hybrid–class II MHC determinants, suggesting that they recognize amino acid sequences of those molecules or a peptide present in their groove [Sainis and Datta, 1988; Datta, 1989]. The recent analysis of the junctional sequences of these autoreactive $CD4^+$ T cells could provide a clue to their fine specificity. Indeed, they were found invariably to express anionic residues in their TCR β-chain junctions (complementary-determining region [CDR] 3) [Adams et al., 1991]. This suggests that they were selected by some cationic peptide presented by the anti-DNA–producing B cells that they help. The cationic autoantigens that could be involved include histones and V regions of the anti-DNA antibodies themselves in the form of endogenous idiopeptides [Adams et al., 1991]. The pathogenicity of the helper $CD4^+$ T-cell clones was confirmed in vivo, since they rapidly induced lupus nephritis after injection in young prenephritic (NZB × SWR) F_1 mice [Adams et al., 1991]. In addition to the $CD4^+$ subset, a set of double negative (DN) ($CD4^-$ $C8^-$) T cells was also found to induce the production of pathogenic autoantibodies in (NZB × SWR) F_1 mice [Datta et al., 1987; Sainis and Datta, 1988]. Interestingly, a significant proportion of these DN cells are leaky T cells expressing forbidden receptors, i.e., TCR specific for endogenous superantigens [Adams et al., 1990]. The reasons why these T cells bearing autoreactive TCR escape thymic deletion are unclear at the present time.

MRL/lpr Mice. MRL mice homozygous for the lpr gene (MRL/lpr) develop a severe autoimmune disease essentially characterized by proliferative glomer-ulonephritis, erosive synovitis, necrotizing medium-sized arteritis, and massive lymphoproliferation [Theofilopoulos and Dixon, 1985]. The latter is due to a progressive infiltration of lymph nodes and, to a lesser extent, of the spleen with $CD4^-$ $CD8^-$ $CD3^+$ cells. These DN T cells, which express B220 and certain other B-cell surface markers, display a number of functional abnormalities [Cohen and Eisenberg, 1991]. Their proliferative responses to mitogens and to TCR ligation are markedly deficient [Igarashi et al., 1988; Davignon et al., 1988] perhaps in relation to their lack of CD2 expression [Shirai et al., 1990].

Moreover, a 26 kD phosphoprotein associated with their TCR and thought to belong to the G-protein family could be responsible for an abnormal transduction pathway [Yokoyama and Gachelin, 1991; Cohen and Eisenberg, 1991]. Interestingly, the DN T cells of MRL/lpr mice spontaneously produce interferon (IFN)-γ [Manolios et al., 1989] as well as several B-cell tropic cytokines. Thus interleukin (IL)-4– and IL-5–like factors were shown to be produced by DN T-cell lines [Rosenberg et al., 1986]. More recently, DN T cells were found constitutively to express very high levels of Eta-1, a newly defined cytokine that induces polyclonal B-cell activation [Lampe et al., 1991]. These observations support the hypothesis that DN T cells are involved in the activation of autoreactive B cells. The therapeutic effect of the *Staphylococcus* enterotoxin B (SEB) superantigen on the autoimmune syndrome of MRL/lpr mice favors this view; indeed, this treatment reduces DN T cells in a rather specific manner by targeting the Vβ8$^+$ TCR that they preferentially express [Kim et al., 1991]. However, there is also evidence that CD4$^+$ T cells play an important role in this model as in vivo administration of an anti-CD4 MoAb inhibits the lymphoproliferation as well as the autoantibody production [Santoro et al., 1988]. It is possible that CD4$^+$ cells are precursors or stimulators of DN T cells. On the other hand, they could also be directly involved in B-cell activation since long-term CD4$^+$ cell lines obtained from MRL/lpr mice were found to be reactive to self-class-II MHC and to produce B-cell proliferation and differentiation factors [Weston et al., 1988; Cohen and Eisenberg, 1991]. The defect in Fas antigen—a cell surface protein that mediates apoptosis—that has already been demonstrated in this mouse strain could well be the primary cause of the emergence of autoreactive T cells by interfering with the process of negative selection in the thymus [Watanabe-Fukunaga et al., 1992].

Allogeneic Diseases

Chronic Stimulatory Graft-Versus-Host Disease. In selected parent–F$_1$ combinations, the graft-versus-host disease (GVHD) induced by the injection of parental lymphocytes into adult unirradiated F$_1$ hybrid mice results in a chronic autoimmune syndrome resembling human SLE. For example, (C57Bl/10 × DBA/2) F$_1$ mice injected with DBA/2 T cells develop hypergammaglobulinema, IgG antibodies to nuclear antigens, erythrocytes, thymocytes, and skin basement membrane, as well as antibody-mediated glomerulonephritis [Gleichmann et al., 1984]. The lack of acute GVHD in this particular model has been related to a functional defect of DBA/2 donor CD8$^+$ cells in the generation of cytotoxic responses to host C57Bl/10 alloantigens [Via and Shearer, 1988].

It was recently shown that a population of host CD8$^+$ cells behaving as veto-like cells are responsible for this inhibition of donor anti-host CD8$^+$ cells [Fast, 1991]. In contrast, donor DBA/2 CD4$^+$ T cells recognizing host class II alloantigens are functional and persistently activate B cells of the host to produce IgG autoantibodies directed against certain self-antigens, including double-stranded DNA and various nuclear and nucleolar proteins such as histones and fibrillarin [Gleichmann et al., 1984; Gelpi et al., 1988; Rozendaal et al., 1990]. These interactions between donor CD4$^+$ T cells and class II–disparate B cells of the host are cognate in nature, as demonstrated by Morris et al. [1990] using double-parental chimeras differing at both Ia and IgH allotypes. The profile of the cytokines produced by the alloreactive donor CD4$^+$ cells rapidly changes during the course of the disease. In the first 2 days after induction of the GVHD, these cells spontaneously proliferate and produce IL-2 [Via, 1991]. Thereafter they develop a profound defect in their proliferative responses and in their ability to secrete IL-2 [Moser et al., 1988] while they produce IL-4 and IL-10 [De Wit et al., 1993] and are possibly also the source of IL-5, IL-6, and B-151-TRF2—another B-cell-tropic cytokine—spontaneously produced by spleen cells [Dobashi et al., 1987; Umland et al., 1992]. IL-4 appears to play an important role in the immunopathological syndrome as in vivo administration of a neutralizing anti-IL-4 monoclonal antibody prevented the development of serum hyper IgE and hyperIgG1 and delayed the glomerular lesions [Doutrelepont et al., 1991; Umland et al., 1992].

Host-Versus-Graft Disease. Allogeneic interactions are involved in another murine model of systemic autoimmunity, namely, the host-versus-graft disease (HVGD) [Simpson et al., 1974; Hard and Kullgren, 1970; Goldman et al., 1983]. In Balb/c mice injected at birth with spleen cells from either (C57Bl/6 × Balb/c) F$_1$ or (A/J × Balb/c) F$_1$ hybrids, the immunopathological syndrome corresponds to an SLE-like disease that is self-limited [Goldman et al., 1983; Florquin et al., 1991; de la Hera et al., 1992]. Pathogenic antibodies are produced by F$_1$ donor B cells that persist in the host [Luzuy et al., 1986]. The lack of rejection of the donor cells is due to a state of tolerance toward donor alloantigens, as demonstrated by a dramatic reduction in the frequency of donor-specific cytolytic T cells and of donor-specific helper T cells secreting IL-2 and IFN-γ [Feng et al., 1983]. However, there is in vivo and in vitro evidence that a subset of CD4$^+$ cells recognizing donor class II MHC remains functional and is responsible for the activation of donor auto-reactive B cells [Merino et al., 1989; Abramowicz et al., 1990b]. These CD4$^+$ cells display a T-helper-2 phenotype [Mossman et al., 1991], as they do not produce T-helper-1-type cytokines but secrete high levels of IL-4 [Abramowicz et al., 1990b]. This latter cytokine plays a central role in the HVGD as indicated by the preferential production of IgG1 and IgE isotypes [Goldman et al., 1988], the increased expression of class II MHC antigens on B cells [Abramowicz et al., 1990a], and the in vivo prevention of the autoimmune features by a neutralizing anti-IL-4 monoclonal antibody [Schurmans et al., 1990].

Besides their role in the induction of donor B-cell activation, host CD4$^+$ cells might also be involved in the maintenance of allotolerance. Indeed, in similar models tolerance of donor skin graft appeared to correlate with increased T- and B-cell activities. [Bandeira et al., 1989], and T cells from tolerant mice were found to suppress the generation of class II–specific cytotoxic T cells [Streilein, 1991]. This suppression could be mediated, at least in part, by IL-10 produced by host antidonor T-helper-2 cells, as we recently detected accumulation of IL-10 mRNA in the spleens of mice undergoing HVGD [Abromowicz et al., 1993].

A ROLE FOR T-HELPER-2 CELLS IN CERTAIN SYSTEMIC AUTOIMMUNE DISEASES?

In the allogeneic diseases described above, the interactions of alloreactive CD4$^+$ cells with corresponding alloantigens lead to their differentiation into T-helper-2 (TH2)-type cells. Several factors are probably involved in the ultimate differentiation of CD4$^+$ cells into TH1 or TH2 cells, including the persistence of the antigen, the nature of the APC, and the cytokine balance during the induction of the immune response [Gajewski et al., 1991; Abbas et al., 1991]. In chronic GVHD and in HVGD, the persistent T-cell stimulation by allogeneic B cells and a default in IFN-γ production due to defective alloreactive CD8$^+$ cells might be important in the skewing of the allogeneic reaction toward a TH2-type response. In both models, alloreactive CD4$^+$ cells initially proliferate—probably in relation with a transient production of IL-2—before differentiating into TH2-type cells [Via, 1991; Schurmans, 1991]. This initial step could correspond to the activation of naive alloreactive T cells (THp), which are known to secrete IL-2 only [Mosman et al., 1991]. This might be important for the further development of the TH2 response, as IL-2 is required for the recruitment of IL-4-producing cells [Seder et al., 1991]. Since there is evidence for an early production of IFN-γ in chronic GVHD [Umland et al., 1992], it is possible that alloreactive CD4$^+$ cells pass through an additional intermediate stage (i.e., TH0) before their final differentiation into TH2 cells.

Similar pathways are probably operative in the pathogenesis of other experimental diseases in which B-cell hyperactivity is associated with defective cell-mediated immunity, such as in chemically induced autoimmunity [reviewed by Goldman et al., 1991] and in the mouse model of AIDS induced by the LP-B-M5 retrovirus [Gazzinelli et al., 1992]. In the latter model, it has been suggested that TH2 cells recognize a virus-encoded superantigen expressed on B cells [Gazzinelli et al., 1992]. Recent studies indicate that similar interactions might occur with bacterial and mycoplasma superantigens, since these substances induce in vitro B-cell activation and autoantibody production by a CD4$^+$ T-cell-dependent mechanism [Tumang et al., 1991; He et al., 1992].

In pathological settings mediated by TH2 cells, IL-10 might play a dual role since this cytokine not only blocks several functions of macrophages, including their ability to induce the production of IFN-γ by T cells [Mosmann, 1991], but is also a potent growth and differentiation factor for B cells [Rousset et al., 1992] (Fig. 1). Neutralization of IL-10 by appropriate monoclonal antibody should allow us to determine whether IL-10 is indeed a crucial mediator of B-cell activation and immunodeficiency in vivo.

The difficulty in designing new therapeutic strategies for systemic autoimmune diseases might be linked to the relative resistance of TH2 cells to suppressive agents. Indeed, TH2 cells proved to be resistant to induction of unresponsiveness by anti-CD3 antibody [Abbas et al., 1991], and they rapidly recover in vivo after total lymphoid irradiation [Bass et al., 1989] or during anti-CD4 monoclonal antibody therapy [Cowdery et al., 1991]. Since TH1 and TH2 clones appear to use different signalling pathways in response to TCR ligation [Gajewski et al., 1990], the characterization of the biochemical events leading to gene transcription in each subset could help to develop therapeutic agents targeting TH2 cells.

RELEVANCE OF EXPERIMENTAL MODELS TO HUMAN SLE

In human SLE too there is good evidence that T cells play a central role in the pathogenesis of the disease, although monocytes and B cells themselves might amplify B-cell hyperactivity via the production of IL-6 [Linker-Israeli

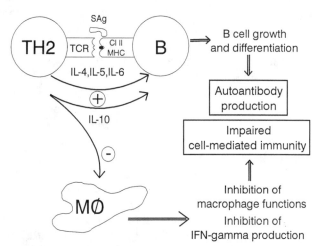

FIGURE 1. Possible role of TH2 cells in systemic autoimmunity associated with immunodeficiency. TH2 cells might be activated by B cells presenting an antigenic peptide (●) within or a superantigen (sAg) outside a class II MHC molecule. TH2 cells produce different B-cell-tropic cytokines (IL-4, IL-5, IL-6) including IL-10, which is also a potent inhibitor of cell-mediated immunity. The possible modulation of macrophage functions by IL-4 and IL-6 and the putative involvement of self-antigens in the activation of autoreactive B cells are not represented.

et al., 1991; Kitani et al., 1992]. A variety of T-cell changes have been reported in SLE patients, the most relevant being the demonstration in their peripheral blood of activated T cells eventually able to induce immunoglobulin hyperproduction by B cells [Volk et al., 1986; Huang et al., 1988]. Additional evidence for an increased in vivo T-cell division and/or survival in SLE was recently provided by assessing the frequency of T cells displaying mutant hprt genes [Gmelig-Meyling et al., 1992]. Interestingly, T cells from SLE patients present an impairment in mitogen-induced IL-2 and IFN-γ production that correlates with spontaneous in vitro IgG hyperproduction [Huang et al., 1988; Linker-Israeli, 1992]. This T-cell dysfunction could be related to a defect in the protein kinase C system [Tada et al., 1991], suggesting that signal transduction pathways might be abnormal in SLE T cells.

The analysis of T-cell lines inducing the production of pathogenic anti-DNA antibodies provided additional information on the T cells responsible for the triggering of autoreactive B cells [Rajagopalan et al., 1990]. Three types of cells were identified: 1) $\alpha\beta$-positive CD4$^+$ cells recognizing self-class-II molecules together with an unknown endogenous peptide; 2) DN CD4$^-$ CD8$^-$ $\alpha\beta^+$ cells that were not restricted to HLA molecules; and 3) DN CD4$^-$ CD8$^-$ $\gamma\delta^+$ T cells that responded to endogenous stress proteins of the HSP 60 family expressed by B cells from lupus patients. Data regarding T-cell receptor usage in SLE are scarce, but recent observations suggest the existence of a susceptibility gene coding for the constant region of the α-chain of the T-cell receptor [Tebib et al., 1990]. As far as the β-chain of the T-cell receptor is concerned, an important observation has recently been made in Sjögren's syndrome, an autoimmune disease related to SLE. By analyzing the repertoire of T cells infiltrating salivary glands, Sumida et al. [1992] found a specific and preferential expression of Vβ-2$^+$ and Vβ-13$^+$ T cells, suggesting the involvement of a superantigen in the process of T-cell activation. Retroviruses that have been shown to be endogenously expressed in murine lupus [Steinberg et al., 1990] could represent one possible source of such superantigen.

Although still fragmentary, these data on T cells in human SLE indicate several similarities with the T-cell changes observed in different models of murine (Table I). As in the mouse, it is likely that the abnormal T–B interactions leading to the production of pathogenic antibodies in man can result

TABLE I. T-cell abnormalities observed in both experimental and human SLE

Increased numbers of activated T cells in vivo
Presence of DN T cells (among T-cell lines in humans)
Autoreactive CD4$^+$ cells responding to self-class-II MHC molecules
Defective production of IL-2 and IFN-γ in vitro
Increased production of B-cell growth and differentiation factors
Defects in TCR-mediated signal transduction

from multiple causes so that SLE should be considered much more as a syndrome than a unique disease entity [Steinberg et al., 1990].

Future advances in the pathobiology of SLE will probably depend on the identification of the fine specificity of the T cells inducing activation of autoreactive B cells. Indeed, the "true" lupus antigens that trigger the autoimmune response might be expressed on B cells either as peptides within class II MHC molecules or as superantigens. Hopefully, the search for such antigens will ultimately lead to more specific treatments of SLE and related autoimmune disorders.

REFERENCES

Abbas AK, Williams ME, Burstein HJ, Chang TL, Bossu P, Lichtman AH (1991): Activation and functions of CD4+ T-cell subsets. Immunol Rev 123:5–22.

Abramowicz D, Doutrelepont JM, Lambert P, Van der vorst P, Bruyns C, Goldman M (1990a): Increased expression of Ia antigens on B cells after neonatal induction of lymphoid chimerism in mice: Role of interleukin-4. Eur J Immunol 20:469–477.

Abramowicz D, Van der vorst P, Bruyns C, Doutrelepont JM, Vandenabeele P, Goldman M (1990b): Persistence of anti-donor allohelper T cells after neonatal induction of allotolerance in mice. Eur J Immunol 20:1647–1653.

Abramowicz D, Durez P, Gérard C, Donckier V, Amraoui Z, Velu T, Goldman M (1993): Neonatal induction of transplantation tolerance in mice is associated with in vivo expression of IL-4 and IL-10 mRNAs. Transplant Proc 25:312–313.

Adams S, Leblanc P, Datta SK (1991): Junctional region sequences of T-cell receptor β genes expressed by pathogenic anti-DNA autoantibody-inducing helper T cells from lupus mice: Possible selection by cationic autoantigens. Proc Natl Acad Sci USA 88:11271–11275.

Adams S, Zordan T, Sainis K, Datta SK (1990): T cell receptor Vβ genes expressed by IgG anti-DNA autoantibody-inducing T cells in lupus nephritis: Forbidden receptors and double-negative T cells. Eur J Immunol 20:1435–1443.

Ando DG, Sercarz EE, Hahn BH (1987): Mechanisms of T and B cell collaboration in the in vitro production of anti-DNA antibodies in the NZB/NZW F₁ murine SLE model. J Immunol 138:3185–3190.

Bandeira A, Coutinho A, Carnaud C, Jacquemart F, Forni L (1989): Transplantation tolerance correlates with high levels of T- and B-lymphocyte activity. Proc Natl Acad Sci USA 86:272–276.

Bass H, Mosmann T, Strober S (1989): Evidence for mouse TH1 and TH2-like helper T cells in vivo. Selective reduction of TH1-like cells after total lymphoid irradiation. J Exp Med 170:1495–1511.

Blaese RM, Grayson J, Steinberg AD (1980): Elevated immunoglobulin secreting cells in the blood of patients with active systemic lupus erythematosis: Correlation of laboratory and clinical assessment of disease activity. Am J Med 69: 345–350.

Casali P, Burastero SE, Nakamura M, Inghirami G, Notkins AL (1987): Human lymphocytes capable of making rheumatoid factor and antibody to ssDNA belong to the Leu1+ B cell subset. Science 236:77–81.

Cohen PL, Eisenberg RA (1991): Lpr and gld: Single gene models of systemic autoimmunity and lymphoproliferative disease. Annu Rev Immunol 9:243–269.

Cowdery JS, Tolaymat N, Weber SP (1991): The effect of partial in vivo depletion of CD4 T cells by monoclonal antibody. Incomplete depletion increases IgG production and augments in vitro thymic-dependent antibody response. Transplantation 51:1072–1075.

Datta SK (1989): A search for the underlying mechanisms of systemic autoimmune disease in the NZB × SWR model. Clin Immunol Immunopathol 51:141–156.

Datta SK, Manny N, Andrzejewski C, Andre-Schwartz J, Schwartz RS (1978): Genetic studies of autoimmunity and retrovirus expression in crosses of New Zealand Black mice. I. Xenotropic virus. J Exp Med 147:854–871.

Datta SK, Patel H, Berry D (1987): Induction of a cationic shift in IgG anti-DNA autoantibodies. Role of T helper cells with classical and novel phenotypes in three murine models of lupus nephritis. J Exp Med 165:1252–1268.

Davignon JL, Cohen PL, Eisenberg RA (1988): Rapid T cell receptor modulation accompanies lack of in vitro mitogenic responsiveness of double negative T cells to anti-CD3 monoclonal antibody in MRL/Mp-lpr/lpr mice. J Immunol 141:1848–1854.

de la Hera M, de la Hera A, Ramos A, Buelta L, Alonso JL, Rodriguez-Valverde V, Merino J (1992): Self-limited autoimmune disease related to transient donor B cell activation in mice neonatally injected with semi-allogeneic F_1 cells. Int Immunol 4:67–74.

Dersimonian H, Schwartz RS, Barret KJ, Stollar BD (1987): Relationship of human variable region heavy chain germ-line genes to genes encoding anti-DNA autoantibodies. J Immunol 139:2496–2501.

De Wit D, Van Mechelen M, Zanin C, Doutrelepont JM, Velu T, Gérard C, Abramowicz D, Scheerlinck JP, De Batselier P, Urbain J, Leo O, Goldman M, Moser M (1993): Preferential activation of TH2 cells in chronic graft-versus-host reaction. J Immunol 150:361–366.

Diamond B, Katz JB, Paul E, Aranow C, Lustgarten D, Scharff M (1992): The role of somatic mutation in the pathogenic anti-DNA response. Annu Rev Immunol 10:731–758.

Dobashi K, Ono S, Murakami S, Takahama Y, Katoh Y, Hamaoka T (1987): Polyclonal B cell activation by a B cell differentiation factor, B151-TRF2. III. B151-TRF2 as a B cell differentiation factor closely associated with autoimmune disease. J Immunol 138:780–787.

Doutrelepont JM, Moser M, Leo O, Abramowicz D, Vanderhaeghen ML, Urbain J, Goldman M (1991): HyperIgE in stimulatory graft-versus-host disease: Role of interleukin-4. Clin Exp Immunol 83:133–136.

Fast LD (1991): In vitro characterization of a murine recipient anti-donor effector cell responsible for the development of chronic graft-versus-host disease. J Immunol 147:1731–1738.

Feng HM, Glasebrook AL, Engers HD, and Louis, J. (1983): Clonal analysis of T cell unresponsiveness to alloantigens induced by neonatal injection of F_1 spleen cells into parental mice. J Immunol 131:2165–2169.

Florquin S, Abramowicz D, de Heer E, Bruijn JA, Doutrelepont JM, Goldman M,

Hoedemaeker P (1991): Renal immunopathology in murine host-versus-graft disease. Kidney Int 40:852–861.

Gajewski TF, Pinnas M, Wong T, Fitch FW (1991): Murine TH1 and TH2 clones proliferate optimally in response to distinct antigen-presenting cell populations. J Immunol 146:1750–1758.

Gajewski TF, Schell SR, Fitch FW (1990): Evidence implicating utilization of different T cell receptor–associated signalling pathways by TH1 and TH2 clones. J Immunol 144:4110–4120.

Gazzinelli RT, Makino M, Chattopadhyay SK, Snapper CM, Sher A, Hugin AW, Morse III RC (1992): CD4$^+$ subset regulation in viral infection. Preferential activation of TH2 cells during progression of retrovirus-induced immunodeficiency in mice. J Immunol 148:182–188.

Gelpi C, Rodriguez-Sanchez JL, Martinez MA, Craft J, Hardin JA (1988): Murine graft vs host disease. A model for study of mechanisms that generate autoantibodies to ribonucleoproteins. J Immunol 140:4160–4166.

Gleichmann E, Pals ST, Rolink AG, Radaskiewicz T, Gleichmann H (1984). Graft-vs-host reactions: Clues to the etiology of a spectrum of immunological diseases. Immunol Today 5:324–332.

Gmelig-Meyling F, Dawisha S, Steinberg AD (1992): Assessment of in vivo frequency of mutated T cells in patients with systemic lupus erythematosus. J Exp Med 175:297–300.

Goldman M, Abramowicz D, Lambert P, Van der vorst P, Bruyns C, Toussaint C (1988): Hyperactivity of donor B cells after neonatal induction of lymphoid chimerism in mice. Clin Exp Immunol 72:79–83.

Goldman M, Druet P, Gleichmann E (1991): TH2 cells in systemic autoimmunity: Insights from allogeneic diseases and chemically-induced autoimmunity. Immunol Today 12:223–227.

Goldman M, Feng HM, Engers H, Hochmann A, Louis J, Lambert PH (1983): Autoimmunity and immune complex disease after neonatal induction of transplantation tolerance in mice. J Immunol 131:251–258.

Hang L, Aguado MT, Dixon FJ, Theofilopoulos AN (1985): Induction of severe autoimmune disease in normal mice by simultaneous action of multiple immunostimulators. J Exp Med 161:423–428.

Hard RC, Kullgren B (1970): Etiology, pathogenesis and prevention of a fatal host-versus-graft syndrome in parent/F$_1$ mouse chimeras. Am J Pathol 59:203–224.

Hayakawa K, Hardy RR, Honda M, Herzenberg LA, Steinberg AD, Herzenberg LA (1984); Ly.1 B cells: Functionally distinct lymphocytes that secrete IgM autoantibodies. Proc Natl Acad Sci USA 81:2494–2498.

He X, Goronzy J, Weyand C (1992): Selective induction of rheumatoid factors by superantigens and human helper T cells. J Clin Invest 89:673–680.

Herron LR, Coffman RI, Kotzin BL (1988): Enhanced response of autoantibody-secreting B cells from young NZB/NZW mice to T cell-derived differentiation signals. Clin Immunol Immunopathol 46:314–327.

Huang YP, Perrin LH, Miescher PA, Zubler RH (1988): Correlation of T and B cell activities in vitro ans serum IL-2 levels in systemic lupus erythematosus. J Immunol 141:827–833.

Igarashi S, Takiguchi M, Kariyone A, Kano K (1988): Phenotypic and functional analyses on T-cell subsets in lymph nodes of MRL/Mp-lpr/lpr mice. Int Arch Allergy Appl Immunol 86:249–255.

Izui S, Lambert PH, Fournié GJ, Turler H, Miescher PA (1977): Features of systemic lupus erythematosus in mice injected with bacterial lipopolysaccharides. Identification of circulating DNA and renal localization of DNA-anti-DNA complexes. J Exp Med 145:1115–1130.

Izui S, McConahey PJ, Dixon FJ (1978): Increased spontaneous polyclonal activation of B lymphocytes with spontaneous autoimmune disease. J Immunol 121:2213–2219.

Jasin HE, Ziff M (1975): Immunoglobulin synthesis by peripheral blood cells in systemic lupus erythematosus. Arthritis Rheum 18:219–228.

Kastner DL, McIntyre TM, Mallett CP, Hartman AB, Steinberg AD (1989): Direct quantitative in situ hybridization studies of Ig VH utilization. A comparison between unstimulated B cells from autoimmune and normal mice. J Immunol 143:2761–2767.

Kim C, Siminovitch KA, Ochi A (1991): Reduction of lupus nephritis in MRL/lpr mice by a bacterial superantigen treatment. J Exp Med 174:1431–1437.

Kincade PW, Lee G, Fernandes G, Moore MAS, Williams N, Good RA (1979): Abnormalities in clonable B lymphocytes and myeloid progenitors in autoimmune NZB mice. Proc Natl Acad Sci USA 76:3464–3468.

Kitani A, Hara M, Hirose T, Harigai M, Suzuki K, Kawakami M, Kawaguchi Y, Hidaka T, Kawagoe M, Nakamura H (1992): Autostimulatory effects of IL-6 on excessive B cell differentiation in patients with systemic lupus erythematosus: Analysis of IL-6 production and IL-6R expression. Clin Exp Immunol 88:75–83.

Klinman DM, Steinberg AD (1987): Systemic autoimmune disease arises from polyclonal B cell activation. J Exp Med 165:1755–1760.

Kofler R, Noonan DJ, Levy DE, Wilson MC, Moller, Niels PH, Dixon FJ, Theofilopoulos AN (1985): Genetic elements used for a murine lupus anti-DNA autoantibody are closely related to those for antibodies to exogenous antigens. J Exp Med 161:805–815.

Kumagai S, Sredni B, House S, Steinberg AD, Green I (1982): Defective regulation of B lymphocyte colony formation in patients with systemic lupus erythematosus. J Immunol 128:258–262.

Lambert PH, Dixon FJ (1968): Pathogenesis of the glomerulonephritis of NZB/W mice. J Exp Med 127:507–522.

Lampe MA, Patarca R, Iregui MV, Cantor H (1991): Polyclonal B cell activation by the Eta-1 cytokine and the development of systemic autoimmune disease. J Immunol 147:2902–2906.

Linker-Israeli M (1992): Cytokine abnormalities in human lupus. Clin Immunol Immunopathol 63:10–12.

Linker-Israeli M, Deans RJ, Wallace DJ, Prehn J, Ozeri-Chen T, Klinenberg JR (1991): Elevated levels of endogenous IL-6 in systemic lupus erythematosus. A putative role in pathogenesis. J Immunol 147:117–123.

Luzuy S, Merino J, Engers H, Izui S, Lambert PH (1986): Autoimmunity after induction of neonatal tolerance to alloantigens: role of B cell chimerism and F_1 donor B cell activation. J Immunol 136:4420–4426.

Manolios N, Schrieber L, Nelson M, Geczy CL (1989): Enhanced interferon-gamma production by lymph node cells from autoimmune (MRL/l, MRL/n) mice. Clin Exp Immunol 76:301–306.

Merino J, Schurmans S, Duchosal MA, Izui S, Lambert PH (1989): Autoimmune syndrome after induction of neonatal tolerance to alloantigens. CD4$^+$ T cells from the tolerant host activate autoreactive F$_1$ B cells. J Immunol 143:2202–2208.

Messina JP, Gilkeson GS, Pisetsky DS (1991): Stimulation of in vitro murine lymphocyte proliferation by bacterial DNA. J Immunol 147:1759–1764.

Morris SC, Cheek RL, Cohen PL, Eisenberg RA (1990): Autoantibodies in chronic graft versus host result from cognate T–B interactions. J Exp Med 171:503–517.

Moser M, Sharrow SO, Shearer GM (1988): Role of L3T4$^+$ and Lyt-2$^+$ donor cells in graft-versus-host immune deficiency induced across a class I, class II, or whole H-2 difference. J Immunol 140:2600–2608.

Mosmann TR, Schumacher JH, Street NF, Budd R, O'Garra A, Fong TAT, Bond MW, Moore KWM, Sher A, Fiorentino DF (1991): Diversity of cytokine synthesis and function of mouse CD4$^+$ T cells. Immunol Rev 123:209–229.

Nakamura M, Burastero SE, Ueki J, Larrick JW, Notkins AL, Casali P (1988): Probing the normal and autoimmune B cell repertoire with Epstein-Barr virus. J Immunol 141:4165–4172.

Prud'homme GJ, Balderas RS, Dixon FJH, Theofilopoulos AN (1983): B cell dependence on and response to accessory signals in murine lupus strains. J Exp Med 157:1815–1827.

Prud'homme GJ, Palfrey NA (1988): Biology of disease: Role of T helper lymphocytes in autoimmune diseases. Lab Invest 59:158–172.

Rajapolan S, Zordan T, Tsokos GC, Datta SK (1990): Pathogenic anti-DNA autoantibody-inducing T helper cell lines from patients with active lupus nephritis: Isolation of CD4$^-$8$^-$ T helper cell lines that express the $\gamma\delta$ T-cell antigen receptor. Proc Natl Acad Sci USA 87:7020–7024.

Rauch J, Murphy E, Roths JB, Stollar BD, Schwartz RS (1982): A high frequency idiotypic marker of anti-DNA autoantibodies in MRL-lpr/lpr mice. J Immunol 129:236–243.

Roitt IM (1991): Principles of autoimmunity. In Brostoff J, Scadding GK, Male D, Roitt IM (eds): "Clinical Immunology." New York: Gower Medical Publishing, pp 4.1–4.12.

Rosenberg YJ, Goldsmith PK, Ohara J, Steinberg AD, Ohriner W (1986): Ia antigen expression and autoimmunity in MRL-lpr/lpr mice. Ann NY Acad Sci 475:251–266.

Rousset F, Garcia E, Defrance T, Péronne C, Vezzio N, Hsu DH, Kastelein R, Moore KW, Banchereau J (1992): Interleukin 10 is a potent growth and differentiation factor for activated human B lymphocytes. Proc Natl Acad Sci USA 89:1890–1893.

Rozendaal L, Pals ST, Gleichmann E, Melief CJM (1990): Persistence of allospecific helper T cells is required for maintaining autoantibody formation in lupus-like graft-versus-host disease. Clin Exp Immunol 82:527–532.

Sainis K, Datta SK (1988): CD4$^+$ T cell lines with selective patterns of autoreactivity as well as CD4$^-$ CD8$^-$ T helper cell lines augment the production of idiotypes shared by pathogenic anti-DNA autoantibodies in the NZB × SWR model of lupus nephritis. J Immunol 140:2215–2224.

Santoro TJ, Portanova JP, Kotzin BL (1988): The contribution of L3T4$^+$ cells to lymphoproliferation and autoantibody production in MRL-lpr/lpr mice. J Exp Med 167:1713–1719.

Schurmans S, Brighouse G, Kramar G, Wen L, Izui S, Merino J, Lambert PH (1991): Transient T and B cell activation after neonatal induction of tolerance to MHC class II or Mls alloantigens. J Immunol 146:2152–2160.

Schurmans S, Heuser C, Qin HY, Merino J, Brighouse G, Lambert PH (1990): In vivo effects of anti-IL-4 monoclonal antibody on neonatal induction of tolerance and on associated autoimmune syndrome. J Immunol 145:2465–2473.

Seder RA, Le Gros G, Ben-Sasson SZ, Urban J, Finkelman FD, Paul WE (1991): Increased frequency of interleukin-4 producing T cells as a result of polyclonal priming. Use of a single-cell assay to detect interleukin-4 producing cells. Eur J Immunol 21:1241–1247.

Shirai T, Abe M, Yagita H, Okumura K, Morse HC, Davidson WF (1990): The expanded populations od CD4$^-$CD8$^-$ T cell receptor $\alpha\beta^+$ T cells associated with the lpr and gld mutations are CD2$^-$. J Immunol 144:3756–3761.

Shoenfeld Y, Isenberg DA, Rauch J, Madaio MP, Stollar BD, Schwartz RS (1983a): Idiotypic cross-reactions of monoclonal lupus autoantibodies. J Exp Med 158:718–730.

Shoenfeld Y, Rauch J, Massicotte H, Datta SK, Andre-Schwartz J, Stollar BD, Schwartz RS (1983b): Polyspecificity of monoclonal lupus antibodies produced by human-human hybridomas. N Engl J Med 308:414–420.

Simpson E, O'Hopp S, Harrison M, Mosier D, Melief K, Cantor H (1974): Immunological disease induced by injecting F$_1$ lymphoid cells into certain parental strains. Immunology 27:989–1007.

Steinberg AD, Krieg AM, Gourley MF, Klinman DM (1990): Theoretical and experimental approaches to generalized autoimmunity. Immunol Rev 118:129–163.

Streilein JW (1991): Neonatal tolerance of H-2 alloantigens. Procuring graft acceptance the "old-fashioned" way. Transplantation 52:1–10.

Sumida T, Yonaha F, Maeda T, Tanabe E, Koike T, Tomioka H, Yoshida S (1992): T cell receptor repertoire of infiltrating T cells in lips of Sjögren's syndrome patients. J Clin Invest 89:681–685.

Tada Y, Nagasawa K, Yamauchi Y, Tsukamoto H, Niho Y (1991): A defect in the protein kinase C system in T cells from patients with systemic lupus erythematosus. Clin Immunol Immunopathol 60:220–231.

Takahashi S, Nose M, Sasaki J, Yamamoto T, Kyogoku M (1991): IgG3 production in MRL/lpr mice is responsible for development of lupus nephritis. J Immunol 147:515–519.

Tebib JG, Alcocer-Varela J, Alarcon-Segovia D, Schur PH (1990). Association between a T cell receptor restriction fragment length polymorphism and systemic lupus erythematosus. J Clin Invest 86:1961–1967.

Theofilopoulos AN, Dixon FJ (1985): Murine models of systemic lupus erythematosus. Adv Immunol 37:269–390.

Theofilopoulos AN, Shawler DL, Eisenberg RA, Dixon FJ (1980): Splenic immunoglobulin secreting cells and their regulation in autoimmune mice. J Exp Med 158:446–466.

Tumang JR, Cherniack EP, Gietl DM, Cole BC, Russo C, Crow MK, Friedman SM (1991): T helper cell-dependent, microbial superantigen-induced murine B cell activation: Polyclonal and antigen-specific antibody responses. J Immunol 147:432–438.

Umland SP, Fei GO, Howard M (1989): Responses of B cells from autoimmune mice to IL-5. J Immunol 142:1528–1535.

Umland SP, Razac S, Nahrebne DK, Seymour BW (1992): Effects of in vivo administration of interferon (IFN)-γ, anti-IFN-γ, or anti-interleukin-4 monoclonal antibodies in chronic autoimmune graft-versus-host-disease. Clin Immunol Immunopathol 63:66–73.

Via CS (1991): Kinetics of T cell activation in acute and chronic forms of murine graft-versus-host disease. J Immunol 146:2603–2609.

Via CS, Shearer GM (1988): T-cell interactions in autoimmunity: Insights from a murine model of graft-versus-host disease. Immunol Today 9:207–213.

Volk HD, Kopp J, Korner J, Jahn S, Grunow R, Barthelmes H, Fiebig H (1986): Correlation between the phenotype and the functional capacity of activated T cells in patients with active systemic lupus erythematosus. Scand J Immunol 24:109–114.

Watanabe-Fukunaga R, Brannan CI, Copeland NG, Jenkins NA, Nagata S (1992): Lymphoproliferation in mice explained by defects in Fas antigen that mediates apoptosis. Nature 356:314–317.

Weston KM, Ju ST, Lu CY, Sy MS (1988): Autoreactive T cells in MRL/Mpr-lpr/lpr mice. Characterization of the lymphokines produced and analysis of antigen-presenting cells required. J Immunol 141:1941–1948.

Wofsy D, Seaman E (1985): Successful treatment of autoimmunity in NZB/W F₁ mice with monoclonal antibody to L3T4. Exp Med 161:378–391.

Yanagi Y, Hirose S, Nagasawa R, Shirai R, Mak TW, Tada T (1986): Does the deletion within T cell receptor beta chain gene of NZW mice contribute to autoimmunity in (NZB × NZW) F₁ mice? Eur J Immunol 16:1179–1182.

Yokoyama K, Gachelin G (1991): An abnormal signal transduction pathway in CD4⁻CD8⁻ double-negative lymph node cells of MRL: lpr/lpr mice. Eur J Immunol 21:2987–2992.

Zouali M, Fournié GJ, Théze J (1991): Quantitative clonal analysis of the B cell repertoire in human lupus. Cell Immunol 133:161–177.

Zouali M, Stollar BD, Schwartz RS (1988): Origin and diversification of anti-DNA antibodies. Immunol Rev 105:137–159.

26

IMMUNODEFICIENCY
AND AUTOIMMUNITY

Fred S. Rosen

*Department of Pediatrics, Harvard Medical School, The Center for Blood
Research and Children's Hospital, Boston, Massachussetts*

INTRODUCTION

Autoimmunity is a prominent feature of certain immunodeficiency states.
From another point of view it might be considered that all autoimmunity is an
expression of immunodeficiency. Jonathan Sprent insightfully noted that
autoimmunity results from an imbalance in the lymphocytes—when there are
too few or too many. X-linked agammaglobulinemia, which is the only pure
B-cell deficiency in humans, is not usually accompanied by autoimmunity.
On the other hand, patients with certain T-cell deficiencies such as the
hyper-IgM syndrome, the Wiskott-Aldrich syndrome, common variable immunodeficiency, and the DiGeorge anomaly frequently have autoimmune
complications. Infants affected with severe combined immunodeficiency do
not survive long enough to provide a record of the incidence of autoimmune
disease; they must be rescued with bone marrow transplants in order to
survive.

Rather surprisingly, deficiency of any of the classic components of the
complement system results in a high frequency of autoimmune disease.
Individuals with a genetically determined deficiency of C1 or C4 almost
invariably develop autoimmune disease. C2 deficiency and C1 inhibitor deficiency are also accompanied by autoimmune phenomena, but to a lesser

Autoimmunity: Physiology and Disease, Pages 423–432
© *1994 Wiley-Liss, Inc.*

extent than is observed in C1 or C4 deficiency. On the other hand, deficiencies of the terminal complement components or of the alternative pathway components are only rarely associated with autoimmune disease.

X-LINKED AGAMMAGLOBULINEMIA

Males affected with X-linked agammaglobulinemia (XLA) have undue susceptibility to recurrent pyogenic infections. Adequate prophylaxis is achieved by repeated intravenous infusions of gammaglobulin. Despite this, affected males exhibit T-cell hyperreactivity to drugs and certain environmental agents such as the toxin of poison ivy [Rosen et al., 1984]. No satisfactory explanation of this increased hypersensitivity has been forthcoming. It is conceivable that an immunosuppressive cytokine, such as interleukin (IL)-10, from B cells is insufficiently produced or that the immunosuppressive effects of anti-idiotypic antibodies are wanting, and this may explain the hypersensitivity. Recently a putative gene for XLA, a tyrosine kinase, was cloned, and this may lead to an understanding of the lymphobiology of XLA [Vetrie et al., 1993; Tsukada et al., 1993].

IMMUNODEFICIENCY WITH NORMAL OR ELEVATED IgM (HIGMX-1)

Of all the primary immunodeficiency syndromes, immunodeficiency with normal or elevated IgM (HIGMX-1) is most consistently associated with autoimmune disease. The underlying genetic cause of this syndrome has only recently been discovered, and this may ultimately provide interesting insights into the pathogenesis of autoimmunity.

HIGMX-1 was first described in male children [Rosen et al., 1961; Burtin, 1961] who had recurrent bacterial infections and exhibited a range of susceptibility to infection that resembled XLA. As a matter of fact, the first case of HIGMX-1 had been mistakenly reported among the first five males to be discovered with XLA. One striking observation among those affected with HIGMX-1 is the frequent occurrence of pneumonia due to *Pneumocystis carinii*. Chronic diarrhea is also a frequent feature of this syndrome, and it has been associated with *Cryptosporidium* infection in some instances. These unusual infections in HIGMX-1 have suggested that a T-cell deficiency may underlie this defect.

Seventy-eight percent of the cases of HIGM are encountered in male children in whom there is proved or presumptive evidence of X-linked inheritance. Other cases are associated with congenital rubella infection or hereditary ataxia telangiectasia. In some instances dominant inheritance of the defect has been shown, and in others the defect is acquired for unknown reasons [Notarangelo et al., 1992]. As is discussed below, the X-linked form of the disease is a heritable defect in the ligand for CD40, which is present on normal activated T cells. The cause of the defect is not yet known in the other non-X-linked forms in which the CD40 ligand appears to be expressed normally or at somewhat decreased levels.

By definition, the serum of patients with HIGMX-1 contains very little IgG, IgA, and IgE. On the other hand, the IgM level may be as high as 1,000 mg/dl. It is always polyclonal. Large amounts of 7S IgM monomers are usually present in the serum, and this may confound the measurement of the IgM level and give more elevated values than exist in reality. The IgD levels are also elevated, and this immunoglobulin class was first identified in the serum of a patient with this syndrome [Rowe and Fahey, 1965]. The IgM fraction contains very high titers of antibody to blood group substances, Forssman antigen, O antigens of gram-negative bacteria, and other lipopolysaccharide antigens.

Almost all patients with this syndrome develop, at one time or another, antibodies to the formed elements of the blood—to granulocytes, red cells, platelets, and lymphocytes, in decreasing order. The most common complication of the syndrome is cyclic neutropenia, but it is sometimes very difficult to detect antibodies to the granulocytes. There appears to be myeloid arrest in the bone marrow, and striking improvement in granulocyte counts have been noted with granulocyte-macrophage colony-stimulating factors. In rare cases lymphocytoxic antibodies cause severe lymphopenia, depressed cell-mediated immunity, and death from opportunistic infections. Tissue-specific antibodies are less frequently encountered in this syndrome, but there are reports of antithyroid antibodies and anticardiolipin antibodies in some cases.

The underlying basis of this syndrome, particularly of the X-linked form, has been perplexing for the past three decades, since the disease was first described. It appeared initially that there was some intrinsic defect in the B cells of these patients that resulted in the failure of isotype switching [Geha et al., 1979; Levitt et al., 1984]. B cells from patients with HIGMX-1, transformed with Epstein-Barr virus, maintained the phenotypic abnormality in long-term culture; the cells secreted only IgM [Schwaber et al., 1981]. Attempts to mix patients' B cells with allogeneic T cells failed to induce isotype switching [Geha et al., 1979]. However, it was subsequently found that the switch regions of the DNA in these patients was normal [Mayer et al., 1986]. Mayer et al. [1986] obtained malignant T cells from a woman with Sezary syndrome. Her activated, malignant T cells were capable of inducing isotype switching in almost a dozen different patients with the hyper-IgM syndrome. These results suggested, in a more definitive way, that the defect in this disease was due to an as yet undetermined factor from T cells.

HIGMX-1 was found to map to Xq24–27 [Mensinck et al., 1987]. In X-linked immunodeficiency diseases examination of the cells of obligate heterozygous females has been useful in determining which cell lineage is affected by the genetic defect, particularly when the defective gene is critical for the development of that cell lineage. For example, in female carriers of

XLA, only the B cells bearing the normal X will multiply and expand. Thus there is nonrandom inactivation of the X chromosome in B-cell populations; all the B cells have the normal X chromosome, and none have the abnormal chromosome. All other cell lines from such women have random X-chromosome inactivation, and this suggests that only the B-cell lineage is affected by the XLA gene. In an extension of these findings, it is apparent that X-linked severe combined immunodeficiency affects both the B and the T cells of obligate female heterozygotes. In the Wiskott-Aldrich syndrome all blood cell lineages are affected. In contrast to these findings, X-chromosome inactivation has been consistently found to be random in obligate female heterozygotes bearing the HIGMX-1 gene [Notarangelo et al., 1992]. These findings suggest that the defective gene is not critical for the development of the cell lineages involved, i.e., the T cells.

The recent discovery of the defect in HIGMX-1 came about from two different approaches, gene mapping and an understanding of the factors involved in isotype switching. CD40 is expressed on B cells and other antigen-presenting cells such as mononuclear phagocytes, follicular dendritic cells, and interdigitating cells. When a cDNA clone was obtained for CD40 it became apparent that it was a member of the tumor necrosis factor (TNF) receptor gene family, and this suggested that there should be a ligand from T cells with homology to TNF-α and -β. Indeed, such a ligand was found, and a cDNA clone was obtained [Hollenbaugh et al., 1992]. It is a membrane protein composed of 261 amino acid residues of type II, that is, the N terminus is cytoplasmic and the C terminus is extracellular. The CD40 ligand has significant homology with TNF-α and TNF-β, and all three proteins have costimulatory effects on B-cell growth. The CD40 ligand was mapped to Xq26.3–27.1 [Graf et al., 1992]. This map location immediately gave rise to the idea that this protein might be defective in HIGMX-1 [Aruffo et al., 1993].

From another approach, it was established that isotype switching to IgE synthesis and the formation of productive gene rearrangements for IgE mRNA production involves two signals, IL-4 and the CD40 ligand. When B cells from HIGMX-1 patients were stimulated with IL-4 and anti-CD40, normal IgE synthesis was induced in vitro. The patients' T cells could not provide this stimulus, and this suggested that the CD40 ligand was defective [Fuleihan et al., 1993]. When the CD40 ligand DNA was sequenced from two patients a 58 base pair deletion was found in one kindred (nucleotides 289–347), and a double mutation was found in the second kindred with a C to A mutation at nucleotide 590 and deletion of the C nucleotide at position 591 [Ramesh et al., 1993]. These findings leave little doubt that the genetic defect in HIGMX-1 is due to an abnormality of the CD40 ligand and provides a splendid opportunity to explore the importance of this molecule in immunity.

The CD40 ligand is expressed transiently on the surface of CD4$^+$ T lymphocytes when they are activated. (A soluble form of the molecule probably also exists.) This ligand acts as an important cofactor in B-cell growth and maturation. As pointed out, together with IL-4 it induces IgE synthesis.

Together with IL-10 and transforming growth factor (TGF)-β it induces IgA synthesis. Anti-CD40 induced the expression of the bcl-2 protein in germinal center B cells [Liu et al., 1991], and the activation of this oncogene (bcl-2) prevents apoptosis of B cells. A B-cell line in culture enters into programmed cell death after stimulation with anti-IgM. The apoptosis can be prevented with anti-CD40 monoclonal antibody [Valentine and Licciardi, 1992]. These observations present some paradoxes in view of what is known about the hyper-IgM syndrome. From the foregoing, it might be predicted that the IgM^+, IgD^+ B cells in these patients would undergo apoptosis. On the contrary there is exuberant lymphoid hyperplasia in these patients, and they often die from the proliferation of these IgM/IgD secreting cells. These IgM-producing plasma cells never undergo malignant transformation, but their proliferation can become so extensive as to have the effects of a malignancy.

It has been observed that administration of large amounts of gamma-globulin by the intravenous route depresses IgM synthesis in these patients. The usual commercial gammaglobulin preparations contain anti-idiotypic antibodies to public determinants on the IgM molecules. It is conceivable that these anti-idiotypes are inducing programmed cell death in the IgM^+ B cells of these patients.

Finally, the overwhelming propensity to produce autoantibodies to the formed elements of the blood in hyper-IgM syndrome suggest that the CD40–CD40 ligand interaction is critical to the induction of B-cell tolerance to these autoantigens.

COMMON VARIABLE IMMUNODEFICIENCY

Common variable immunodeficiency (CVID), formerly called *acquired agammaglobulinemia,* may be expressed in several variations. However, most of these patients have normal numbers of B lymphocytes that do not function normally; the reason for this is unknown. The most frequent age of onset of this immunodeficiency is in the second decade of life, but it may occur at any age and affects males and females equally. In addition to increased susceptibility to pyogenic infections there is a high frequency of autoimmune disease in this population. Approximately 50% of CVID patients develop pernicious anemia with chronic atrophic gastritis. Recently the auto-antibodies to the parietal cells have been shown to be directed against the proton pump. Patients with CVID lack antiparietal cell antibodies, and it remains to be shown if they have T-cell reactivity to this antigen [Gleeson and Toh, 1991]. Other organ-specific autoimmunity is encountered in these patients with great frequency. Curiously, first-degree relatives also have a high frequency of autoimmune disease and IgA deficiency. Furthermore CVID and IgA deficiency have been associated with the fixed MHC haplotype HLA-B8, HLA-DR3 and the complotype SC01, where S represents the slow form of factor B, C the common form of C2, 0 an absence of the C4A allele, and 1 the isoform of C4B. Thus there appears to be a spectrum of immunodeficiency from CVID at one end to isotype deficiencies at the other that are associated with the MHC [Schaffer et al., 1989; Alper et al., 1993]. It is not clear what genes in the MHC affect these immunodeficiencies. These patients have a subtle T-cell defect that is not completely understood and may be the underlying basis of their frequent autoimmune disease.

WISKOTT-ALDRICH SYNDROME

The Wiskott-Aldrich syndrome (WAS) is an X-linked simple Mendelian trait. The gene has been mapped to Xp11.22 [Kwan et al., 1991]. Affected males have the early onset of bloody diarrhea or excessive bleeding from other sites. Their platelets are small and very few in number. In infancy, affected males develop eczema. Subsequently they exhibit increasing susceptibility to opportunistic and pyogenic infections [Rosen et al., 1984].

The precise gene defect is not yet known. The white blood cells and platelets of affected males lack the major surface sialoglycoprotein CD43 [Remold and Rosen, 1990]. The gene encoding CD43 has been mapped to the short arm of chromosome 16 and thus is not the basic defect in the disease [Shelley et al., 1989]. The T cells and platelets of WAS patients are markedly abnormal as studied by scanning electron microscopy [Kenney et al., 1986]. T cells from WAS patients, maintained in long-term cell culture, are also grossly abnormal and exhibit blebbing, abnormal forms, aborted mitosis, and so forth [Molina et al., 1992]. Recently Yonemura et al. [1993] have shown that CD43, during cytokinesis, is colocalized in the cleavage furrow and is associated with actin filaments. From these findings, it appears that a cytoskeletal abnormality is present in the lymphocytes of WAS. The resulting T-cell defect is subtle and is manifest by failure of signal transduction to bring about normal T-cell activation (Molina et al., unpublished data).

Patients with WAS frequently make autoantibodies to the formed elements of the blood, particularly to platelets and B cells. Indeed, Brouet et al. [1980] found that seven of nine WAS patients made autoantibody to a subset of normal B cells. They also have a high incidence of chronic glomerulonephritis.

THE DiGEORGE ANOMALY

The DiGeorge anomaly is an embryonic field defect in the cephalic portion of the neural crest and the derivatives of the branchial pouches. The defect is congenital, but only rarely does it appear to be hereditary. As a result of the malformation, the facies are peculiar and marked by low-set ears, shortened filtrum of the upper lip, and hypertelorism. The thymus and the parathyroids are abnormally formed. Truncal defects of the heart result in tetralogy of Fallot, abnormalities of the aorta, and other cardiac abnormalities. In many cases there is monosomy of chromosome 10p or 22q. Neonatal tetany from hypocalcemia and the cardiac abnormalities frequently overwhelm what may be a subtle T-cell deficiency in these patients. Consequently open heart surgery and the administration of unirradiated blood leads to graft-versus-host disease. The T-cell deficiency may be very variable in affected infants [Hong, 1991].

The CD4/CD8 ratio in the DiGeorge anomaly is usually high, as there is a relative deficiency of CD8 cells [Reinherz et al., 1981]. Graves' disease and other autoimmune phenomena have been observed with increased frequency in the DiGeorge anomaly as the patients get older [Ham Pong et al., 1985].

DEFICIENCIES OF THE CLASSICAL COMPLEMENT COMPONENTS

The genes encoding the second (C2) and the fourth (C4) components of complement are located in the major histocompatibility complex. Heterozygous deficiency of C2 is found in 1%–1.5% of the normal population, and 1 in 10,000 individuals are homozygous for the deficiency. Lupus erythematosus, discoid lupus, dermatomyositis, Henoch-Schoenlein purpura, and glomerulonephritis are encountered with great frequency in the population deficient in C2. Among patients with lupus 5.9% are heterozygous for C2 deficiency, and among patients with juvenile rheumatoid arthritis 3.7% are heterozygous for C2 deficiency [Glass et al., 1976].

There are two sets of alleles for C4: C4A and C4B. As many as 35% of all populations do not express one of the four alleles, and 11% do not express two. Only 1% of the population does not express three alleles. The homozygous complete deficiency of C4 is thus very rare. Almost 20 individuals who totally lack C4 have been reported. These patients have an extraordinarily high incidence of lupus-like disease; they are usually ANA negative. Many have died, however, of immune complex disease and renal failure. They frequently have anti-SSA (Ro) antibodies but never anti-SSB (La) antibodies [Hauptmann et al., 1988].

The gene encoding C1q maps to the long arm of chromosome 1. The two genes encoding C1r and C1s are located at the terminus of the short arm of chromosome 12 and the deficiency of these two subcomponents usually occurs together. Of the two dozen patients reported with C1q or C1r and C1s deficiency almost all have had a lupus-like disease such as is encountered in C2 and C4 deficiencies [Reid, 1989].

C1 inhibitor deficiency is associated with the prominent symptoms of angioneurotic edema. Several of these patients have also been noted to have a lupus-like syndrome as is encountered in the other classic component deficiencies but at a much lower frequency than is encountered in C1, C2, and C4 deficiencies.

When these observations were first made they were quite surprising because it was not anticipated that the classic complement pathway played such a vital role in preventing immune complex disease. It became apparent that large immune complexes were destroyed by complement and that the classic pathway was critical to the uptake of these complexes by complement receptor 1 (CR1) [Schifferli et al., 1986]. In this regard it has been observed that patients with classic forms of lupus have a deficiency of CR1, and the reasons for this appear to be complex [Kazatchkine and Fearon, 1990]. Efficient antibody formation is dependent on the classic pathway. C4-deficient guinea pigs do not respond to ϕX 174 unless they are reconstituted with C4A; C4B has no effect [Finco et al., 1992].

REFERENCES

Alper CA, Marcus-Bagley D, Awdeh Z, Kruskall MS, Eisenbarth GS, Brink SJ, Katz AJ, Hauser SL, Ahmed AR, Bing DH, Yunis EJ, Schur PH (1993): Many individuals who carry the [HLA-B8, SC01, DR3] conserved extended haplotype have immunoglobulin deficiencies. Submitted.

Aruffo A, Farrington M, Hollenbaugh D, et al. (1993): The CD40 ligand, gp39, is defective in activated T cells from patients with X-linked hyper-IgM syndrome. Cell 72:291–300.

Brouet JC, Grillot-Courvalin C, Seligmann M (1980): Human antibody reacts with a B-cell subset in man to induce B-cell differentiation. Nature 283:668–669.

Burtin P (1961): Un example d'agammaglobulinemie atypique (un cas de grande hypogammaglobulinemie avec augmentation de la beta2-macroglobuline). Rev Fr Etud Clin Biol 6:286–289.

Finco O, Li S, Cuccia M, Rosen FS, Carroll MC (1992): Structural differences between the two human complement C4 isotypes affect the humoral immune response. J Exp Med 176:867–874.

Fuleihan R, Ramesh N, Loh R, Jabara H, Rosen FS, Chatila T, Fu SM, Stamenkovic I, Geha RS (1993): Defective expression of the CD40 ligand in X-linked immunoglobulin deficiency with normal or elevated IgM (HIGMX-1). Proc Natl Acad Sci USA 90:2170–2173.

Geha RS, Hyslop N, Alami S, Farah F, Schneeberger EE, Rosen FS (1979): Hyper immunoglobulin M immunodeficiency (dysgammaglobulinemia). J Clin Invest 64:385–391.

Glass D, Raum D, Gibson D, Stillman JS, Schur P (1976): Inherited deficiency of the second component of complement: Rheumatic disease association. J Clin Invest 58:853–861.

Gleeson PA, Toh B-H (1991): Molecular targets in pernicious anemia. Immunol Today 12:233–238.

Graf D, Korthauer U, Mages HW, Senger G, Kroczek RA (1992): Cloning of TRAP, a ligand for CD40 on human T cells. Eur J Immunol 22:3191–3194.

Ham Pong AJ, Cavallo A, Holman GH, Goldman AS (1985): Di George syndrome: Long term survival complicated by Grave's disease. J Pediatr 106:619–620.

Hauptmann G, Tappeiner G, Schifferli JA (1988): Inherited deficiency of the fourth component of complement. Immunodef Rev 1:3–22.

Hollenbaugh D, Grosmaire LS, Kullas CD, Chalupny NJ, Braesch-Andersen S, Noelle RJ, Stamenkovic I, Ledbetter JA, Aruffo A (1992): The human T cell antigen gp39, a member of the TNF gene family, is a ligand for the CD40 receptor: Expression of a soluble form of gp39 with B cell costimulatory activity. EMBO J 11:4313–4321.

Hong R (1991): The DiGeorge anomaly. Immunodef Rev 3:1–4.

Kazatchkine MD, Fearon DT (1990): Deficiencies of human C3 complement receptors type 1 (CR1, CD35) and type 2 (CR2, CD21). Immunodeficiency Rev 2:17–42.

Kenney DM, Cairns L, Remold-O'Donnell E, Peterson J, Rosen FS, Parkman R (1986): Morphological abnormalities in the lymphocytes of patients with Wiskott-Aldrich syndrome. Blood 68:1329–1332.

Kwan S-P, Lehner T, Hagemann T, Lu B, Blaese M, Ochs H, Wedgwood R, Ott J, Craig I, Rosen FS (1991): Localization of the gene for the Wiskott-Aldrich syndrome between two flanking markers TIMP and DXS255 on Xp11.22–11.3. Genomics 10:29–33.

Levitt D, Haver P, Rich K, Cooper MD (1984): Hyper IgM immunodeficiency. A primary dysfunction of B lymphocytes isotype switching. J Clin Invest 72:1650–1657.

Liu Y-J, Mason DY, Johnson GD, Abbot S, Gregory CD, Hardie DL, Gordon J, MacLennan ICM (1991): Germinal center cells express bel-2 protein after activation by signals which prevent their entry into apoptosis. Eur J Immunol 21:1905–1910.

Mayer L, Kwan S-P, Thompson C, Ko HS, Chiorazzi N, Waldmann T, Rosen FS (1986): Evidence for a defect in "switch" T cells in patients with immunodeficiency and hyperimmunoglobulinemia M. N Engl J Med 314:409–413.

Mensinck EJBM, Thompson A, Sandkuyl LA, Kraakman MEM, Schot JDL, Espanol T, Schuurman RKB (1987): X-linked immunodeficiency with hyperimmunoglobulinemia M appears to be linked to the DXS42 restiction fragment length polymorphism locus. Hum Genet 76:96–99.

Molina IJ, Kenney DM, Rosen FS, Remold-O'Donnell E (1992): T cell lines characterize events in the pathogenesis of the Wiskott-Aldrich syndrome. J Exp Med 176:867–874.

Notarangelo LN, Duse M, Ugazio AG (1992): Immunodeficiency with hyper-IgM. Immunodef Rev 3:101–122.

Ramesh N, Fuleihan R, Ramesh V, Sharma S, Rosen FS, Geha RS (1993): Deletions in the ligand for CD40 in X-linked immunoglobulin deficiency with normal or elevated IgM (HIGMX-1). International Immunol 5(7):769–773.

Reid KBM (1989): Deficiency of the first component of human complement. Immunodef Rev 1:247–260.

Reinherz EL, Cooper MD, Schlossman SF, Rosen FS (1981): Abnormalities of T cell maturation and regulation in human beings with immunodeficiency disorders. J Clin Invest 68:699–705.

Remold-O'Donnell E, Rosen FS (1990): Sialophorin (CD43) and the Wiskott-Aldrich syndrome. Immunodef Rev 2:151–174.

Rosen FS, Cooper MD, Wedgwood RJP (1984): The primary immunodeficiencies. I. N Engl J Med 311:235–242.

Rosen FS, Kevy SV, Merler E, Janeway CA, Gitlin D (1961): Recurrent bacterial infections and dysgammaglobulinemia: Deficiency of 7S gammaglobulins in the presence of elevated 19S gamma-globulins. Pediatrics 28:182–195.

Rowe DS, Fahey J (1965): A new class of human immunoglobulins: Normal serum IgD. J Exp Med 121:185–199.

Schaffer FM, Palermos J, Zhu ZB, Berger BO, Cooper MD, Volanakis JE (1989): Individuals with IgA deficiency and common variable immunodeficiency share polymorphisms of the major histocompatibility complex class III genes. Proc Natl Acad Sci USA 86:8015–8019.

Schifferli JA, Ng YC, Peters DK (1986): The role of complement and its receptor in the elimination of immune complexes. N Engl J Med 315:488–495.

Schwaber JF, Lazarus H, Rosen FS (1981): IgM restricted production of immuno-globulin by lymphoid cell lines from patients with immunodeficiency with hyper IgM (dysgammaglobulinemia). Clin Immunol Immunpathol 29:91–97.

Shelley CS, Remold-O'Donnell E, Davis AE III, Bruns GAP, Rosen FS, Carroll MC, Whitehead AS (1989): Molecular characterization of sialophorin (CD43), the lymphocyte surface sialoglycoprotein defective in Wiskott-Aldrich syndrome. Proc Natl Acad Sci USA 86:2819–2823.

Tsukuda S, Saffran DC, Rawlings DJ, Parolini O, Allen RC, Klisak I, Sparkes RS, Kubagawa H, Mohandas T, Quan S, Belmont JW, Cooper MD, Conley ME, Witte ON (1993): Deficient expression of a B cell cytoplasmic tyrosine kinase in human X-linked agammaglobulinemia. Cell 72:279–290.

Valentine MA, Licciardi KA (1992): Rescue from anti-IgM-induced programmed cell death by the B cell surface proteins CD20 and CD40. Eur J Immunol 22:3141–3148.

Vetrie D, Vorechovsky I, Sideras P, Sideras P, Holland J, Davies A, Flinter F, Hammarstrom L, Kinnon C, Levinsky P, Bobrow M, Smith CIE, Bentley DR (1993): The gene involved in X-linked agammaglobulinemia is a member of the src family of protein-tyrosine kinases. Nature 361:226–233.

Yonemura S, Nagafuchi A, Sato N, Tsukita S (1993): Concentration of an integral membrane protein, CD43 (leukosialin, sialophorin), in the cleavage furrow through the interaction of its cytoplasmic domain with actin-based cytoskeletons. J Cell Biol 120:437–449.

27

AUTOIMMUNITY TOMORROW

Antonio Coutinho and Michel D. Kazatchkine

*Unité d'Immunobiologie, Institut Pasteur (A.C.); Unité d'Immunopathologie,
Hôpital Broussais (M.D.K.), Paris, France*

Autoimmunity today continues to be a set of questions, embodying many doubts and alternatives. It is possible today for equally serious scientists to express quite opposite opinions on very basic issues. In our minds, however, the very fact that conventional views currently are questioned is already an index of progress, for this will stimulate reflection and debate and hopefully a more critical analysis of ideas and experiments that otherwise would be accepted readily, as has been the case in the past. This was precisely our original intention when choosing the topics and the authors for this volume.

It is difficult to predict the directions that a rapidly moving area will take tomorrow; here we present some of the possible scenarios in basic and clinical research in autoimmunity and autoimmune disease. We define autoimmune disease as a set of sustained organ-specific or systemic clinical symptoms and signs associated with altered immune homeostasis that is manifested by qualitative and/or quantitative defects of expressed autoimmune repertoires. Regardless of the nature of the triggering events—e.g., microbial infection, tissue damage, primary immunodeficiency—the defect in selecting appropriate immune repertoires is the failure of basic mechanisms that ensure homeostasis of molecular shapes (configurations) in a healthy individual. A major difficulty with autoimmune disease continues to be the fact that we are unable to recognize those failures (i.e., to identify

Autoimmunity: Physiology and Disease, Pages 433–437
© *1994 Wiley-Liss, Inc.*

altered immune repertoires) before the target structure or its function is damaged beyond possibilities for restoration by immune intervention. Thus, in contrast to other areas in modern medicine, this results in our current inability to provide prophylaxis and successful immunological treatment of the autoimmune patient. That is to say, even if we had appropriate and efficacious treatments for autoimmune disease, we could not use them optimally, for we lack diagnostic tools and criteria for presymptomatic immunological alterations of autoimmune disease.

In a clonal perspective of disease, it is obviously impossible to recognize immune dysfunction when the disease is "only immunological," since this would require a search for all putatively altered reactivities to any body component. On the other hand, systemic views, advocating that alterations in the structure or dynamic behavior of any component necessarily will reflect on many others, predict that it should be possible to identify signs of repertoire alterations, provided that the appropriate means for global analysis are available. As circulating natural antibodies represent the totality of the operation of the immune system, it is possible that appropriate study of the reactivities and/or kinetics of natural autoantibodies will bring new, as yet unsuspected, possibilities for diagnosis. We refer to the analyses of epitope specificities, of antibody diversity and mutual interactions, rather than the genetic and molecular structure of "isolated" antibody molecules. Thus, as repeatedly discussed in several sections of this volume, the extensive work on "structure–function" correlates of V regions has yielded little: Similar reactivities may be encoded by a variety of genetic elements, and, conversely, the same genes may be used in the construction of V regions with quite different functional properties. If immune repertoires and dynamics exist at equilibrium with the somatic self, it also follows that the potential diagnostic value of natural autoantibody analyses would help to identify other dysfunctions in the body. In our view, this is one of the identifiable areas in which research is urgently needed.

On the experimental side, one of the current problems is the unavailability of animal models of induced chronic autoimmune disease. In most available systems, the initial symptomatic phase following immunization rapidly and spontaneously remits into a phase of increased resistance to disease induction when the same protocol is repeated. In other words, a normal individual shows a remarkable ability to control pathogenic autoreactivities, even when these are specifically and forcefully activated experimentally. This is probably why that individual is normal to start with! It would appear, therefore, that autoimmune disease indeed results from the breakdown of this competence, and this is actually what we are most interested in understanding. In other words, experimental models should probably aim primarily at identifying the humoral and cellular mechanisms that confer resistance and/ or transient expression of autoimmune disease in healthy individuals, rather than pursuing the dissection of autoreactive clones and their effector functions. Thus the current preoccupation with the mechanisms of tissue destruction can only be useful for the design of symptomatic therapies. In addition, current efforts to identify putative autoantigens and the ways by which these may drive abnormal clonal expansions can only be of curative therapeutic potential if these are based on the postulate that autoantigens in autoimmune disease are structurally altered. In this view, the immune system of an autoimmune patient is normal: Autoimmune disease would actually be an autoantigen disease.

The fact that the course of autoimmune disease characteristically exhibits intercalating exacerbations and remissions or complete recovery indicates that associated symptoms, or the disease itself, may resolve through the activity of the immune system, even after periods of profound dysfunction. This indicates that autoimmune disease may be appropriately corrected by natural immunological "reagents" that participate in the selection of structural and functional V region repertoires under physiological conditions. To us, this also indicates that the future of autoimmune disease therapy is on the utilization of normal components of the system (or appropriate substitutes) rather than on further refined immunosuppressive measures. This view is compatible with a general tendency in modern medical practice to restore health by strategies developed from the understanding of physiology and using biological components, rather than by combating disease with empirically derived active drugs. This is particularly pertinent to autoimmune disease. Thus, unless one is a strong believer in forbidden clones, it is difficult to conceive of a single drug that will restore the fine intricacies of a complex system's operation. Furthermore, if autoimmune disease is associated with a failure in mechanisms controlling an underlying, potentially pathogenic autoreactivity, the indiscriminate utilization of immunosuppressive therapies may aggravate disease, even if symptomatic improvement can be obtained in the short term. Actually, if autoimmune disease is a primary or secondary immune deficiency, then the general strategy of therapy should be substitution or restoration of normal immunocompetence.

An area that likely will be active in the future thus should be the search for reagents and interventions aimed at immune restoration through biological means. This constitutes a wide spectrum of possibilities, ranging from bone marrow transplantation to single cytokine administration. The increasing use of IVIg for the treatment of autoimmune disease in the last 10 years constitutes the first and best example of these new strategies. The fact that such preparations contain 1) specific components reactive with the clonal products directly implicated in the pathogenic process, 2) a very large V-region diversity that optimally addresses the level of complexity required for the system's restoration, and 3) structures that might account for other modifications in the recipient (e.g., Fc-mediated anti-inflammatory effects) make them therapies with multiple potentialities. Thus far, the diversity in IVIg preparations and the doses utilized in clinical practice seem to cover discretely the limitations in our current understanding of the pathogenesis of autoimmune disease. However, for network views of IVIg action in autoimmune disease, it is actually essential that such large "nonspecific" pools are used. Ironically for those who aim at component analyses, however, such treatments possibly will only work as long as we do not attempt to develop new preparations enriched for the "appropriate" antibodies. It is likely, we think, that "second generation" therapeutic immunoglobulin preparations will in any case include a wide V-region repertoire, possibly selectively enriched in those "connected" immunoglobulin molecules that are directly involved in controlling, and that result from, the activity of the autoimmune network. This emerging notion of connectivity is indeed an important concept for the global organization of immune components that provides for natural tolerance. We would not be surprised if future therapeutic interventions in autoimmune disease aim predominantly at reestablishing physiological connectivity.

We believe that regulation of T-cell effector function or, more generally, class regulation of immune activities should be another area for targeted research efforts. Already by the 1970s it was established that cell-mediated reactions are opposed polarly to simultaneous antibody responses. More recently, the concept of two distinguishable classes of T-cell effector functions has been established and rapidly adopted in models aimed at explaining the origin of autoimmune disease. This oversimplification notwithstanding, that autoimmune disease can be classified into two groups (Th1 and Th2) of diseases is important, first of all from the conceptual point of view. Thus, autoreactivity, rather than normally being deleted or inactivated, is now accepted as physiologic, provided that class regulation controls effector functions into nonaggressive types. If ontogenic development and/or local conditions of activation of autoreactive cells impose and maintain nonaggressive effector functions, autoimmune disease could represent the failure of this type of regulation. This hypothesis is compatible with the experimental possibility of inducing autoimmune disease symptoms in healthy individuals, because disease induction would correspond to deviation in class regulation of productive autoreactivities present in normal individuals. The concept of class regulation also has implications for therapeutic strategies. Given that the process of class regulation relies on positive feedback loops (previous or concomitant Th1 or Th2 activities lead to reinforcement of the respective class), it is conceivable to envisage a rationale for "vaccination against autoimmune disease" by imposing the nonaggressive type of response. This opens novel, active strategies in therapeutics of autoimmune disease that go beyond the specific antiidiotypic immunity against the "pathogenic clones" that has been attempted thus far.

On a highly speculative basis, one may conceive that "autoimmunity tomorrow" could extend the field of immunointervention beyond that of autoimmune disease. Thus if the immune system exists at equilibrium with all other structures in the body, and if natural antibodies contribute to molecular complementarities in the organism, it follows that dysfunctions in other biological systems (coagulation, hormonal, neuronal, and so forth) might be corrected by manipulating the dynamics of expression and production of specific sets of natural antibodies. This cannot be done by conventional immunization and specific immune responses, since the respective dynamics are not at equilibrium, and since current protocols for immunization have been developed for provoking aggressive effector functions. If we knew, however, how to alter the concentrations and /or the oscillatory dynamics of natural antibodies, it would be conceivable that we would be in a position to compensate for an excess of a hormone or a deficit in a particular receptor expression. In other words, the future of clinical immunology could include the possibility of using the immune system to correct diseases that are not of an immunological nature.

INDEX

ABO histoblood group
  B cell tolerance and, 182, 183–184
  IgM-elevated immunodeficiency
      and, 425
Abortion, clonal, 191
Acanthosis nigricans, 131, 135
Acetylcholine receptors, 108
  and disease, 131, 268–283, 286–290
  See also Myasthenia gravis
Acinar cells, 212
Actin, 109
Acute phase proteins, 14
Addison's disease, 131, 219
Adhesion molecule(s), 14, 327–328
  blockade, 387
  retinal antigens and, 378, 383, 385
Adjuvant arthritis, 378
Adjuvants
  basic protein, 14, 204
  self-nonself nondifferention of,
      14–15
  See also Infection
Adrenalitis, 219
  autoantibodies, 212
  endocrine function and, 318
Adrenergic receptors, 277
Adrenocortical cells, 212
Affinity maturation, 29
Aging
  natural autoantibodies and, 112–113
  organ-specific disease and, 219, 220
  thymus and, 162
AIDS, cytomegalovirus retinitis and,
      391
  See also Immunodeficiency
Albumin, 109

Amino acids
  antigen receptor genes and, 29–30,
      37–38, 272–274
  peptide binding and, 36–38, 272,
      340–343
  thyroglobulin and, 316
Anchor residues, 36
Anemia, hemolytic, 131, 135
  and B cell anergy, 182
  CD5 B cells and, 96
  chaos-type unpredictability and, 185
  germline V genes and, 176
  pharmacological triggers, 367
Anemia, pernicious, 131, 204, 217, 219,
      318
  immunodeficiency and, 427–428
Anergy
  B cell, 182, 184
  clonal, 4, 40, 97, 198–199, 229
  peripheral T cell, 161–169, 191–199,
      366, 369, 371
  self-tolerance and, 14, 184, 205–212
  T cell, 40, 132, 170, 184, 191–199
Animals, laboratory
  B-1 cell population in, 59, 60–61,
      65–69, 76
  disease inducement in, 131, 136,
      150–151, 197–198, 204,
      214–215, 217, 248–252,
      269–280, 339–348, 354–360,
      370
  foreign antigens and, 13, 14, 131,
      193–194
  and gene manipulation, 60, 148,
      196–197
  germ-free, 244

Ig-secreting cells and, 53–54, 110, 182, 408
lymphocyte activation in, 46, 50, 51, 62–69, 94–99, 148, 152–153, 217
and lymphocyte population(s), 143–146, 148, 150–151, 162–168
myasthenia gravis and, 269–280
ocular experiments and, 377–391
and rheumatoid factor, 248–252
and severe combined immunodeficiency (SCID), 65, 98, 149, 165, 167
T cell expression and, 162–168, 204, 217, 340–343
thyroiditis in, 340–343
Torpedo receptor and, 275
vaccination, 389
Ankylosing spondylitis, 36
Anterior chamber associated immune deviation (ACAID), 380–381, 384, 385, 389–390
Antiacetylcholine receptor (AChR) antibodies, 22
Antibodies
  acetylcholine receptors and, 268–295
  anti-idiotypic, 20, 97, 136–138, 273–274, 276, 280–286, 283–286, 288, 289, 292, 293, 307–308, 311, 321, 330, 342–346, 348, 388–389, 424
  antineutrophil cytoplasm (ANCA), 307–311
  B cells and, 14–15, 20, 48, 50–54, 57–80, 89–102, 107–120, 175, 179–182, 282
  connective, 94–99, 135
  disease and, 131–132, 175, 177–178, 180–182, 268, 342–346, 348
  foreign antigens and, 12, 16, 109–110, 130–138, 181, 182
  germline genes and, 19–30, 51, 61, 73–76, 176, 253, 280
  and light chain mutation, 26–29
  monoclonal, 51, 70, 101, 108–109, 109–111, 113–114, 194, 248–252, 254–258, 273–274, 276, 280–286, 292–294, 340–343, 340–348, 387

monoreactive, 77–78
myasthenia gravis, 273, 274–280, 285–295
natural, 58, 62, 69–72, 89–102, 107–120, 176, 237
polyreactive, 22, 58, 69, 71, 77–79, 109–111, 176, 177–178, 184, 250–252
production of, 46–52, 57–80, 89–102, 130–138, 175, 179–182, 237, 268–295
thyroidism and, 342–346, 348
thyroid microsomal (antithyroid peroxidase), 321
See also Autoantibodies
Anticoagulation disease(s), 135, 408
Anti-DNA antibodies, 30, 61, 110, 114, 132, 176, 178, 408
Antigen-presenting cells (APC), 47, 109, 174, 333
  adhesion molecules and, 327–328, 383, 385
  anergic T cells and, 194
  autoreactive lymphocytes and, 183–185, 230–239, 327–331, 408
  hormone-producing cells and, 324–327
  self-reactive T cells and, 204, 215, 217–220
  suppression and, 383, 389–391
  x-linked immunodeficiency and, 426
Antigen(s)
  ABO histoblood group, 180, 182
  acetycholine receptors and, 272–274, 276–277
  allergic encephalomyelitis, 354–360
  antibody production and, 58, 61, 76–79, 108–109, 131–132, 176
  antithymocyte surface, 61
  autoantibodies and, 26–29, 108, 109, 131–132, 134–136, 177–178
  basic protein adjuvants and, 14, 109, 204
  B cell activation and, 46–47, 48–49, 76–79, 180
  cell-surface-, 212
  and homunculus organization, 15
  myelin basic protein, 354–360
  nuclear, 407–408

organ-specific disease and, 204,
217–220, 221, 378–396
primal immune system and, 11
reactivity, 4, 76–79, 91–102,
108–120, 131–132, 192–195,
217–220, 272–274, 357–359,
389–391
recognition, 12, 13, 14–15, 16, 20,
108–109, 183–184, 217–220,
318, 378–385, 389–391, 393
retinal, 378–379, 380–381, 389–391,
393–394
self-nonself recognition of, 12–16,
58, 61, 77–79, 109–111, 131,
136–138, 192, 217–220
system interpretation of, 13–15, 16,
192
T cells and, 35–40, 46–47, 108, 132,
161, 161–169, 166–169,
173–174, 175, 181, 192–195,
217–220, 272–274
See also Autoantigen(s); Foreign
antigen(s); Self-antigen(s)
Antimyelin-associated glycoprotein, 114
Antineutrophil cytoplasm antibodies
(ANCA), 307–311
Antirabies virus antibodies, 178
Antithyroglobulin (Tg) antibodies, 22,
112, 131
and B cell production, 176
cross-reactive idiotypes and,
114–115
Arthritis. See Adjuvant arthritis;
Rheumatoid arthritis
Ataxia telangectasia, 131, 424
Autoantibodies
acetylcholine receptors and,
267–272, 274–295
anti-idiotypic, 136–138, 230,
276–280, 285–287, 291,
307–311, 342–346, 348
characterization of, 22–26, 91–102,
107–120, 134–138, 176, 244,
267–272, 274–295
disease and, 22–25, 73–76, 99–101,
109, 114–115, 131–132,
134–136, 176, 177–178,
180–182, 212, 214–215,
267–295, 307–311, 407–409
dysteological, 3

gene function and, 19–22, 26–30,
68–69, 73–76, 89–102,
214–215, 274, 409–413
Ig and, 61, 66, 89–102, 108, 109–111,
114, 115–116, 175–176, 178,
180, 181, 247–248, 274, 408
mutation of, 26–29
natural, 107–120, 134–136, 176
pathogenetic, 136–137, 409–411
polyreactive, 109–111, 250–252, 408
production of, 61, 66, 67, 68–69, 70,
72, 73, 89–102, 108–111,
113–114, 130–138, 180, 181,
212, 214–215, 248–252,
254–258, 274–295, 370,
407–409
regulatory function of, 134–136
See also Autoreactivity, antibody;
individual antibody type by
name
Autoantigen(s)
acetylcholine receptors and, 271,
273, 274–280, 285–295
hyper-IgM syndrome and, 427
lymphocyte clone specificity and,
3–4, 11
T cell autoreactivity and, 39–40, 369
thyroid function and, 318–320,
342–346, 348
v-region genes and, 243–246
See also Self-antigens
Autocrine stimulation, 40
Autoimmune
polyendocrinopathy-candidiasis-
ectodermal dystrophy
(APECED), 220
Autoimmunity, 433–437
acetylcholine receptors and, 267–295
antigen recognition and, 15–16, 132,
136–137, 174–185, 354–358
autoantibody production and, 20–30,
22–26, 73–76, 109, 130–138,
176, 177–178, 180–182, 212,
267–295
cellular competition model and,
152–154
disease [types] and, 16, 22, 73, 109,
131–132, 135, 152–154,
173–185, 205–221, 318–321,
340–348, 365–372, 407–416

idiotypic network and, 136–138,
191–192, 229–239, 273,
274–280, 285–295, 340–348,
388–389, 424
IgG infusion and, 290–292
IgM and, 424–427
immunodeficiency and, 423–430
ocular, 377–397
peripheral anergy and, 170, 191–198,
214–215, 369–372
thymus and, 145, 150, 162–164,
192–195, 203–221
thyroid function and, 318–320,
332–333, 339–348
v-region genes and, 243–246,
354–358, 360
Autoreactivity, antibody, 20–30,
107–120, 243–246, 288
anergy and, 182, 184, 191–199, 366
B cells and, 91–102, 107–120, 132,
173, 174–185, 244, 366, 415
disease and, 100–101, 114, 131–132,
135, 137, 173–185, 204–221,
229–230, 237, 239, 379–380,
414–416
gene abnormalities and, 217–220,
415
healthy individuals and, 108–109,
114, 204, 229, 379–380
historical theories and, 3–5
idiotypic network and, 136–138,
191–192, 229–239, 273,
274–280, 285–295, 342–346,
348, 388–389
light chain genes and, 22–25, 30
myasthenia gravis and, 268, 268–295
T cell expression and, 173–174, 175,
184, 191–199, 204–221, 246,
273–274, 366–372, 379–380,
414–416
thyroidism and, 342–346, 348
v-gene segments and, 243–246
See also Autoantibodies
Azoospermia, 131

B-1 (CD5$^+$) cells, 57–80
antibody specificity and, 61–62, 66,
67, 68–69, 72, 73, 78–79,
178–179

and B cell ontogeny, 112, 134
distribution of, 100
natural autoantibodies and, 111,
178–179
origin of, 58–69, 77–79
Bacterium
antibody production and, 58
and antigen recognition, 13, 14–15
B cell induction and, 48–49, 99,
413–414
enteric, 13
gram-negative, 425
and heat shock proteins, 174
mycobacterium laprae, 16
streptococci, 13
and thyroid autoantigens, 326
Basic protein (BP), 13, 16
adjuvants, 14, 204
immunization, 204
B cell(s)
anergy, 182, 184
and antibody production, 14, 30, 46,
52, 57, 61–62, 66, 67, 68–69,
72, 73, 78–79, 89–102,
107–120, 177–184, 282, 307
autoreactivity, 111–120, 132,
151–154, 173, 174–184, 244,
250, 250–251, 318, 366–367,
371, 407–409, 413–414, 415
B-1 CD5$^+$ clonotypes, 57–80, 111
culture assays, 174–175
differentiation, 47, 52, 65, 68–69,
89–102, 134, 150–151
environmental pathogens and, 366
Epstein-Barr virus and, 22, 108,
118–119, 175, 408
foreign antigens and, 12, 14–15, 20,
173, 174–184, 180, 181
generation of, 20, 46–52, 65–69,
77–79, 90–100, 107–120,
145–151
and Grave's disease, 323–324
in healthy individuals, 4, 46, 60–61,
108–109, 114, 132, 307
lifespan, 53, 145, 146–151
in lymphoid organs, 20, 132, 150
and natural autoantibodies, 107–120,
408
polyclonal, 175, 407–409

population(s), 143–146, 151–154
receptors, 4, 12, 20, 52, 59, 68–69,
    108
rheumatoid factor and, 248, 250
selectivity, 154, 177–184, 407–416
stimulation of, 45–54, 92–102, 154,
    250–251
and T cell interaction, 51, 69, 77,
    152, 175, 181, 182, 183, 184,
    340–343, 366–367, 413–414
thymus-independent antigens and,
    48–49
thyroiditis and, 340–343
tissue distribution of, 60–61
tolerance induction and, 38,
    107–120, 151–154, 177–184
types and subsets, 46–47, 48, 49–50,
    57–80, 94–99, 111, 134,
    151–154
x-linked immunodeficiency and,
    423, 426–427
Bee venom phospholipase, 182
Behcet's disease, 391
Bernard, Claude, 203
Bible [Genesis], 10
Binarism, 133–134, 139
Biopsy, retinal, 391–392
Blast cells, 46–47
    lipopolysaccharides and, 49–50
Blastogenesis, 59
Blocking antibody, 15
Blocking antigen, 14–15
Blood cells
    acetylcholine receptors and, 281
    adhesion molecules and, 319, 383,
        385
    and antiplatelet antibodies, 132
    gene defect and, 428
    lupus autoantibodies and, 408
    peripheral mononuclear, 273
    polyreactive antibodies and, 112
    retinal antigens and, 379
    T cell populations and, 161, 168
    See also ABO blood groups
Blood-retinal barrier, 378, 379,
    381–384, 392
Bone marrow
    B-1 cells and, 65, 77
    B cells and, 20, 49–50, 52, 59

lymphocyte production and,
    145–146, 150
transplantation, 59, 169, 197, 210,
    423
Brain, 391
    and boundary interpretation, 15–16
    lesions, 353–354, 361
Bromelain, proteolytic enzyme, 61
Burkitt-type lymphoma, 75
    See also Lymphoma(s)
Burnetian clonal selection, 229, 237
    See also Clonal selection theory

C3 nephritic factors (C3NeF), 22
Cancer, 219
    See also Malignancy
Cardiac abnormalities, 219
    See also Heart
Cataracts, 219
Causality paradigms, 5
    autoantibodies and, 134–136,
        267–295
    genetic abnormalities and, 216–220,
        424–428
    and myasthenia gravis, 267–268
    self vs. nonself, 12, 130–138, 348
    thyroid activity and, 315–333,
        340–348
CD4-TH1 T cells, 14
    and Grave's disease, 321, 322,
        329–331
    and IgG infusion, 290–292
    monoclonal antibodies and, 292–294
    peripheral tolerance and, 205–212
    retinal antigens and, 377, 394
    See also T cells
CD4-Th2 T cells, 14
    See also T cells
CD8 T cells, 14
    and diabetes mellitus, 365–372
    See also T cells
Cell type specificity
    acetylcholine receptors and,
        272–274, 281–283
    antibodies and, 131–132, 178–184
    B cell transformation, 22, 38, 47–54,
        67–69, 92–102, 107–120,
        152–153, 177–184, 340–343,
        366, 407–416

division/maturity, 146–149, 168–169, 219, 414–416
gene abnormalities and, 217–220
infection triggers and, 14–15, 36, 217–220, 318–320, 365–372
integrated unity and, 139, 152–153
and lifespan, 46, 53, 145, 146–151, 168–169
and lymphocyte population(s), 143–146, 151–154, 161–170, 205–212
retinal, 377, 381, 392, 394
selective/competitive behavior model and, 152–153, 177–184
stimulation and, 45–54, 107–120, 151–154, 168–169, 177–184
T cell activation and, 16, 35–40, 152–153, 161–170, 205–212, 217–220, 272–274, 340–343, 354–357, 366–367, 378–381, 388, 389, 390, 394
therapy and, 3–4, 245, 290–292, 386, 386–387, 389–391, 395–396, 414
thyroid function and, 114–115, 131, 204, 205, 315–333, 316–317, 339–348
See also individual cell type by name
Cell walls, 14
Central immune system, 230
See also Immune response
Chagas' disease, 135
Cholinesterase, 269
Chromosome(s)
autoantibody production and, 20–30, 90–91
B cells and, 426
and blood lymphoid cells, 168
complement components, 429–430
gene deficiency and, 429–430
and lpr mutant mouse, 153
rubella virus and, 219
See also X-linked immunodeficiency
Chronicity, disease, 137
autoreactive clonal specificities and, 244–246, 411–413
immunodeficiency and, 424
thymus/T cell aberration and, 218–219, 359

Chronic lymphocytic leukemia (CLL), 61
B-1 cells and, 75
monoclonal immunoglobulin, 108
rheumatoid factor and, 177, 250
Cirrhosis, primary biliary, 131
Clinical models, autoimmune disease and, 5, 391–396
Clonal selection theory, 3–4, 229
autoreactive lymphocytes and, 183–185, 229–239, 340–348, 407–409
and cellular competition model and, 153–154
cellular maturity/division and, 146–149, 150–151, 152–153
and homunculus set, 16, 16–17
natural autoantibodies and, 107–120, 134–136, 138, 178
self-nonself separability and, 10–11, 78, 132–133, 138, 348, 408
Clone(s)
anergic, 4, 40, 97, 191–199, 229
autoreactive lymphocytes, 3, 112, 132–133, 152–153, 174–185, 230, 236, 340–348, 379–380, 407–409
B cell generation and, 20, 49–50, 52, 57–80, 92–102, 112, 229, 407–409
cellular maturity/cell division and, 146–149
deletion, 4, 20, 185, 191, 198, 209, 212, 221, 229, 379, 380, 410
expansion, 20, 40, 60–61, 164–166, 179–180, 206, 210–211, 244, 378
idiotypic network and, 138, 229–239, 273, 274–280, 285–295, 342–346, 348, 388–389, 408
and lpr mutant mouse, 152–153
ocular antigens and, 378–395, 379
and somatic mutation, 20, 26–29, 111
T cell response and, 16, 40, 152–153, 174, 183–184, 191–199, 206, 210–211, 274, 340–343, 378–395, 409
Cold agglutinins (CA), 22, 30
Common variable immunodeficiency, 423, 427–428

Complement components, 14, 429–430
Connectivity
   of antibodies, 94–99, 348
   defects, 244
   idiotypic, 233–234, 348
   v-gene segments and, 243–246
Consciousness, 16
Control, clonal, 4
Control systems, 5
Conversion, gene, 22
   See also Gene(s)
Costimulatory signal, 40
   anergy and, 194
   See also T cell(s)
Coxsackie B virus, 366
Cryoglobulinemia, 75
   rheumatoid factor and, 248–252
Cryptic epitopes, 37
Cyclosporin A fungal metabolite, 212,
   385–386
Cytokine secretion, 14, 333, 414
   adhesion molecules and, 319, 326
   inhibition, 372
   interferon and, 387
   interleukin (IL)-2 and, 386, 424
   therapy, 246
Cytomegalovirus, 213–214, 219
   retinal, 391
Cytoskeleton proteins, self-antigens
   and, 108, 109
Cytostatic drug therapy, 3–4, 147

Dante, 162
Deafness, 219
Death, cell, 46, 145, 146–151
   B lymphocytes and, 53
Definition(s), 10
   of activation, 46
   of autoantibodies, 108
   of autoimmunity, 423
   See also Separation, conceptual
      perception
Deletion, clonal, 4, 185
   self-antigen lymphocytes and, 20,
      229
   T cells and, 191, 198, 209, 212, 221,
      379, 380, 410
de Lima, Angelo, 143
Deoxynucleotidyltransferase activity,
   terminal, 79

Descartes, Rene, 134
Desire clonotypic antibody, 196, 199
Diabetes mellitus
   Desire mice and, 196–197
   endocrine function and, 318
   insulin dependent, 36, 178, 204, 205,
      217, 219, 274, 365–372
   insulin resistant, 131, 135
   Type I, 131
Diagnostics, clinical, 392
Differentiation, cell
   autoantibodies and, 134–136
   B-1 cell, 65, 68, 78, 134
   B lymphocytes and, 89–102,
      107–120, 134, 150–151, 427
   and inhibition, 52
   lineage hypothesis and, 58, 67–68
   T lymphocytes and, 132, 138,
      143–144, 151, 153, 192–195,
      208–209, 212
Differentiation pathway hypothesis, 58
   B-1 cells and, 68–69, 78
   natural autoantibodies and, 89–102
DiGeorge anomaly, 423, 428–429
Disease
   acetylcholine receptors and,
      268–283, 268–295, 286–290
   antigen recognition and, 16, 135,
      136–138, 204, 208–211,
      217–220, 378–381, 389–391,
      393–394
   antilymphocyte activity and, 99–100
   autoantibodies and, 22–25, 74–76,
      99–100, 114, 131–132,
      134–136, 274–279, 283,
      286–290
   B-1 cells and, 61, 73–76
   CD4$^+$ T cells and, 205–212, 290–294
   congenital, 219–221, 428–429
   environmental variables and,
      211–214, 217, 218–220,
      365–366
   idiotypic network and, 138, 229–230,
      239, 273, 274–280, 285–295,
      307–308, 311, 342–346, 348,
      355, 388–389
   IgH enhancer transgenes and,
      215–216
   MHC genes and, 215–218, 409–413
   ocular antigens and, 377–397

organ-specific, 204, 215–216,
    217–218, 221, 244, 267–295,
    315–333, 365–372, 377–397,
    407–416
peptide binding and, 36–38, 204,
    340–343
peripheral anergy and, 170, 191–199
rheumatoid factor and, 248–252,
    254–258
self-reactive lymphocytes and,
    173–185, 204, 205–212,
    217–220, 318, 322–327,
    340–348, 368–371
statistics, 219, 268–269, 309,
    317–318, 327, 427
T cell activation and, 36, 152–153,
    191–199, 203–221, 309,
    368–371, 378
thyroid activity and, 315–333, 348
See also individual diseases by name
DNA [antibodies]
anti-, 61, 110, 114, 132, 176, 178, 408
antigen receptor genes and, 29–30,
    177
autoantibodies and, 108, 114–115,
    132, 177, 179–180, 181,
    407–409
cell division and, 147
cellular competition model and, 153
denatured, 180
perception and, 15
probes, 48
self-antigens and, 108, 132
SLE disease and, 132
synthesis, 147, 163
Double negative T cells, 14
See also T cells
Double positive T cells, 14
See also T cells
Dual gene hypothesis, 217–218
Duality, 133–134, 139
Duplication, gene, 21, 22
See also Gene(s)
Dysteological autoantibodies, 3

EAU. *See* Uveoretinitis, experimental
    autoimmune
Ecosystem, 139
Eczema, 428

Eels, electric, 268, 269
See also Myasthenia gravis
Electrophorus electricus, 268
ELI-Spot Assay (ESA), 48
Encephalomyelitis, autoimmune, 14
allergic [experimental], 353–361
T cells and, 204
Endoplasmic reticulum
peptide chains and, 36
Enteric bacteria, 13
See also Bacterium
Enteroviruses, 366
Epstein-Barr virus (EBV), 22
acetylcholine receptors and, 280,
    282–283
B cell activation and, 22, 108,
    118–119, 175, 408
IgM antibodies and, 118–119, 177
monoclonal antibodies and, 108, 252
rheumatoid factor and, 252
Erythrocytes, antibody production
    and, 58
Escher, M.C., 9–10, 11–16
See also Immunological homunculus
    theory
Escherichia coli, 175
Eukaryotic cells, 49
Evolution, vertebrate, 5
and somatic perception, 15
Exons, secretory, 50–51
Expansion, clonal, 20
B cells and, 51, 60–61, 179–180
costimulatory signal and, 40, 194
retinal antigens and, 378
T cell(s), 164–166, 167–168, 204,
    205–212, 206, 210–211, 219,
    244
Eye function abnormalities, 317,
    331–332, 377–397
and ocular antigen tolerance,
    378–380, 389–391, 393–394
See also Grave's disease; Ocular
    autoimmunity

Factor VIII, 109
Families, gene, 21–25
abnormalities, 217–220, 423–430
and B cell development, 90–100,
    150–151

and disease resistance, 215–216
and germline mutation, 28–29
v-gene segments and, 114
See also Gene(s)
Fetus
  B cells and, 60, 65, 77, 79, 90, 111–112
  eye development in, 379
  T cells and, 206
  thyroid gland and, 315–316
Filler cells, thymus, 49–50
Foreign antigen(s), 10–15, 229
  antigen recognition and, 12–16,
      136–138, 173–185, 192,
      193–195, 209
  genetic germlines and, 14, 19–20,
      218–220
  and individual somatic experience,
      14–15
  and reactivity, 14–15, 130, 193, 209
  self-nonself nondifferention of,
      14–15, 130–138, 173–174, 184,
      192
  See also Antigen(s)
Freund's adjuvant, 204, 269, 377
Fungi, antibody production and, 58

Gammaglobulin therapy, 424
Gastritis, autoimmune, 204, 205, 214,
    219
  autoantibodies, 212
  host genes and, 217
  pernicious anemia and, 427
Gene(s), 19–30
  acetylcholine receptors and, 280
  autoantibody production and, 20–30,
      73–76, 89–102, 113–114,
      136–137, 176, 214–215,
      248–252, 409
  B cell stimulation and, 50–54, 58–59,
      68–69, 133, 150–151, 176,
      426–427
  chromosomal loci and, 20–29,
      90–91, 153, 428
  defects, 130, 199, 216–218
  and disease resistance, 215–216
  germline encoded, 19, 51, 61, 74–76,
      77, 92–102, 113–114, 133, 176,
      214–215, 248–252, 253
  HLA, 130, 396, 427–428

and Ig-secreting cells, 50–51, 50–54,
    61, 73–76, 89–102, 177,
    215–216, 248–252, 424–427
and lymphocyte population(s),
    143–146, 148, 150–151,
    166–169
MHC/non-MHC, 216–218
mutation, 60, 73–76
ocular antigens and, 383, 385, 396
peptide binding and, 36–38
rheumatoid factor and, 248–252, 253
and self-tolerance, 37–38, 77–79,
    130, 176, 195–197, 199
T cell receptor, 204, 214–215,
    216–218, 274, 322, 354–357,
    409–413
X-linked immunodeficiency, 60, 423,
    428
See also Families, gene; V-gene
    segments
Germline(s), 14–15
  abnormalities, 217–220
  acetylcholine receptors and, 280
  autoantibodies and, 19, 26–29,
      74–76, 92–102, 113–114, 176
  and human light chain genes, 20–21,
      26–30
  and knock-out technique, 50, 51
  rheumatoid factor and, 248–252, 253
  and T cell receptor genes, 214–215
  v-gene segments, 176, 248–252
  See also Gene(s)
Glomerular basement membrane, 109
Glomerulonephritis, immune complex
    mediated, 210
Glycoprotein, 196, 354
Goiter, 321
  See also Grave's disease;
      Hyperthyroidism
Golgi vesicle, post-, 36
Goodpasture's syndrome, 132, 135
Graft(s)
  ocular antigens and, 378–379
  skin, 193–194, 196–197
  See also Transplant(s)
Graft-versus-host disease, 411–413
Grave's disease, 36, 131, 135, 274, 315,
    316–333
  and adhesion molecules, 327–328

and autoimmunity, 318–320
cellular interactions in, 320–327
epidemiology, 317–318
and eye-muscle disturbance, 317,
331–332
and thyroid-stimulating hormone
(TSH), 320

Haemophilus influenzae, 177
Hashimoto's disease, 131, 204, 279,
316, 317, 340
cytotoxic CD8 cells and, 321, 329
See also Thyroiditis
Healthy patients/individuals. *See*
Normalcy
Heart
defects, 219
-muscle antigens, 276
Heart block, congenital, 135
Heat shock proteins, 13, 174
and infection resistance, 15
Heavy chain gene sequences
acetylcholine receptors and, 280
antigen receptors and, 29, 77
autoantibody production and, 26,
69–70, 89–102
and B cell differentiation, 52, 89–102
and T cell germline alteration,
214–215
Henoch-Schoenlein purpura, 429
Hepatitis, 174
Heredity, 396, 428
ataxia telangiectasia and, 424
Histones, 407–408
HIV. *See* Human Immunodeficiency
Virus
HLA genes, 130
common variable immunodeficiency
and, 427–428
and Grave's disease, 318
and organ-specific diseases, 220, 396
uveitis disease and, 396
See also Gene(s)
Homeostasis, immune potential and, 5
Homology, gene sequence, 21–30
and germline mutation, 28–29
See also Gene(s)
Homunculus. *See* Immunological
homunculus

Hormone(s), 58
antibody production and, 58
pituitary, 316
thyroid, 315–316, 317, 324–327
Host-versus-graft disease, 412–413
Human Immunodeficiency Virus
(HIV), 180
immunoglobulin antibodies and, 181
Hybridomas
B cell activation and, 175, 176,
340–343
cytotoxic T cell, 340, 340–343, 357,
371
monoclonal antibodies and, 108
polyreactive autoantibodies and, 176
V-gene segments and, 100
Hydroxyurea, 147
See also Cytostatic drug therapy
Hypergammaglobulinemia, 153, 154
Hyper-IgM syndrome, 423, 427
Hyperplasia, 269
acetylcholine receptors and, 272
Grave's disease and, 317
IgM/IgD and, 427
Hyperthyroidism, 320
See also Grave's disease
Hypervariability, 36–37
Hypoparathyroidism, idiopathic, 131
Hypothalamus, 316
Hypothyroidism, 316, 329
experimentally-induced, 339–348

Idiotypic network interactions, 4
allergic encephalomyelitis and, 355,
359
antineutrophil cytoplasm antibodies
(ANCA) and, 307–311
binarism and, 133
and Grave's disease, 330–331
lymphocyte reactivity and, 191–192,
230, 236
myasthenia gravis autoantibodies
and, 273–274, 276, 280–286
ocular uveitis and, 388–389
self-antiself and, 136–138, 229–239,
340–348
thyroidism and, 342–346, 348
IgA antibodies
acetylcholine receptors and, 288

B-1 cells and, 61
immunodeficiency and, 425, 427
IgD antibodies
and B-1 cells, 59, 62, 66, 67, 68
and B cells, 48, 50, 51
and lymphoid hyperplasia, 427
IgE antibodies, immunodeficiency and, 425
IgG antibodies
acetylcholine receptors and, 280, 282–283, 288, 290–292
ANCA and, 308
B-1 cells and, 61
idiotypic network and, 330
immunodeficiency and, 425
lupus autoantibodies and, 408
monoreactive, 408
natural autoantibodies and, 109–110, 112, 114, 116, 177
rheumatoid factor and, 177, 247–248, 252–253, 258, 408
and T cells, 108–109, 112
and *yersinia enterocolitica*, 326–327
IgH enhancer antibodies, 215–216
IgM antibodies
ABO histoblood group amd, 182
acetylcholine receptors and, 280, 282–283, 288
ANCA and, 308
and antigen self-reactivity, 108, 109–110, !80, 237, 330
and B-1 cells, 61, 65–67, 68
B cell stimulation and, 48, 50–51, 54, 91–92, 94, 96–97, 108–109, 175–177, 408
coxsackie B virus and, 366
idiotypic network and, 330
immunodeficiency and, 424–427
monoclonal, 114
natural autoantibodies and, 109–110, 114, 116, 176
polyreactive, 178, 408
rheumatoid factor and, 177, 248, 252–253, 258
and thyroid autoantigens, 318
Immune response
aging and, 112–113, 162, 219
antigen interpretation vs. recognition, 15–16, 108–109, 136–138, 173–185, 218–220
autoaggressive, 3, 130, 140, 191, 193, 319, 379
autoantibody production and, 22, 26, 61, 66, 67, 68–69, 70, 72, 73, 90–100, 107–120, 134–136, 177–178
basic protein adjuvants and, 14, 204
B lymphocyte activation and, 45–54, 57–80, 89–120, 151–152, 154, 340–343, 371, 407–416
cellular competition model and, 152–154
delayed-type sensitivity and, 380, 381
germline genes and, 19–30, 204, 214–215, 218–220
humoral, 393
idiotypic network and, 136–138, 191–192, 229–239, 273, 274–280, 285–295, 307–311, 330–331, 342–346, 348, 388–389
IgG infusion and, 290–292
lymphocyte population(s) and, 143–146, 151–154
ocular antigens and, 378–380, 381–396
primal, 11
rheumatoid factor, 248–252, 254–258
self-nonself differentiation and, 12–16, 36–38, 58, 77–79, 108–111, 130–138, 173–185, 192, 217–220, 348
T cell receptor specificity and, 35–40, 45–47, 112, 152–154, 191–199, 204, 214–215, 217–220, 309, 340–343, 371–372, 388
thyroid activity and, 315–333, 339–348
Immunization
antibody production and, 58, 76–79, 98–99, 136, 138, 177, 178, 274–280
autoimmune disease and, 4, 136, 138, 152–154, 204
electric eels/rays and, 268, 269–270
idiotypic network and, 136–138, 273, 274–280, 285–295, 342–346, 348, 388–389

immunoglobulin and, 98–99,
150–151, 177, 178, 268
Pasteur antirabies vaccine, 353–354
rheumatoid factor and, 248, 248–252
T cells and, 194, 204, 214–215,
340–343, 378, 385–387, 389
thyroiditis and, 340–348
Immunodeficiency, 423–430
IgM and, 424–427
x-linked, 60, 423, 424
See also AIDS
Immunoendocrinopathy syndrome, 219
Immunoglobulin gene complex, 19–30
antibody production and, 59–62, 66,
67, 68–70, 72, 78, 90–100, 177,
237, 276, 280, 425
autoantibodies and, 26–29, 108, 109,
112, 114, 115–116, 117, 130,
134, 177, 214–215, 247–248,
249–252
B cells and, 20, 48, 50–54, 59–62,
66, 67, 68–70, 72, 78, 91–92,
94, 96–97, 150–151, 154, 230
idiotypic clonal network and,
229–239, 273, 274, 280,
285–295, 307–308, 311, 330
and lymphocyte lifespan(s), 53, 145,
146–151
and *myasthenia gravis*, 288, 290–292
natural autoantibodies and, 89–102,
177, 237
rheumatoid factor and, 247–248, 258,
259
T cell receptor genes and, 214–215,
217–220, 274, 425
thyroid epithelial cells and, 324–327
See also individual Ig antibody by
name
Immunological homunculus theory, 11,
12–13, 15, 16
Immunology
binarism and, 133–134
historical theories and, 3–5, 267–268
idiotypic clonal network and,
229–239, 273, 274–280,
285–295, 342–346, 348,
388–389
self-nonself differentiation and,
10–11, 36–38, 77–79, 130–138,
340–348

Immunosuppression
adaptation to pathogens and, 5,
132–138, 211–214
AIDS and, 391
autoreactivity and, 4–5, 132,
212–213, 371–372
B cells and, 97, 424
lymphocytes and, 3–4, 211–214
ocular inflammation and, 382–393
strategies, 246
T cells and, 4, 46, 132, 211–214,
380–381, 388
See also Cytokine(s)
Infection
basic protein adjuvants and, 14, 36,
204
B cell connectivity and, 97, 175
environmental pathogens and,
365–366
germline and, 14–15
Grave's disease and, 332–333
protein recognition and, 36, 318–320
pyogenic, 424
rheumatoid factor and, 248
system interpretation and, 13–15
T cells and, 199, 218–221, 424
Inflammation
adhesion molecule blockade and,
387
germline and, 14–15
humoral immunity and, 393
immunogenic, 383
intraocular, 377, 379, 387, 391, 392,
393, 395
monoclonal antibodies and, 294
self-antigens and, 16
Instinct, 15
Insulin, 13
autoantibodies and, 108, 178
resistance, 131
Insulitis, 204, 214
host genes and, 217
Interferon
adhesion molecules and, 319, 383,
385
B-1 cells and, 60
cytokine network and, 387
and lymphocyte lifespan(s), 144–145
T cells and, 414
tolerance induction and, 194

Interleukin(s)
  anti-Ig antibodies and, 51
  IL-2, 40, 47, 175, 194, 197–198, 382, 386–387, 424
  IL-4, 16, 412
  IL-5, 59
  IL-6, 68
  receptor(s), 59
  T cells and, 40, 47, 414
Interphotoreceptor retinoid-binding protein (IRBP), 377, 381, 392, 394
Interpretation, antigen, 13–15
  recognition facility and, 16
Intrinsic factor, 109
Iodine, 316
Iodotyrosines, 316
Irradiation, high dose, 213, 414
Isotype(s)
  of gene segments, 21–22
  switching, 61

Jung, Carl, 15

Kadishman, Menashe, 7–11
Kant, Immanuel, 134
Killer cells, natural, 14
k locus, 20–30
  See also Gene(s)

Langherhans islet cells, 212
Leprosy, lepromatous, 16
Leukemia
  B-1 cells and, 61
  rheumatoid factor and, 177, 250
  See also Chronic lymphocytic leukemia (CLL)
Leukocyte common antigen (LCA), 59
Leukocytes
  polymorphonuclear, 14
  retinal antigens and, 378
Ligand(s), 133
  antigen-presenting cells and, 357
  cholinergic, 271, 276
  defect, 424–425
  environmental, 153
  lymphocyte differentiation and, 152–153
Light chain variable region gene locus, 20–30
  acetylcholine receptors and, 280

and autoantibody mutation, 26–29, 89–102
and B cell differentiation, 52, 89–102
rheumatoid factor and, 250
  See also Gene(s)
Lineage hypothesis, 58, 59
  B-1 cells and, 67–68, 72, 78
  B cell, 90–93, 107–120
Lipopolysaccharides (LPS), 14, 47
  and B cell stimulation, 49–50, 52
  and cell death, 53
Lupus erythematosus, systemic, 13, 61, 73, 132, 178, 204, 308, 318
  antilymphocytic activity and, 99–100, 217
  autoantibodies and, 177–178
  cellular/molecular interactions, 407–416
  gene abnormalities and, 217, 220, 409–413, 429–430
  humoral immunity and, 393
  immunoglobulin secretion and, 180, 408
  and lpr mutant mouse, 152–153
  pharmacological triggers, 367
  rheumatoid factor and, 248
Ly-1$^+$ B cells, 57–58
Lymphadenopathy, 153
Lymph nodes
  myasthenia gravis and, 268
  T cells and, 161–162
Lymphocyte(s)
  acetylcholine receptors and, 272–274, 281–283
  adhesion molecules and, 319, 327–328, 383, 385
  antibody production and, 22, 30, 47–52, 57–80, 89–102, 130–138, 244, 408
  antigen recognition and, 11, 61, 108–109, 136–138, 161, 166–169, 173–185, 193–195, 230, 236, 408
  and autoimmune disease, 75, 107–120, 131–132, 173–185, 199, 205–221, 230, 236, 323–324, 340–348, 407–416
  deficiency, 423–429
  differentiation, 19–20, 67–69, 94–99, 151–154, 414–416

lifespan(s), 145, 146–151, 168–169
natural antibodies and, 62–64, 66,
    69–72, 89–102, 107–120,
    130–138
population(s), 143–146, 151–154,
    161–170, 206
reactivity, 76–79, 91–102, 107–120,
    130–138, 151–154, 173–185,
    191–199, 230, 236, 340–348,
    366–372, 371, 378–379,
    407–416
stimulation, 45–54, 152–153,
    177–184, 407–409
stress and, 144–145, 146–147, 327
suppression of, 3–4, 20, 132,
    380–385, 396
and tolerance induction, 193–195,
    198–199, 205–212, 230, 236,
    340–348, 366–367
See also B cell(s); T cell(s)
Lymphocytic choriomeningitis virus
    (LCMV), 196
Lymphoid cells
adhesion molecules and, 319, 383,
    385
chromosome breaks and, 168
DNA precursors and, 163
and Grave's disease, 322
malignant, 382–383
SCID mice and, 167
Lymphoid organs
B cells and, 20, 100
ionizing radiation and, 213
lymphocyte production and,
    145–146, 150
T cells and, 212
Lymphokine production, 59–60, 208
retinal antigens and, 378, 385–386
Lymphoma(s)
autoantibody gene segments and, 30,
    75–76
B-1 CD5$^+$ cells and, 57, 59–60,
    61, 75

Macrolides, 385–386
interleukin (IL)-2 and, 386–387
Macrophages, 14, 387
ACAID-inducing potential and, 390
T-helper cells and, 414

Major histocompatibility complex
    (MHC)
adhesion molecules and, 319,
    327–328, 383, 385
allogeneic signals and, 14, 409–413
B cells and, 150–151, 184, 230
foreign antigens and, 14–15, 216–218
IgH enhancer genes and, 215–216
IgM antibodies and, 183
ocular antigens and, 383, 385, 396
self-antigen tolerance and, 195–197,
    218–220, 230–239, 324–327
self-peptides and, 174
T cells and, 35–40, 174, 184,
    191–192, 193, 215–216,
    218–220, 230, 330
uveitis and, 396
v-region genes and, 357–358
Malarial B cells, 180
Malignancy
B-1 cells and, 58, 73–76, 108
IgM and, 427
natural autoantibodies and, 113
ocular inflammation and, 382–
    383
T cells and, 425
thyroid and, 317
Mast cell(s)
inhibitors, 382
ocular tissue, 382
retinal antigens and, 378
Measles, 213, 219
Memory, immune, 230
Mental retardation, 219
Metabolic activity
blast cells and, 46–47
thyroid gland and, 315–316
Mice, lab
autoreactivity and, 107–108, 110,
    182, 204, 250, 408
disease inducement in, 131, 136,
    150–151, 197–198, 204, 206,
    214–215, 269–280, 339–348,
    354–360, 370
foreign antigens and, 13, 131,
    193–194
gene manipulation in, 60, 148,
    196–197
homunculus sets in, 15

IGg infusion and, 290–292
lpr mutant, 152–153
and lymphocyte population(s),
        143–146, 148, 152–153,
        162–168
myasthenia gravis and, 269–280,
        290–292
natural autoantibodies and, 100–101,
        107–108, 110, 408
ocular mast cells in, 382
rheumatoid factor and, 250
SCID and, 65, 98, 149, 165, 167
and thyroiditis, 340–343
and T-lymphotropic virus (MTLV),
        214, 215–216, 218–219, 220
Torpedo receptor and, 275, 276
See also Animals, laboratory
Mind, 140
Mitogen
B cells and, 46–47, 49–50, 52, 175
idiotypic network and, 138
polyclonal, 4
Molecular mimicry, 220, 221
Monoclonal antibodies
B cells and, 51, 70, 101, 108–109
and CD4$^+$ T cells, 292–294
interleukin (IL)-2 and, 387
myasthenia gravis autoantibodies
        and, 273–274, 276, 280–286
natural autoantibodies and, 109–111,
        113–114
rheumatoid factor, 248–252, 254–258
T cells and, 194
therapy, 414
and thyroiditis, 340–343
Müller cells, 382–393, 395
Multiple sclerosis, 16, 131, 274, 359
allergic encephalomyelitis and,
        353–361
lesions, 353
v-genes and, 360–361
Mumps, 219
Muramyldipeptide, 14
Murid herpesvirus, 214
Muscle(s), *myasthenia gravis*, 268–269
antigens, 276–277
autoantibodies, 274–280
Mutation
autoantibodies and, 26–29, 61

clonal, 20, 26–29
gene abnormalities and, 217–220
genes and, 60, 61, 66
somatic, 26, 30, 71, 111
Myasthenia gravis, 131, 135, 267–295,
        308, 318
experimental, 269–280
human, 268–269, 280–295
pharmacological triggers, 367
Mycobacterium leprae, 16
See also Bacterium
Mycoplasma, 51
Myelin basic protein(s), 204, 354, 366
antigen-specific suppression and,
        390–391
Myeloma, 22
Myelomonocytic lineage, 59
See also Lineage hypothesis
Myoglobin, 109

Natural antibodies
B-1 cells and, 62, 78
B cell differentiation and, 89–102,
        107–120
polyreactive, 58, 69–72, 109–111,
        176
and self-nonself recognition,
        134–136, 237, 340–348
See also Antibodies; Autoantibodies
Neoantigens, 367
Neonate
B cells and, 60, 65, 77, 79, 90,
        111–112
and maternal Grave's disease,
        320–321
maternal immunoglobulin and, 98–99
thymus, 205
Neurological homunculus, 11
Neuromuscular disease, 267
See also Myasthenia gravis
Neutrophil cytoplasmic antigens, 109
Nonreactivity. *See* Anergy
Nonsuppressive therapy, 4–5
Normalcy
autoantibodies and, 114, 252–253
autoreactive lymphocytes and, 4,
        45–54, 108–109, 132, 174, 177,
        183–185, 204, 229, 244, 246,
        252–253, 318

B-1 cells and, 60–61, 108–109
healthy individuals, 4, 11, 36, 46,
   108–109, 114, 132, 180,
   183–185, 204, 229, 244, 246,
   252–253, 274, 281, 307, 379
self-antigens and, 11, 36, 108–109,
   132–133, 136–138, 204, 229,
   318, 330
N-segment addition. *See*
   Deoxynucleotidyltransferase
   activity, terminal
Nucleic acids, 13, 14–15
antibody production and, 58, 69, 73
See also Viral agent(s)
Nucleoprotein, 196
Nucleotides
B-1 cells and, 74
germline genes and, 28, 30
V-region segment and, 100

Ocular autoimmunity, 377–397
Oligoclonal antibodies, 407, 409
Ontogeny, 4, 58
B-1 cell, 76–79
B cell, 90–93, 107, 112, 366
of extrajunctional receptors, 271
of self-reactive clones, 229
T cell, 162–169, 215, 366, 379
Oophoritis, 205
autoantibodies, 212, 214
Ophthalmia, sympathetic, 379
Orchitis, 205, 206
autoantibodies, 212, 214
Organ-specific disease(s), 204, 221
acetylcholine receptor and, 267–295
autoreactive clonal specificities and,
   244–246
environmental variables and,
   211–214, 217, 218–220,
   365–366
gene abnormalities and, 217–220,
   396
IgH enhancer genes and, 215–216
ocular autoimmunity and, 377–397
Orphon gene segments, 20–26
See also Gene(s)
Ovarian disease, 318
Ovarian failure, premature, 131

Pancreas, 196, 217, 365
See also Diabetes mellitus
Paraproteins, monoclonal, 22
Parathyroid disease, 318
Pemphigus, 131, 135
Peptide chains
and T cell activation, 35–40, 174,
   359, 385, 389, 414
thyroglobulin and, 340
thyroiditis and, 340–343
Peptide motif, 36
Peptons, 193
Perception, 7–11
autoantibodies and, 130
duality and, 133–134, 139
somatic response and, 15
Peripheral immune system, 230
T cell anergy and, 161–169, 170,
   191–199, 204, 205–212, 217–220
See also Immune response
P. falciparum, 180
Phagocytosis, 139
Phospholipids
antibody production and, 58, 69, 73,
   408
Photoreceptor cell(s)
retinal antigens and, 378–395
Pineal gland, 378
and ocular antigens, 379
Pituitary hormone, 316
Plaque-forming cell (PFC), 48
Plasma cells, 53
Ig-secretion and, 50
Plummer's disease, 317
Pneumocystis carinii, 424
Poison ivy, 424
Polyclonal B cell activators, 48–49,
   407–409, 425
Polyclonal mitogen, 4
Polyclonal T cell(s), 272
Polyglandular autoimmune syndrome
   (PGA), 219, 220
Polymiositis, 132
Polymorphism
gene duplication and, 21
major histocompatibility complex
   molecules and, 36–37
T cell receptor(s) and, 274, 322
Polymorphonuclear leukocytes, 14

Polyreactive antibodies (PR), 22, 58, 109–111, 177–178
  ABO histoblood group and, 182
  B-1 cells and, 61, 66, 69, 71, 77–79, 178–179
  hybridomas and, 176
  lupus autoantibodies, 408
  rheumatoid factor and, 250–252
Polysaccharides, 69
  hemophilus, 97
  and Ig-secreting cells, 177, 252
  pneumococcal, 96
  See also Lipopolysaccharides
Polyvinyl pyrrolidone (PVP), 77
Protein(s)
  actin, 109
  acute phase, 14
  adhesion molecules and, 319, 383, 385
  albumin, 109
  antibody production and, 58, 69, 108, 272
  basic, 13, 14, 204
  cytoskeleton, 108, 109
  gene sequencing and, 21–22
  IgG antibodies and, 326, 408
  interphotoreceptor retinoid binding-, 377, 381, 392, 394
  intraocular, 381
  myelin, 354, 366, 390–391
  myoglobin, 109
  para-, 22
  peptide fragments of, 35, 36, 272
  plasmid, 326–327
  ribosomal, 108
  T cell activation and, 35–40, 108, 174, 272
  thyroglobulin, 315–316
  transferrin, 108, 109
  tubulin, 109
Proteolytic enzymes, 316
Protozoa, 58
Pseudogenes, 20–21
  gene segments and, 22
  See also Gene(s)
Purified protein derivative (PPD), 47

Rabies
  anti-, vaccine, 353–354
  IgM and, 178

Radiation
  chromosome damage and, 168–169
  ionizing, 213
  x-ray, 205
Rays, electric, 268
  See also Myasthenia gravis
Reality, self-nonself, 7–16, 130–138
Receptors, cellular
  acetylcholine, 108, 267–295
  adrenergic, 277
  antibodies and, 3, 22, 59, 68–69, 89–102, 131–132, 268–295
  antigen recognition and, 11, 12, 20, 29–30, 133, 193–194, 354–357
  B cell, 4, 12, 20, 52, 59, 76–79, 97, 173, 174–185, 340–343
  gene segments and, 29–30, 89–94, 204, 214–215, 245, 280, 354–357
  monoreactive, 77–78
  polyreactive, 77–78, 110
  retinal, 377, 381, 389, 392, 394
  T cell, 4, 12, 35–40, 161–169, 173–174, 175, 181, 192–195, 204, 214–215, 245, 322, 340–343, 354–357, 359–360, 366, 368–371, 389, 409–413
  Torpedo marmorata, 276, 277
  v-gene segment, 245, 354–357
Renal disease, 221, 429–430
Retina
  and line vision, 15
  photoreceptor cell proteins, 377, 381, 392, 394
  See also Antigens, retinal
Rheumatoid arthritis, 29, 61, 73, 111, 204
  autoantibodies and, 114, 132, 408
  characterization of, 247–248
  host genes and, 217, 429
  T clones and, 174
Rheumatoid factors (RF), 247–248
  anti-IgG, 61
  autoantibody reactivity and, 29, 30, 61, 132, 177, 247–259
  and B cell activation, 175–177, 180
  in healthy individuals, 252–253
  and Ig-secreting cells, 177, 247–250, 252, 257–258

lpr mutant mouse and, 153
monoclonal, 22, 248–252, 254–258
Ribonucleoproteins, 407–408
Ribosomes
lymphocyte activation and, 46
self-antigens and, 108
RNA
SLE disease and, 132, 407–408
transcription, 197
Rubella, 213, 219–220
x-linked inheritance and, 424

Salivary glands, 212
Salk, Jonas, 129
Self-antigens
anti-Ptc, 77
autoantibodies and, 108, 109–111,
134–138, 412
B cell types and, 58, 61, 65, 75–76,
89–102, 107–120, 340–343,
366–367, 408
essence and origin of, 13–16, 68–69,
77–79, 108, 136–138, 193, 209
genetic germlines and, 19–20, 75–76,
77, 91–102, 204, 217–220
idiotypic clonal network and,
229–239, 273, 274–280,
285–295, 330, 342–346, 348,
388–389
and immunization, 136–138, 204
reactivity of, 14–15, 16, 76–79,
91–102, 107–120, 184,
192–195, 204, 205–212, 215,
217–220, 229–239, 366, 408
substance of, 12, 108–109
T cells and, 192–195, 204–221, 246,
340–343, 366–367, 368–371,
412
v-region genes and, 243–246
See also Antigen(s); Foreign
substance; V-gene segments
Self-nonself distinguishability, 7–16,
130–138, 192
antibody reactivity and, 77–79,
108–111, 130–138, 184, 348
autoreactive lymphocytes and,
173–185, 243–246
germline genes and, 19–20, 77–79,
217–220
Grave's disease and, 320

major histocompatibility complex
and, 36–38, 217–220
thyroiditis and, 348
Semiology, 133
Separation
conceptual perception and, 7–11
self-nonself and, 7–16, 36–38, 77–79,
130–138, 173–185, 217–220,
348
Serum proteins
antibody production and, 58
Sialoadenitis
autoantibodies, 212, 214
host genes and, 217
Side chain theory, 3
Sjogren's syndrome, 111, 132
rheumatoid factor and, 248
Skeletal muscle endplate(s), 268
acetylcholine receptors and, 272–280
antigens, 276–277
See also Myasthenia gravis
Skin disease
antibodies and, 131, 132
grafting and, 193–194, 196–197
T cells and, 162
vitiligo, 131, 318
SLE. *See* Lupus erythematosus,
systemic
Somatic response, individual, 14–15
B cell mutation and, 20, 61–62, 71
germline genes and, 19–20, 26–30,
217–220
Specificity. *See* Cell type specificity
Specific pathogen free (SPF)
conditions, 46
Sperm, 212
Spleen
B cells and, 59, 60, 68, 90
fetal, 60
ocular uveitis and, 379
suppressor cells, 380
T cells and, 161–162, 206, 209
Sprent, Jonathan, 423
Staphylococcus aureus, 41, 175
Steroids
and lymphocyte lifespan(s), 144
and uveitis therapy, 386
Streptococci, 13
renal disease and, 221
See also Bacterium

Stress
  Grave's disease and, 327
  and lymphocyte depletion, 144–145,
      146–147
Striational antibodies (SA), 22
  antigen receptor genes and, 29–30
Stromal cell(s), 49–50
  See also Bone marrow
Subject-ground conflict, 7–16
Suppression
  B cells and, 97
  T cells and, 20, 46, 132, 371–372,
      380–381, 388
  therapy, 3–4, 386–387, 389–391
  types of, 14–15
  See also Immunosuppression;
      Nonsuppressive therapy
Systemic lupus erythematosus. *See*
    Lupus, erythematosus, systemic

T cell(s)
  acetylcholine receptors and, 272–274
  allogeneic, 4, 164–166, 409–413
  anergy, 40, 132, 170, 184, 191–199
  anti-, drugs, 385–386
  and antigen reactivity, 12, 14–15,
      131, 132, 139, 161–169,
      173–174, 181, 183, 183–185,
      184, 192–195, 204, 209, 215,
      217–220, 272–274, 329–331,
      354–357, 378
  autoreactive, 173–174, 175, 184,
      191–199, 204–221, 246,
      272–274, 318, 329, 329–331,
      366–367, 371, 413–414, 427
  differentiation, 47, 52, 151, 152, 153,
      165–166, 167–168, 192–195,
      208–209, 212
  and disease generation, 203–221,
      272–274, 309, 340–343,
      354–357, 368–371, 378,
      414–416
  environmental pathogens and,
      211–214, 217–220, 365–366
  expansion, 205–212, 219
  generation of, 20, 46–52, 145–151,
      205, 340–343
  genetic abnormalities and, 217–220,
      409–413, 428
  in healthy individuals, 4, 36, 46, 132

  lifespan(s), 145, 146–151, 168–169
  myelin basic protein and, 354–357,
      359, 360
  natural autoantibodies and, 108–109,
      112, 131, 137
  peripheral, 161–169, 191–198, 204,
      211–214, 217–220, 366–367
  polyclonal, 272
  population(s), 143–146, 152,
      152–153, 161–170, 206
  receptors, 4, 12, 35–40, 45–47,
      161–169, 192, 217–220, 245,
      274, 340–343, 354–357,
      368–371, 409–413
  and response specificity, 16, 35–40,
      131, 137, 194, 217–220,
      340–343, 354–357
  selectivity, 152–154, 161, 166–169,
      181, 212, 217–220
  stimulation of, 45–54, 152–154,
      168–169
  and suppression/cytotoxicity, 20, 46,
      193, 205, 211–214, 219–220,
      318, 321, 340–343, 380–381,
      385–387, 388, 414–416
  tolerance induction and, 193–195,
      205–212, 217–220
  types of, 14–15, 46–47, 166, 193,
      205–212, 272, 290–294, 322,
      329–331, 340–343, 365, 378,
      413–414
  uveitogenic, 378–395
  X-linked immunodeficiency genes
      and, 60, 423, 425, 426
Tdt enzyme activity
  antibody production and, 30
Testicular disease, 318
Tetanus toxoid, 180
T-helper cell(s), 51, 181
  acetylcholine receptors and, 272
  autoreactive lymphocytes and,
      183–184, 413–414
  B-1 cells and, 69, 777
  CD4$^+$ T cells and, 205
  Grave's disease and, 321
  uveitogenic, 378
Therapy
  cytostatic regimen, 3–4, 147
  gammaglobulin, 424
  IgG infusion, 245, 290–292

interleukin (IL)-2, 386–387
monoclonal antibody, 414
peripheral anergy and, 170
retinal antigen, 389–391
SCID marrow treatment, 169
uveitis, 386, 395–396
Thoracic duct, 161
Thrombocytopenia, 367
Thrombocytopenic purpura, idiopathic, 132
Thymic necrosis virus, 214
Thymocytes, 153, 162, 212
Thymus
    and cortex-medulla, 162
    environmental pathogens and,
        211–214, 217, 218, 218–220
    filler cells of, 49–50
    lymphocyte production and,
        145–146, 150
    MHC genes and, 216–218
    myasthenia gravis and, 268–269, 274
    ocular antigens and, 379
    resting cells and, 46, 49–50
    self-tolerance and, 192–195,
        205–212, 370
    T cell [receptors] and, 40, 151, 153,
        162–164, 192, 211–214,
        216–218, 274
Thymus-independent (TI) antigens,
    48–49
Thyroglobulin, 13, 315–316, 340
    autoantibodies, 109, 131, 212, 330,
        369
    degradation of, 316
    immunization, 204
    self-antigens and, 108
Thyroid gland, 315–316, 331–332
    and T cell infiltration, 339–340, 341,
        370
Thyroiditis, autoimmune, 114–115, 131,
    316–317
    adhesion molecules and, 327–328
    autoantibodies, 212, 214, 276–277
    B cells and, 340–343
    cytotoxic CD8 cells and, 321
    experimental, 339–348
    host genes and, 217
    T cells and, 204, 205, 340–343, 370
Thyroid-stimulating hormone (TSH),
    316, 319, 320, 322, 331

Thyrotoxicosis, 316, 318, 320–321, 329
Thyrotropin-releasing hormone (TRH),
    316
Thyroxine hormone, 316
Tolerance
    B cell differentiation and, 20,
        107–120, 151–154, 182, 427
    clonal, 4, 20, 198–199, 229–239, 318
    competitive selectivity and, 151–154
    cryptic epitopes and, 37
    genetic germlines and, 19–20,
        196–197, 199
    immunization and, 136, 204, 339–348
    interleukin (IL)-2 and, 197–198
    pathogens and, 5, 133–136, 139, 182,
        193–194
    peripheral, 366–367, 368–371
    retinal antigens and, 378–380, 385,
        389–391, 393–394
    self-nonself antigens and, 14–15, 16,
        19, 77–79, 107–120, 130–138,
        174–185, 193–195, 229–239,
        340–348, 366
    T cell expression and, 161, 166–169,
        191–198, 205–212, 221, 359
Toxoplasmosis, 391
Transferrin, self-antigens and, 108, 109
Transfusion(s)
    IgG, 290–292
    immunoglobulin, 268
    lymph, 268
Transplants
    bone marrow, 59, 169, 197, 210, 423
    retinal, 380
    T cell rejection of, 193
Triiodothyronine hormone, 316
Tubulin, 109
Tumor(s)
    -specific antigens, 380
    TSH-producing, 317

Uveitis, 378, 395–396
    adhesion molecule blockade and, 387
    and genetic implications, 396
    humoral immunity and, 393
    retinal antigen, 389–391
    therapy, 386, 395–396
Uveoretinitis, 131
Uveoretinitis, experimental
    autoimmune (EAU), 377–391

Vasculitis, systemic, 307–311
V-gene segments
    allergic encephalomyelitis and,
        354–358, 360
    autoimmune disease and, 114–115,
        135, 137, 153, 243–246,
        354–357
    hybridomas and, 100
    lymphocyte lifespan(s) and, 150–151
    and multiple sclerosis, 360
    polyreactive autoantibodies and,
        112, 113–114, 176, 178
    and rheumatoid factor, 176, 248–252,
        253
    T cell receptors and, 274, 354–357
    See also Gene(s); Germline(s)
Viral agent(s), 14–15
    adhesion molecules and, 326, 383,
        385
    antibody production and, 58, 178
    antigen-presenting cells and, 199
    autoantibody reactivity and, 22,
        409–413

and disease causation, 213–214,
        218–220, 353–354, 365–372
    experimental encephalomyelitis,
        353–354
    genetic abnormalities and, 271–280
Vitiligo, 131
    endocrine function and, 318
Vogt-Koyanagi-Harada syndrome, 391

Waldenstrom's macroglobulinemia
    IgM and, 108
Wegener's granulomatosis, 310
Wiskott-Aldrich syndrome, 423, 426,
        428

X-linked immunodeficiency, 60, 423
    agammaglobulinemia, 423, 424, 427
    IgM and, 424–427
    and Wiskott-Aldrich syndrome, 428
X-ray irradiation, low-dose
    self-reactive T cells and, 205

Yersinia enterocolitica, 326